Heart Disease: Multidisciplinary Approach

Editorial Advisor

JOEL J. HEIDELBAUGH

ELSEVIER

1600 John F. Kennedy Boulevard • Suite 1800 • Philadelphia, Pennsylvania, 19103-2899

http://www.theclinics.com

CLINICS COLLECTIONS
ISSN 2352-7986, ISBN-13: 978-0-443-12939-1

Editor: John Vassallo (j.vassallo@elsevier.com)

Clinics Collections (ISSN 2352-7986) is published by Elsevier Inc., 360 Park Avenue South, New York, NY 10010-1710. Business and editorial offices: 1600 John F. Kennedy Boulevard, Suite 1800, Philadelphia, PA 19103-2899. **POSTMASTER:** Send address changes to *Clinics Collections*, Elsevier Health Sciences Division, Subscription Customer Service, 3251 Riverport Lane, Maryland Heights, MO 63043. **Customer Service: Telephone: 1-800-654-2452** (U.S. and Canada); **1-314-447-8871** (outside U.S. and Canada). **Fax: 314-447-8029. E-mail: journalscustomerserviceusa@elsevier.com** (for print support); **journalsonlinesupport-usa@elsevier.com** (for online support).

Reprints. For copies of 100 or more of articles in this publication, please contact the Commercial Reprints Department, Elsevier Inc., 360 Park Avenue South, New York, NY 10010-1710. Tel.: 212-633-3874; Fax: 212-633-3820; E-mail: reprints@elsevier.com.

Contributors

EDITOR

JOEL J. HEIDELBAUGH, MD, FAAFP, FACG
Clinical Professor, Departments of Family Medicine and Urology, Director of Medical Student Education and Clerkship Director, Department of Family Medicine, University of Michigan Medical School, Ann Arbor, Michigan, USA

AUTHORS

AARON W. ADAY, MD, MSc
Vanderbilt Translational and Clinical Cardiovascular Research Center, Division of Cardiovascular Medicine, Vanderbilt University Medical Center, Nashville, Tennessee, USA

FEDERICA AMODIO, MD
Department of Translational Medical Sciences, University of Campania "Luigi Vanvitelli," Naples, Italy

MARCELLO ARCA, MD
Professor of Medicine, Department of Translational and Precision Medicine, University of Rome, Sapienza, Italy

JONATHAN P. ARIYARATNAM, MB BChir
Centre for Heart Rhythm Disorders, The University of Adelaide and Royal Adelaide Hospital, Adelaide, Australia

MAURIZIO AVERNA, MD
Professor of Medicine, University of Palermo, Italy

NICHOLAS J. BARONE, BS
Office of the Medical Director, Montefiore Medical Center, Bronx, New York, USA

ESSRAA BAYOUMI, MD
Cardiovascular Disease Fellow, MedStar Washington Hospital Center, Georgetown University, VA Medical Center, Washington, DC, USA

SHALENDER BHASIN, MB, BS
Professor of Medicine, Harvard Medical School, Director, Research Program in Men's Health: Aging and Metabolism, Director, Boston Claude D. Pepper Older Americans Independence Center for Function Promoting Therapies, Brigham and Women's Hospital, Boston, Massachusetts, USA

MICHAEL J. BLAHA, MD, MPH
Division of Cardiology, Department of Medicine, Ciccarone Center for the Prevention of Cardiovascular Disease, Johns Hopkins School of Medicine, Baltimore, Maryland, USA

NUNZIA BORRELLI, MD
Department of Translational Medical Sciences, University of Campania "Luigi Vanvitelli,"
Naples, Italy

BIYKEM BOZKURT, MD, PhD
Michael E. DeBakey VA Medical Center, Winters Center for Heart Failure Research,
Cardiovascular Research Institute, Baylor College of Medicine, Houston, Texas, USA

MARTINA CAIAZZA, MD
Inherited and Rare Cardiovascular Disease Unit, Department of Translational Medical
Sciences, University of Campania "Luigi Vanvitelli," AORN dei Colli, Monaldi Hospital,
Naples, Italy

PAOLO CALABRÒ, MD, PhD
Department of Translational Medical Sciences, University of Campania "Luigi Vanvitelli,"
Naples, Italy; Division of Cardiology, A.O.R.N. "Sant'Anna e San Sebastiano," Edificio C –
Cardiologia Universitaria, Caserta, Italy

SILVIA CASTELLETTI, MD, PhD
Istituto Auxologico Italiano, IRCCS-Center for Cardiac Arrhythmias of Genetic Origin,
Milan, Italy

ALBERICO CATAPANO, MD, PhD
Professor of Pharmacology, Department of Pharmacological and Biomolecular Sciences,
Universita' degli Studi di Milano, Milan, Italy; IRCCS MultiMedica, Sesto San Giovanni, Italy

HONG Y CHOI, PhD
Research Institute of the McGill University Health Centre, Montreal, Quebec, Canada

ANNAPAOLA CIRILLO, MD, PhD
Inherited and Rare Cardiovascular Disease Unit, Department of Translational Medical
Sciences, University of Campania "Luigi Vanvitelli," Naples, Italy

DIEGO COLONNA, MD
Department of Translational Medical Sciences, University of Campania "Luigi Vanvitelli,"
Naples, Italy

MARIA ROSA COSTANZO, MD, FACC, FAHA, FESC
Medical Director, Heart Failure Research, Advocate Heart Institute, Medical Director,
Edward Hospital Center for Advanced Heart Failure, Naperville, Illinois, USA

PETER N. DEAN, MD
Division of Pediatric Cardiology, Department of Pediatrics, University of Virginia,
Charlottesville, Virginia, USA

LAURA D'ERASMO, MD, PhD
Department of Translational and Precision Medicine, University of Rome, Sapienza, Italy

JOSEPH A. DIAMOND, MD
Associate Professor of Medicine, Donald and Barbara Zucker School of Medicine at
Hofstra/Northwell, Director of Nuclear Cardiology, Department of Cardiology, Long Island
Jewish Hospital, Northwell Health, New Hyde Park, New York, USA

KATHERINE E. DI PALO, PharmD, FAHA
Office of the Medical Director, Montefiore Medical Center, Bronx, New York, USA

BARBARA D'ONOFRIO, MD
Inherited and Rare Cardiovascular Disease Unit, Department of Translational Medical
Sciences, University of Campania "Luigi Vanvitelli," AORN dei Colli, Monaldi Hospital,
Naples, Italy

FABRIZIO DRAGO, MD, PhD
The European Reference Network for Rare, Low Prevalence and Complex Diseases of the Heart - ERN GUARD-Heart, Pediatric Cardiology and Arrhythmia/Syncope Units, Department of Paediatric Cardiology and Cardiac Surgery, Bambino Gesu' Children's Hospital and Research Institute, IRCSS, Rome, Italy

ALVIS COLEMAN HEADEN, BS
Perelman School of Medicine, University of Pennsylvania, Philadelphia, Pennsylvania, USA

SAVITRI FEDSON, MD, MA
Michael E. DeBakey VA Medical Center, Center for Medical Ethics and Health Policy, Baylor College of Medicine, Houston, Texas, USA; Winters Center for Heart Failure Research

FABIO FIMIANI, BSc
Unit of Inherited and Rare Cardiovascular Diseases, A.O.R.N. Dei Colli "V. Monaldi," Pediatric Cardiology Unit, Monaldi Hospital, Department of Translational Medical Sciences, University of Campania "Luigi Vanvitelli," Naples, Italy

CHRISTOPHER FOX, MD, CAQ-SM
Assistant Professor, University of Missouri-Kansas City, School of Medicine, Physician, Department of Community and Family Medicine, Truman Medical Centers, Kansas City, Missouri, USA

GIULIA FRISSO, MD, PhD
Dipartimento di Medicina Molecolare e Biotecnologie Mediche, Universita' di Napoli Federico II, CEINGE Advanced Biotechnologies, CEINGE Biotecnologie Avanzate, Scarl, Naples, Italy

ADELAIDE FUSCO, MD
Inherited and Rare Cardiovascular Disease Unit, Department of Translational Medical Sciences, University of Campania "Luigi Vanvitelli," Naples, Italy

JACQUES GENEST, MD
Research Institute of the McGill University Health Centre, Montreal, Quebec, Canada

EARL GOLDSBOROUGH III, BS
Johns Hopkins School of Medicine, Baltimore, Maryland, USA

J. ANTONIO GUTIERREZ, MD, MHS
Division of Cardiology, Department of Medicine, Duke University Health System, Durham, North Carolina, USA

AZIZ HAMMOUD, MD
Section of Cardiovascular Medicine, Department of Internal Medicine, Wake Forest University School of Medicine, Winston-Salem, North Carolina, USA

MARK HENDERSON, MD MACP
Professor and Vice Chair for Education, Department of Internal Medicine, University of California, Davis School of Medicine, Sacramento, California, USA

IULIA IATAN, PhD, MD
Research Institute of the McGill University Health Centre, Montreal, Quebec, Canada

CARMEN LOK TUNG HO, BSc
Section of Endocrinology and Investigative Medicine, Imperial College London, United Kingdom

TARA A. HOLDER, MD
Division of Cardiovascular Medicine, Vanderbilt University Medical Center, Nashville, Tennessee, USA

PARDIS HOSSEINZADEH, MD
Section of Reproductive Endocrinology and Infertility, Department of Obstetrics and Gynecology, University of Oklahoma Health and Sciences Center, Oklahoma City, Oklahoma, USA

HAISAM ISMAIL, MD
Assistant Professor of Medicine, Donald and Barbara Zucker School of Medicine at Hofstra/Northwell, Electrophysiologist, Department of Cardiology, Long Island Jewish Hospital, Northwell Health, New Hyde Park, New York, USA

LANIER B. JACKSON, MD
Division of Pediatric Cardiology, Department of Pediatrics, Medical University of South Carolina, Charleston, South Carolina, USA

CHANNA N. JAYASENA, MA, PhD, MRCP, FRCPath
Section of Endocrinology and Investigative Medicine, Reader, Imperial College London, Consultant in Reproductive Endocrinology and Andrology, Hammersmith Hospital, London, United Kingdom

BOBBY JOHN, MBBS, MD, DM, PhD, FHRS
Associate Professor, James Cook University, Townsville, Australia; Townsville University Hospital, Douglas, Queensland, Australia; Christian Medical College, Vellore, India

JEFFERY CHAD JOHNSON, MD
Department of Surgery, Division of Cardiothoracic Surgery, Naval Medical Readiness and Training Center Portsmouth, Portsmouth, Virginia, USA

HOWARD M. JULIEN, MD, MPH, ML
Assistant Professor of Clinical Medicine, Perelman School of Medicine, University of Pennsylvania, Philadelphia, Pennsylvania; Penn Cardiovascular Outcomes, Quality, and Evaluative Research Center, Penn Cardiovascular Center for Health Equity and Social Justice

JONATHAN M. KALMAN, MBBS, PhD
Department of Cardiology, Royal Melbourne Hospital, Department of Medicine, University of Melbourne, Melbourne, Australia

PAMELA KARASIK, MD
Chief, Medical Service VA Medical Center, Professor of Medicine, The George Washington University Medical Center, Washington, DC, USA

MI-NA KIM, MD, PhD
Division of Cardiology, Department of Internal Medicine, Korea University Medicine, Korea University Anam Hospital, Seoul, Republic of Korea

JOHN LANDEFELD, MD MS
Assistant Clinical Professor, Department of Internal Medicine, University of California, Davis School of Medicine, Sacramento, California, USA

CHU-PAK LAU, MD
Honorary Clinical Professor, Department of Medicine, Queen Mary Hospital, The University of Hong Kong, Central, Hong Kong

DENNIS H. LAU, MBBS, PhD
Department of Cardiology, Centre for Heart Rhythm Disorders, The University of Adelaide, Royal Adelaide Hospital, Adelaide, Australia

GIUSEPPE LIMONGELLI, MD, PhD, FESC
Inherited and Rare Cardiovascular Disease Unit, Department of Translational Medical Sciences, University of Campania "Luigi Vanvitelli," AORN dei Colli, Monaldi Hospital, Naples, Italy; Division of Cardiology, A.O.R.N. "Sant'Anna and San Sebastiano," Caserta, Italy Institute of Cardiovascular Sciences, University College of London and St. Bartholomew's Hospital, London, United Kingdom

MICHELE LIONCINO, MD
Inherited and Rare Cardiovascular Disease Unit, Department of Translational Medical Sciences, University of Campania "Luigi Vanvitelli," Naples, Italy

EMANUELE MONDA, MD
Inherited and Rare Cardiovascular Disease Unit, Department of Translational Medical Sciences, University of Campania "Luigi Vanvitelli," AORN dei Colli, Monaldi Hospital, Naples, Italy

ASHLEY E. NEAL, MD
Associate Professor, Department of Pediatrics, University of Louisville School of Medicine and Norton Children's, Louisville, Kentucky, USA

CAMERON K. ORMISTON, BS
Division of Cardiovascular Medicine, Department of Medicine, University of California, San Diego, San Diego, California, USA

NGOZI OSUJI, MD, MPH
Division of Cardiology, Department of Medicine, Ciccarone Center for the Prevention of Cardiovascular Disease, Johns Hopkins School of Medicine, Baltimore, Maryland, USA

ROBERTA PACILEO, MD
Department of Translational Medical Sciences, University of Campania "Luigi Vanvitelli," Naples, Italy

SEONG-MI PARK, MD, PhD
Division of Cardiology, Department of Internal Medicine, Korea University Medicine, Korea University Anam Hospital, Seoul, Republic of Korea

ANDREW M. REITTINGER, MD
Division of Pediatric Cardiology, Department of Pediatrics, University of Virginia, Charlottesville, Virginia, USA

ASHLEY ROSANDER, BS
Division of Cardiovascular Medicine, Department of Medicine, University of California, San Diego, San Diego, California, USA

MARTA RUBINO, MD
Inherited and Rare Cardiovascular Disease Unit, Department of Translational Medical Sciences, University of Campania "Luigi Vanvitelli," AORN dei Colli, Monaldi Hospital, Naples, Italy

MARIA GIOVANNA RUSSO, MD, PhD
Department of Translational Medical Sciences, University of Campania "Luigi Vanvitelli," Department of Pediatric Cardiology, AORN dei Colli, Monaldi Hospital, Naples, Italy

PRASHANTHAN SANDERS, MBBS, PhD
Centre for Heart Rhythm Disorders, The University of Adelaide and Royal Adelaide
Hospital, Adelaide, Australia

BERARDO SARUBBI, MD, PhD
Adult Congenital Heart Diseases Unit, AORN dei Colli, Monaldi Hospital, Department of
Translational Medical Sciences, University of Campania "Luigi Vanvitelli," Naples, Italy

MICHAEL SCOTT, DO
Pediatric Resident, Department of Pediatrics, University of Louisville, Office of Medical
Education, School of Medicine, Louisville, Kentucky, USA

MICHAEL D. SHAPIRO, DO, MCR
Fred M. Parrish Professor of Cardiology and Molecular Medicine, Section of
Cardiovascular Medicine, Department of Internal Medicine, Wake Forest University
School of Medicine, Center for Prevention of Cardiovascular Disease, Winston-Salem,
North Carolina, USA

ANDREW SIAW-ASAMOAH, BA, MPhil
Perelman School of Medicine, University of Pennsylvania, Philadelphia, Pennsylvania,
USA

ERIC FRANCIS SULAVA, MD
Department of Emergency Medicine, Naval Medical Readiness and Training Center
Portsmouth, Portsmouth, Virginia, USA

LISA R. TANNOCK, MD
Professor of Internal Medicine, Division of Endocrinology, Diabetes, and Metabolism,
University of Kentucky, Department of Veterans Affairs, Lexington, Kentucky, USA

PAM R. TAUB, MD, FACC
Division of Cardiovascular Medicine, Department of Medicine, University of California,
San Diego, California, USA

PAUL D. THOMPSON, MD
Chief of Cardiology – Emeritus, Hartford Hospital, Hartford, Connecticut; Professor of
Medicine, University of Connecticut, USA

JONATHAN A. TOBERT, MD, PhD
Academic Visitor, Nuffield Department of Population Health, University of Oxford, Oxford,
United Kingdom

MELODY TRAN-REINA, MD
Assistant Clinical Professor, Department of Internal Medicine, University of California,
Davis School of Medicine, Sacramento, California, USA

ROBERT WILD, MD, MPH, PhD
Section of Reproductive Endocrinology and Infertility, Department of Obstetrics and
Gynecology, University of Oklahoma Health and Sciences Center, Oklahoma City,
Oklahoma, USA

ALBERTO ZAMBON, MD, PhD
Associate Professor of Medicine, Department of Medicine - DIMED, University of Padova,
Padova, Italy

Contents

Most children with congenital heart disease (CHD) survive to adulthood, owing largely to significant advances in the diagnosis and management of CHD over the past few decades. Primary care providers are essential partners in the recognition and management of these patients in our current medical environment. This article reviews the role of the primary care physician in detecting fetuses, infants, and children with possible CHD. Furthermore, this article discusses common primary care issues arising for patients with CHD, including growth and development, mental illness, dental care, and the transition to adult primary care.

Pediatric hypertension is becoming of increasing concern as the incidence rate increases alongside pediatric obesity. Practitioners need to be aware of the screening recommendations for early recognition and management of this disorder. Lifestyle modifications should be addressed early and specialty referral considered if the child is not improving. Further workup to rule out secondary causes of pediatric hypertension should also be considered in any child with stage 2 hypertension and in those with persistently elevated blood pressures. Early recognition and management are key to not only preventing present complications but also future cardiovascular disease in adulthood.

Each year millions of children and adolescents undergo sports preparticipation evaluations (PPEs) before participating in organized sports. A primary aim of the PPE is to screen for risk factors associated with sudden cardiac death. This article is designed to summarize the current thoughts on the PPE with a specific slant toward the pediatric and early adolescent evaluation and how these evaluations may differ from those in adults.

> Sudden unexplained death (SUD) is a tragic event for both the family and community, particularly when it occurs in young individuals. Sudden cardiac death (SCD) represents the leading form of SUD and is defined as an unexpected event without an obvious extracardiac cause, occurring within 1 hour after the onset of symptoms. In children, the main causes of SCD are inherited cardiac disorders, whereas coronary artery diseases (congenital or acquired), congenital heart diseases, and myocarditis are rare. The present review examines the current state of knowledge regarding SCD in children, discussing the epidemiology, clinical causes, and prevention strategies.

Adult Heart Disease

> Assessment of atherosclerotic cardiovascular disease (ASCVD) risk is the cornerstone of primary ASCVD prevention, enabling targeted use of the most aggressive therapies in those most likely to benefit, while guiding a conservative approach in those who are low risk. ASCVD risk assessment begins with the use of a traditional 10-year risk calculator, with further refinement through the consideration of risk-enhancing factors (particularly lipoprotein(a)) and subclinical atherosclerosis testing (particularly coronary artery calcium (CAC) testing). In this review, we summarize the current field of ASCVD risk assessment in primary prevention and highlight new guidelines from the Endocrine Society.

> A modern approach to mitigating the impact of cardiovascular disease on Americans demands not only an understanding of modifiable conditions that contribute to its development but also a greater appreciation of the heterogeneous distribution of these conditions based on race. As race is not a biological construct, further research is needed to fully elucidate the mechanisms that contribute to these differences. The consequences of the differential impact of modifiable risk factors on cardiovascular disease outcomes among black Americans compared with white Americans cannot be understated.

> Cardiovascular disease is the major cause of death in women. Older women remain at risk for coronary artery isease/cardiovascular disease,

but risk-modifying behavior can improve outcomes. Women have a different symptom profile and have been underdiagnosed and under-treated as compared with men. Although older women are underrepre-sented in trials, clinicians should be more attuned to the prevention, diagnosis, and treatment of cardiovascular disease in older women.

Significant drug interactions contribute to hospitalizations, mortality, and health care costs. They often are preventable with a basic understanding of pharmacokinetics and pharmacodynamics. More than quarter of Amer-icans above the age of 40 years take a statin, the most commonly used lipid-lowering therapy in modern times. Because of their pharmacoki-netics, statins interact with numerous other drugs and substances, often in a manner that differs from statin to statin. This article provides an over-view of important drug interactions for the most commonly used medica-tions in preventive cardiology, with an emphasis on clinically significant interactions involving statins.

 Video content accompanies this article at http://www.medical. theclinics.com.

This review highlights the key components of a heart-healthy diet and presents an evidence-based overview of recent research. Diets that in-crease plant-based food sources and healthy unsaturated fats consumption and limit foods that are processed and/or high in sodium, refined sugar, and saturated fat are recommended. Dietary modification can be supplemented with lifestyle-based therapies (eg, exercise, time-restricted eating) to maximize clinical benefit and achieve the "cardiometabolic jackpot." Physicians should take into account cul-tural preferences, affordability and accessibility of foods, and their pa-tients' cultural values or expectations when recommending dietary interventions.

The cardiovascular epidemiologist, Jeremy Morris, called physical activity "the best bargain in public health," but few clinicians use exercise and physical activity in their practice. Clinicians should routinely inquire about physical activity and recommend that patients achieve the minimal levels recommended by the 2018 Physical Activity Guidelines for Americans. Clinician should avoid unnecessary testing that discourages patients from an active lifestyle. Patients after myocardial infarction, cardiac sur-gery, or the diagnosis of heart failure or claudication should be referred to an exercise-based cardiac rehab program. Physical activity and exer-cise training may be a clinical bargain, but as with all medical interventions, it must be used to be effective.

Obstructive sleep apnea (OSA) presents as repetitive interruptions of ventilation >10 seconds during sleep as a result of upper airway obstruction resulting in increased respiratory effort. Intermittent hypoxia causes physiologic changes resulting in increased catecholamine production, increased total peripheral resistance, tachycardia, and increased venous return, leading to increased cardiac output, hypertension, tachyarrhythmias, left ventricular hypertrophy, and heart failure. OSA causes an abnormal dip on 24-hour ambulatory blood pressure monitoring. Definitive diagnosis is made by polysomnography. Continuous positive airway pressure (CPAP) remains the first-line treatment. Effective treatment using CPAP reduces blood pressure and is indispensable for proper management of atrial fibrillation.

Most endocrine disorders are chronic in nature, and thus even a minor effect to increase risk for cardiovascular disease can lead to a significant impact over prolonged duration. Although robust therapies exist for many endocrine disorders (eg suppression of excess hormone amounts, or replacement of hormone deficiencies), the therapies do not perfectly restore normal physiology. Thus, individuals with endocrine disorders are at potential increased cardiovascular disease risk, and maximizing strategies to reduce that risk are needed. This article reviews various endocrine conditions that can impact lipid levels and/or cardiovascular disease risk.

Managing dyslipidemia over a women's life, including a focus on pregnancy, contraception, and atherosclerotic cardiovascular disease risk prevention can decrease the burden of cardiovascular disease.

Atherosclerotic cardiovascular disease (ASCVD) continues to represent a growing global health challenge. Despite guideline-recommended treatment of ASCVD risk, including antihypertensive, high-intensity statin therapy, and antiaggregant agents, high-risk patients, especially those with established ASCVD and patients with type 2 diabetes, continue to experience cardiovascular events. Recent years have brought significant developments in lipid and atherosclerosis research. Several lipid drugs owe their existence, in part, to human genetic evidence. Here, the authors briefly review the mechanisms, the effect on lipid parameters, and safety profiles of some of the most promising new lipid-lowering approaches that will be soon available in our daily clinical practice.

Combinations of lipid-lowering agents can often bring LDL cholesterol down to around 40 mg/dL (1 mmol/L). Randomized controlled trials indicate that this reduces the risk of atherosclerotic vascular events with minimal adverse effects. This has raised the question of whether there is any concentration of LDL cholesterol below which further lowering is futile and/or a source of new adverse effects. This article examines several lines of evidence that lead to the conclusion that there is no known threshold below which lowering LDL cholesterol is harmful, but reduction of LDL cholesterol below 25 mg/dL may provide little if any further benefit.

Decades of research have shown that high-density lipoprotein cholesterol (HDL-C) levels in humans are associated with atherosclerotic cardiovascular disease (ASCVD). This association is strong and coherent across populations and remains after the elimination of covariates. Animal studies show that increasing HDL particles prevent atherosclerosis, and basic work on the biology of HDL supports a strong biological plausibility for a therapeutic target. This enthusiasm is dampened by Mendelian randomization data showing that HDL-C may not be causal in ASCVD. Furthermore, drugs that increase HDL-C have largely failed to prevent or treat ASCVD.

Heart failure with preserved ejection fraction (HFpEF) is a significantly symptomatic disease and has a poor prognosis similar to that of heart failure with reduced ejection fraction (HFrEF). Contrary to HFrEF, HFpEF is difficult to diagnose, and the recommended diagnostic algorithm of HFpEF is complicated. Several therapies for HFpEF have failed to reduce mortality or morbidity. HFpEF is thought to be a complex and heterogeneous systemic disorder that has various phenotypes and multiple comorbidities. Therefore, therapeutic strategies of HFpEF need to change depending on the phenotype of the patient. This review highlights the pharmacologic and nonpharmacologic treatment of HFpEF.

Telehealth presents opportunities for enhanced care and benefits to patients with heart failure. As technology develops, telehealth is increasingly being integrated into the standard care of heart failure. Telehealth can help enhance timely access and follow-up, facilitate care coordination for diagnostic and management strategies, individualize management, increase opportunities for multidisciplinary care, help implement complementary management strategies, and improve outcomes. Telehealth commonly includes clinician-to-clinician communication; patient interaction with mobile health technologies including remote monitoring, and clinician-to-patient interaction modalities. Despite all the potential benefits of expanded access, telehealth may have limitations especially for vulnerable populations, who are at risk for less access to telehealth modalities and infrastructure. Clinicians and health networks should examine strategies to incorporate telehealth in the management of patients with heart failure. Health care systems should invest in technologies and provide equipment and connectivity to ensure that telehealth does not widen health disparities.

Abnormal fluid handling leads to physiologic abnormalities in multiple organ systems. Deranged hemodynamics, neurohormonal activation, excessive tubular sodium reabsorption, inflammation, oxidative stress, and nephrotoxic medications are important drivers of harmful cardiorenal interactions in patients with heart failure. Accurate quantitative measurement of fluid volume is vital to individualizing therapy for such patients. Blood volume analysis and pulmonary artery pressure monitoring seem the most reliable methods for assessing fluid volume and guiding decongestive therapies. Still the cornerstone of decongestive therapy, diuretics' effectiveness decreases with progression of heart failure. Extracorporeal ultrafiltration, an alternative to diuretics, has been shown to reduce heart-failure events.

Preface

Cardiovascular disease across the lifespan remains perhaps the most prominent thread of commonality in disease prevention and need for recognition in primary care practices. It comprises a significant burden of illness and requires well-orchestrated collaboration and follow-up with specialty colleagues. According to 2021 data from the Centers for Disease Control and Prevention, the life expectancy for both men and women in the United States continues to decrease annually, now at 73.2 and 79.1 years, respectively, with cardiovascular disease being the number one cause of death for both genders. Of course, the COVID-19 pandemic has provided a substantial, negative impact on life expectancy.

This *Clinics Collections* was a privilege to conceive, as our main objective was to provide readers with an overview of the highest-quality and most current evidence for addressing common cardiovascular conditions in both pediatric and adult populations. The issue commences with overviews of congenital heart disease, pediatric hypertension, and guidance on preparticipation screening and risk of sudden cardiac death in children. The aim of these articles is to guide primary care clinicians in appropriate screening practices and to foster timely diagnosis and management across primary and specialty care practices.

The adult heart disease section comprises most of the issue, highlighting articles that detail the most commonly encountered cardiac conditions in our practices. While many articles are centered on the disease process, this issue provides insight into many ancillary factors and elements related to heart disease outcomes, including diet, exercise, the impact of social determinants on race and gender, and the role of telehealth in disease management. Current guidelines on hypertension, lipid management, coronary artery disease, atrial fibrillation, and heart failure are presented with salient references and practical key points. The controversial topic of testosterone replacement therapy and its relationship to cardiovascular health is also explored.

We hope that this *Clinics Collections* dedicated to heart disease will provide readers with useful information to augment their daily practice of medicine. We thank you all for being loyal readers of our series, and for providing outstanding medical care for our patients.

Joel J. Heidelbaugh, MD, FAAFP, FACG
Departments of Family Medicine and Urology
Department of Family Medicine
University of Michigan Medical School
Ann Arbor, MI, USA

Ypsilanti Health Center
200 Arnet Street, Suite 200
Ypsilanti, MI 48198, USA

E-mail address:
jheidel@umich.edu

Clinics Collections 13 (2023) xvii
https://doi.org/10.1016/j.ccol.2023.04.001
2352-7986/23/© 2023 Published by Elsevier Inc.

Pediatric Heart Disease

Congenital Heart Disease

Michael Scott, DO[a], Ashley E. Neal, MD[b],*

KEYWORDS

- Congenital heart disease • Pediatric cardiology • CHD • Screening
- Patent ductus arteriosus

KEY POINTS

- Most children with congenital heart disease (CHD) survive to adulthood.
- The genetic cause of CHD continues to be elucidated; thus, consultation with a pediatric geneticist or pediatric cardiologist may be useful in children with genetic syndromes when the cardiac implications are unclear.
- Because the availability and accuracy of prenatal screening for certain cardiac lesions varies, pediatricians must remain vigilant for neonates presenting with symptoms that suggest CHD.
- Children with CHD need comprehensive pediatric care that considers the increased risk of growth issues, developmental delay, and mental health disorders in this population.

INTRODUCTION

Congenital heart disease (CHD) is the most common birth defect, affecting 8 to 10 per 1000 newborns in the United States and 17.9 per 1000 newborns worldwide. Fortunately, the mortality rate for CHD has decreased by 34.5% globally between 1990 and 2017, due largely to rapid advances in diagnostic imaging, medications, catheter techniques, and surgical interventions.[1] Recent estimates suggest about 2.4 million adults in the United States and 12 million adults globally are survivors of CHD.[1,2] For children with CHD, the pediatric primary care provider and pediatric cardiologist collaborate to identify CHD, monitor for symptoms, counsel about necessary interventions, and ultimately provide optimal transitions to adult providers. These children, who often have multiple comorbidities, receive the best care through a team-based approach coordinated by the primary care physician, establishing a medical home.[3]

This article originally appeared in *Primary Care: Clinics in Office Practice*, Volume 48 Issue 3, September 2021.

[a] Department of Pediatrics, University of Louisville, Office of Medical Education, School of Medicine, 571 South Floyd, Suite 412, Louisville, KY 40202, USA; [b] Department of Pediatrics, University of Louisville School of Medicine and Norton Children's, 571 South Floyd Street, Suite 113, Louisville, KY 40202, USA
* Corresponding author.
E-mail address: ashley.neal.1@louisville.edu

CAUSE OF CONGENITAL HEART DISEASE

The cause of CHD is multifactorial with both environmental and genetic influences. Thus, it is useful for primary care providers, geneticists, obstetricians, and pediatric cardiologists to have a basic understanding of these risk factors. Although the association between genetic factors and CHD was first recognized in the late 1940s, the precise relationship between specific genetic mutations and CHD remains quite complex.[4] Rarely, a single gene has been linked to a specific lesion. More frequently, genetic syndromes are associated with a diverse array of cardiac lesions as shown in **Table 1**.[4] New genes correlated with CHD or cardiomyopathy continue to be identified on a regular basis, making the rote memorization of all genes potentially associated with cardiac pathology an impossible undertaking. It would be practical to reference Online Mendelian Inheritance in Man (OMIM)[5] or consult a pediatric geneticist or pediatric cardiologist when a genetic abnormality or syndrome is suspected and the cardiac implications are unclear. Many congenital heart defects are identified prenatally, with one indication for a fetal echocardiogram being suspicion of a genetic condition by cell-free fetal DNA testing.[6] Environmental risk factors also contribute to the development of CHD. Reported prenatal risk factors include maternal ingestion of ethanol or prescription medications such as sodium valproate, retinoic acid, lithium, nonsteroidal antiinflammatory drugs, angiotensin-converting enzyme inhibitors, and paroxetine. During pregnancy, maternal infections such as rubella and cytomegalovirus and poorly controlled maternal diabetes are also well-described environmental risk factors associated with subsequent development of CHD.[6,7] Environmental risk factors may also prompt referral for fetal echocardiogram and subsequent prenatal detection of CHD (**Table 2**).

PRENATAL DIAGNOSIS OF CONGENITAL HEART DISEASE

The care of many children with CHD begins prenatally with maternal referral for a fetal echocardiogram. Referral may be based on findings from the obstetric evaluation or other predisposing conditions as noted in **Table 2**. This testing is considered cost-effective when risk of CHD exceeds 3%.[6] Comprehensive fetal echocardiograms, which often include additional views of cardiac structures and color Doppler imaging, can increase detection rates of CHD from less than 50% to nearly 90% of serious CHD when compared with routine obstetric ultrasounds.[6,8–10] When CHD is identified prenatally, families can receive appropriate counseling and delivery plans can be adjusted accordingly, reducing preoperative mortality.[11] Unfortunately, even within the United States, large disparities exist in prenatal detection of CHD, with diagnosis rates among states ranging from 11.8% to 53.4%.[12] Remote interpretation of fetal echocardiograms coupled with sonographer training can improve prenatal CHD detection rates. However, this strategy has only been implemented in limited regions of the country.[13] Therefore, normal prenatal assessments do not exclude structural heart disease. Even when a comprehensive fetal echocardiogram has been performed, some aspects of the fetal circulation differ from the postnatal circulation, limiting the diagnostic accuracy of fetal examinations for certain lesions. For example, a patent ductus arteriosus (PDA) would be a normal finding during fetal life. Therefore, predicting whether or not a child will develop heart failure from a PDA postnatally is nearly impossible based on prenatal imaging.

NORMAL FETAL AND TRANSITIONAL CIRCULATION

During fetal life, most of the gas exchange occurs at the placenta, with only 10% to 25% of the blood ejected by the right ventricle making it to the fetal lungs.[14] The

Table 1
Examples of genetic syndromes commonly associated with cardiac disease

Genetic Syndrome [associated gene(s)]	Extracardiac Features	Associated Cardiac Disease
Trisomy 21	Brachycephaly, small ears, upslanting palpebral fissures, epicanthal folds, duodenal atresia, imperforate anus, Hirschsprung disease, leukemia	AVSD, VSD, ASD, PDA, TOF, pulmonary hypertension
Trisomy 18	Micrognathia, short sternum, rocker-bottom feet, omphalocele, renal anomalies, severe intellectual disability	ASD, VSD, PDA, TOF, DORV, TGA, valve abnormalities
Trisomy 13	Cleft lip and palate, hypotelorism, coloboma, holoprosencephaly, deafness, severe intellectual disability, polydactyly, omphalocele, cryptorchidism	ASD, VSD, PDA, valve abnormalities
Turner syndrome	Short stature, early loss of ovarian function, lymphedema, webbed neck, renal anomalies	Coarctation of the aorta, aortic stenosis, BAV
CHARGE syndrome (CHD7, SEMA3E)	Coloboma, choanal atresia, genital hypoplasia, ear abnormalities, hearing loss, developmental delay, growth retardation, intellectual disability	ASD, VSD, TOF
DiGeorge syndrome, velocardiofacial syndrome (TBX1)	Myopathic facies, tubular nose with bulbous nasal tip, immunodeficiency, hypocalcemia, intellectual disability	TOF, IAA, TA, VSD
Holt-Oram syndrome (TBX5)	Absent thumb, radius hypoplasia/limb defects, triphalangeal thumb	ASD, VSD, PDA, AVSD, conduction defects
Alagille syndrome (JAGGED1, NOTCH2)	Prominent forehead, hypertelorism, intellectual disability, liver failure, ophthalmologic problems, butterfly vertebrae, renal defects	Peripheral pulmonary stenosis, PS, TOF
Noonan syndrome (PTPN11, KRAS, SOS1, SOS2, RAF1, BRAF, MEK1, HRAS, NRAS, SHOC2, CBL, NF1)	Short stature, hypertelorism, ptosis, pectus deformity, bleeding disorder, chylothorax, cryptorchidism, lymphatic abnormalities	PS, ASD, TOF, VSD, PDA, hypertrophic cardiomyopathy

(continued on next page)

Table 1
(continued)

Genetic Syndrome [associated gene(s)]	Extracardiac Features	Associated Cardiac Disease
Williams syndrome (ELN)	Short stature, flat midface, epicanthal folds, long philtrum, sensorineural hearing loss, thick lips, intellectual disability, sociable, hypercalcemia	Supravalvular AS, peripheral PS, VSD, ASD
Marfan Syndrome (Fibrillin)	Arm span to height >1.05, disproportionate tall stature, long narrow face, ectopia lentis, pectus excavatum, pectus carinatum, high-arched palate	Aortic aneurysm, mitral valve prolapse, dilated pulmonary artery
Kabuki syndrome (KMT2D, KDM6A)	Growth deficiency, wide palpebral fissure, intellectual disability, fetal finger pads	ASD, VSD, TOF, coarctation of aorta, BAV, TGA, HLHS
Ellis-van Creveld (EVC, EVC2)	Short upper lip, natal teeth, enamel hypoplasia, polydactyly	ASD, common atrium

Abbreviations: AS, aortic stenosis; ASD, atrial septal defect; AVSD, atrioventricular septal defect; BAV, bicuspid aortic valve; DORV, double outlet right ventricle; HLHS, hypoplastic left heart syndrome; IAA, interrupted aortic arch; PDA, patent ductus arteriosus; PS, pulmonary stenosis; TA, truncus arteriosus; TGA, transposition of the great arteries; TOF, tetralogy of Fallot; VSD, ventricular septal defect.
Data from Refs.[4,5,15]

Table 2
Indications for fetal echocardiogram

Screening Indicated	May be Considered	Not Indicated
Maternal Indications		
• Uncontrolled (Hgb A1C >6) pregestational diabetes mellitus (DM) • DM diagnosed in 1st trimester • Uncontrolled phenylketonuria • Anti-Ro (SSA)/anti-La (SSB)+ autoantibodies with a previously affected child • Retinoic acid use (third trimester) • Nonsteroidal antiinflammatory drug (NSAID) use (third trimester) • ubella (first trimester)	• Anti-Ro (SSA)/anti-La (SSB)+ autoantibodies without a previously affected child • Angiotensin-converting enzyme inhibitor use • Anticonvulsant use • Lithium use • Vitamin A use • Paroxetine use • NSAIDs (first/second trimester) • Pregnancy resulting from assisted reproduction technology	• Gestational DM with Hgb A1c <6% • Vitamin K agonist use • Selective serotonin reuptake inhibitor use (other than paroxetine) • Maternal infection other than rubella with seroconversion only
Fetal Indications		
• Suspected fetal cardiac abnormality by obstetric ultrasound • Extracardiac abnormality identified by obstetric ultrasound • Infection with suspicion of fetal myocarditis • Suspected or confirmed chromosome abnormality • Fetal tachycardia, bradycardia, or frequent or persistent irregular heart rhythm • Increased nuchal thickness >99% (≥3.5 mm) • Increased nuchal thickness >95% (≥3 mm) with abnormal ductus venosus flow • Monochorionic twinning • Fetal hydrops or effusions	• Increased nuchal thickness >95% (≥3 mm) • Abnormality of the umbilical cord • Abnormality of the placenta • Abnormality of intraabdominal venous anatomy	
Family History		
• CHD in 1st degree relative of the fetus • Relative with disorder with mendelian inheritance that has a CHD association	CHD in a second degree relative of the fetus	Isolated CHD in a relative other than first or second degree

Data from Donofrio MT, Moon-Grady AJ, Hornberger LK et al. American Heart Association Adults With Congenital Heart Disease Joint Committee of the Council on Cardiovascular Disease in the Young and Council on Clinical Cardiology, Council on Cardiovascular Surgery and Anesthesia, and Council on Cardiovascular and Stroke Nursing. Diagnosis and treatment of fetal cardiac disease: a scientific statement from the American Heart Association. Circulation. 2014 May 27;129(21):2183-242.

PDA allows blood oxygenated in the placenta to travel from the pulmonary artery to the descending aorta, bypassing the fetal lungs.[14–16] During fetal life, pulmonary vascular resistance (PVR) is elevated, leading to right-to-left shunting at the PDA. Following delivery of the newborn, oxygen tension increases, and the newborn lungs expand, forcing amniotic fluid from the alveolar sacs. These changes dramatically decrease the PVR, which combined with a concomitant increase in the systemic vascular resistance, results in shunting across the PDA becoming left-to-right (from the aorta to the pulmonary artery). The PDA begins to functionally close at approximately 10 to 15 hours of life and is anatomically closed by around 2 to 3 weeks in most infants in response to persistently increased arterial oxygen tension and decreased prostaglandin (PGE) levels.[14] Over the first 6 to 8 weeks of life, the PVR continues to decrease to normal adult levels.[15] These physiologic changes are important to consider when evaluating a patient with confirmed or suspected CHD as will be discussed in subsequent sections.

PULSE OXIMETRY SCREENING

Acknowledging the limitations of prenatal testing and dynamic aspects of neonatal cardiovascular physiology, providers caring for newborns must remain vigilant for children who develop signs or symptoms that may suggest CHD. In conjunction with a comprehensive history and physical examination, predischarge pulse oximetry has an overall sensitivity of 76.3% and specificity of 99.9% in detecting critical CHD.[17–19] This screening should be performed no sooner than 24 hours of life and, ideally, as close to newborn nursery discharge as possible. For this assessment, oxygen saturation is measured in the right arm and a foot. When the oxygen saturation is greater than or equal to 95% in either the right arm or a foot with less than or equal to 3% difference between measured saturations, no additional screening is indicated. Otherwise, the infant requires repeat pulse oximetry measurement. With persistently abnormal findings, noncardiac causes of hypoxia ought to be excluded. In the absence of a noncardiac cause of hypoxia, the child should undergo a pediatric echocardiogram to evaluate for CHD.[18,20]

NEONATAL PRESENTATIONS OF CONGENITAL HEART DISEASE

The timing and symptomatology of neonatal presentations of CHD can best be understood in the context of the physiologic changes that occur with the transition from fetal to postnatal life (**Fig. 1**). Some of the more common forms of CHD, emphasizing key physical examination findings and lesions that may require intervention, are briefly discussed.

NEONATAL CONGENITAL HEART DISEASE REQUIRING EMERGENT INTERVENTION
Total Anomalous Pulmonary Venous Return

- Brief overview: the connection of all 4 pulmonary veins is abnormal and/or obstructed.
- Presentation: may develop cyanosis, respiratory distress, and symptoms of low cardiac output within the first few hours of life, as newborn lung perfusion increases significantly.
- Treatment: urgent surgical correction

This is one of the few surgical emergencies in pediatric cardiology. Importantly, it is also a lesion in which PGE may cause further deterioration by increasing pulmonary blood flow, worsening pulmonary edema. Children most at risk for decompensation

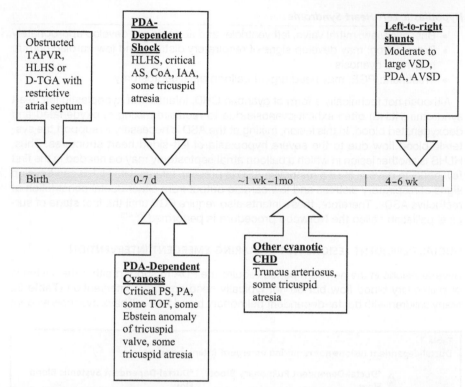

Fig. 1. Neonatal presentations of CHD. AS, aortic stenosis; ASD, atrial septal defect; AVSD, atrioventricular septal defect; CoA, coarctation; D-TGA, D-transposition of the great arteries; HLHS, hypoplastic left heart syndrome; IAA, interrupted aortic arch; PA, pulmonary atresia; PDA, patent ductus arteriosus; PS, pulmonary stenosis; TAPVR, Total anomalous pulmonary venous return; TOF, tetralogy of Fallot; VSD, ventricular septal defect.

with this lesion have infracardiac total anomalous pulmonary venous return (TAPVR), in which the pulmonary venous return travels through the liver. Of note, in the absence of pulmonary venous obstruction, infants with TAPVR may have minimal symptoms.[21,22]

D-Transposition of the Great Arteries

- Brief overview: systemic and pulmonary circulation occur in parallel with the aorta arising from the right ventricle and the pulmonary artery from the left ventricle.
- Presentation: may present either at birth or in the first few days of life with variable degree of cyanosis, may develop acidosis
- Treatment: PGE; may need urgent balloon atrial septostomy

In D-transposition of the great arteries (D-TGA), although the PDA may permit some oxygenated blood to reach the body, a minimally restrictive atrial level shunt is required to adequately support the systemic circulation. Children with D-TGA and restrictive atrial septal defects (ASDs) may present either at birth or in the first few days of life with profound cyanosis and acidosis, requiring an emergent interventional cardiology procedure called a balloon atrial septostomy to enlarge the ASD. Children with adequate atrial mixing may have mild-to-moderate cyanosis at birth and typically require PGE until definitive surgical repair is performed in the first week of life.[22,23]

Hypoplastic Left Heart Syndrome

- Brief overview: mitral valve, left ventricle, and aorta do not develop appropriately
- Presentation: may develop signs of respiratory distress and low cardiac output, may have cyanosis
- Treatment: PGE; may need urgent balloon atrial septostomy

Although not technically a form of cyanotic CHD, infants with hypoplastic left heart syndrome (HLHS) often exhibit cyanosis due to requisite mixing of oxygenated and deoxygenated blood. In this lesion, mixing at the ASD is necessary to support the systemic blood flow due to the severe hypoplasia of left-sided heart structures. Thus, HLHS is another lesion in which a balloon atrial septostomy may be needed in the first few hours to days of life if a restrictive ASD is present. Infants with HLHS can develop signs of respiratory distress and low cardiac output from either ductal constriction or restrictive ASDs. Therefore, these infants also require PGE until the first stage of surgical palliation called the Norwood procedure is performed.[24–26]

DUCTAL-DEPENDENT LESIONS NOT REQUIRING EMERGENT INTERVENTION

Several lesions in the newborn period require the PDA to support either the systemic or pulmonary blood flow but do not typically need emergent intervention (**Table 3**). Many children with ductal-dependent pulmonary blood flow will have cyanosis evident

Table 3 Ductal-dependent lesions not requiring emergent intervention		
	[a]Ductal-Dependent Pulmonary Blood Flow	[a]Ductal-Dependent Systemic Blood Flow
Lesion and Key Points	**Critical pulmonary stenosis (PS)** • Loud murmur • +PGE	**Hypoplastic left heart syndrome (HLHS)** • May require emergent intervention • Requires unrestrictive ASD and PDA • +PGE
	Pulmonary atresia • +PGE	**Critical aortic stenosis** • Loud murmur • +PGE
	Tetralogy of Fallot (TOF), some forms • Loud murmur • Cyanosis may be progressive/risk for "Tet" spells • +/−PGE • Consider 22q11 testing	**Critical coarctation of the aorta (CoA)** • More likely to be missed with pulse oximetry screen • May present with shock first week of life • +PGE
	Ebstein anomaly of tricuspid valve (severe forms) • Loud murmur • Marked cardiomegaly on chest radiograph • +/−PGE	**Interrupted aortic arch** • More likely to be missed with pulse oximetry screen • May present with shock first week of life • +PGE • Consider 22q11 testing
	Tricuspid atresia (some forms) • +/−PGE	**Tricuspid atresia (some forms)** • May present with shock first week of life if VSD restrictive • +/−PGE

Abbreviations: ASD, atrial septal defect; PDA, patent ductus arteriosus; PGE, prostaglandin; VSD, ventricular septal defect.
[a] See notes in text regarding decision-making related to initiation of PGE in these lesions.

clinically or by pulse oximetry in the first hours to days of life. Although some lesions in this category will require PGE until an intervention is performed, close monitoring for development of marked cyanosis with PDA closure may be needed to determine whether other lesions are truly ductal dependent. It is worth noting that infants with tetralogy of Fallot (TOF) are at risk for the development of progressive subpulmonary stenosis. This subpulmonary stenosis usually worsens at a few months of age, creating a substrate for hypercyanotic episodes or "tetralogy spells." In these episodes, the infant's murmur may become inaudible due to a significant decrement in pulmonary blood flow as deoxygenated blood flows right to left across the ventricular septal defect and out the aorta. To abort episodes, the infant should be soothed, given oxygen, and the knees pushed toward the chest among other maneuvers to favor pulmonary over systemic blood flow. Once hypercyanotic episodes have been observed, an infant with TOF warrants urgent surgical intervention.[27,28]

Lesions that require the PDA to support systemic blood flow (see **Table 3**) may not be adequately identified by prenatal ultrasound or newborn pulse oximetry and may present in shock with ductal closure in the first week of life.[29] Thus, one should have a high index of suspicion for possible ductal-dependent CHD in the neonate presenting with shock in the first few weeks of life and a low threshold for initiation of PGE. Although tricuspid atresia is considered a form of cyanotic CHD, it is a complex lesion that presents with a variable degree of cyanosis and can present with shock if systemic blood flow becomes compromised due to a restrictive ventricular septal defect.[27,30]

OTHER NEONATAL CONGENITAL HEART DISEASE PRESENTATIONS
"Cyanotic" Congenital Heart Disease: Tricuspid Atresia and Truncus Arteriosus

Tricuspid atresia is a highly variable and complex, cyanotic single ventricle CHD lesion. Some infants with this lesion require PGE to maintain pulmonary or systemic blood flow depending on the relative position of the great vessels (eg, D-transposition). Other infants with tricuspid atresia, normal position of the great arteries, and a large ventricular septal defect will develop pulmonary edema over the first few weeks of life and may require a surgical procedure called a pulmonary artery band to restrict pulmonary blood flow if they develop tachypnea, tiring with feeds, sweating with feeds, and poor growth that suggest heart failure.[27,30] Truncus arteriosus is another CHD lesion typically included with cyanotic CHD lesions due to obligate mixing of oxygenated and deoxygenated blood at an unrestrictive ventricular septal defect and a single outflow supplying the body and lungs. However, many infants with truncus arteriosus will have nearly normal oxygen saturations. Clinically, children with this lesion usually develop pulmonary edema, tachypnea, and signs of heart failure within the first few weeks of life.[27]

Left-To-Right Shunts

As the PVR normalizes over the first 6 to 8 weeks of life, infants with moderate-to-large left-to-right shunts develop symptoms of pulmonary overcirculation. This category includes infants with a ventricular septal defect, atrioventricular canal defect, patent ductus arteriosus, or ASD. However, ASDs rarely cause symptoms in infancy. Infants with significant left-to-right shunts may initially be asymptomatic, have soft murmurs with large ventricular septal defects, or have more obvious murmurs with some large PDAs. However, in the first 1 to 2 months of life, these infants may demonstrate a gradual decline in growth percentiles or develop progressive tachypnea, worsening reflux, sweating with feeds, and/or tiring with feeds. These symptoms of heart failure may respond to increased caloric intake and initiation of diuretics, but consultation with a pediatric cardiologist is recommended. In contrast, many types of asymptomatic CHD are also identified in the neonatal period. For example, infants with small, isolated ventricular septal defects may have readily apparent murmurs prompting evaluation, but these defects would not be expected to cause symptoms and may spontaneously resolve in the first few years of life. In addition, mild valve abnormalities or dysfunction (ie, bicuspid aortic valve) may also be identified during the newborn period.[31]

Childhood Presentations of Congenital Heart Disease

Many types of CHD requiring intervention are recognized in newborns. During childhood and adolescence, pediatric cardiologists often see children for acquired forms of heart disease such as Kawasaki disease and cardiomyopathy or nonstructural concerns such as arrhythmia. Two relatively common CHD lesions presenting in childhood or adolescence are ASD and noncritical CoA. Although ASDs are generally asymptomatic, many are diagnosed incidentally as part of a murmur evaluation. Careful auscultation in children with these lesions may demonstrate a fixed, split S2 or pulmonary flow murmur. An electrocardiogram may demonstrate right axis deviation or right ventricular hypertrophy. A high index of suspicion is needed for detection of this lesion because symptoms and physical examination findings may be subtle.[32] One should consider expert consultation for additional diagnostic testing if an abnormality is suspected by physical examination or electrocardiogram. Noncritical CoA, in which patency of the ductus arteriosus is not required to maintain cardiac output, becomes evident in childhood or adolescence. Children with noncritical CoA may have upper-extremity hypertension, femoral pulses occurring after radial pulses (radial-femoral delay), intermittent claudication, or a systolic murmur at the left lower sternal border radiating to the back.[25,26] Thus, in children with hypertension, blood pressure in all 4 extremities and femoral pulses should be assessed.

LONGITUDINAL FOLLOW-UP ISSUES IN THE CHILD WITH CONGENITAL HEART DISEASE
Growth and Development

The child with CHD may have associated anomalies or comorbidities related to chronic illness, prior interventions, and prolonged hospitalizations. Approximately, 25% of infants with CHD have a noncardiac anomaly and about 15% have multiple congenital anomalies.[7] Those caring for children with CHD should have a low threshold to obtain genetic testing or consultation as well as diagnostic tests to evaluate for extracardiac comorbidities. Understanding whether or not a genetic abnormality is present may help determine the likelihood and expected magnitude of developmental delay (DD), which might be seen for the child.

Factors in children with CHD that increase risk of DD are as follows[33,34]:

- History of heart surgery in infancy
- Cyanotic lesions not requiring open heart surgery
- Premature birth
- Known genetic anomaly associated with DD
- History of mechanical support (ie, extracorporeal membrane oxygenation or ventricular assist device)
- History of heart transplantation
- History of cardiopulmonary resuscitation
- History of prolonged hospitalization (>2 weeks)

- Perioperative seizures
- Significant abnormalities on brain imaging

Any child or adolescent with CHD and developmental concern should be referred for formal developmental evaluation to optimize neurodevelopmental outcomes and quality of life.[33,34] In addition to developmental concerns, growth issues in infants and children with CHD are prevalent. In early childhood, even children with nonsurgical and repaired CHD may demonstrate poor relative growth.[35] However, in later childhood, rates of combined obesity and overweight in children with CHD mirror the general population at about 29%.[36] Some parents may restrict physical activity inappropriately in a child with repaired CHD or continue to provide excess calories when supplementation is not needed.[36] Thus, children with CHD may need specific counseling about physical activity and nutrition throughout childhood and adolescence. Overweight and obese children with CHD, as all children, require screening for development of associated comorbidities such as hypertension, diabetes, obstructive sleep apnea, and nonalcoholic fatty liver disease.[35]

Mental Illness

As noted earlier, children with CHD are at increased risk for developmental delay, specifically issues with executive function and attention, which may predispose them to subsequent development of mental illness in adolescence and adulthood.[37] In a recent Colorado statewide survey, 20% of adolescents with CHD had mental illness including anxiety disorders, attention disorders, conduct disorders, and impulse control disorders. Not surprisingly, those with a genetic diagnosis and a higher number of recent cardiac procedures had an increased risk of mental illness.[38] When evaluating adolescent CHD patients with single ventricle lesions, the lifetime risk of psychiatric diagnosis was ~65%, with anxiety disorders and attention disorders seen most frequently.[39] Thus, screening and addressing any psychiatric comorbidity in this population is crucial to improving overall quality of life and general well-being.

Dental Care

Another important aspect of primary care for children with CHD, as other pediatric patients, is encouraging routine dental visits. Although CHD is a known risk factor for developing infective endocarditis, recent guidelines suggest only a limited number of high-risk lesions require antibiotic prophylaxis before invasive dental procedures.[40] Children who need prophylaxis include those with

- Prosthetic cardiac valve or valve material,
- Previous endocarditis,
- Unrepaired or palliated cyanotic CHD,
- Completely repaired CHD with prosthetic material or device in the first 6 months after repair,
- Repaired CHD with residual defect near patch or device, or
- Valvulopathy developing after heart transplant.[40]

Transitions

Yet another critical aspect of caring for the adolescent with CHD is enabling a successful transition to adult providers. This process should ideally be initiated in early adolescence and completed by age 21 years. Although changes in insurance coverage and emotional attachment to a pediatric provider may create barriers, these are not insurmountable. Factors such as adolescents attending appointments without parents and the current primary care provider offering a recommendation for an adult provider can help facilitate these transitions.[41,42] In fact, ensuring the adult with CHD remains in a medical home and is not lost to follow-up may be one of the most valuable services a pediatric primary care provider can offer.

SUMMARY

Even children born with complex CHD and multiple extracardiac anomalies may survive to adulthood due to recent advances in the fields of pediatric cardiology and congenital heart surgery. Optimizing the growth, development, and quality of life for these children remains a challenge for primary care providers and pediatric subspecialists alike. Providers should continue to collaborate to meet the health care needs of this growing population. In addition, pediatric primary care providers and pediatric cardiologists should strive to prepare these children for a seamless transition to adulthood and adult care providers.

CLINICS CARE POINTS

- Consider discussion of any newly identified genetic abnormality in a child or child's first-degree relative with a geneticist or pediatric cardiologist if the cardiac implications are unclear.
- Recommend fetal echocardiogram screening to families when appropriate, as this screening has improved mortality in critical CHD.
- Do not assume that normal prenatal screening excludes CHD. This screening is not well standardized and still has limitations in detecting some forms of CHD.
- Do not assume that normal newborn pulse oximetry screening excludes CHD. Newborn hospitalization duration varies and the transition from fetal to postnatal circulation occurs at a variable rate.
- The timing of symptom emergence can help refine the list of potential diagnoses in children with suspected CHD.
- Have a low threshold to refer children with CHD for formal developmental assessment due to the increased risk of developmental delay.
- Carefully monitor growth in children with CHD, as the risk of obesity and obesity-related comorbidities is similar to the general population.
- Screen for psychiatric comorbidities in children and adolescents with CHD due to the increased risk of mental illness.
- Encourage children with CHD and repaired CHD to have regular dental care; however, only a limited number of these children require endocarditis prophylaxis based on current guidelines.
- Plan how and when to transition children with CHD to adult providers so they are not lost to follow-up.

DISCLOSURE

The authors have nothing to disclose.

REFERENCES

1. Collaborators GCHD. Global, regional, and national burden of congenital heart disease, 1990-2017: a systematic analysis for the Global Burden of Disease Study 2017. Lancet Child Adolesc Health 2020;4(3):185–200.

2. Burchill LJ, Gao L, Kovacs AH, et al. Hospitalization trends and health resource use for adult congenital heart disease-related heart failure. J Am Heart Assoc 2018;7(15):e008775.
3. Lantin-Hermoso MR, Berger S, Bhatt AB, et al. The care of children with congenital heart disease in their primary medical home. Pediatrics 2017;140(5): e20172607.
4. Pierpont ME, Brueckner M, Chung WK, et al. Genetic basis for congenital heart disease: revisited: a scientific statement from the American Heart Association. Circulation 2018;138(21):e653–711.
5. Online Mendelian Inheritance in Man, OMIM. Available at: https://omim.org. Accessed January 30, 2020.
6. Donofrio MT, Moon-Grady AJ, Hornberger LK, et al. Diagnosis and treatment of fetal cardiac disease: a scientific statement from the American Heart Association. Circulation 2014;129(21):2183–242.
7. Stoll C, Dott B, Alembik Y, et al. Associated noncardiac congenital anomalies among cases with congenital heart defects. Eur J Med Genet 2015;58(2):75–85.
8. Stümpflen I, Stümpflen A, Wimmer M, et al. Effect of detailed fetal echocardiography as part of routine prenatal ultrasonographic screening on detection of congenital heart disease. Lancet 1996;348(9031):854–7.
9. Yagel S, Weissman A, Rotstein Z, et al. Congenital heart defects: natural course and in utero development. Circulation 1997;96(2):550–5.
10. Pinto NM, Henry KA, Grobman WA, et al. Physician barriers and facilitators for screening for congenital heart disease with routine obstetric ultrasound: a national united states survey. J Ultrasound Med 2020;39(6):1143–53.
11. Holland BJ, Myers JA, Woods CR. Prenatal diagnosis of critical congenital heart disease reduces risk of death from cardiovascular compromise prior to planned neonatal cardiac surgery: a meta-analysis. Ultrasound Obstet Gynecol 2015; 45(6):631–8.
12. Quartermain MD, Pasquali SK, Hill KD, et al. Variation in prenatal diagnosis of congenital heart disease in infants. Pediatrics 2015;136(2):e378–85.
13. Brown J, Holland B. Successful fetal tele-echo at a small regional hospital. Telemed J E Health 2017;23(6):485–92. https://doi.org/10.1089/tmj.2016.0141.
14. Finnemore A, Groves A. Physiology of the fetal and transitional circulation. Semin Fetal Neonatal Med 2015;20(4):210–6.
15. Kliegman R, St. Geme J, Blum N, et al. Nelson textbook of pediatrics. 21st edition. Philadelphia, PA: Elsevier; 2020. p. 2.
16. Rios DR, Bhattacharya S, Levy PT, et al. Circulatory insufficiency and hypotension related to the ductus arteriosus in neonates. Front Pediatr 2018;6:62.
17. Kemper AR, Mahle WT, Martin GR, et al. Strategies for implementing screening for critical congenital heart disease. Pediatrics 2011;128(5):e1259–67.
18. Mahle WT, Newburger JW, Matherne GP, et al. Role of pulse oximetry in examining newborns for congenital heart disease: a scientific statement from the American Heart Association and American Academy of Pediatrics. Circulation 2009; 120(5):447–58.
19. Plana MN, Zamora J, Suresh G, et al. Pulse oximetry screening for critical congenital heart defects. Cochrane Database Syst Rev 2018;3:CD011912.
20. Mahle WT, Martin GR, Beekman RH, et al, Committee SoCaCSE. Endorsement of health and human services recommendation for pulse oximetry screening for critical congenital heart disease. Pediatrics 2012;129(1):190–2.
21. Files MD, Morray B. Total anomalous pulmonary venous connection: preoperative anatomy, physiology, imaging, and interventional management of postoperative

pulmonary venous obstruction. Semin Cardiothorac Vasc Anesth 2017;21(2): 123–31.

22. Kliegman R, St. Geme J, Blum N, et al. Nelson textbook of pediatrics. 21st edition. Philadelphia, PA: Elsevier; 2020. p. 13.
23. Puri K, Allen HD, Qureshi AM. Congenital heart disease. Pediatr Rev 2017;38(10): 471–86. https://doi.org/10.1542/pir.2017-0032.
24. Kliegman R, St. Geme J, Blum N, et al. Nelson textbook of pediatrics. 21st edition. Philadelphia, PA: Elsevier; 2020. p. 9.
25. Nguyen L, Cook SC. Coarctation of the aorta: strategies for improving outcomes. Cardiol Clin 2015;33(4):521–30, vii.
26. Dijkema EJ, Leiner T, Grotenhuis HB. Diagnosis, imaging and clinical management of aortic coarctation. Heart 2017;103(15):1148–55.
27. Kliegman R, St. Geme J, Blum N, et al. Nelson textbook of pediatrics. 21st edition. Philadelphia, PA: Elsevier; 2020. p. 12.
28. Villafañe J, Feinstein JA, Jenkins KJ, et al. Hot topics in tetralogy of Fallot. J Am Coll Cardiol 2013;62(23):2155–66.
29. Lannering K, Bartos M, Mellander M. Late diagnosis of coarctation despite prenatal ultrasound and postnatal pulse oximetry. Pediatrics 2015;136(2):e406–12.
30. Anderson RH, Cook AC. Morphology of the functionally univentricular heart. Cardiol Young 2004;14(Suppl 1):3–12.
31. Kliegman R, St. Geme J, Blum N, et al. Nelson textbook of pediatrics. 21st edition. Philadelphia, PA: Elsevier; 2020. p. 7.
32. Saito T, Ohta K, Nakayama Y, et al. Natural history of medium-sized atrial septal defect in pediatric cases. J Cardiol 2012;60(3):248–51.
33. Marino BS, Lipkin PH, Newburger JW, et al. Neurodevelopmental outcomes in children with congenital heart disease: evaluation and management: a scientific statement from the American Heart Association. Circulation 2012;126(9): 1143–72.
34. Ryan KR, Jones MB, Allen KY, et al. Neurodevelopmental outcomes among children with congenital heart disease: at-risk populations and modifiable risk factors. World J Pediatr Congenit Heart Surg 2019;10(6):750–8.
35. Daymont C, Neal A, Prosnitz A, et al. Growth in children with congenital heart disease. Pediatrics 2013;131(1):e236–42.
36. Pinto NM, Marino BS, Wernovsky G, et al. Obesity is a common comorbidity in children with congenital and acquired heart disease. Pediatrics 2007;120(5): e1157–64.
37. Calderon J, Bonnet D, Courtin C, et al. Executive function and theory of mind in school-aged children after neonatal corrective cardiac surgery for transposition of the great arteries. Research Support, Non-U.S. Gov't. Dev Med Child Neurol 2010;52(12):1139–44.
38. Khanna AD, Duca LM, Kay JD, et al. Prevalence of mental illness in adolescents and adults with congenital heart disease from the colorado congenital heart defect surveillance system. Am J Cardiol 2019;124(4):618–26.
39. DeMaso DR, Calderon J, Taylor GA, et al. Psychiatric disorders in adolescents with single ventricle congenital heart disease. Pediatrics 2017;139(3):e20162241.
40. Wilson W, Taubert KA, Gewitz M, et al. Prevention of infective endocarditis: guidelines from the American Heart Association: a guideline from the American Heart Association Rheumatic Fever, Endocarditis, and Kawasaki Disease Committee, Council on Cardiovascular Disease in the Young, and the Council on Clinical Cardiology, Council on Cardiovascular Surgery and Anesthesia, and the Quality of

Care and Outcomes Research Interdisciplinary Working Group. Circulation 2007; 116(15):1736–54.

41. Everitt IK, Gerardin JF, Rodriguez FH, et al. Improving the quality of transition and transfer of care in young adults with congenital heart disease. Congenit Heart Dis 2017;12(3):242–50.

42. Reid GJ, Irvine MJ, McCrindle BW, et al. Prevalence and correlates of successful transfer from pediatric to adult health care among a cohort of young adults with complex congenital heart defects. Pediatrics 2004;113(3 Pt 1):e197–205.

Pediatric Hypertension

Christopher Fox, MD, CAQ-SM[a,b],*

KEYWORDS

- Hypertension • Pediatric hypertension • Elevated blood pressure
- Pediatric screening • Pediatric management

KEY POINTS

- The incidence rate of pediatric hypertension is between 2% and 4%; however, it is as high as 24% in obese children.
- There is strong evidence linking pediatric hypertension to cardiovascular disease in adults.
- Early recognition and intervention are key to prevent long-term complications.

INTRODUCTION
Epidemiology

Hypertension in the pediatric population has been an increasing concern over the last decade. Recent epidemiologic studies have shown an incidence rate in children and adolescents from 0.8% to as high as 4% and up to 24% in obese children.[1–3] The national average for obesity in the pediatric population is 35%, which has quadrupled in the last 40 years.[2,4] Rates of pediatric hypertension show an increasing linear relationship to increasing adiposity.[2] Boys have consistently shown a higher prevalence than girls.[2,5] There is also a higher prevalence among Hispanic and non-Hispanic African Americans.[2,5] Children classified as obese (body mass index [BMI] 95% to 98%) had a twofold increase in hypertension compared with healthy weight children, and severely obese (BMI >99%) have a fourfold increase.[3]

The American Heart Association (AHA) and the American Academy of Pediatrics (AAP) recently updated guidelines for diagnosing pediatric hypertension. The national prevalence has consistently been around 2% to 4%; however, with the recent change, the incidence of diagnosing prehypertension has increased.[1] A study by Bell and colleagues in the Houston area found a 1.5% increase in the prevalence of elevated blood pressure or previously labeled prehypertension in their study population by reclassifying to the new AAP criteria.[1]

This article originally appeared in *Primary Care: Clinics in Office Practice*, Volume 48 Issue 3, September 2021.

[a] University of Missouri-Kansas City, School of Medicine, Kansas City, MO, USA; [b] Department of Community and Family Medicine, Truman Medical Centers, Kansas City, MO, USA
* 600 NE Adams Dairy Pkwy, Blue Springs, MO 64014, USA.
E-mail addresses: chrisfox.m@gmail.com; Christopher.fox@tmcmed.org

There have been numerous studies that show that elevated blood pressure in childhood increases the risk for adult hypertension and other comorbidities.[2,6] This highlights the importance of making an early diagnosis but also in identifying the steps for early intervention.

Definitions

The definition of pediatric hypertension was recently updated by the AAP in 2017. Previously the Fourth Report (2004) defined normal blood pressure as systolic (SBP) and diastolic blood pressure (DBP) reading less than 90 percentile based on age, sex, and height normograms. Prehypertension was defined as blood pressure greater than 120/90 (or 90th) to 95th percentile. Hypertension was defined as SBP and/or DBP greater than the 95th percentile.[7,8]

The AAP updated these definitions as follows: for children over 13 years of age, the definition for hypertension remains the same as the 2017 AHA adult classification.[2,7,9] The term prehypertension has also been reclassified as elevated blood pressure. The definitions of elevated blood pressure under the age of 13 years remains SBP and/or DBP in the 90th to 94th percentiles. Stage 1 hypertension is defined as blood pressure readings in the 95th to 99th percentiles, and stage 2 hypertension is defined as blood pressure readings greater than the 95th percentile plus 12 mm Hg.

The AAP has developed tables based on normative data of blood pressure in healthy children. These tables factor in the child's height, age, and sex and allow comparison of blood pressure readings to these normative classifications in order to determine if a child's blood pressure is elevated. The normative tables were also updated, which removed the values of children who were overweight or obese (BMI >85th percentile).[2] Studies looking at these updated normograms have shown remarkably high sensitivities of 99.9%; however, specificity was around 84%.[10] The rates of hypertension have remained steady; however, there has been an increase in the diagnosis of elevated blood pressure as previously discussed.[1] These normative tables can be found on the AAP's Web site for clinical use.

https://pediatrics.aappublications.org/content/140/3/e20171904/tab-figures-data.

Screening Recommendations

Currently the AAP recommends that all children be screened for hypertension starting at the age of 3 years, and this should be continued yearly (Grade C recommendation). If the child has obesity, renal disease, coarctation of the aorta, diabetes, or is on a medication that can increase blood pressure, then it is recommended that he or she has his or her blood pressure measured at every health care encounter (Grade C recommendation). Children under the age of 3 years who have medical conditions making them higher risk for hypertension such as prematurity, low birth weight, kidney dysmorphia, or a maternal history of smoking should also have the blood pressure monitored at their routine wellness visits.[2] The latest United States Preventive Services Task Force (USPSTF) update from 2020 determined there was insufficient evidence to recommend screening for primary hypertension in asymptomatic children and adolescents.[11–14]

ETIOLOGY AND RISK FACTORS FOR DEVELOPMENT
Primary versus Secondary

Pediatric hypertension can further be classified as either primary (essential) hypertension or secondary hypertension. Secondary hypertension is hypertension that develops secondary to another identifiable cause. Primary hypertension that does not have an identifiable secondary cause is therefore a diagnosis of exclusion.

There are some identified risk factors for the development of primary pediatric hypertension. A family history of hypertension or cardiovascular disease is a known risk factor for the development of hypertension, especially in older children.[15] Male gender, Hispanic decent, and African American decent are also known risk factors for the development of primary hypertension.[2,16–18] This is suggestive of a genetic basis for the development of primary hypertension that is, poorly understood.[2,15–17]

Overweight and obese children also have an increased risk of developing primary hypertension as discussed in the introduction. Insulin resistance and sleep disorders are both chronic conditions that have independently shown an increased risk for the development of hypertension. Sleep disorders that are associated with pediatric hypertension include obstructive sleep apnea, snoring, and fragmented sleep.[16,18] Chronic kidney disease, low birth weight, or a maternal history of smoking are also additional risk factors.[18] Studies show breastfeeding has a protective relationship with hypertension and may be linked to lower systolic pressures later in life.[16,18,19] There have also been several studies looking at the correlation between uric acid levels and the development of pediatric hypertension. Studies have shown a positive relationship between uric acid levels greater than 5.5 mg/dL and elevated blood pressure in adolescents.[16,20] (**Box 1**).

Secondary hypertension can be caused by several different underlying medical pathologies that need to be excluded prior to the diagnosis of primary hypertension (**Table 1**).

EVALUATION
Blood Pressure Measurement

Any child over the age of 3 years with obesity or other risk factors known to predispose them to the development of hypertension should have their blood pressure measured at every health care encounter.[2] It is also recommended to have multiple readings during the same visit and across additional office visits to evaluate children whose blood pressure is reading elevated. There is a wide degree of variability in pediatric blood pressure readings, and outside influences such as stress and anxiety can cause those blood pressure readings to be momentarily elevated.[2]

Box 1
Risk factors for the development of primary hypertension in children and adolescents

1. Family history of hypertension or cardiovascular disease
2. Male gender
3. Hispanic decent
4. African American decent
5. Overweight/obesity
6. Insulin resistance
7. Sleep disorders
8. Low birth weight
9. Maternal history of smoking
10. Chronic kidney disease
11. Elevated uric acid levels

Table 1
Etiologies of secondary hypertension in children

Etiology	History	Physical Examination	Diagnostic Tests
Coarctation of the aorta	Family history	Diminished femoral pulses, Difference in blood pressure between right and left arms	Echocardiogram
Cushing syndrome	Family history	Acne, hirsutism, obesity, moon facies	Cortisol levels
Renal artery stenosis	History of umbilical catheterization	None	Renin, aldosterone, renal Doppler
Drug-induced	Medication history, illicit drug use	Tachycardia Diaphoresis	Urine drug screen
Hyperthyroidism	Family history, weight loss, diaphoresis	Tachycardia, exophthalmos, thyromegaly	Thyroid function tests
Congenital adrenal hyperplasia	Family history	Ambiguous genitalia	Aldosterone, renin, hypokalemia
Obstructive sleep apnea	Snoring, obesity	Mallampati score, tonsillar hypertrophy	Sleep study
Pheochromocytoma	Flushing, sweating, tremors, palpitations	Diaphoresis, tachycardia, pallor	Plasma and urine catecholamines
Renal parenchymal disease	Family history, enuresis	Hematuria, edema	Blood urea nitrogen, creatinine, urinalysis, renal ultrasound
Autoimmune disease	Family history Joint pain, fevers, weight loss	Synovitis, hematuria, mallor rash	Complete blood cell count, basic metabolic panel, inflammatory markers, autoimmune laboratory testing

Data from Refs.[2,18,31]

The child's blood pressure can be measured by either using an oscillometric automated device or by an auscultatory method.[2] When measuring a child's blood pressure, selection of the appropriate cuff is critical. If a cuff that is too large or too small for the child's arm is used, it will not yield an accurate reading. The current recommendations by the AAP are to use the midarm circumference to determine the appropriate cuff size. This location is the midpoint between the acromion of the scapula and the olecranon of the elbow.

After measurement of the child's blood pressure, the pressure should be compared with the normograms discussed in the definitions section. If the blood pressure is above the 90th percentile for that child, then a minimum of 2 more measurements should be taken at that office visit and the average of all 3 measurements determined. This should then be the blood pressure used to determine the child's blood pressure category[2] (**Fig. 1**).

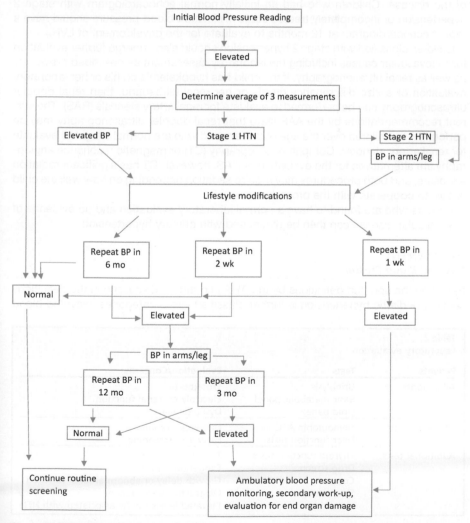

Fig. 1. Pediatric hypertension evaluation.

Primary versus Secondary

After the determination of the child's blood pressure category, the child may require additional work-up to determine the etiology of his or her hypertension. Children found to be in stage 2 hypertension are at higher risk for having secondary hypertension. These children should undergo further laboratory evaluation to rule out renal or endocrine causes of their hypertension (**Table 2**).

A diagnosis of stage 2 hypertension also warrants further evaluation to rule out of end organ damage. Echocardiography was determined by the Fourth Report to be the recommended tool for evaluation of left ventricular hypertrophy (LVH) associated with pediatric hypertension. Studies have shown an independent relationship of LVH to adverse cardiac outcomes as an adult.[2] The AAP currently recommends an echocardiogram be performed on children in consideration for pharmacologic management of hypertension. Children found to have LVH on their initial echocardiogram should have a repeat echocardiogram in 6 to 12 months to evaluate for progression of the disease. Children who had an initially normal echocardiogram with stage 2 hypertension or incompletely treated stage 1/elevated blood pressure should have a repeat echocardiogram at 12 months to evaluate for the development of LVH.

Children classified with stage 2 hypertension should also undergo further evaluation for renovascular causes including the laboratory assessment as described previously as well as renal ultrasonography. If the child has hypokalemia on his or her laboratory evaluation or a size discrepancy on his or her renal ultrasound, then renal doppler ultrasonography can be performed to evaluate for renal artery stenosis (RAS). The current recommendations by the AAP state that renal doppler ultrasonography may be performed on children over the age of 8 years and who are normal weight to evaluate for renal artery stenosis. Computed tomography (CT) or magnetic resonance angiography are alternatives for the evaluation of RAS; however, CT has significant radiation exposure, and both procedures may require sedation depending on how well the child is able to cooperate with the procedure.[2]

Patients who are found to have a normal laboratory evaluation and no evidence of renovascular disease can then be diagnosed with primary hypertension.

MANAGEMENT
Elevated Blood Pressure

Based on the updated definitions by the AHA and further discussed in the definitions section, pediatric hypertension is further classified into 3 categories: elevated blood

Table 2		
Laboratory evaluation		
Patients	**Tests**	**Evaluation/Concerns**
All patients	Urinalysis	Proteinuria
	Basic metabolic panel	Electrolytes, renal function
	Lipid panel	Dyslipidemia
Obese patients	Hemoglobin A1C	Diabetes screening
	Liver function tests	Fatty liver screening
Additional tests	Thyroid function tests	Thyroid function
	Drug screen	Exogenous causes
	Complete blood count	Growth delay or abnormal renal function
	Sleep study	Obstructive sleep apnea
	Uric acid	Elevated levels can be associated with HTN

Data from Refs.[2,16]

pressure (formerly prehypertension), stage 1 hypertension, and stage 2 hypertension.[2,21] If a child's blood pressure falls into the elevated blood pressure category during his or her routine screening, the blood pressure should be measured again during the visit. If it then normalizes, the child can continue routine follow-ups with yearly blood pressure screening (see **Fig. 1**).

Children whose blood pressure remains greater than the 90% percentile but less than the 95% percentile on repeat measurement are considered to have elevated blood pressure. The first recommended intervention is lifestyle modifications. These can include:

- Decreasing dietary sodium
- Healthier eating habits
- Weight loss
- Nutrition management or consultation with a registered dietician
- Encouragement of physical activity (guidelines can be discussed)
- Promotion of healthy sleep patterns

These children should have their blood pressure measured again in 6 months by auscultation.[2] If their blood pressure remains elevated at 6 months, then repeating the measurement in both arms and a lower extremity is recommended to evaluate for aortic coarctation. Lifestyle changes and weight management should be discussed again, and referrals may be warranted. The child should then be followed again in 6 months. If blood pressure remains elevated after 12 months, ambulatory blood pressure monitoring and further work-up should be considered to rule out secondary causes. In children whose blood pressure continues to fail to normalize after conservative management, pharmacologic management can be considered and is discussed further in the stage 2 hypertension management section (see **Fig. 1**).

Stage 1 Hypertension

Stage 1 hypertension is diagnosed when a child's (<13 year old) blood pressure remains over the 95% percentile but less than the 99% percentile. For an adolescent (>13 year old), this is defined as a blood pressure between 130/80 and 139/89.

A diagnosis of stage 1 hypertension in an asymptomatic child can initially be treated with lifestyle changes, conservative management, and close monitoring/follow-up. It is currently recommended that any child initially diagnosed with stage 1 hypertension be followed in 1 to 2 weeks and have his or her blood pressure rechecked by auscultation.[2]

Recheck blood pressure in both arms and a lower extremity if elevated readings persist. Should there be difficulty implementing lifestyle changes, then a nutrition consultation may be warranted with follow-up in 3 months.

Initiate ambulatory blood pressure monitoring and pharmacologic treatment if the child's blood pressure remains elevated after 3 visits. Subspecialty referral can be considered to nephrology or cardiology for the child with persistently elevated blood pressures.

Stage 2 Hypertension

Stage 2 hypertension is defined as a blood pressure greater than the 95% + 12 mm Hg or greater than 140/90, whichever is lower.

For a child or adolescent diagnosed with stage 2 hypertension, it is recommended that the blood pressure measurement be repeated in both upper and a lower extremity at that visit. The child should be referred to nutrition or weight management.

Follow-up measurements of blood pressure should occur within 1 week. If the child remains in the stage 2 hypertension category at follow-up, then ambulatory blood pressure monitoring should be performed, further laboratory and imaging evaluations ordered, and pharmacologic treatment initiated.2,21 A subspecialty referral can be considered in patients with both stage 1 and stage 2 hypertension.

Any child who presents with stage 1 or 2 hypertension and is symptomatic should be referred to the emergency room for acute blood pressure management. These symptoms could include seizures, lethargy, vision changes, altered mental status, headache, nausea, pulmonary edema, or other symptoms of congestive heart failure.[9] A study by Hamby and colleagues demonstrated that, on average, years passed prior to a child being referred to a nephrologist for hypertension despite remaining elevated at multiple visits.[22] It is important for clinicians to recognize these elevated blood pressures in order to make a timely diagnosis and referral if needed (see **Fig. 1**).

Pharmacologic Management

When considering starting a child diagnosed with primary hypertension on an anti-hypertensive medication much thought and discussion should go into the decision. Lifestyle modifications should fully be maximized prior to consideration of initiating pharmacologic therapy. However, if a child's blood pressure is staying in the stage 2 category, he or she has LVH on echocardiography, or he or she is symptomatic, then a pharmacologic agent should be initiated. For children started on pharmacologic management, follow-up every 4 to 6 weeks is recommended initially for dose titration and then every 3 to 6 months for monitoring.[21]

Anti-hypertensives have been less studied in children; therefore less is known about the long-term outcomes of these medications compared with adults. Many of these medications are considered off-label use in the pediatric population.[23] Initial treatment is recommended with an angiotensin-converting enzyme (ACE) inhibitor or angiotensin receptor blocker (ARB), long-acting calcium channel blocker, or thiazide diuretic. Beta blockers are not recommended as initial agents.[2] In adolescents, careful attention needs to be paid to a sexual history in girls, as ACE inhibitors and ARBs are contra-indicated during pregnancy. In children with hypertension and chronic kidney disease, proteinuria, or diabetes, an ACE inhibitor or ARB is recommended as first-line treatment.[2]

There has also been an association found between elevated uric acid levels and primary hypertension. Treatment of these uric acid levels with a uric acid-lowering agent may help in reducing blood pressure; however, more studies are needed to clarify the utility.[2,16,23]

DISCUSSION
Long-Term Complications

The development of hypertension in a child can have long-term implications, especially if elevated blood pressures persist. Persistently elevated blood pressures can damage the small vessels, creating target organ damage including involvement of the eyes, kidneys, heart, brain, and arteries in children.[10] There have also been studies showing a correlation between pediatric hypertension and the development of cardiovascular disease as an adult.[2] Epidemiologic studies have shown that elevated blood pressures in children as young as age 12 may increase the incidence of adult cardiovascular disease.[24]

LVH is a known complication of pediatric hypertension. This occurs as the left ventricular mass is increased in response to elevated blood pressures. A study by Conkar and colleagues of 82 children with pediatric hypertension showed rates of target organ damage including retinopathy (35%), microalbuminuria (26%), and increased left ventricular mass (17%).[24] LVH is a known surrogate marker for morbidity and mortality associated with pediatric hypertension.[10] The prevalence of LVH in children and adolescents has been difficult to determine given the multiple definitions that are used. In essential hypertension, severe LVH with left ventricular mass index (LVMI) above 51g has been estimated to be 10% to 15%.[10] The presence of LVH in children with hypertension should prompt treatment with the goal of LVH reversal. Hypertension remains a rare cause of heart failure in children.[10]

The development of chronic kidney disease is another potential long-term complication of persistent uncontrolled hypertension in children. Microalbuminuria is a marker of potential development of hypertensive kidney injury in children, and a positive test should prompt pharmacologic treatment.[2,16] Treatment in adults with an ACE inhibitor or ARB has been shown to effectively reduce microalbuminuria, and improvement in microalbuminuria has been associated with reduced cardiovascular risk; however, these studies have not been successfully reproduced in a pediatric population.[2,10]

Damage to the microvasculature affecting the retina is another known complication of pediatric hypertension.[16] The rates of retinopathy associated with pediatric hypertension have been estimated as high as 8% to 35%.[24,25] A formal retinal examination should be considered for children diagnosed with hypertension, especially stage 2 hypertension. There has also been evidence of impaired cognition in children diagnosed with hypertension and documented improvement with treatment.[16,26]

Many of these long-term complications do lead to permanent organ damage and morbidity and mortality as an adult; however, it has also been demonstrated that if hypertension is controlled some of the target organ damage may be reversible.

Prevention

The incidence of primary hypertension in pediatrics has closely mirrored the increasing rates of obesity in the pediatric population. Currently around one-third of children in the Unites States are affected by overweight or obesity, and the rates increase with age.[27] When discussing prevention of pediatric hypertension, the discussion of pediatric obesity must be at the center.

Physical activity is a key component to the prevention of pediatric obesity and hypertension and one of the first recommended lifestyle modifications for those diagnosed with elevated blood pressure or hypertension. Currently the CDC recommend a goal of 60 minutes of moderate-to-vigorous physical activity daily for children ages 6 to 17 years; however, only about 33% are achieving this goal.[2,16,28] The recommendations for children under 6 year old is to be active throughout the day. Adults should help find activities to keep children active and encourage the children to remain engaged in these activities.[29]

Nutrition management and sleep hygiene are also key components to prevention and lifestyle modifications. There have been studies showing evidence of an association between shortened sleep duration and childhood obesity.[27] A detailed sleep history and input from parents can help identify poor sleep patterns. A sleep study can also be considered for a child with a history of snoring.

Sports Clearance/Preparticipation Examinations

All athletes participating in organized sports are required to undergo a preparticipation exam (PPE) to determine if they can safely participate in sport. The overarching goal of the PPE is to promote an environment of safety in athletics and provide a screening opportunity for injuries and underlying medical conditions that could predispose the athlete to an adverse outcome.[30]

Hypertension is one of the most commonly encountered pathologies at the PPE, and screening for hypertension is recommended for every PPE.[30] According to the PPE Monograph in association with the AAP, children with severe or stage 2 hypertension should not be initially cleared and undergo further work-up or specialty consultation. These athletes should avoid heavy intensity static exercises such as powerlifting and bodybuilding. Once the investigation is complete and blood pressure is controlled, then participation should be re-evaluated. Those with stage 1 hypertension or elevated blood pressure may be cleared for participation with the condition that the child follow-up for further evaluation of his or her elevated blood pressure.[30] Determining and ensuring parent and child understanding of the need for further work-up and any restrictions placed on the athlete are important. Discussing provisional clearance can be important to help with parent and athlete compliance. If an athlete fails to follow-up or complete the requested work-up, removal of the provisional clearance may be needed to ensure the continued safety of that athlete.

CLINICS CARE POINTS

- The incidence of pediatric hypertension is increasing in a linear relationship to the increasing rates of childhood obesity.
- Blood pressure should be measured at every well child examination starting at the age of 3 years and at every office visit for children who are at higher risk.
- Practitioners need to be aware of the pediatric normograms for comparison of blood pressures in the office and to assist in early diagnosis of pediatric hypertension.
- Multiple measurements of blood pressure should be made during an office visit if a child has an elevated blood pressure and the average used to determine blood pressure classification.
- Lifestyle modifications are first-line management for all asymptomatic patients; however, secondary causes and end organ damage need to be excluded in patients with stage 2 hypertension or persistently elevated blood pressure despite lifestyle modifications.
- Children with symptomatic hypertension should be evaluated in the emergency room for more prompt evaluation and management.

DISCLOSURE

The author has nothing to disclose.

REFERENCES

1. Bell CS, Samuel JP, Samuels JA. Prevalence of hypertension in children. Hypertension 2019;73(1):148–52.
2. Flynn JT, Kaelber DC, Baker-Smith CM, et al. Clinical practice guideline for screening and management of high blood pressure in children and adolescents. Pediatrics 2017;140(3). https://doi.org/10.1542/peds.2017-1904.
3. Parker ED, Sinaiko AR, Kharbanda EO, et al. Change in weight status and development of hypertension. Pediatrics 2016;137(3):e20151662.
4. Fryer C. Products - health E stats - prevalence of overweight and obesity among children and adolescents aged 2–19 years: United States, 1963–1965 through 2013–2014. 2016. Available at: https://www.cdc.gov/nchs/data/hestat/obesity_child_13_14/obesity_child_13_14.html. Accessed September 29, 2020.

5. Kit BK, Kuklina E, Carroll MD, et al. Prevalence of and trends in dyslipidemia and blood pressure among US children and adolescents, 1999-2012. JAMA Pediatr 2015;169(3):272–9.
6. Bucher BS, Ferrarini A, Weber N, et al. Primary hypertension in childhood. Curr Hypertens Rep 2013;15(5):444–52.
7. Genovesi S, Parati G, Giussani M, et al. How to apply European and American guidelines on high blood pressure in children and adolescents. A position paper endorsed by the Italian Society of Hypertension and the Italian Society of Pediatrics. High Blood Press Cardiovasc Prev 2020. https://doi.org/10.1007/s40292-020-00369-y [Review].
8. National High Blood Pressure Education Program Working Group on High Blood Pressure in Children and Adolescents. The fourth report on the diagnosis, evaluation, and treatment of high blood pressure in children and adolescents. Pediatrics 2004;114(2 Suppl 4th Report):555–76.
9. Baracco R. A practical guide to the management of severe hypertension in children. Paediatr Drugs 2020;22(1):13–20.
10. Zhang Y, Yang L, Hou Y, et al. Performance of the simplified American Academy of Pediatrics table to screen elevated blood pressure in children. JAMA Pediatr 2018;172(12):1196–8.
11. Moyer V. Screening for primary hypertension in children and adolescents: U.S Preventive Services Task Force recommendation statement. Pediatrics 2013; 132(5):907–14.
12. Unites States Preventative Services Task Force. High blood pressure in children and adolescents: screening. Available at: https://www.uspreventiveservicestaskforce.org/uspstf/recommendation/blood-pressure-in-children-and-adolescents-hypertension-screening#fullrecommendationstart. Accessed December 15, 2020.
13. Whelton PK, Carey RM, Aronow WS, et al. 2017 ACC/AHA/AAPA/ABC/ACPM/AGS/APhA/ASH/ASPC/NMA/PCNA guideline for the prevention, detection, evaluation, and management of high blood pressure in adults: a report of the American College of Cardiology/American Heart Association Task Force on Clinical Practice Guidelines. Circulation 2018;138(17):e484–594.
14. Woroniecki RP, Kahnauth A, Panesar LE, et al. Left ventricular hypertrophy in pediatric hypertension: a mini review. Front Pediatr 2017;5:101.
15. Matossian D. Pediatric Hypertension. Pediatr Ann 2018;47(12):e499–503.
16. Ahern D, Dixon E. Pediatric hypertension: a growing problem. Prim Care 2015; 42(1):143–50.
17. Guzman-Limon M, Samuels J. Pediatric hypertension: diagnosis, evaluation, and treatment. Pediatr Clin North Am 2019;66(1):45–57 [Review].
18. Riley M, Hernandez AK, Kuznia AL. High blood pressure in children and adolescents. Am Fam Physician 2018;98(8):486–94.
19. Owen CG, Whincup PH, Gilg JA, et al. Effect of breast feeding in infancy on blood pressure in later life: systematic review and meta-analysis. BMJ 2003;327(7425): 1189–95.
20. Raj M. Essential hypertension in adolescents and children: Recent advances in causative mechanisms. Indian J Endocrinol Metab 2011;15(Suppl 4):S367–73.
21. Sinha R, Saha A, Samuels J. American Academy of Pediatrics clinical practice guidelines for screening and management of high blood pressure in children and adolescents: what is new? Indian Pediatr 2019;56(4):317–21.
22. Hamby T, Pueringer MR, Noorani S, et al. Time to referral to a nephrology clinic for pediatric hypertension. Pediatr Nephrol 2020;35(5):907–10.

23. Misurac J, Nichols KR, Wilson AC. Pharmacologic management of pediatric hypertension. Paediatr Drugs 2016;18(1):31–43.
24. Conkar S, Yılmaz E, Hacıkara Ş, et al. Is daytime systolic load an important risk factor for target organ damage in pediatric hypertension? J Clin Hypertens (Greenwich) 2015;17(10):760–6.
25. Foster BJ, Ali H, Mamber S, et al. Prevalence and severity of hypertensive retinopathy in children. Clin Pediatr (Phila) 2009;48(9):926–30.
26. Taylor-Zapata P, Baker-Smith CM, Burckart G, et al. Research gaps in primary pediatric hypertension. Pediatrics 2019;143(5). https://doi.org/10.1542/peds.2018-3517.
27. Kumar S, Kelly AS. Review of childhood obesity: from epidemiology, etiology, and comorbidities to clinical assessment and treatment. Mayo Clin Proc 2017;92(2): 251–65.
28. Foster C, Moore JB, Singletary CR, et al. Physical activity and family-based obesity treatment: a review of expert recommendations on physical activity in youth. Clin Obes 2018;8(1):68–79.
29. Centers for Disease Control and Prevention. Youth physical activity guidelines. Centers for Disease Control and Prevention; 2019. Available at: www.cdc.gov/healthyschools/physicalactivity/guidelines.htm.
30. Bernhardt DT, Roberts WO. PPE: preparticipation physical evaluation. Itasca (IL): American Academy of Pediatrics; 2019.
31. Saida K, Kamei K, Hamada R, et al. A simple refined approach for renovascular hypertension in children: a ten-year experience. Pediatr Int 2020.

Preparticipation Cardiac Evaluation from the Pediatric Perspective

Andrew M. Reittinger, MD[a], Lanier B. Jackson, MD[b],
Peter N. Dean, MD[a],*

KEYWORDS

- Preparticipation examination • Sudden cardiac death • Sports cardiology • Pediatric
- Adolescent

KEY POINTS

- The sports preparticipation examination is an opportunity to screen for risk factors for sudden cardiac death (SCD).
- Evaluation of the pediatric population presents different considerations and challenges compared with adults.
- A normal preparticipation or cardiac examination does not mean that it will be normal in perpetuity, as the age of onset of certain cardiac disorders predisposing to SCD present at varying times during development.

INTRODUCTION

Each year millions of children and adolescents undergo sports preparticipation evaluations (PPEs) before participating in organized sports. The clinicians who evaluate these patients have a wide range of expertise and experience performing sports PPEs and/or evaluating pediatric and adolescent patients. This article is designed to summarize the current thoughts on the PPE with a specific slant toward the pediatric and early adolescent evaluations and how they may differ from those in adults.

CASES

1. An 11-year-old boy presents for sports clearance to play high school basketball. He has a family medical history of hypertrophic cardiomyopathy (HCM) in his father.

This article originally appeared in *Cardiology Clinics*, Volume 41, Issue 1, February 2023.
[a] Division of Pediatric Cardiology, Department of Pediatrics, University of Virginia, 1204 West Main Street, Battle Building, 6th Floor, Charlottesville, VA 22903, USA; [b] Division of Pediatric Cardiology, Department of Pediatrics, Medical University of South Carolina, 10 McClennan Banks Drive, MSC 915, Charleston, SC 29425, USA
* Corresponding author.
E-mail address: PND8J@hscmail.mcc.virginia.edu

Clinics Collections 13 (2023) 29–48
https://doi.org/10.1016/j.ccol.2023.02.021
2352-7986/23/

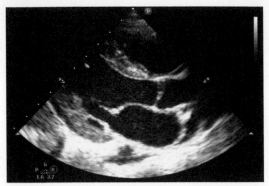

Fig. 2. Initial echocardiogram of an 11-year-old boy from Case 1 with a family history of HCM. This is a parasternal long axis image in 2D showing normal left ventricular and interventricular septal dimensions.

His father has not had genetic testing. **Figs. 1** and **2** show his normal electrocardiogram (ECG) and normal echocardiogram. What do you do next?

2. A 10-year-old boy presents for clearance before youth league soccer. When asked about a history of syncope or unresponsive spells, his mother reports he had a recent syncopal episode. She reports that he was running to the school bus with his siblings when she noticed that he started to lag behind his siblings, fell to his knees, screamed, and then fell on his face. He was noted to be unconscious for a period of about 15 seconds and did not require any resuscitative measures. He was noted to have significant abrasions on his face. When he recovered, he apologized for the fact that "his legs stopped working." His mother recounts that 2 months earlier she received a call from school after he fell while running on the track during gym class. This event was also associated facial abrasions. His mother attributed the inability to catch himself during his fall to prevent facial injury to what she described as general clumsiness and his history of mild gross motor delay. What do you do next?

3. An 18-year-old male college baseball player presents to a mass preparticipation screening clinic. He reports a history of Kawasaki disease (KD) and is currently taking aspirin and dipyridamole. There is no access to outside medical records. What do you do next?

WHAT IS THE PURPOSE OF PREPARTICIPATION EVALUATION?

The purpose of preparticipation screening is to identify individuals who may be at risk for adverse health effects such as illness or injury secondary to sports participation. The most serious potential adverse event is sudden cardiac arrest (SCA) or sudden cardiac death (SCD). As SCA and SCD can sometimes be the first presentation of an underlying cardiac condition, the PPE is an attempt to catch underlying cardiac diseases that predispose individuals to SCA and SCD.

Although studies have called into question the efficacy of the PPE and in particular the screening tools for SCA risk factors,[1] the PPE is still viewed as an avenue to encourage non-acute primary care visits.[2] This gives the opportunity to provide counseling on not only sports-related physical concerns but also mental health topics, diet, high-risk behaviors, and medication, supplement illicit drug use.

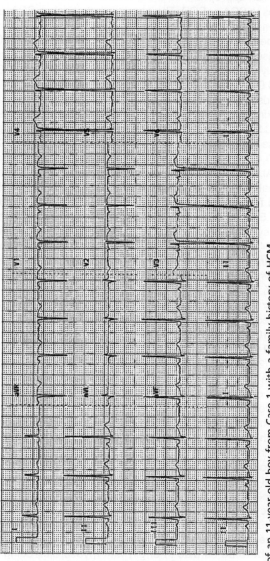

Fig. 1. Initial ECG of an 11-year-old boy from Case 1 with a family history of HCM.

Although overall the evaluation is similar to the adult population, there are some differences and particular challenges in the pediatric population. The authors intend to focus on these in this article.

DIFFERENCES IN INCIDENCE AND CAUSES OF SUDDEN CARDIAC ARREST

In order to perform an appropriate PPE the clinician should know the conditions that predispose athletes to SCA or SCD. The conditions that cause SCA are one of the differences in children and adolescents compared with adults.

Overall, the incidence of SCA in adults is approximately 135 per 100,000,[3] with coronary artery disease accounting for 75% to 80% of SCD in the United States and Europe. Fortunately, in the young adult population, the rate of SCD is significantly lower (0.7 per 100,000 person-years in 18–35 year old group and 13.7 per 100,000 person-years in those over 35 years of age).[4]

Specifically looking at athletes, the incidence of sports-related sudden death in young athletes is 0.5 to 2.1 per 100,000 people per year.[4] This is higher in elite athletes. The incidence of SCD over a 4-year collegiate athletic career in the United States in any sport is 1:13,425 based on data gathered from the National Collegiate Athletic Association (NCAA). The risk seems to be higher in males and black athletes. Basketball (male and female) was the sport with the highest rate of SCD, followed by men's soccer and men's football. Division I male basketball players had the highest incidence of SCD at 1:5200 athlete years. The common causes of SCD in the NCAA population were autopsy-negative sudden unexplained death (25%), verified or suspected cardiomyopathy (24%; 8% confirmed HCM), coronary artery anomalies or disease (21%), and myocarditis (10%). In total, SCD comprised 15% of sudden death in NCAA athletes, whereas the combination of accidents, homicide, and suicide accounted for 68%.[5]

A recent study by Burns and colleagues looked into the incidence and cause of sudden death in the pediatric population. The 2020 study found the incidence of sudden death was 1.9 per 100,000 in children between 1 and 17 years of age. The lowest incidence was in 6 to 9 year olds (1.1/100,000 children), and the highest incidence was in 14 to 17 year olds (2.4/100,000). Unfortunately, it was difficult to determine the cause of sudden death in a significant number of cases (43% of the cases were "unexplained"). Cardiac causes accounted for 16% of the "explained" cases and were the second most common cause (behind respiratory). Only a small percentage of all sudden death events occurred cases occurred during exertional activities (13%).[6] These findings highlight that medical providers should be thinking of the variety of causes of sudden in all pediatric patients and not just "athletes."

Another epidemiologic study out of Denmark published in 2014 reports that the incidence of confirmed or suspected SCD in children 1 to 18 year old is 1.1 per 100,000 person-years (0.8 per 100,000 when suspected cases are excluded). In children older than 1 year, the incidence of SCD death increased to its highest levels in the 13 to 18 year old age group.[7] Of the SCDs, only 23% had previously diagnosed cardiac disorders, and 61% were not known to have any health conditions. After autopsy, 70% of deaths were thought to be cardiac in origin with myocarditis being the highest incidence at 9%. In this population, only 59% of patients experienced symptoms before the SCD.[7]

DIFFERENCES IN PHENOTYPE PRESENTATION

Another significant difference between adults and pediatric patients is pediatric patients are more likely to be evaluated before their phenotype has presented. Although some cardiac conditions that predispose to SCA will be present at birth (Wolff–Parkinson–White, long QT syndrome [LQTS], anomalous origin of a coronary artery, aortic valve stenosis, and so forth), there are others that cannot be diagnosed early in life even with appropriate or extensive cardiac testing.

HCM is a leading cause of sudden death in young athletes,[8] but screening for HCM can be difficult at young ages because sometimes the phenotype is not present until adulthood.[9] Patients at risk for developing HCM may have normal testing early in childhood and then develop HCM and be at risk for SCD later in adolescents. Owing to this, it is recommended that children who are asymptomatic who have a first-degree relative with HCM should be screened with an ECG and echocardiogram every 1 to 3 years.[9]

Marfan syndrome is similar to HCM in that individuals can have relatively normal physical examinations and normal sized aortic roots in childhood but develop significant aortic dilation throughout adolescence and young adulthood, predisposing them to aortic root dissection and rupture. Recent studies looking at the phenotypes of patients with pathologic genetic mutations for Marfan syndrome showed that only 56% of 10 to 18 year olds will meet the clinical diagnostic criteria for Marfan[10] compared with 79% of adults.[11]

Arrhythmogenic right ventricular cardiomyopathy (ARVC) is another cause of SCA that has variable ages of presentation. ARVC is particularly challenging to diagnosis in the pediatric population as there is typically a "concealed phase," during which no structural or electrocardiographic abnormalities are identifiable but malignant arrhythmias with sports or physical activity can occur.[12] Studies have demonstrated that pediatric patients are more likely than adults to have SCA as their presenting symptom for this reason.[13,14] Unfortunately, diagnosis can be challenging.[15] In a recent study, even pediatric patients who were thought to have definitive ARVC after a cardiac MRI rarely had abnormal ECGs (4%) and none had abnormal echocardiograms.[16]

Because of the variable presentations of many cardiac diseases over time, providers evaluating patients in early or mid-childhood need to understand the limits of their screening and consider repeat testing later in adolescence or young adulthood, regardless of whether the initial screening included cardiac testing. Similarly, providers should be cognizant of the fact that in some circumstances, the parents or other first-degree relatives of a young athlete are themselves of an age at which potential cardiac disorders have not clinically presented.

Providers need to stress to patients and families that a "normal cardiac screen" demonstrates that there is no evidence of cardiac disease at that specific point in time. This designation does not last in perpetuity and new cardiac symptoms or concerns should be reevaluated. Patients under the assumption that their heart is "normal" may not seek medical care for otherwise concerning cardiac symptoms.

This is highlighted by a recent article that showed that the rate of SCD in 11,168 adolescent soccer players was still 6.8 per 100,000 despite extensive cardiac screening (history, examination, ECG, and echocardiogram) before participation. The reason for the relatively high number of SCD was related to cardiomyopathies that were not detected by screening. The mean age of screening was 16.4 ± 1.2 years, and the time between the screening and the episode of SCD was 6.8 years.[17] Although it is certainly unknown whether athletes would have had detectable abnormalities around the time of the SCD, this suggests that serial screening may be indicated. In a response to a Letter to the Editor, the investigators of the study state that the English Football Association has recently recommended initial screening at

16 years of age as part of a fitness assessment before signing a professional contract and repeat screening 18, 20, and 25 year old (**Table 1**) greater than.[17]

WHO SHOULD BE EVALUATED AND WHEN SHOULD IT START?

As most adults are not still participating in competitive sports as they age, it seems easier to describe an adult as a competitive athlete, a recreational athlete, or a nonathlete. This is more difficult in the pediatric population, as sport intensity varies greatly and participation varies from year to year. Owing to this, it seems as though categorizing elementary school students or junior high students as an "athlete" or "nonathlete" is not a medically important classification. This is in line with the recent American Academy of Pediatrics (AAP) policy statement on the topic of screening for sudden death.[18] In that statement, they recommend screening patients every 2 to 3 years without any differentiation between athlete and nonathlete. It also suggests that screening should be performed starting at age six. They recommend four specific questions:

1. Have you ever fainted, passed out, or had an unexplained seizure suddenly and without warning, especially during exercise or in response to sudden loud noises, such as doorbells, alarm clocks, and ringing telephones?
2. Have you ever had exercise-related chest pain or shortness of breath?
3. Has anyone in your immediate family (parents, grandparents, siblings) or other, more distant relatives (aunts, uncles, cousins) died of heart problems or had an unexpected sudden death before age 50? This would include unexpected drownings, unexplained auto crashes in which the relative was driving, or sudden infant death syndrome (SIDS).
4. Are you related to anyone with HCM or hypertrophic obstructive cardiomyopathy, Marfan syndrome, arrhythmogenic cardiomyopathy, LQTS, short QT syndrome, Brugada Syndrome, or catecholaminergic polymorphic ventricular tachycardia or anyone younger than 50 years with a pacemaker or implantable defibrillator?[15]

The first two questions are likely not useful for children under 6 year old, but the last two questions, regarding family history are important at any age. LQTS and HCM are

Table 1
Possible differences between pediatric and young adult/adult preparticipation cardiac screening

Pediatric Specific Screening	Young Adult and Adult Screening
More likely to have vague or unclear symptoms	Better able to communicate symptoms
Likely requires repeat screening as adolescent and/or young adult	More likely to have already expressed the phenotype of specific cardiac disease
Parents too young to demonstrate phenotype	Older parents with more detail about family history
Pediatric providers are less experienced in ECGs	Family physicians and adult providers more experienced interpreting ECGs
More likely to have undiagnosed congenital heart disease	Less likely to have undiagnosed congenital heart disease
More likely to have history of Kawasaki disease	
Suboptimal criteria for ECG abnormalities	

causes of SIDS or death in early childhood, so obtaining a detailed family history is important even in infancy. The authors believe that primary care physicians should be asking those questions or similar questions starting at the well-child visits soon after birth.

As adolescents enter high school and college, the line between athletes and nonathletes becomes better demarcated, but it still is not completely clear. Most of the sports participation is likely sanctioned through the school, but some elite-level or "travel" sports participants do not play on their corresponding school-sanctioned teams. Beyond this, there are certainly other physically demanding sports and activities undertaken by the teenager or young adult that are similar in their potential to cause SCA (hiking, climbing, mountain biking, skiing, trampolining, and so forth). Owing to this, primary care physicians should be asking questions about physical activity, cardiac symptoms with exertion, and family history regardless of whether or not there is an official "school preparticipation form" to sign. In a similar fashion, ECG screening programs, if offered, should be offered to any adolescent, regardless of their "athlete" status.

WHERE DO PREPARTICIPATION EVALUATIONS OCCUR?

Current PPE guidelines recommend yearly screening at least 6 weeks before the first sports practice or workout.[18] Ideally, these visits would occur with the patient's primary care provider, but there are other settings where evaluations occur, including mass screening events or urgent care offices. Most states require that a medical doctor, doctor of osteopathic medicine, nurse practitioner, or physician's assistant provide the clearance, but there is typically no discussion on experience or specific specialty of the provider.

The preferred provider is the patient's primary care provider. This allows for centralization of a patient's care, access to patient's past medical records, more nuanced understanding of the patient's medical, family, and social histories, and the ability to have consistent longitudinal follow-up. It also provides appropriate follow-up of referrals to ensure they are performed and recommendations are followed.

Although they are time efficient and allow for improved access to medical providers, mass screening events such as those in a school gymnasium can be problematic. These potential problems are (1) difficulty maintaining patient privacy and a safe space for patient to bring concerns to physician, (2) suboptimal environment for physical examination, (3) lack of access to patient's medical records, (4) lack of time and space for appropriate counseling when an abnormality or suspected abnormality is found, and (5) difficulty ensuring appropriate follow-up/referrals when abnormalities are found. The concept of mass PPE events promotes efficiency, but could also unintentionally create the feeling of being rushed, which may alter a provider's typical practice or athlete's willingness to disclose symptoms. The potential problems with mass screenings are not a reason to avoid doing them, but they should be addressed.[18]

THE COMPONENTS OF THE PREPARTICIPATION EVALUATION

Typically, PPEs are based on the PPE monograph that has been developed and endorsed by the AAP, American Academy of Family Physicians, the American College of Sports Medicine, and American Medical Society for Sports Medicine for the past 40 years (AMSSM).[118] There is also an American Heart Association (AHA) 14-point questionnaire that has a similar format and questions.[19]

The PPE has three, and possibly four, main parts: history, family history, and examination and sometimes an ECG.

History

A medical history, encompassing both past medical history and cardiac symptoms, is an essential part of any patient encounter and should be carried out in any PPE. Cardiac symptoms with exercise should prompt further investigation. In addition, other odd or suspicious symptoms such as seizures, syncope, or extensive breath holding spells should be considered as potential signs of malignant arrhythmias. Any known or previously diagnosed cardiac pathology, including congenital heart disease, cardiac arrhythmia or channelopathies, cardiomyopathy, history of myocarditis, or coronary artery anomalies, including those caused by KD, should be evaluated by a cardiologist before clearance.

Studies have shown that complete agreement between athlete and parental reports of medical history on the PPE is less than 20%. The cardiovascular section, along with neurologic, musculoskeletal, and weight sections, accounted for nearly 60% of the discrepancies.[20] This highlights the importance of involving parents or primary caregivers in the history.

How to Respond When a History of Cardiac Disease Is Reported

Typically, when a patient reports a history of cardiac disease, they should be cleared by the cardiologist caring for that patient.

Providers evaluating pediatric athletes are more likely to be confronted with known congenital heart disease or undiagnosed congenital heart disease. Often these congenital heart defects, repaired or unrepaired, do not have significant impact on sports participation. Examples of these include small atrial septal defects, small patent ductus arteriosus, mild pulmonary valve stenosis, repaired ventricular septal defects, among others. Sometimes the congenital heart disease is significant and can have significant implications for sports participation. Given this, when an athlete has congenital heart disease, they should be evaluated by a pediatric or congenital cardiologist before participation.

KD is an inflammatory disease of early childhood that can cause coronary artery aneurysms and subsequent coronary artery thrombus and stenosis. The huge majority of patients recover without significant coronary sequelae but some will have residual disease that may impact exercise and sports participation. As KD was only fully described in the mid to late 1970s and most patients recover without residual heart disease, providers who do not routinely care for pediatric patients may have limited experience. No exercise restrictions are indicated if patients did not have coronary artery abnormalities during the acute phase of KD or if they have had complete resolution of coronary aneurysms. If the athlete has persistent coronary artery aneurysms, antiplatelet or anticoagulation treatment is likely indicated and they are at risk for developing coronary artery stenosis, both of which can impact decisions regarding sports participation.[21]

How to Respond to a History of Cardiac Symptoms

A report of cardiac symptoms by a patient is important because it can be a signal for the provider that cardiac disease is present. Reporting of symptoms can be challenging for any patient, but it can be especially difficult for children and adolescents. Owing to a lack of experience, a lack of vocabulary, and an intimidating environment, young patients are more likely to report vague symptoms or not fully understand or remember the situation when they had symptoms. Owing to these difficulties, providers asking and evaluating these symptoms should be experienced in interviewing pediatric and adolescent patients.

Chest pain

Chest pain is an extremely common complaint in the pediatric population—fortunately, only 0.2% to 1% of reported chest pain is cardiac in nature in the pediatric and adolescent population.[22] Red flags for cardiac chest pain include exertional pain and pain associated with palpitations or syncope (**Table 2**).

Syncope

Pre-syncope and syncope are frequently encountered in pediatric and adolescent patients. Although it can be a difficult task, it is vital to attempt to distinguish between different etiologies of pre-syncope and syncope and to know when further workup and evaluation are indicated. Obtaining a detailed history about the circumstances of the event is the most useful way to determine whether further workup is required. Typically, an ECG is required in the evaluation and many times it is the only test required.[23] Red flags for cardiac-related syncope are syncope with exertion or exercise, a lack of prodromal symptoms before the syncope, other associated cardiac symptoms, head or body injury at the time of syncope, and abnormal examination or ECG findings. Even if the baseline ECG is normal, concerning syncopal episodes with exertion require further workup, often including echocardiogram, cardiac ambulatory monitor, exercise stress test, extensive family history, and in some instances CT angiogram and/or cardiac MRI (**Table 3**).

Palpitations

A positive screen for palpitations means that a patient can be experiencing rapid, irregular, or prominent-feeling heart beats. Often this can be attributed to sinus tachycardia; however, atrial or ventricular dysrhythmias need to be ruled out. Children will often describe their heart as "pounding," "racing," "fluttering," "starting and stopping," or "beeping." Palpitations can be associated with pain, dizziness, shortness of breath, diaphoresis, nausea or vomiting, or syncope. Palpitations with exercise raise the level of concern. Typically, patients require an ECG and exercise stress test if the symptoms occur with exercise. Sometimes cardiac event monitors and echocardiograms can be helpful.

History of viral upper respiratory tract infection (COVID-19, influenza, rhinovirus, and so forth)

Even before the emergence of the COVID-19 infection related to the SARS-CoV-2 virus, there was a concern for myocarditis and sports participation. The primary reason for this is that myocarditis is well known to be a cause of SCD in athletes. At the beginning of the pandemic, there was a significant concern that COVID-19 was going to cause increased rates of myocarditis and put athletes at increased risk of SCA or SCD. Fortunately, overtime, this has found to not be true and the risk of myocarditis associated with COVID-19 is very low.[24,25] Owing to this, most patients can be cleared to return to sports after they have recovered from COVID-19 similar to the way they are cleared after other viral infection. Athletes with a history of myocardial injury or myocarditis or abnormal cardiac testing during an acute viral infection should have cardiac testing before participation. Athletes should also have a cardiac evaluation if they have cardiac symptoms during the acute illness or after returning to exercise (**Fig. 3**).

Family Medical History

Genetic heritability is an aspect of many diseases that confer an increased risk of SCD, such as cardiomyopathies, channelopathies, conduction abnormalities, and congenital heart disease to name a few. Providers will often find that the three family

Table 2
Common causes of cardiac and noncardiac pediatric chest pain

Causes	Features
Cardiac chest pain	
Myocarditis	Nonspecific symptoms ranging from mild to signs of shock, often mimicking sepsis. Tachycardia and hypotension on vitals. ECG with diffuse ST-segment and T-wave abnormalities and often low voltages, particularly in precordial leads
Pericarditis	Retrosternal chest pain alleviated by leaning forward, often associated with fever or viral illness, friction rub on auscultation, ST-segment elevation, and PR depression on ECG
Aortic stenosis (AS)/coarctation (CoA)	Fatigue, dyspnea, angina, and syncope can be presenting symptoms, but only in more moderate to severe disease, blood pressure differentials (R arm > L arm in AS, R arm > either leg in CoA). Systolic murmur may be heard. Decreased lower extremity pulses in CoA
Ischemia	Anginal chest pain due to increased myocardial demand or decreased ability to supply the myocardium with its metabolic needs includes atherosclerotic coronary anomalies and acquired coronary artery disease from inflammatory causes such as Kawasaki disease and multisystem inflammatory syndrome in children
Mitral valve prolapse	May present with chest pain, anxiety, palpitations, or shortness of breath. Found in patients with connective tissue disorder. Associated with a mid-to-late systolic click with a high-pitched late systolic murmur
Arrhythmia	Supraventricular tachycardia or ventricular ectopy/tachycardia can cause chest pain, palpitations, diaphoresis, anxiety, shortness of breath, exercise intolerance, or pre-syncopal or syncopal symptoms. Will be tachycardic
Noncardiac chest pain	
Costochondritis	Reproducible pain on palpation and the costochondral junction
Precordial Catch	Sharp, localized pain that is brief and can be exacerbated with inspiration. Can often occur at test
Musculoskeletal	Associated with trauma or overuse. Can be seen frequently in athletes or those with recent respiratory infection featuring frequent cough
Asthma	Chest tightness and can be exercise-induced. Have trouble with inhalation and can have associated respiratory or allergic symptoms
Gastroesophageal reflux/esophagitis	Epigastric pain with burning sensation. Can have associated regurgitation or metallic taste in the mouth. Symptoms worsened by certain types of food or exertion shortly after eating

Table 3
Common causes of cardiac and noncardiac pediatric syncope

Causes	Features
Cardiac syncope	
Structural	Occurs without warning
• Coronary artery anomalies	No pre-syncopal prodrome
• Severe great vessels outflow obstruction	Event occurred during physical exertion
• Hypertrophic cardiomyopathy	Severe chest pain
Arrhythmia	Palpitations
• Atrioventricular block	Syncopal episode leading to need for
• Long QT Syndrome	resuscitative measures
• Short QT Syndrome	
• Wolff–Parkinson–White syndrome	
• Catecholaminergic polymorphic ventricular tachycardia	
Myocardia dysfunction	
• Cardiomyopathy (dilated, restrictive)	
• Myocarditis	
Noncardiac syncope	
Vasovagal	Pre-syncopal prodrome of lightheadedness or visual changes is common. Can have frequent pre-syncope without loss of consciousness. Associated with abrupt positional changes. Loss of consciousness is often <1 min
Autonomic dysfunction/orthostatic hypotension	Associated with marked increase in heart rate without hypotension on assuming an upright position. More common in females 5.1. Pre-syncopal symptoms with rare syncope. Associated with chronic fatigue and other vague systemic symptoms
Seizure	Tonic-clonic movements, tongue biting, or incontinence can be seen. prolonged period of confusion or postictal state after the event
Non-epileptic seizures	Associated with occurring at in predictable situations or when certain observers are present. Often occur during times of stress or high emotions. Episodes can be prolonged with abnormal movements not typical of seizures with epileptiform neural activity. Frequently during adolescent years. Often not a conscious act, but can be. This is typically a diagnosis of exclusion

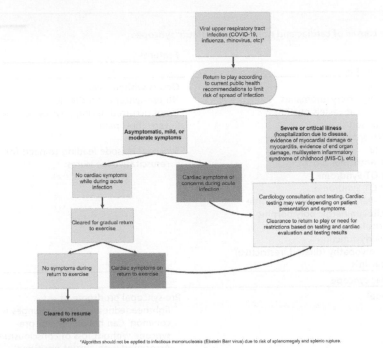

Fig. 3. Return to play algorithm after viral upper respiratory tract infection (COVID-19, influenza, rhinovirus, etc).

history questions in the AHA 14-point PPE need further explanation or examples to help patients give the most accurate history. Providing examples of sudden premature death (SIDS, unexplained drowning, or single-car accident of unknown cause) may aid in reducing ambiguity in the question. Many patients may be more comfortable using layman's terms, such as "enlarged heart" to represent cardiomyopathy. In other cases, patients and caregivers may be more familiar with interventions a family member may have had rather than a diagnosis. Asking about pacemaker insertion, implantable defibrillator devices, and heart transplant history can give clues about the underlying disease and whether it is applicable to the patient. This is another case in which it is likely important to have a parent or caregiver available to supplement the history, as they may have more knowledge of the family's medical history than the patient.

How to Respond to an Abnormal Family History

When an athlete or family reports a positive family history of a cardiac disorder, efforts should be made to determine details regarding the exact diagnosis and whether or not genetic testing is available. These details will help guide the athlete's required evaluation and need for follow-up. Depending on the history, sports and exercise restriction may be required until details and cardiac testing is obtained.

Physical Examination

A detailed physical examination can uncover cardiovascular disease that may warrant further evaluation before sports participation clearance. The importance of vital signs, specifically blood pressure, should not be ignored. Elevated blood pressure is common. It can be a sign of underlying cardiac disease (eg, coarctation of the aorta) or undiagnosed hypertension and can predispose a patient to SCD/SCA. If a patient has upper extremity hypertension, careful attention should be paid to femoral pulses and blood pressure gradient between right arm and leg.

General examination is important to identify features that could be suspicious for certain syndromes. Providers should specifically physical stigmata of Marfan syndrome, such as abnormalities of spinal curvature, pectus deformities, hyperextensible joints, arm span to height ratio, myopia, and other characteristic facial features. The revised Ghent criteria can be used to determine the likelihood of Marfan syndrome or another connective tissue disorder. If there is any concern, then an echocardiogram is required to evaluate the aortic root, ascending aorta and mitral valve before sports participation.[19] Patients with findings consistent with Turner syndrome such as neck webbing, short stature, a low hairline, or low-set ears should also be evaluated with an echocardiogram given their risk of bicuspid aortic valve, coarctation of the aorta, and aortic aneurysms and dissections.

There should be a focus on identifying pathologic heart murmurs, abnormal or extra heart sounds, or rhythm irregularity. Benign murmurs are common in pediatrics, and it can be a challenge to differentiate between benign and pathologic. Benign murmurs typically are soft, systolic ejection murmurs that resolve with standing and do not radiate. Malignant murmurs are typically holosystolic, radiate to the back or neck, occur in diastole, or increase with standing.

Electrocardiogram Screening

There continues to be debate regarding whether or not ECGs should be added to the typical PPE. The European Society for Cardiology recommends including ECG for competitive athletes[26] and some countries mandate ECGs at various ages.[27–29] The most recent guidelines from the American College of Cardiology (ACC), AHA, and AMSSM suggest that ECG may be performed but did not recommend universal ECG screening.[19,30] There have been recent articles examining the utility of adding the ECG to the typical PPE.[31,32]

Advocates of ECG screening argue that the ECG is an inexpensive test, and with the use of new guidelines[33] and experienced interpreting physicians, the sensitivity and specificity are appropriate.[34]

Those who argue against ECG programs contend that resources should be focused elsewhere because ECGs have not been shown to save lives or prevent SCD, they add significant cost, and they lead to unnecessary, sometimes invasive, testing and procedures.

Interpretation of ECGs in pediatric patients can also be challenging. First, childhood ECGs are not as good at diagnosing cardiac pathology using typical standard criteria created for adults. A recent article from Japan, where ECG screening has been mandated for all students in 1st, 7th, and 10th grade since 1973, demonstrated that the sensitivity of ECGs at diagnosing HCM using typical HCM criteria (pathologic Q waves, T-wave inversions, ST depression) was poor at 9% in first grade students. Sensitivity improved to 84% in the 7th grade group and 76% in 10th grade group.[35]

Second, as suggested earlier in this article, a single ECG in childhood or adolescence does not mean the patient will not develop an abnormal ECG or cardiac pathology later in childhood.

Last, the availability of experienced interpreting physicians may be limited. In general, pediatric primary providers are less experienced at ordering and

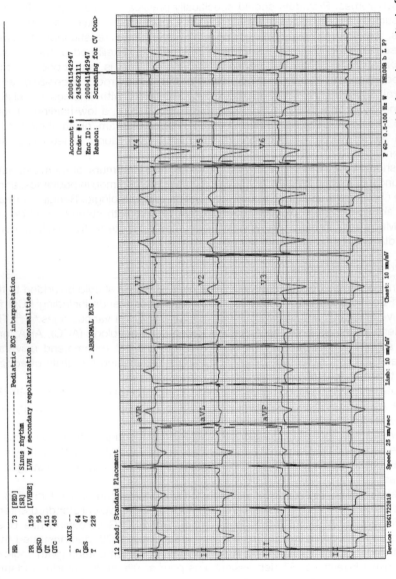

Fig. 4. Follow-up ECG of a now 15-year-old boy from Case 1 with a family history of HCM. This ECG is notable for voltage criteria for left ventricular hypertrophy and T-wave inversion in the inferolateral limb leads.

interpreting ECGs compared with their adult counterparts. There are also significantly fewer pediatric cardiologists in the country and world compared with adult cardiologists.

Despite scientific evidence not being definitive, there will likely always be patient-led and family-led programs that offer ECG screening for pediatric and adolescent athletes. These programs should not be taken lightly and there should be significant thought into how the ECGs will be performed and interpreted as well as how abnormal results are communicated and further evaluated.

What Is Required If ECG Screening Is Pursued

1. Adequate training and experience of interpreting physicians
2. Appropriate privacy for performing of ECG and counseling (of patient and family) after ECG
3. An avenue for cardiologist evaluation and cardiac testing to be performed quickly and fully (ideally at the time of the screening, but if not, a few days later)

Other Nonroutine Modalities of Cardiac Evaluation

There have been studies evaluating the use of echocardiograms and exercise stress testing in PPEs. There has also been suggestion of using genetics[36] and [37] MRIs in preparticipation screening. These modalities certainly have advantages over the history, physical examination, and ECG, but given the cost and resources required for this type of testing and interpretation, widespread use of these modalities seems unlikely.

Return to the Cases

1. Adolescent with family history of HCM:

As the patient was 11 year old at the time of his initial normal cardiac evaluation, it was recommended that he return to clinic in 4 years for repeat evaluation. At that visit, he reports that he has been participating in competitive sports without problems and has no cardiac symptoms. He has a normal physical examination with murmurs. His routine ECG (**Fig. 4**) shows left ventricular hypertrophy and significant T-wave inversions throughout the inferolateral leads (significantly different compared with initial

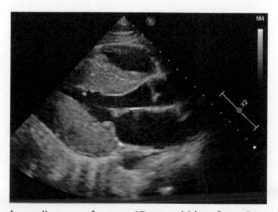

Fig. 5. Follow-up echocardiogram of a now 15-year old boy from Case 1 with a family history of HCM. This is a parasternal long axis image in 2D showing significant left ventricular hypertrophy and interventricular septal thickening to (1.6 cm, Z-score = 6.0), consistent with a diagnosis of hypertrophic cardiomyopathy).

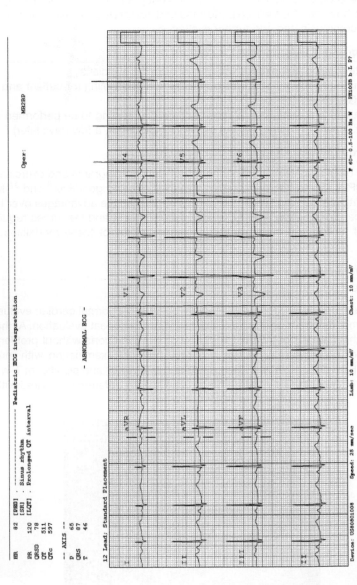

Fig. 6. ECG from patient in Case 2 showing a prolonged QT segment with a calculated QTc of 597 ms, consistent with a diagnosis of LQTS.

ECG at 11 years of age, **Fig. 1**). His echocardiogram (**Fig. 5**) shows significant concentric hypertrophy of the left ventricle (ventricular septal thickness of 16 mm) and dynamic flow acceleration in the left ventricular outflow tract consistent with the diagnosis of HCM. This case highlights the importance of repeated screening in the pediatric population.

2. School-age child with an episode of syncope:

The 10-year-old patient with syncope underwent further cardiac evaluation due to the history of atypical nature of the syncope and the association with exercise. An ECG (**Fig. 6**) is notable for a correct QT duration of 597 ms. Laboratory testing does not reveal a secondary cause of prolonged QT interval. There is no family history of LQTS or other dysrhythmia. His routine echocardiogram is normal. The patient will be started on a beta blocker to reduce the risk of cardiac events and genetic testing demonstrated a pathogenic mutation in the KCNQ1 gene, which is associated with LQTS type 1. This case emphasizes the need to seriously consider all suspicious exercise-related events or symptoms, especially in school-age children who may not be able to communicate their symptoms as well. Syncope during exertion should always raise concern for cardiac pathology.

3. A collegiate baseball player with a history of KD:

As most patients with KD do not have significant residual coronary artery pathology, they do not require long-term antiplatelet or anticoagulation. The fact that the athlete remains on aspirin and dipyridamole should be a sign that he has residual coronary artery pathology and review of his past medical records and possible repeat cardiac testing is required before "clearance." On further review of this patient's history, it is determined that he was diagnosed with KD at the age of 3 years and at that time he had large coronary artery aneurysms. The coronary aneurysms have subsequently decreased in size to medium-sized coronary artery aneurysms (**Fig. 7**). The persistent aneurysms place him at risk for thrombus, so he has

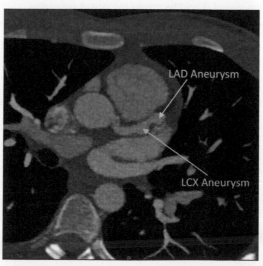

Fig. 7. CT angiogram showing 10 mm aneurysms of both the left anterior descending (LAD) and left circumflex (LCX) coronary arteries in a 15-year-old boy with a history of Kawasaki disease (KD).

continued antiplatelet therapy.[21] Persistent coronary aneurysms related to KD require cardiology follow-up every 6 to 12 months and regular stress testing for inducible myocardial ischemia, both of which should be normal before sports clearance. As this patient enters adulthood, he should be considered for cardiac MRI to monitor for function and signs of ischemia and CT angiogram to monitor for coronary artery stenosis and calcification. This athlete has had those tests and they have been reassuring without evidence of inducible ischemia. The most recent ACC/AHA guidelines[19] allow him to participate in low to moderate static and dynamic competitive sports because he has no evidence of inducible ischemia. Baseball is not a collision sport so there should be no restrictions related to his antiplatelet medications.

SUMMARY

While imperfect, the current sports preparticipation examination guidelines provide a solid framework for ensuring the safe engagement in physical activity for teenagers and children. It is also an important piece of health surveillance and maintenance in the pediatric population. As pediatric patients grow and develop quickly, so too does the need to regularly evaluate their health needs and risks. Informed and appropriately applied principles of the sports PPE will help providers give their patients the ability to be physically active with confidence.

CLINICS CARE POINTS

- Cardiac disease can present differently in children than in adults.
- Careful family history and symptom history is important when clearing pediatric patients prior to sports paticipation.
- Cardiac symptoms with exercise or exertion should have cardiac testing prior to participation.
- Exact type of testing should should be driven by patient symptoms.

DISCLOSURES

The authors have no relevant commercial or financial conflicts of interest in producing this article.

REFERENCES

1. Erickson CC, Salerno JC, Berger S, et al. Sudden death in the young: Information for the primary care provider. Pediatrics 2021;148(1). https://doi.org/10.1542/peds.2021-052044.
2. LaBotz M, Bernhardt DT. Preparticipation physical examination: is it time to stop doing the sports physical? Br J Sports Med 2017;51(3):152.
3. Gajewski KK, Saul JP. Sudden cardiac death in children and adolescents (excluding Sudden Infant Death Syndrome). Ann Pediatr Cardiol 2010;3(2):107–12.
4. Katritsis DG, Gersh BJ, Camm AJ. A clinical perspective on sudden cardiac death. Arrhythmia Electrophysiol Rev 2016;5(3):177–82.

5. Harmon KG, Asif IM, Maleszewski JJ, et al. Incidence, cause, and Comparative frequency of sudden cardiac death in National collegiate athletic association athletes: a decade in review. Circulation 2015;132(1):10–9.
6. Burns KM, Cottengim C, Dykstra H, et al. Epidemiology of sudden death in a population-based study of infants and children. J Pediatr X 2020;2. https://doi.org/10.1016/j.ympdx.2020.100023.
7. Winkel BG, Risgaard B, Sadjadieh G, et al. Sudden cardiac death in children (1-18 years): symptoms and causes of death in a nationwide setting. Eur Heart J 2014;35(13):868–75.
8. Maron BJ, Doerer JJ, Haas TS, et al. Sudden deaths in young competitive athletes analysis of 1866 deaths in the United States, 1980-2006. Circulation 2009; 119(8):1085–92.
9. Maron BJ, Seidman JG, Seidman CE. Proposal for contemporary screening strategies in families with hypertrophic cardiomyopathy. J Am Coll Cardiol 2004; 44(11):2125–32.
10. Faivre L, Masurel-Paulet A, Collod-Béroud G, et al. Clinical and molecular study of 320 children with Marfan syndrome and related type I fibrillinopathies in a Series of 1009 probands with pathogenic FBN1 mutations. Pediatrics 2009;123(1): 391–8.
11. Faivre L, Collod-Beroud G, Child A, et al. Contribution of molecular analyses in diagnosing Marfan syndrome and type I fibrillinopathies: an international study of 1009 probands. J Med Genet 2008;45(6):384–90.
12. Corrado D, Fontaine G, Marcus FI, et al. Arrhythmogenic right ventricular Dysplasia/cardiomyopathy. Circulation 2000;101(11). https://doi.org/10.1161/01.CIR.101.11.e101.
13. te Riele ASJM, James CA, Sawant AC, et al. Arrhythmogenic right ventricular Dysplasia/cardiomyopathy in the pediatric population. JACC: Clin Electrophysiol 2015;1(6):551–60.
14. DeWitt ES, Chandler SF, Hylind RJ, et al. Phenotypic Manifestations of arrhythmogenic cardiomyopathy in children and adolescents. J Am Coll Cardiol 2019;74(3): 346–58.
15. Steinmetz M, Krause U, Lauerer P, et al. Diagnosing ARVC in pediatric patients Applying the revised task Force criteria: importance of imaging, 12-lead ECG, and genetics. Pediatr Cardiol 2018;39(6). https://doi.org/10.1007/s00246-018-1875-y.
16. Etoom Y, Govindapillai S, Hamilton R, et al. Importance of CMR within the task Force criteria for the diagnosis of ARVC in children and adolescents. J Am Coll Cardiol 2015;65(10):987–95.
17. Malhotra A, Dhutia H, Finocchiaro G, et al. Outcomes of cardiac screening in adolescent soccer players. N Engl J Med 2018;379(6):524–34.
18. Miller SM, Peterson AR. The sports preparticipation evaluation practice gaps. Available at: http://pedsinreview.aappublications.org/.
19. Maron BJ, Zipes DP, Kovacs RJ. Eligibility and Disqualification recommendations for competitive athletes with cardiovascular abnormalities: Preamble, principles, and general considerations. Available at: http://www.elsevier.com/about/.
20. Carek PJ, Futrell M, Hueston WJ. The preparticipation physical examination history: who has the correct answers? Clin J Sport Med 1999;9(3). https://doi.org/10.1097/00042752-199907000-00002.
21. McCrindle BW, Rowley AH, Newburger JW, et al. Diagnosis, treatment, and long-term Management of Kawasaki disease: a scientific statement for health professionals from the American heart association. Circulation 2017;135(17):e927–99.

22. Barbut G, Needleman JP. Pediatric chest pain Education gaps. Available at: http://pedsinreview.aappublications.org/.
23. Cannon B, Wackel P. Syncope Educational Gap. Available at: http://pedsinreview.aappublications.org/.
24. Martinez MW, Tucker AM, Bloom OJ, et al. Prevalence of inflammatory heart disease among professional athletes with prior COVID-19 infection who received systematic return-to-play cardiac screening. JAMA Cardiol 2021;6(7):745–52.
25. Moulson N, Petek BJ, Drezner JA, et al. SARS-CoV-2 cardiac Involvement in young competitive athletes. Circulation 2021;144(4):256–66.
26. Corrado D, Pelliccia A, Bjørnstad HH, et al. Cardiovascular pre-participation screening of young competitive athletes for prevention of sudden death: proposal for a common European protocol. Consensus statement of the study group of sport cardiology of the working group of cardiac Rehabilitation and exercise Physiology and the working group of myocardial and Pericardial diseases of the European Society of cardiology. Eur Heart J 2005;26(5). https://doi.org/10.1093/eurheartj/ehi108.
27. Corrado D, Basso C, Pavei A, et al. Trends in sudden cardiovascular death in young competitive athletes after implementation of a preparticipation screening program. JAMA 2006;296(13). https://doi.org/10.1001/jama.296.13.1593.
28. Steinvil A, Chundadze T, Zeltser D, et al. Mandatory electrocardiographic screening of athletes to reduce their risk for sudden death: Proven fact or wishful thinking? J Am Coll Cardiol 2011;57(11):1291–6.
29. HANEDA N, MORI C, NISHIO T, et al. Heart diseases discovered by mass screening in the schools of Shimane prefecture over a period of 5 years. Jpn Circ J 1986;50(12). https://doi.org/10.1253/jcj.50.1325.
30. Drezner JA, O'Connor FG, Harmon KG, et al. AMSSM position statement on cardiovascular preparticipation screening in athletes: current evidence, knowledge gaps, recommendations and future directions. Br J Sports Med 2017;51(3): 153–67.
31. Petek BJ, Baggish AL. Current controversies in pre-participation cardiovascular screening for young competitive athletes. Expert Rev Cardiovasc Ther 2020; 18(7):435–42.
32. Orchard JJ, Neubeck L, Orchard JW, et al. ECG-based cardiac screening programs: Legal, ethical, and logistical considerations. Heart Rhythm 2019;16(10): 1584–91.
33. Sharma S, Drezner JA, Baggish A, et al. International recommendations for electrocardiographic interpretation in athletes. Eur Heart J 2018;39(16). https://doi.org/10.1093/eurheartj/ehw631.
34. Harmon KG, Zigman M, Drezner JA. The effectiveness of screening history, physical exam, and ECG to detect potentially lethal cardiac disorders in athletes: a systematic review/meta-analysis. J Electrocardiol 2015;48(3):329–38.
35. Yoshinaga M, Horigome H, Ayusawa M, et al. Electrocardiographic diagnosis of hypertrophic cardiomyopathy in the pre- and Post-diagnostic phases in children and adolescents. Circ J 2021. https://doi.org/10.1253/circj.CJ-21-0376. CJ-21-0376.
36. Magavern EF, Badalato L, Finocchiaro G, et al. Ethical considerations for genetic testing in the context of mandated cardiac screening before athletic participation. Genet Med 2017;19(5):493–5.
37. Angelini P, Muthupillai R, Lopez A, et al. Young athletes: Preventing sudden death by adopting a modern screening approach? A critical review and the opening of a debate. Int J Cardiol Heart Vasc 2021;34:100790.

The Risk of Sudden Unexpected Cardiac Death in Children
Epidemiology, Clinical Causes, and Prevention

Emanuele Monda, MD[a], Michele Lioncino, MD[a],
Marta Rubino, MD[a], Martina Caiazza, MD[a],
Annapaola Cirillo, MD[a], Adelaide Fusco, MD[a],
Roberta Pacileo, MD[a], Fabio Fimiani, MD[a], Federica Amodio, MD[a],
Nunzia Borrelli, MD[a], Diego Colonna, MD[a],
Barbara D'Onofrio, MD[a], Giulia Frisso, MD, PhD[b],
Fabrizio Drago, MD, PhD[c], Silvia Castelletti, MD, PhD[d],
Berardo Sarubbi, MD, PhD[a], Paolo Calabrò, MD, PhD[a],
Maria Giovanna Russo, MD, PhD[a],
Giuseppe Limongelli, MD, PhD[a,e,*]

KEYWORDS

• Sudden cardiac death • Children • Cardiomyopathies • Channelopathies

KEY POINTS

• In children, the main causes of sudden cardiac death (SCD) are inherited cardiac disorders, whereas coronary artery diseases, congenital heart diseases, and myocarditis are rare.
• The identification of inherited cardiac disorders that predispose to SCD is required to prevent future cardiac events both in the proband and affected family members.
• Hypertrophic cardiomyopathy is the major cause of SCD among cardiomyopathies, followed by arrhythmogenic cardiomyopathy.
• Channelopathies represent among the leading cause of sudden arrhythmic death syndrome (sudden unexplained death with negative pathologic and toxicologic assessment).

This article originally appeared in *Heart Failure Clinics*, Volume 18, Issue 1, January 2022.
[a] Department of Translational Medical Sciences, University of Campania "Luigi Vanvitelli", Via L. Bianchi, 80131 Naples, Italy; [b] Department of Molecular Medicine and Medical Biotechnologies, University of Naples Federico II, Via Pansini 5, 80131 Naples, Italy; [c] Istituto Auxologico Italiano, IRCCS-Center for Cardiac Arrhythmias of Genetic Origin, Via Pier Lombardo 22, 20135 Milan, Italy; [d] Istituto Auxologico Italiano, IRCCS-Center for Cardiac Arrhythmias of Genetic Origin, Milan, Italy; [e] Institute of Cardiovascular Sciences, University College of London and St. Bartholomew's Hospital, Grower Street, London WC1E 6DD, UK
* Corresponding author. Inherited and Rare Cardiovascular Diseases, Department of Translational Medical Sciences, University of Campania "Luigi Vanvitelli", AO Colli - Monaldi Hospital - ERN Guard Heart Member, 80131 Naples, Italy.
E-mail address: limongelligiuseppe@libero.it

INTRODUCTION

Sudden unexplained death (SUD) is a tragic event for both the family and community, particularly when it occurs in young individuals. The term SUD is used to refer to an unexpected and sudden death that occurs in an individual older than 1 year. On the other part, sudden death occurring in the first year of life is defined as sudden unexplained death in infancy.[1]

Sudden cardiac death (SCD) represents the leading form of SUD[2] and is defined as an unexpected event without an obvious extracardiac cause, occurring within 1 hour after the onset of symptoms.[3] SCD in children often occurs without warning symptoms, manifesting as the first presentation of an underlying cardiac disease.[4] In children, the main causes of SCD are inherited cardiac disorders,[5–9] whereas coronary artery diseases (congenital or acquired), congenital heart diseases, and myocarditis are rare (**Table 1**). The identification of inherited cardiac disorders that predispose to SCD is a fundamental step to prevent future cardiac events both in the proband and affected family members.[4,10]

The present review examines the current state of knowledge regarding SCD in children, discussing the epidemiology, clinical causes, and prevention strategies.

EPIDEMIOLOGY

SCD is an uncommon event in childhood. Several population-based studies investigated the incidence of SCD in young individuals, reporting an incidence ranging from 0.7 to 7.4 per 100.000 person-years.[5–9,11] Several factors were associated with the variability of the SCD incidence, such as age, sex, country, comorbidities, and participation in athletic activity. The rate of SCD was less than in the adult population and was age dependent, with an initial period of higher risk in infants (<1 year old), a lower rate in children aged 6 to 10 years old, and a progressive increase in risk in children older than 10 years.[6,12,13] Men showed an increased risk, which was twice that of women.[5,14]

CAUSES

Several conditions have been associated with SCD. They can be classified into cardiomyopathies (CMPs), primary arrhythmia syndromes (channelopathies), congenital heart diseases, coronary artery diseases, aortic diseases, and myocarditis. In children who died suddenly, the underlying cardiac cause may be known or in the preclinical phase, and the proportion of the detected risk of SCD varies by age and diagnosis.

Table 1
Causes of sudden cardiac death in children categorized into structural and arrhythmogenic causes

	Structural Causes	Arrhythmogenic Causes
Common	Arrhythmogenic cardiomyopathy Hypertrophic cardiomyopathy Myocarditis	Brugada syndrome Catecholaminergic polymorphic ventricular tachycardia Long QT syndrome
Uncommon	Aortic disease Congenital heart disease Coronary artery disease Dilated cardiomyopathy Restrictive cardiomyopathy	Early repolarization syndrome Progressive cardiac conduction disease Short QT syndrome Wolff-Parkinson-White syndrome

In the following paragraphs, the authors describe the main causes of SCD in children and the related known risk factors for single cause.

Cardiomyopathies

SCD in children with CMPs depends on age, gender, and phenotype. Male patients and children older than 10 years show a higher risk of SCD. Hypertrophic cardiomyopathy (HCM) is the major cause of SCD among CMPs, followed by arrhythmogenic cardiomyopathy (ACM). SCD due to dilated cardiomyopathy, restrictive cardiomyopathy, or left ventricular (LV) noncompaction is a rare event.[8,15]

Hypertrophic cardiomyopathy

The prevalence of SCD rates in children with HCM varies widely, with reported rates ranging from 1% to 7.2% per year.[16–20] The clinical course of patients with HCM can be extremely variable,[21–28] and the identification of young patients at high risk of SCD is often challenging. Both the European Society of Cardiology and the American Heart Association–American College of Cardiology guidelines recommend implantable cardioverter-defibrillator (ICD) implantation in children with more than 1 risk factor, including unexplained syncope, massive left ventricular hypertrophy (LVH), nonsustained ventricular tachycardia (NSVT), or family history of HCM-related SCD.[29,30] However, a consensus on SCD risk stratification for children with HCM is not currently available. A recent systematic review identified several risk factors for SCD, categorizing them into major and minor risk factors.[31] Major risk factors included previous aborted cardiac arrest or sustained ventricular tachycardia, extreme LVH, syncope, and NSVT, whereas minor risk factors included family history of SCD, age at presentation or diagnosis, electrocardiogram (ECG) changes, abnormal blood pressure response to exercise, LV outflow tract obstruction, left atrial size, restrictive physiology, and abnormal 24-hour blood pressure monitoring. Moreover, 2 different risk prediction models for SCD in children with HCM have been recently proposed. Norrish and colleagues[32] developed a 5-year SCD risk prediction model from a retrospective cohort study of 1024 consecutive patients aged 16 years or younger with HCM, with the final model including unexplained syncope, NSVT, left atrial diameter z-score, LV maximal wall thickness z-score, and LV outflow tract gradient. Similarly, Miron and colleagues[33] developed and validated a 5-year SCD risk prediction model from 572 consecutive patients aged 18 years or younger with HCM. Risk predictors included age at diagnosis, NSVT, unexplained syncope, septal diameter z-score, LV posterior wall diameter z score, left atrial diameter z score, peak LV outflow tract gradient, and presence of a pathogenic variant. Interestingly, both models showed a discrete prediction accuracy, with the potential to improve the application of clinical practice guidelines and shared decision-making for ICD implantation. On the contrary, no ECG abnormalities, either in isolation or combined in the previously described ECG risk score,[34] have been found to be associated with 5-year SCD risk in a large multicenter retrospective cohort of children with HCM.[35]

Arrhythmogenic cardiomyopathy

ACM is a common cause of SCD in children[5,9] and among the most important in young athletes.[36–42] However, there are few studies focused on children with ACM, and, as a consequence, SCD risk factors in those patients are poorly known. Furthermore, no guideline or consensus document provides specific recommendations for risk stratification and ICD implantation in children with ACM. DeWitt and colleagues[43] evaluated 32 children aged 21 years or younger with ACM. Cardiac arrest and ventricular tachycardia occurred in 15% and 31% of patients, and predominant right ventricular disease was significantly associated with both the events. Moreover, they were more likely to occur in probands. Similarly, Riele and colleagues[44] identified 75 patients with pediatric-onset disease (<18 years of age) and found that 15% of pediatric patients presented with SCD and 11% with sudden cardiac arrest (SCA). In most of the patients, SCD occurred during exercise activity. In ACM, participation in high-intensity activity can favor the disease progression and trigger life-threatening arrhythmias. Therefore, avoidance from competitive sports should be recommended.[45]

Channelopathies

Channelopathies represent among the leading cause of sudden arrhythmic death syndrome (SADS), a term used to describe an individual with SUD who shows negative pathologic and toxicologic assessment (autopsy-negative SUD). In particular, long QT syndrome (LQTS) and catecholaminergic polymorphic ventricular tachycardia (CPVT) are the most common causes of SADS, followed by Brugada syndrome (BrS).[4,46–50]

Long QT syndrome

LQTS is a cause of SUD in up to 20% of victims younger than 30 years.[47,49] Furthermore, about 10% of infants (<1 year) who died suddenly carry a disease-causing mutation in an LQTS-related gene, and a prolonged QT interval in newborns increased the risk of SCD.[50–52] In addition, an episode of SCA during infancy is associated with a very high risk for subsequent SCD during the next 10 years of life.[52]

The risk of SCD in patients with LQTS is influenced by age, gender, genotype, and environmental or genetic modifiers.[53] Men carry an increased risk of SCD during childhood and preadolescence,[54–56] whereas the gender-related risk reverses after childhood, and women show higher risk than men during adolescence and adulthood[56]; the reason of this gender-related risk is unknown. Moreover, other major risk factors in children include the history of syncope, QTc duration greater than 500 ms, and episodes of T wave alternans.[54,57,58] In LQTS there is a strong genotype-phenotype correlation with the most important correlation evidenced for the specific trigger for life-threatening arrhythmias: patients with LQT1 are at increased risk during emotional or physical stresses, conditions characterized by increased sympathetic activity[59]; patients with LQT2 are at increased risk when exposed to sudden noises[59]; patients with LQT3 are at risk during asleep or when they are at rest.

Catecholaminergic polymorphic ventricular tachycardia

CPVT is among the most frequent cause of SADS,[47,60] especially when the death occurred during exertional activity. CPVT can manifest at any age. However, the most common presentation occurs during the first 2 decades of life, with fast palpitations, presyncope, syncope, SCA, or SCD under adrenergic stress.[61] Hayashi and colleagues[62] identified younger at diagnosis, absence of beta-blocking therapy, and history of aborted cardiac arrest as independent predictors for cardiac events. Unfortunately, to date, there is no risk stratification protocol in patients with CPVT.

Brugada syndrome

BrS is a rare cause of SUD. It is mostly diagnosed during adulthood and, given the rarity of BrS in the pediatric population, risk stratification in children and young patients is very difficult. Andorin and colleagues[63] reported that the risk of life-threatening arrhythmias was related to 2 clinical parameters: spontaneous ECG type 1 Brugada pattern and syncope. Subsequently, a clinical score model to predict lethal events in patients younger than or equal to 19 years with BrS was proposed. This model includes 4 main clinical variables: SCD or syncope, spontaneous type 1 ECG pattern, sinus node dysfunction and/or atrial tachycardia, and conduction abnormality.[64] However, an important limitation of these studies was the small sample size of the cohort, which limits the generalization of the results. Indeed, considering the high rate of complication associated with ICD implantation in children, the patient selection requires attention to avoid unnecessary implantation. Interestingly, Mazzanti and colleagues[65] showed that in a cohort of 129 pediatric patients, only 3 of them experienced a life-threatening arrhythmic event and no patients who had presented with syncope experienced a cardiac arrest during follow-up, suggesting that a more conservative approach may be indicated in the pediatric population.

PREVENTION

The prevention of SCD in children can be categorized into 3 different sections: the identification of patients at risk for SCD and the implementation of strategies to prevent the event (primary prevention); the identification of the underlying cause in SCA survivors and the implementation of strategies to prevent further events (secondary prevention); and the identification of family member at risk for SCD.

Identification of Children at Risk for Sudden Cardiac Death

Cardiac arrest is often the first manifestation of an underlying inherited cardiac disease. Thus, cardiovascular screening represents an important prevention strategy to avoid SCD in children. Several screening programs have been proposed for different populations and subgroups, such as athletes, to early detect the patients at risk.[66] Furthermore, children with cardiac inherited disorders can be identified for other reasons, such as family screening (discussed later) or the presence of warning symptoms (eg, syncope or presyncope).[67,68]

In these patients, several interventions should be started, such as lifestyle modification, medical treatment, and ICD implantation in primary prevention for those at high risk.[69,70] The possible lifestyle modification would be avoiding dehydration and electrolyte imbalance for children with channelopathies; avoiding hyperthermia from febrile illnesses for patients with BrS; avoiding strenuous physical activity in patients with HCM, ACM, LQTS, and CPVT; avoiding certain drugs for patients with LQTS or BrS, and so forth.[71] Medical treatment varies according to the underlying cardiac condition.[21,22,69,72–74] For example, beta-blockers play a role in SCD prevention in patients with LQTS and CPVT,[69] whereas their role is uncertain in children with HCM.[70] Finally, in patients considered at high risk for SCD, ICD implantation should be considered. However, as discussed earlier, risk stratification is often difficult in children with CMPs or channelopathies due to the paucity of data in the literature.

Investigations in Sudden Cardiac Arrest Survivors

In children who experienced an SCA, the identification of the underlying cause is mandatory to start appropriate treatment and identify family members at risk. Thus, a comprehensive clinical and instrumental evaluation is required[10] (**Fig. 1**): the information on age, sex, symptoms, and family history activity at the time of SCA. For example, children with BrS or LQT3 generally experience SCA during sleep or at rest, whereas ACM, LQT1, and CPVT during emotional or physical stress.[59,61,63] Baseline investigations should include blood testing, standard 12-lead ECG, high precordial lead ECG, signal-average ECG, echocardiography, and cardiac magnetic resonance (CMR).[75–78] Coronary imaging may be considered in selected cases. Baseline investigation can be helpful to diagnose most overt acquired or genetic cardiac

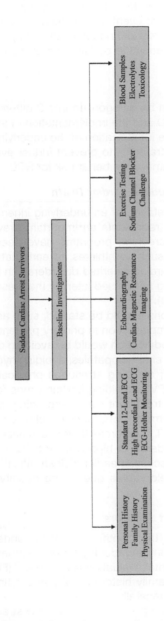
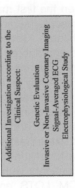

Fig. 1. Investigation of sudden cardiac arrest survivors.

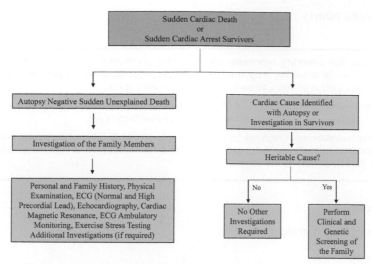

Fig. 2. Identification of family members at risk for sudden cardiac death.

diseases. However, these conditions can be concealed, and provocative maneuvers are sometimes required to obtain a final diagnosis. For example, sodium channel blocker challenge can be useful for the diagnosis of Brugada syndrome,[79] exercise testing may support the diagnosis of CPVT or ACM,[69,80] and so forth. Finally, genetic testing should be considered in patients with a diagnosis or strong suspect for inherited cardiac disease, in particular when the results are likely to influence the management and to guide family screening.[4,81–84] Of importance, for children who experience an SCA, the prevention of further episodes is mandatory, and, except for selected cases, survivors should undergo ICD implantation.

Identification of Family Members at Risk

Two different strategies can be used to detect family members at risk. If the proband obtained a final diagnosis and showed positive genetic testing for a disease-causing mutation (either obtained in SCA survivors with the genetic testing or in patients who died suddenly with the molecular autopsy), the cascade screening is the best strategy to early identify other family members who may carry the genetic mutation (**Fig. 2**). Family members who result negative for that implicated variant can be dismissed, whereas those positive will require disease-specific surveillance and therapy.

On the other hand, when the cause of SCD is not identified, either because there was no postmortem examination or because the autopsy was negative, the identification of family members at risk is more difficult and requires a comprehensive screening of first-degree relatives of the SCD victim. Baseline investigations include family history, physical examination, standard 12-lead ECG, high precordial lead ECG, echocardiography, CMR, exercise testing, and sodium channel blocker challenge.[10,85]

SUMMARY

SCD is a tragic and often unexpected event, especially if it is the sentinel manifestation of the disease in a family. Clinical and genetic evaluation of survivors and family members plays a key role in diagnosing the underlying inherited cardiac disease in the family in order to start appropriate prevention strategies.

CLINICS CARE POINTS

- Cardiovascular screening represents an important prevention strategy to avoid SCD in children. Several screening programs have been proposed for different populations and subgroups, such as athletes, to early detect the patients at risk.

- In children who experienced an SCA, the identification of the underlying cause is mandatory to start appropriate treatment and identify family members at risk.

- In patients considered at high risk for SCD, ICD implantation should be considered. However, risk stratification is often difficult in children with cardiomyopathies or channelopathies due to the paucity of data in the literature.

DISCLOSURE

The authors have nothing to disclose.

REFERENCES

1. Mitchell EA, Krous HF. Sudden unexpected death in infancy: a historical perspective. J Paediatr Child Health 2015;51(1):108–12.
2. Risgaard B, Lynge TH, Wissenberg M, et al. Risk factors and causes of sudden noncardiac death: a nationwide cohort study in Denmark. Heart Rhythm 2015; 12(5):968–74.
3. Fishman GI, Chugh SS, Dimarco JP, et al. Sudden cardiac death prediction and prevention: report from a National Heart, Lung, and Blood Institute and Heart Rhythm Society Workshop. Circulation 2010;122(22):2335–48.
4. Monda E, Sarubbi B, Russo MG, et al. Unexplained sudden cardiac arrest in children: clinical and genetic characteristics of survivors. Eur J Prev Cardiol 2020. 2047487320940863.
5. Winkel BG, Holst AG, Theilade J, et al. Nationwide study of sudden cardiac death in persons aged 1-35 years. Eur Heart J 2011;32:983–90.
6. Bagnall RD, Weintraub RG, Ingles J, et al. A prospective study of sudden cardiac death among children and young adults. N Engl J Med 2016;374:2441–52.
7. Winkel BG, Risgaard B, Sadjadieh G, et al. Sudden cardiac death in children (1-18 years): symptoms and causes of death in a nationwide setting. Eur Heart J 2014;35:868–75.
8. Eckart RE, Shry EA, Burke AP, et al. Sudden death in young adults: an autopsy based series of a population undergoing active surveillance. J Am Coll Cardiol 2011;58:1254–61.
9. Wisten A, Krantz P, Stattin EL. Sudden cardiac death among the young in Sweden from 2000 to 2010: an autopsy-based study. Europace 2017;19:1327–34.
10. Stiles MK, Wilde AAM, Abrams DJ, et al. 2020 APHRS/HRS expert consensus statement on the investigation of decedents with sudden unexplained death and patients with sudden cardiac arrest, and of their families. Heart Rhythm 2021;18(1):e1–50.
11. Martens E, Sinner MF, Siebermair J, et al. Incidence of sudden cardiac death in Germany: results from an emergency medical service registry in Lower Saxony. Europace 2014;16(12):1752–8.
12. Mellor G, Raju H, de Noronha SV, et al. Clinical characteristics and circumstances of death in the sudden arrhythmic death syndrome. Circ Arrhythm Electrophysiol 2014;7:1078–83.

13. Papadakis M, Raju H, Behr ER, et al. Sudden cardiac death with autopsy findings of uncertain significance: potential for erroneous interpretation. Circ Arrhythm Electrophysiol 2013;6:588–96.
14. Meyer L, Stubbs B, Fahrenbruch C, et al. Incidence, causes, and survival trends from cardiovascular-related sudden cardiac arrest in children and young adults 0 to 35 years of age: a 30-year review. Circulation 2012;126(11):1363–72.
15. Harmon KG, Asif IM, Klossner D, et al. Incidence of sudden cardiac death in National Collegiate Athletic Association athletes. Circulation 2011;123(15):1594–600.
16. Kaski J, Tome´ Esteban MT, Lowe M, et al. Outcomes after implantable cardioverter-defibrillator treatment in children with hypertrophic cardiomyopathy. Heart 2007;93:372–4.
17. McKenna W, Deanfield J, Faruqui A, et al. Prognosis in hypertrophic cardiomyopathy: role of age and clinical, electrocardiographic and hemodynamic features. Am J Cardiol 1981;47:532–8.
18. McKenna WJ, Deanfield JE. Hypertrophic cardiomyopathy: an important cause of sudden death. Arch Dis Child 1984;59:971–5.
19. Ostman-Smith I, Wettrell G, Keeton B, et al. Age- and gender-specific mortality rates in childhood hypertrophic cardiomyopathy. Eur Heart J 2008;29:1160–7.
20. Yetman AT, Hamilton RM, Benson LN, et al. Long-term outcome and prognostic determinants in children with hypertrophic cardiomyopathy. J Am Coll Cardiol 1998;32:1943–50.
21. Monda E, Palmiero G, Rubino M, et al. Molecular basis of inflammation in the pathogenesis of cardiomyopathies. Int J Mol Sci 2020;21(18):6462.
22. Monda E, Limongelli G. The hospitalizations in hypertrophic cardiomyopathy: "The dark side of the moon". Int J Cardiol 2020;318:101–2.
23. Limongelli G, Monda E, Tramonte S, et al. Prevalence and clinical significance of red flags in patients with hypertrophic cardiomyopathy. Int J Cardiol 2020;299:186–91.
24. Esposito A, Monda E, Gragnano F, et al. Prevalence and clinical implications of hyperhomocysteinaemia in patients with hypertrophic cardiomyopathy and MTHFR C6777T polymorphism. Eur J Prev Cardiol 2020;27(17):1906–8.
25. Caiazza M, Rubino M, Monda E, et al. Combined PTPN11 and MYBPC3 gene mutations in an adult patient with noonan syndrome and hypertrophic cardiomyopathy. Genes (Basel) 2020;11(8):947.
26. Monda E, Kaski JP, Limongelli G. Editorial: paediatric cardiomyopathies. Front Pediatr 2021;9:696443.
27. Monda E, Rubino M, Lioncino M, et al. Hypertrophic cardiomyopathy in children: pathophysiology, diagnosis, and treatment of non-sarcomeric causes. Front Pediatr 2021;9:632293.
28. Limongelli G, Monda E, D'Aponte A, et al. Combined effect of mediterranean diet and aerobic exercise on weight loss and clinical status in obese symptomatic patients with hypertrophic Cardiomyopathy. Heart Fail Clin 2021;17(2):303–13.
29. Elliott PM, Anastasakis A, Borger MA, et al. 2014 ESC guidelines on diagnosis and management of hypertrophic cardiomyopathy: the task force for the diagnosis and management of hypertrophic cardiomyopathy of the European Society of Cardiology (ESC). Eur Heart J 2014;35(39):2733–79.
30. Ommen SR, Mital S, Burke MA, et al. 2020 AHA/ACC guideline for the diagnosis and treatment of patients with hypertrophic cardiomyopathy: a report of the American College of Cardiology/American Heart Association Joint Committee on

Clinical Practice Guidelines [published correction appears in Circulation. 2020 Dec 22;142(25):e633]. Circulation 2020;142(25):e558–631.

31. Norrish G, Cantarutti N, Pissaridou E, et al. Risk factors for sudden cardiac death in childhood hypertrophic cardiomyopathy: a systematic review and meta-analysis. Eur J Prev Cardiol 2017;24(11):1220–30.

32. Norrish G, Ding T, Field E, et al. Development of a novel risk prediction model for sudden cardiac death in childhood hypertrophic cardiomyopathy (HCM Risk-Kids). JAMA Cardiol 2019;4(9):918–27.

33. Miron A, Lafreniere-Roula M, Steve Fan CP, et al. A validated model for sudden cardiac death risk prediction in pediatric hypertrophic cardiomyopathy. Circulation 2020;142(3):217–29.

34. Östman-Smith I, Sjöberg G, Rydberg A, et al. Predictors of risk for sudden death in childhood hypertrophic cardiomyopathy: the importance of the ECG risk score. Open Heart 2017;4(2):e000658.

35. Norrish G, Topriceanu C, Qu C, et al. The role of the electrocardiographic phenotype in risk stratification for sudden cardiac death in childhood hypertrophic cardiomyopathy [published online ahead of print, 2021 Mar 27]. Eur J Prev Cardiol 2021;zwab046.

36. Maron BJ. Sudden death in young athletes. N Engl J Med 2003;349(11):1064–75.

37. Maron BJ, Epstein SE, Roberts WC. Causes of sudden death in competitive athletes. J Am Coll Cardiol 1986;7(1):204–14.

38. Thiene G, Nava A, Corrado D, et al. Right ventricular cardiomyopathy and sudden death in young people. N Engl J Med 1988;318(3):129–33.

39. Barretta F, Mirra B, Monda E, et al. The hidden fragility in the heart of the athletes: a review of genetic biomarkers. Int J Mol Sci 2020;21(18):6682.

40. Monda E, Frisso G, Rubino M, et al. Potential role of imaging markers in predicting future disease expression of arrhythmogenic cardiomyopathy. Future Cardiol 2021;17(4):647–54.

41. Limongelli G, Nunziato M, D'Argenio V, et al. Yield and clinical significance of genetic screening in elite and amateur athletes [published online ahead of print, 2020 Jul 2]. Eur J Prev Cardiol 2020. 2047487320934265.

42. Limongelli G, Nunziato M, Mazzaccara C, et al. Genotype-phenotype correlation: a triple DNA mutational event in a boy entering sport conveys an additional pathogenicity risk. Genes (Basel) 2020;11(5):524.

43. DeWitt ES, Chandler SF, Hylind RJ, et al. Phenotypic manifestations of arrhythmogenic cardiomyopathy in children and adolescents. J Am Coll Cardiol 2019;74(3):346–58.

44. Te Riele ASJM, James CA, Sawant AC, et al. Arrhythmogenic right ventricular dysplasia/cardiomyopathy in the pediatric population: clinical characterization and comparison with adult-onset disease. JACC Clin Electrophysiol 2015;1(6):551–60.

45. Pelliccia A, Solberg EE, Papadakis M, et al. Recommendations for participation in competitive and leisure time sport in athletes with cardiomyopathies, myocarditis, and pericarditis: position statement of the Sport Cardiology Section of the European Association of Preventive Cardiology (EAPC). Eur Heart J 2019;40(1):19–33.

46. Behr ER, Dalageorgou C, Christiansen M, et al. Sudden arrhythmic death syndrome: familial evaluation identifies inheritable heart disease in the majority of families. Eur Heart J 2008;29(13):1670–80.

47. Tester DJ, Medeiros-Domingo A, Will ML, et al. Cardiac channel molecular autopsy: insights from 173 consecutive cases of autopsy-negative sudden

unexplained death referred for postmortem genetic testing. Mayo Clin Proc 2012; 87(6):524–39.

48. Skinner JR, Crawford J, Smith W, et al. Prospective, population-based long QT molecular autopsy study of postmortem negative sudden death in 1 to 40 year olds. Heart Rhythm 2011;8(3):412–9.

49. Tester DJ, Ackerman MJ. Postmortem long QT syndrome genetic testing for sudden unexplained death in the young. J Am Coll Cardiol 2007;49(2):240–6.

50. Schwartz PJ, Stramba-Badiale M, Crotti L, et al. Prevalence of the congenital long-QT syndrome. Circulation 2009;120(18):1761–7.

51. Schwartz PJ, Stramba-Badiale M, Segantini A, et al. Prolongation of the QT interval and the sudden infant death syndrome. N Engl J Med 1998;338(24):1709–14.

52. Spazzolini C, Mullally J, Moss AJ, et al. Clinical implications for patients with long QT syndrome who experience a cardiac event during infancy. J Am Coll Cardiol 2009;54(9):832–7.

53. Schwartz PJ, Ackerman MJ, Antzelevitch C, et al. Inherited cardiac arrhythmias. Nat Rev Dis Primers 2020;6(1):58.

54. Goldenberg I, Moss AJ, Peterson DR, et al. Risk factors for aborted cardiac arrest and sudden cardiac death in children with the congenital long-QT syndrome. Circulation 2008;117(17):2184–91.

55. Locati EH, Zareba W, Moss AJ, et al. Age- and sex-related differences in clinical manifestations in patients with congenital long-QT syndrome: findings from the International LQTS Registry. Circulation 1998;97(22):2237–44.

56. Zareba W, Moss AJ, Locati EH, et al. Modulating effects of age and gender on the clinical course of long QT syndrome by genotype. J Am Coll Cardiol 2003;42(1): 103–9.

57. Priori SG, Schwartz PJ, Napolitano C, et al. Risk stratification in the long-QT syndrome. N Engl J Med 2003;348(19):1866–74.

58. Schwartz PJ, Malliani A. Electrical alternation of the T-wave: clinical and experimental evidence of its relationship with the sympathetic nervous system and with the long Q-T syndrome. Am Heart J 1975;89(1):45–50.

59. Schwartz PJ, Priori SG, Spazzolini C, et al. Genotype-phenotype correlation in the long-QT syndrome: gene-specific triggers for life-threatening arrhythmias. Circulation 2001;103(1):89–95.

60. Tester DJ, Spoon DB, Valdivia HH, et al. Targeted mutational analysis of the RyR2-encoded cardiac ryanodine receptor in sudden unexplained death: a molecular autopsy of 49 medical examiner/coroner's cases. Mayo Clin Proc 2004;79(11): 1380–4.

61. Priori SG, Napolitano C, Tiso N, et al. Mutations in the cardiac ryanodine receptor gene (hRyR2) underlie catecholaminergic polymorphic ventricular tachycardia. Circulation 2001;103(2):196–200.

62. Hayashi M, Denjoy I, Extramiana F, et al. Incidence and risk factors of arrhythmic events in catecholaminergic polymorphic ventricular tachycardia. Circulation 2009;119(18):2426–34.

63. Andorin A, Behr ER, Denjoy I, et al. Impact of clinical and genetic findings on the management of young patients with Brugada syndrome. Heart Rhythm 2016; 13(6):1274–82.

64. Gonzalez Corcia MC, Sieira J, Pappaert G, et al. A clinical score model to predict lethal events in young patients (≤19 Years) with the brugada syndrome. Am J Cardiol 2017;120(5):797–802.

65. Mazzanti A, Ovics P, Shauer A, et al. Unexpected risk profile of a large pediatric population with brugada syndrome. J Am Coll Cardiol 2019;73(14):1868–9.

66. Mont L, Pelliccia A, Sharma S, et al. Pre-participation cardiovascular evaluation for athletic participants to prevent sudden death: position paper from the EHRA and the EACPR, branches of the ESC. Endorsed by APHRS, HRS, and SOLAECE. Eur J Prev Cardiol 2017;24(1):41–69.
67. Drezner JA, Fudge J, Harmon KG, et al. Warning symptoms and family history in children and young adults with sudden cardiac arrest. J Am Board Fam Med 2012;25(4):408–15.
68. Wisten A, Messner T. Symptoms preceding sudden cardiac death in the young are common but often misinterpreted. Scand Cardiovasc J 2005;39(3):143–9.
69. Priori SG, Blomström-Lundqvist C, Mazzanti A, et al. 2015 ESC Guidelines for the management of patients with ventricular arrhythmias and the prevention of sudden cardiac death: the task force for the management of patients with ventricular arrhythmias and the prevention of sudden cardiac death of the European Society of Cardiology (ESC). Endorsed by: Association for European Paediatric and Congenital Cardiology (AEPC). Eur Heart J 2015;36(41):2793–867.
70. Al-Khatib SM, Stevenson WG, Ackerman MJ, et al. 2017 AHA/ACC/HRS guideline for management of patients with ventricular arrhythmias and the prevention of sudden cardiac death: a report of the American College of Cardiology/American Heart Association Task Force on Clinical Practice Guidelines and the Heart Rhythm Society [published correction appears in Circulation. 2018 Sep 25;138(13):e419-e420]. Circulation 2018;138(13):e272–391.
71. Ackerman MJ, Zipes DP, Kovacs RJ, et al. American heart association electrocardiography and arrhythmias committee of council on clinical cardiology, council on cardiovascular disease in young, council on cardiovascular and stroke nursing, council on functional genomics and translational biology, and American College of Cardiology. Eligibility and disqualification recommendations for competitive athletes with cardiovascular abnormalities: task force 10: the cardiac channelopathies: a scientific statement from the American Heart Association and American College of Cardiology. Circulation 2015;132(22):e326–9.
72. Antzelevitch C, Yan GX, Ackerman MJ, et al. J-Wave syndromes expert consensus conference report: emerging concepts and gaps in knowledge. J Arrhythm 2016;32(5):315–39.
73. Towbin JA, McKenna WJ, Abrams DJ, et al. 2019 HRS expert consensus statement on evaluation, risk stratification, and management of arrhythmogenic cardiomyopathy. Heart Rhythm 2019;16(11):e301–72.
74. Ammirati E, Contri R, Coppini R, et al. Pharmacological treatment of hypertrophic cardiomyopathy: current practice and novel perspectives. Eur J Heart Fail 2016; 18(9):1106–18.
75. Papadakis M, Papatheodorou E, Mellor G, et al. The diagnostic yield of Brugada syndrome after sudden death with normal autopsy. J Am Coll Cardiol 2018;71: 1204–14.
76. Krahn AD, Healey JS, Chauhan V, et al. Systematic assessment of patients with unexplained cardiac arrest: Cardiac Arrest Survivors with Preserved Ejection Fraction Registry (CASPER). Circulation 2009;120:278–85.
77. White JA, Fine NM, Gula L, et al. Utility of cardiovascular magnetic resonance in identifying substrate for malignant ventricular arrhythmias. Circ Cardiovasc Imaging 2012;5:12–20.
78. Rodrigues P, Joshi A, Williams H, et al. Diagnosis and prognosis in sudden cardiac arrest survivors without coronary artery disease: utility of a clinical approach using cardiac magnetic resonance imaging. Circ Cardiovasc Imaging 2017;10: e006709.

79. Govindan M, Batchvarov VN, Raju H, et al. Utility of high and standard right pre-cordial leads during ajmaline testing for the diagnosis of Brugada syndrome. Heart 2010;96:1904–8.
80. Perrin MJ, Angaran P, Laksman Z, et al. Exercise testing in asymptomatic gene carriers exposes a latent electrical substrate of arrhythmogenic right ventricular cardiomyopathy. J Am Coll Cardiol 2013;62:1772–9.
81. James CA, Bhonsale A, Tichnell C, et al. Exercise increases age-related pene-trance and arrhythmic risk in arrhythmogenic right ventricular dysplasia/cardiomyopathy-associated desmosomal mutation carriers. J Am Coll Cardiol 2013;62:1290–7.
82. van Rijsingen IA, van der Zwaag PA, Groeneweg JA, et al. Outcome in phospho-lamban R14del carriers: results of a large multicentre cohort study. Circ Cardio-vasc Genet 2014;7:455–65.
83. van Rijsingen IA, Arbustini E, Elliott PM, et al. Risk factors for malignant ventric-ular arrhythmias in Lamin A/C mutation carriers: a European cohort study. J Am Coll Cardiol 2012;59:493–500.
84. De Ferrari GM, Dusi V, Spazzolini C, et al. Clinical management of catecholamin-ergic polymorphic ventricular tachycardia: the role of left cardiac sympathetic denervation. Circulation 2015;131:2185–93.
85. Gray B, Ackerman MJ, Semsarian C, et al. Evaluation after sudden death in the young: a global approach. Circ Arrhythm Electrophysiol 2019;12(8):e007453.

Adult Heart Disease

Assessment of Cardiovascular Disease Risk: A 2022 Update

Earl Goldsborough III, BS[a], Ngozi Osuji, MD, MPH[a,b],
Michael J. Blaha, MD, MPH[b],*

KEYWORDS

- Risk assessment • Primary prevention • Atherosclerosis • Cardiovascular disease
- Cardiovascular risk • Family history • Coronary artery calcium • Lipoprotein(a)

KEY POINTS

- ASCVD risk assessment is critical for personalizing preventive therapy, targeting the most aggressive interventions to those most likely to benefit, while allowing conservative therapy approaches for those who are low risk.
- The first step in ASCVD risk assessment is the use of a traditional 10-year risk calculator, for example, the Pooled Cohort Equations or the SCORE2 algorithm.
- Next, risk-enhancing factors (otherwise unaccounted for factors that raise risk estimates) should be considered, such as family history.
- Subclinical atherosclerosis testing, notably using coronary artery calcium (CAC), can further personalize risk particularly in borderline to intermediate-risk individuals.
- Lipoprotein(a) is perhaps the most promising serum biomarker and should be considered for one-time measurement in most patients with risk attributable to family history or dyslipidemia.
- 2020 guidelines from the Endocrine Society focus on traditional 10-year risk assessment, risk-enhancing factors, CAC, and lipoprotein(a) testing in clinical practice. Most other tests, including advanced lipid testing and stress testing, are considered much less helpful for routine clinical practice.

INTRODUCTION

Cardiovascular diseases (CVDs) are the leading cause of death worldwide, with atherosclerotic cardiovascular disease (ASCVD) being the dominant cause of total CVD mortality.[1–3] From 1993 to 2019, the global prevalence of CVD nearly doubled[4] and is projected to continue increasing through 2024.[5] In the United States (US), ASCVD is the predominant cause of morbidity and health care expenditure.[6] As

This article originally appeared in *Endocrinology and Metabolism Clinics*, Volume 51, Issue 3, September 2022.
[a] Johns Hopkins University School of Medicine, 600 North Wolfe Street, Baltimore, MD 21287, USA; [b] Division of Cardiology, Department of Medicine, Ciccarone Center for the Prevention of Cardiovascular Disease, Johns Hopkins University School of Medicine, Baltimore, MD, USA
* Corresponding author. Blalock 524D1 JHH, 600 N Wolfe Street, Baltimore, MD 21287.
E-mail address: mblaha1@jhmi.edu

such, clinical ASCVD risk assessment is instrumental in constructing a holistic view of patient health. However, this assessment is particularly imperative for patients with a diagnosis of, or under suspicion for, dyslipidemia as these patients portend an increased risk of developing ASCVD.[7–11]

Primary prevention is directed at either the level of the population or the individual,[12] depending on the degree of predisposing risk. Preventive strategies directed at the population emphasize lifestyle modifications (eg, diet improvement, regular exercise, and avoidance of tobacco and secondhand smoke exposure) and are generally indicated for individuals regardless of predisposing risk.[13] Through general recommendations and/or public policy approaches, population-centered approaches focused on mitigating the effect of modifiable risk factors can eschew some risk and derive a net cardiovascular benefit for the general population. However, this generalizability can come at the expense of selectively identifying high-risk groups with prodigious vascular aging who may gain larger benefits and exclusion of very low-risk patients for whom strict adherence to such recommendations would derive little to no net benefit.

Statins are an example of a therapy that may straddle the boundaries between population and individual-level prevention. For example, a meta-analysis on statin efficacy yielded data suggesting that statin use poses minimal risks while significantly reducing ASCVD risk,[14] leading some to propose statin use for almost everyone over the age of 50.[15] While expansion in statin use may be a step forward, it is incomplete. There are individuals in their 40s with predisposing factors for whom statin therapy would be of greater benefit, and there are individuals more than 50 for whom the risk-benefit ratio of initiating statin therapy would not substantiate lifelong preventive therapy. Thus, while general population-level preventive guidelines are an important first step, in routine clinical practice there is a need for guidance at the level of the individual.

Formal ASCVD risk assessments aid in identifying individuals at increased risk of developing ASCVD, stratifying risk into clinically actionable categories, and concomitantly guiding the clinical decision-making process.[16–18] The primary objectives of this review are to:

1. Describe the commonly used ASCVD risk calculators and elucidate ASCVD risk score interpretation.
2. Highlight the role of risk-enhancing factors and family history in interpreting patient risk.
3. Discuss the role of inflammatory markers, coronary artery calcium (CAC) scoring, and lipoprotein A (Lp(a)) in risk assessment.
4. Provide additional context to the most recent Endocrine Society guidelines on Lipid Management in Patients with Endocrine Disorders.

ATHEROSCLEROTIC CARDIOVASCULAR DISEASE RISK ASSESSMENT

Clinical risk assessment can be facilitated via many modalities, with traditional risk calculators, imaging, hybrid risk calculators, serum biomarkers, polygenic risk scores (PRS), and stress testing predominating. However, the gold standard for initial clinical risk assessment remains the traditional risk calculators—notably, the Pooled Cohort Equations (PCE) in the U.S.[13] and the Systemic COronary Risk Evaluation (SCORE) in Europe.[19]

TRADITIONAL ATHEROSCLEROTIC CARDIOVASCULAR DISEASE RISK CALCULATORS

Traditional risk calculators are the recommended first steps for facilitating a clinical risk assessment for individuals with no known ASCVD (ie, no known acute coronary syndrome (ACS), myocardial infarction (MI), stable angina, unstable angina, coronary revascularization, arterial revascularization, stroke, transient ischemic attack (TIA), or peripheral artery disease (PAD) of atherosclerotic etiology).[19,20] Risk calculators are mathematical equations that stratify individuals by prognosticated likelihood of experiencing an atherosclerotic event in future years (eg, 10-year or lifetime estimation). These risk assessments are generally most validated and beneficial in the risk stratification of middle-aged adults.

ASCVD risk calculators are derived from data pooled from multiple cohort studies in the population or populations for which they are indicated. The score derived from the calculator relates to an estimated likelihood of an atherosclerotic event over a defined time period and is concomitant with delegation into an absolute risk category. From this risk stratification, the most appropriate preventive strategy can be identified. These preventive strategies range from risk discussion to lifestyle modifications concurrent with pharmacotherapy.[13]

Pooled Cohort Equations

Since its introduction in 2013, the American College of Cardiology and American Heart Association (ACC/AHA) have endorsed the PCE for primary clinical risk assessment.[13] The PCE is a race- and sex-specific traditional risk calculator, developed and validated by the Working Group of the ACC/AHA, and it is derived from the data of 5 large US cohort studies.[21] It is used in primary risk assessment for non-Hispanic African American and White adults aged 40 to 79 years and in some non-Hispanic African American and White adults as young as 20 years (**Fig. 1**).[20] The PCE should only be used for individuals with no known ASCVD.

It estimates the 10-year risk of developing a first hard ASCVD event (eg, nonfatal MI, stroke death, coronary heart disease (CHD) death) for non-Hispanic African American and White adults aged 40 to 79 years.[21] Additionally, it can estimate the lifetime risk of developing a first hard ASCVD event in non-Hispanic African American and White adults aged 20 to 59 years.[21] For other racial/ethnic groups, it is recommended that the equation for non-Hispanic White adults be used to assess risk and that results be cautiously interpreted.[21]

The risk factors operationalized include chronologic age, sex, total cholesterol (TC), high-density lipoprotein cholesterol (HDL-C), systolic blood pressure (SBP), blood pressure treatment, diabetes mellitus (DM), and current smoking status.[21] Scores are delegated into one of the 4 absolute risk categories: low (<5%), borderline (5%–7.4%), intermediate (7.5%–19.9%), and high (≥20%).[13]

Systemic Coronary Risk Evaluation (Score)

The SCORE has been endorsed by the European Society of Cardiology (ESC) for primary clinical risk assessment in European adults[22] aged 45 to 64 years and is further endorsed by the European Atherosclerosis Society (EAS).[19] SCORE was developed through pooled data from 12 diverse European cohort studies[23] and functions as a country- and sex-specific calculator which estimates the 10-year risk of an incident fatal atherosclerotic event[23] in European adults aged 45 to 64 years.[23] Additionally, it can be used to assess total cardiovascular risk[19] (ie, 10-year risk of both fatal and nonfatal ASCVD events) by multiplying the 10-year cardiovascular mortality SCORE risk by 3.[23]

The risk factors operationalized include age, sex, TC, HDL-C, SBP, smoking status, and nationality. The SCORE differentially uses either a high- or low-risk chart (**Figs. 2 and 3**),[24] dependent on the patient's nationality.[23] SCORE risk is delegated into one of the 4 absolute risk categories: low (<1%), moderate (1 to <5%), high (5 to <10%), and

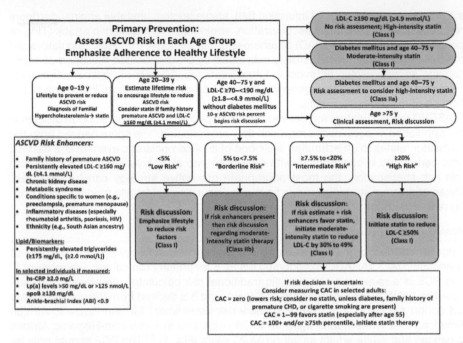

Fig. 1. Primary prevention algorithm in the AHA/ACC Guideline on the Management of Blood Cholesterol. (*From* Grundy SM, Stone NJ, Bailey AL, Beam C, Birtcher KK, Blumenthal RS, Braun LT, de Ferranti S, Faiella-Tommasino J, Forman DE, Goldberg R, Heidenreich PA, Hlatky MA, Jones DW, Lloyd-Jones D, Lopez-Pajares N, Ndumele CE, Orringer CE, Peralta CA, Saseen JJ, Smith SC Jr, Sperling L, Virani SS, Yeboah J. 2018 AHA/ACC/AACVPR/AAPA/ABC/ACPM/ADA/AGS/APhA/ASPC/NLA/PCNA Guideline on the Management of Blood Cholesterol: Executive Summary: A Report of the American College of Cardiology/American Heart Association Task Force on Clinical Practice Guidelines. J Am Coll Cardiol. 2019 Jun 25;73(24):3168-3209.)

very high ($\geq$10%).[23] An additional, unofficial very high-risk group exists for several countries. For these countries, results must be cautiously interpreted, as both low- and high-risk charts are likely to underestimate actual risk.[25]

The 2019 ESC/EAS Guideline on the management of dyslipidemia[19] was published before the development and validation of SCORE2,[26] a revision of the original SCORE.[23] Unlike SCORE, SCORE2 is derived from data of 13 diverse European cohort studies, has more inclusive study endpoints (eg, 10-year incident fatal and nonfatal CVD event), and has an extended age range of 40 to 69 years.[26] Since August 2021, the ESC has recommended the use of SCORE2 for primary risk assessment in the 40 to 69-year groups.[27] **Fig. 1** shows a sample SCORE2 chart.[26]

Other Traditional Atherosclerotic Cardiovascular Disease Risk Calculators

There are numerous traditional risk calculators which have been validated and are used in distinct populations. Notably, the Reynolds CVD Risk Scores for Women[28] and Men[29] can be used in the clinical risk assessment of 10-year incident cardiovascular event (eg, MI, ischemic stroke, coronary revascularization, cardiovascular mortality) for American women and men, more than 45 and 50 years, respectively.[28,29] Both risk scores incorporate lipid profiling and inflammatory markers in their

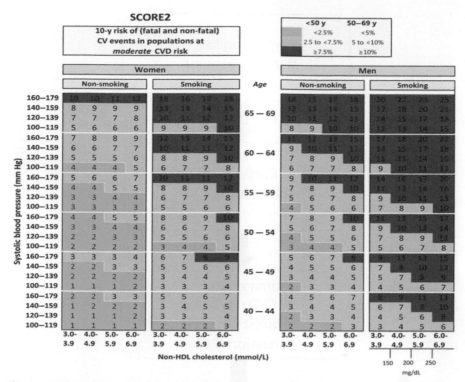

Fig. 2. SCORE2 ASCVD risk calculator for populations with moderate CVD risk. (*Adapted from* SCORE2 working group and ESC Cardiovascular risk collaboration. SCORE2 risk prediction algorithms: new models to estimate 10-year risk of cardiovascular disease in Europe. *Eur Heart J.* 2021;42(25):2439-2454.)

assessment of risk, with the Risk Score for Women having more extensive incorporation of lipid profiling.[28,29] Additionally, multiple QRISK calculators exist for estimating 10-year incident CVD event likelihood (eg, MI, CHD, stroke, TIA) in specific countries such as the United Kingdom.[30–32] The most recent QRISK, the QRISK3, is indicated for British adults as young as 25 years and additionally incorporates atrial fibrillation, chronic kidney disease, and erectile dysfunction in the clinical assessment of ASCVD risk.[32] **Table 1** shows a summary of ASCVD risk calculators.

Specific Populations

A limitation of the PCE and SCORE is their unvalidated utility for clinical risk assessment in adults under the age of 40. To account for this, the ACC recommends measuring traditional risk factors every 4 to 6 years, beginning at age 20 (but without formal global risk assessment)[13]; meanwhile, the ESC/EAS recommends risk factor screening and lipid profiling for men beginning at age 40 and for women beginning at either age 50 or after menopause.[19] This still leaves European adults under the age of 45 without a clinical risk assessment when using SCORE[23] and European adults under the age of 40 bereft of a clinical risk assessment using SCORE2.[26]

Additionally, the ESC/EAS endorse the risk assessment tool, SCORE2-Older Persons (SCORE2-OP) for patients more than 70 years[33] and the ADVANCE and DIAL risk scores and models for patients living with diabetes.[19]

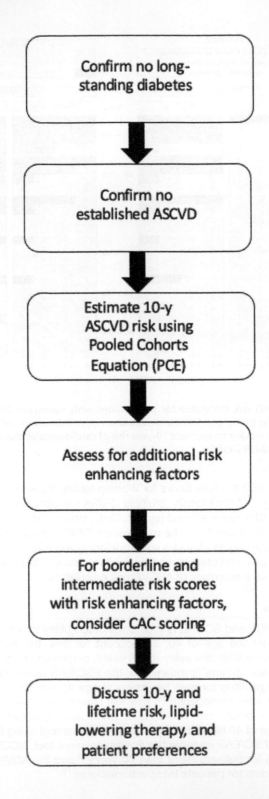

RISK-ENHANCING FACTORS
Underrepresented Risk-Enhancing Factors

Several risk-enhancing factors (newer risk factors that may elevate risk in particular clinical situations) are not traditionally represented in risk calculators. Some of these include infrequent exercise,[13] unhealthy diet,[13] dyslipidemia,[19] elevated TC in the elderly (ie, >70–75 y),[19,34] family history of premature ASCVD, metabolic syndrome, aspects of the lipid and inflammatory biomarker profiles, and chronic inflammatory conditions (**Table 2**).[20]

Risk Assessment in Specific Populations

Diabetes mellitus

Adults with DM are considered a higher-risk population for developing ASCVD but are no longer considered a "ASCVD risk equivalent."[20] Consequently, for adults aged 40 to 75 years with a diagnosis of DM, while the initiation of statin therapy is indicated before a clinical ASCVD assessment, further risk assessment is required for other decision-making.[20] For example, the intensity of statin and other nonstatin lipid-lowering therapy should match the accumulation of risk factors. Notably, there are DM-specific, independent risk factors that must also be considered in the clinical risk assessment for this population. These include the duration of DM ($\geq$10 y for type 2 DM; $\geq$20 y for type 1 DM), albuminuria ($\geq$30 mcg/mg creatinine); eGFR less than 60 mL/min/1.73 m²,[2] retinopathy, neuropathy, and ankle-brachial index (ABI) < 0.9.[20]

Endocrine diseases

Various non-DM endocrine diseases, such as persistent Cushing syndrome or untreated thyroid disorders, influence lipid levels, often increasing ASCVD risk. The 10-year ASCVD risk should still be calculated using a traditional risk calculator such as the PCE. However, assessing risk-enhancing factors (ie, insulin-resistance-related risk factors such as metabolic syndrome) is especially salient in adjudicating risk, and when assessing subclinical atherosclerosis, CAC is preferred. Measuring lipoprotein a (Lp(a)) may further enhance short-term and lifetime ASCVD risk prediction and inform the indication and intensity of low-density lipoprotein C (LDL-C) lowering therapy when in addition to an endocrine disorder there is a personal history of ASCVD or a family history of either ASCVD or high Lp(a).[35]

Women

Clinical risk assessment for women must assess sex-specific disparities in predisposition, exposure, and access to care. Some risk-enhancing factors are sex-specific and include a history of premature menopause (<40 y), preeclampsia,[20] previous preterm delivery,[36] hypertensive pregnancy disorders, depression, and autoimmune diseases such as systemic lupus erythematosus (SLE) and rheumatoid arthritis (RA).[37] Further, traditional risk factors such as DM, obesity, and smoking pose a greater risk of developing ASCVD in women, when compared with men of the same age.[37] Thus, clinical risk assessment in women should not be limited to assessment via traditional risk-enhancing factors but should involve a holistic assessment of individual risk.

Fig. 3. Steps in initial ASCVD risk assessment. (*Adapted from* Newman CB, Blaha MJ, Boord JB, Cariou B, Chait A, Fein HG, Ginsberg HN, Goldberg IJ, Murad MH, Subramanian S, Tannock LR. Lipid Management in Patients with Endocrine Disorders: An Endocrine Society Clinical Practice Guideline. J Clin Endocrinol Metab. 2020 Dec 1;105(12):dgaa674.)

Table 1
ASCVD traditional risk calculators

Risk Calculator	Indicated Population	Risk-Enhancing Factors Included	Endpoint(s)	Validation	Benefits	Limitations
ASSIGN[116]	Scotland, 30–74 y/o	Age, cigarettes/d, DM, family hx of CHD or stroke, HDL-C, SBP, sex, SIMD score, SS, TC	1—year CVD mortality; incident CHD; incident cerebrovascular disease; coronary artery intervention	No	Incorporates social deprivation to address disproportionate burden; cigarette use is a quantitative variable	Not validated; limited applicable population
China-PAR[117]	Chinese, 35–74 y/o	Women: DM, GR, HDL-C, SBP, SS, WC Men: + family hx ASCVD, urbanization	10-y first nonfatal MI, stroke, stroke death, or CHD death	Yes	Validated in Chinese population; equation for women (C-statistic = 0.811); equation for men (C-statistic = 0.794); predicted rates comparable to observed rates (women [P = .17]; men [P-0.16])	Only uses hard ASCVD outcomes as endpoint; does not incorporate CAC scoring; does not incorporate lipid-lowering therapy
Framingham General CVD Risk Score[118]	United States, 30–74 y/o	Age, anti-HTN tx, DM, HDL-C, SBP, SS, TC	Incident CVD (CHD, cerebrovascular disease, peripheral vascular disease, HF)	Yes	Good discrimination (0.763 for men; 0.793 for women)	Data from noncontemporary studies
JBS3[119–122]	Great Britain, >40 y/o	Age, BMI, ethnicity, HDL-C, SBP, sex, Townsend deprivation	10-y and lifetime incident CVD	Yes	Quick; most information is readily available through normal screening	No indication for younger age groups

Score	Population/Age	Variables	Outcome	Validated	Advantages	Limitations
MESA[104]	United States, 45–84 y/o	Age, anti-HTN tx, CAC, DM, family hx of MI, HDL-C, lipid-lowering tx, race/ethnicity, SBP, sex, SS, TC	10-y incident CHD	Yes	Incorporation of CAC increases accuracy (0.80 vs 0.75, $P < .0001$); multi-ethnic, highly powered cohort for the derivation of equation; can identify subclinical CVD	No indication for younger age groups
PCE[13]	United States, non-Hispanic African American, and Whites, 40–79 y/o	Age, anti-HTN tx, DM, HDL-C, race, SBP, sex, SS, TC	10-y (40–79 y/o) or lifetime (20–59 y/o) incident hard ASCVD event	Yes	Quick; reliable; online version is free	Limited age range; limited racial/ethnic representation; data from noncontemporary studies
QRISK[30]	United Kingdom, 35–74 y/o	Age, anti-HTN tx, area measure of deprivation, BMI, family hx of CHD in first-degree relative < 60 y, HDL-C, SBP, sex, SS, TC	10-y first CVD event (MI, CHD, stroke, TIA)	Yes	Incorporates deprivation in risk assessment; incorporates family hx of CHD; better discrimination than Framingham and ASSIGN	Not racial/ethnic specific
QRISK 2[31]	England and Wales, 35–74 y/o	Afib, age, anti-HTN tx, BMI, ethnicity, family hx of CHD in first-degree relative < 60 y, HDL-C, renal disease, RA, SBP, sex, SS, T2DM, Townsend deprivation	10-y incident CVD event (CHD, stroke, TIA)	Yes	Ethnic specific; incorporates more risk-enhancing factors than QRISK; better discrimination of high-risk individuals	Does not use MI as an endpoint, unlike in QRISK; validation in a population with similar demographic composition to the population used to derive the equation

(continued on next page)

Table 1
(continued)

Risk Calculator	Indicated Population	Risk-Enhancing Factors Included	Endpoint(s)	Validation	Benefits	Limitations
QRISK 3[32]	England, 25–84 y/o	Afib, age, anti-HTN tx, atypical antipsychotic tx, BMI, CKD, ethnicity, ED ± tx, family hx of CHD in first-degree relative < 60 y, HDL-C, HIV/AIDS, migraine status, RA, renal disease, SBP, SBP sd, severe mental illness, sex, SLE, SS, steroid tablets, T2DM, TC, Townsend deprivation	Incident CVD (CHD, stroke, TIA)	Yes	Good discrimination (Harrell's C statistical of 0.88 for women, 0.86 for men); additional variables better identify high-risk individuals; expanded age range	Validation in a population with similar demographic composition to the population used to derive the equation; limited applicable population; does not incorporate MI as an endpoint
Reynolds CVD Risk Score for Women[28]	United States, women, ≥45 y/o	Age, Apo A1, Apo B-100, hsCRP, parental hx of MI < 60y, SBP, SS HbA1c if DM, Lp(a) if Apo B-100 ≥ 100 mg/dL	10-y incident CV event (MI, ischemic stroke, coronary revascularization, CV mortality)	Yes	Good discrimination (C-statistic = 0.809); incorporates conditional variables for increased sensitivity	Limited ethnic- and SES-diversity of cohort population used to derive the equation; BP data was self-reported
Reynolds CVD Risk Score for Men[29]	United States, men, ≥50 y/o	Age, HDL-C, hsCRP, parental hx of MI < 60 y, SBP, SS, TC	10-y incident CV event (nonfatal MI, nonfatal stroke, coronary revascularization, CV death)	Yes	Larger C-index compared with traditional model (P < .001); improved accuracy among reclassified individuals	Limited ethnic- and SES-diversity of cohort population used to derive the equation; BP data were self-reported

SCORE[23,26,120]	Europeans, 45–64 y/o	Age, HDL-C, SBP, sex, SS, TC	10-y cardiovascular mortality	Yes	Low-risk and high-risk charts for different European countries; data pooled from 12 European cohort studies	Only uses CV mortality as endpoint; minimizes international differences by stratifying country risk categories by geography; data are from cohorts before 1986
SCORE 2[26]	Europeans, 40–69 y/o, no previous CVD or diabetes	Age, HDL-C, SBP, sex, SS, TC	10-y first fatal and nonfatal CVD event	Yes	Data pooled from cohort studies in 13 European countries; includes nonfatal endpoints; uses more recent data than SCORE; moderate-to-good discrimination in external validation (C-indices from 0.67 to 0.81)	High-risk CVD countries had smaller contribution to developing the equation; does not incorporate family hx, medication status, ethnicity, or SES

Abbreviations: Afib, atrial fibrillation; Apo, apolipoprotein; BMI, body mass index; CAC, coronary artery calcium; CHD, coronary heart disease; CKD, chronic kidney disease; ED, erectile dysfunction; GR, geographic region; HbA1c, hemoglobin A1c; HDL-C, high-density lipoprotein-cholesterol; hsCRP, high-sensitivity C-reactive protein; HTN, hypertension; hx, history; Lp(a), lipoprotein a; MI, myocardial infarction; RA, rheumatoid arthritis; SBP, systolic blood pressure; sd, standard deviation; SIMD, Scottish Index of Multiple Deprivation; SLE, systemic lupus erythematosus; SS, smoking status; T2DM, type 2 diabetes mellitus; TC, total cholesterol; TIA, transient ischemic attack; tx, therapy; WC, waist circumference

Table 2
Risk-enhancing factors for ASCVD

Family History	Patient Comorbidities	Lipid Testing and Serum Biomarkers
1. Premature ASCVD (eg, males <55 y; females <65 y) 2. High-risk race/ethnicity (eg, S. Asian)	1. Primary hypercholesterolemia 2. Metabolic syndrome 3. Chronic kidney disease 4. Chronic inflammatory conditions (eg, rheumatoid arthritis, HIV/AIDS) 5. Premature menopause 6. Pregnancy-associated conditions which increase the risk of ASCVD (eg, pre-eclampsia)	1. Primary persistent hypertriglyceridemia 2. Elevated hsCRP 3. Elevated Lp(a) 4. Elevated apoB 5. Ankle-brachial index (ABI) < 0.9

Adapted from Grundy SM, Stone NJ, Bailey AL, Beam C, Birtcher KK, Blumenthal RS, Braun LT, de Ferranti S, Faiella-Tommasino J, Forman DE, Goldberg R, Heidenreich PA, Hlatky MA, Jones DW, Lloyd-Jones D, Lopez-Pajares N, Ndumele CE, Orringer CE, Peralta CA, Saseen JJ, Smith SC jr, Sperling L, Virani SS, Yeboah J. 2018 AHA/ACC/AACVPR/AAPA/ABC/ACPM/ADA/AGS/APhA/ASPC/NLA/PCNA Guideline on the Management of Blood Cholesterol: Executive Summary: A Report of the American College of Cardiology/American Heart Association Task Force on Clinical Practice Guidelines. J Am Coll Cardiol. 2019 Jun 25;73(24):3168-3209.

Low socioeconomic status

Low socioeconomic status (SES) as well as poor neighborhood socioeconomic factors are associated with poorer cardiovascular health and increased ASCVD adverse events.[20,38,39] The mechanism mediating the increased risk associated with these 2 factors is not well known.[38] Incorporating annual household income to the PCE yielded a modest increase in discrimination (C-Index of 0.739 vs 0.743).[40]

Chronic inflammatory conditions

Chronic inflammatory conditions predispose an individual to increased risk of atherothrombogenesis[41] and ASCVD.[20] It is unclear whether this association is causal or related to shared risk factors, genetic profile, or exposures.[42] Conditions such as inflammatory bowel disease (IBD), periodontitis, RA, psoriasis, and SLE increase the risk of developing ASCVD.[43]

Human immunodeficiency virus

Human immunodeficiency virus (HIV) infection is associated with an increased risk of developing ASCVD in adults ≥19 years.[44] For individuals with a low CD4 count (<350 cells/mm^3), it is important to note that a calculated risk may underestimate actual risk.[45]

Race/ethnicity

Race can portend an increased risk of developing ASCVD. A South Asian ancestry is associated with an increased risk of developing ASCVD,[20] incident stroke rates for African Americans are almost twice that of White Americans, and there are many other relationships between race/ethnicity and ASCVD.[46] However, race/ethnicity alone may not account for these differences. Rather, these effects may be further mediated by habitus and lifestyle (eg, exercise). Thus, race/ethnicity-specific guidance should additionally address the habitus and lifestyle of the individual.

Young (<40) and elderly (>75)

Young adults aged less than 40 years are underrepresented in major risk calculators and often considered to be at nonsignificant levels of risk. However, prevalent coronary atherosclerosis as measured using the CAC scoring is considerable in high-risk young adults, with a graded increased odds with increasing risk factor burden.[47] Prevalent CAC is estimated as high as 34.4% in young adults aged 30 to 49 years who are classified as low-risk by a 10-year ASCVD assessment.[48] Imaging seems to be the gold standard for detecting premature coronary atherosclerosis in those younger than the indicated age for traditional calculators. A recent CAC Percentile Calculator for adults aged 30 to 45 years calculates the estimated probability of a CAC greater than 0 for a given age, sex, and race as well as a CAC percentile ranking with the additional input of an observed CAC score.[49]

For those greater than 75 years, the ACC/AHA only recommends the discussion of preventive therapies appropriate to comorbidities and life expectancy.[13] Moving forward, concise guidelines for initiating or continuing preventive therapy in the elderly are needed.

Family History

Assessment of a family history can improve risk estimation and assist in adjudicating preventive therapy in patients for whom risk stratification is uncertain.[13,50] A family history assessment can be a brief yet invaluable tool. Data suggest only asking about a history of (CHD) in first-degree relatives was as predictive of ASCVD risk as more intensive assessments. Any family history of CHD in a first-degree relative has been associated with an increased relative risk of incident ASCVD[50,51] and CVD mortality.[52] Additionally, it has been shown to be an independent risk factor for ASCVD and to have additive associations with elevated plasma Lp(a).[53] Alone, a family history significant for CHD can indicate benefit from advanced risk assessment. However, it does not substantiate the benefit of high-intensity statin therapy or prophylactic aspirin therapy.[54] Nearly half of the patients in the MESA cohort with a family history significant for CHD had a CAC = 0. However, for those with a significant family history and a nonzero CAC, CAC was a good estimate of ASCVD risk.[54] A family history of CAD was shown to be associated with markers of subclinical atherosclerosis.[55] The ACC/AHA acknowledges a family history of premature ASCVD (eg, male, <55 y; female, <65 y) as a risk-enhancing factor and recommends using such information to revise the 10-year risk estimation.[13] Thus, the assessment of family history can increase the likely benefit from CAC scoring[54] and enhance risk estimation[13] but, alone, should not dictate the intensity of preventive therapy.[13]

Summary of Traditional Risk Atherosclerotic Cardiovascular Disease Assessment

Traditional ASCVD risk calculators are invaluable tools in primary risk assessment. They function to identify and stratify risk, especially in middle-aged adults. Most calculators are readily available online, brief, and of no cost. A universal limitation of these traditional risk calculators is that they are only intended for clinical risk assessment in the population for which they are indicated. As with the PCE, estimated risk from use outside of non-Hispanic African American and White populations should be cautiously interpreted,[21] epitomizing this limitation. Modified versions of the PCE have been developed to address this. In 2020, a Modified PCE were developed and validated for use in American Indian populations.[56] Nonetheless, the original PCE still carry dubious applicability outside strict racial/ethnic categories. Further, the 10-year PCE risk estimation has been shown to be overestimated by approximately 20% across all risk groups.[57] Moreover, the PCE is liable to underestimate risk in select younger populations, on the predication that the accumulation of risk at an early age (eg, <40 y) is not substantial enough to warrant pharmacologic therapy.[58,59] This presumption is often at the expense of those at increased risk for the rapid accumulation of risk factor exposure. Such high-risk groups include those who have a genetic disposition (eg, familial hypercholesterolemia, phytosterolemia, and lipodystrophy), social strain (eg, SES[40,60]), or predisposing medical conditions (eg, HIV,[61] chronic inflammatory disease[62]).

Overall, these calculators are crucial in primary risk assessment, but they should be used as the first step in risk assessment, identifying those who may benefit from advanced risk stratification. **Fig. 2** provides step by step approach to ASCVD risk assessment.[35]

ATHEROSCLEROSIS IMAGING
Coronary Artery Calcium Scoring

Coronary artery calcium (CAC) scoring was first introduced in 1990 as a means of measuring subclinical coronary atherosclerosis burden and, therefore, assessing ASCVD risk[63] through noncontrast computed tomography (CT). As then, multiple studies have substantiated CAC scoring as an effective assessment of ASCVD risk. The Multi-Ethnic Study of Atherosclerosis (MESA) data suggest CAC can effectively stratify CHD risk.[64] In response to the ESC and the American Stroke Association's (ASA) push for the inclusion of stroke in the holistic risk assessment of CVD,[65,66] another study validated CAC as an effective predictor of CVD, rather than solely CHD.[67] Currently, the Endocrine Society strongly endorses CAC in assessing subclinical atherosclerosis.[35]

CAC scoring has been shown to effectively stratify CVD risk in asymptomatic middle-aged-to-elderly men and women with dyslipidemia[68] and to reclassify risk even in patients with LDL-C ≥190 mg/dL.[69] It is more predictive of CVD risk than traditional and novel estimators.[70,71] A CAC ≥1000 has been shown to be a unique identifier of increased ASCVD risk and benefit from highly aggressive preventive therapy.[72] While the CAC score predicts absolute cardiovascular risk, the CAC score percentile tracks the lifetime risk trajectory.[73] CAC score percentiles are calculated using the MESA CAC Reference Tool and estimate age-, sex-, and race/ethnicity-specific lifetime risk of ASCVD for individuals greater than 45 years.[73]

The ACC/AHA indicate the use of CAC in adjudicating the utility of initiating statin therapy in patients for whom the initial risk assessment, and benefit from statin therapy, derived from the PCE is uncertain (see **Fig. 1**.)[20] In individuals with baseline CAC = 0 whereby an initial conservative approach to prevention is chosen, evidence suggests repeating a CAC scan after 5 to 7 years in low-risk patients, 3 to 5 years in borderline-to-intermediate-risk patients, and in 3 years for high-risk patients or those with diabetes.[74] **Table 3** provides a guide for optimizing absolute CAC scoring versus CAC percentile scoring.[75]

CAC scoring is recommended to aid decision making regarding statin or aspirin initiation in borderline- or intermediate-risk patients for whom the indication to recommend therapy is unclear.[75] The CAC "Agatston" score can either buttress (eg, high CAC score) or weaken (eg, CAC = 0) the indication for initiating statin therapy.[13]

CAC imaging seems to be the most promising means of assessing risk and statin benefit due to its overall increased ability to personalize risk, especially in middle-aged and intermediate-risk populations.[76]

Other Atherosclerosis Imaging Techniques

Carotid ultrasound imaging allows the measurement of the amount of carotid plaque and carotid intima-media thickness (CIMT) to estimate risk.[12] An 8-study meta-

Table 3
Utility of CAC score and CAC percentile in ASCVD risk assessment

CAC Assessment	Population(s) with Unique Perceived Benefit	Unique Benefit
CAC Score	Middle-aged and intermediate-risk patients	Enhanced risk stratification and prognostication of benefit from statin therapy
CAC Percentile	Youth (eg, <40 y)	Prognostication of risk with subclinical risk factor accumulation

Data from Hecht H, Blaha MJ, Berman DS, Nasir K, Budoff M, Leipsic J, Blankstein R, Narula J, Rumberger J, Shaw LJ. Clinical indications for coronary artery calcium scoring in asymptomatic patients: Expert consensus statement from the Society of Cardiovascular Computed Tomography. J Cardiovasc Comput Tomogr. 2017 Mar-Apr;11(2):157-168.

analysis demonstrated a 10% to 15% increased risk of MI with every 0.1-mm increase in CIMT[77] and a 2021 study demonstrated the relationship between the amount of carotid plaque and increased risk of chronic CHD and incident CAC.[78] Cardiac computed tomographic angiography (CCTA) can be used to assess risk through identifying and estimating the extent of coronary atherosclerosis, specifically including noncalcified plaque, as well as the degree of coronary stenosis in asymptomatic patients.[12,79] Despite the availability of other atherosclerosis imaging techniques, currently, only CAC scoring is endorsed by the ACC/AHA for clinical risk assessment by imaging due to its excellent performance, low cost, wide availability, and low intrascan variability.[13]

Functional Tests that Imply Atherosclerosis – Stress Testing

Noninvasive cardiac stress testing can be used to enhance risk stratification in intermediate-risk patients. Additionally, when paired with imaging, stress testing can be diagnostic of CAD.[80,81] However, the American Society of Echocardiography indicates its use only for symptomatic patients.[82] Stress testing in asymptomatic individuals reduces its sensitivity and specificity to 45% to 60%.[83]

Plaque burden has been shown to be the main predictor of cardiovascular events and death.[84] This explains the paradigm shift away from the assessment of stenosis severity and ischemia toward the ascertainment of plaque burden by direct subclinical atherosclerosis imaging modalities for risk assessment. Therefore, the role of stress testing in primary prevention is extremely limited.

Summary of Atherosclerosis Imaging for Risk Prediction

Imaging is increasingly favored in clinical risk assessment due to its aptitude in highly personalizing risk assessment. Unlike traditional risk calculators, imaging estimates the accumulated ASCVD risk from both known and unknown risk factors and risk-enhancing factors. By addressing both known and unknown risk factors, imaging offers a more personalized assessment of risk.

However, imaging is much less accessible than traditional risk calculators. Not all health plans cover the cost of CAC scoring,[85] as these are often considered screening examinations.[86] Consequently, the out-of-pocket cost can range from $100 to $400 in the US.[85] Additionally, there is risk from imaging. On average, patients are exposed to 1 to 2 mSv of ionizing radiation during CAC scoring[87] and 5 mSv during CT angiography.[88] This is comparable to the ionizing radiation exposure of a mammogram (<0.3 mSv)[88] and less than the annual background radiation exposure in the US

(3.1 mSv).[89] Additionally, there is a risk of a hypersensitivity reaction when using contrast, as in CCTA, presenting CCTA as a less favorable imaging modality for primary prevention.[90] Therefore, imaging has not superseded traditional risk calculators, and remains the preferred "second step" in risk assessment. Stress testing has little to no role for risk assessment in primary prevention.

ADVANCED LIPID TESTING
Overview

Lipid profiling can optimize the adjudication of risk by contributing additional input data as well as assessing atherogenic potential, especially in high-risk asymptomatic individuals. Advanced lipid testing may include the direct measurement of low-density lipoprotein particle number (LDL-P), low-density lipoprotein particle size, apolipoprotein B (apoB), and Lp(a).[91] While such advanced testing is helpful for the diagnosis of genetic dyslipidemias, current guidelines suggest that most tests offer minimal additional benefit for the primary assessment of risk beyond the standard lipid profile.[92] Lp(a) testing is the only advanced lipid test that should be considered for routine use in primary prevention.

Apolipoprotein B

Apolipoprotein B (apoB), a major protein in all atherogenic lipoproteins (eg, chylomicron remnants, VLDL, IDL, LDL, Lp(a))[93] and the major component of LDL and VLDL, is a strong portent of atherogenicity.[20] A meta-analysis using data from 12 studies, demonstrated that apoB was the most potent lipid marker of cardiovascular risk.[94] Measuring apoB levels may be particularly salient in assessing risk in patients with hypertriglyceridemia.[95] It is suggested that apoB be measured if triglycerides ≥200 mg/dL, with apoB ≥130 mg/dL being a risk-enhancing factor favoring statin therapy.[13,96]

Lipoprotein(a) (Lp(a))

Lp(a) is a largely genetically determined independent risk factor for premature CHD, and an elevated Lp(a) is tantamount to the attributable risk of TC ≥240 mg/dL or HDL-C ≤35 mg/dL.[24,25,96] Lp(a) ≥50 mg/dL is considered a risk-enhancing factor with risk ascending with Lp(a) concentration.[13] Lp(a) has shown risk-enhancing attributes, especially in women with hypercholesterolemia[97] and those of intermediate- or high-CVD/CHD risk.[98] The ACC/AHA recommend measuring Lp(a) when family history is significant for premature ASCVD.[13] Here, it can be used to enhance 10-year risk estimation. Serum Lp(a) is a good predictor of incident ASCVD for middle-aged adults, with a similar associated risk across racial subgroups[99] and is shown to have additive effects with elevated CAC (ie, <100) on the development of incident ASCVD.[100] Elevated Lp(a) in asymptomatic individuals with a family history of premature ASCVD has been associated with increased CAC score[101] and may increase the benefit of CAC scoring in this population. As Lp(a) testing is helpful for the assessment of familial risk, and levels do not change much over one's lifetime, it does not need to be repeated if previously measured in childhood or early adulthood.

Inflammatory Biomarkers – High-Sensitivity C-Reactive Protein

Plasma high-sensitivity C-reactive protein (hsCRP) ≥2 mg/dL is a risk-enhancing factor. hsCRP is particularly salient for those at intermediate risk.[13] However, recent data suggest that hsCRP predicts increased ASCVD risk for all PCE risk categories and is independent of atherogenic lipid levels.[102] hsCRP ≥2 mg/dL is also a consistent portent of residual inflammatory risk.[103] Following lipid-lowering therapy, hsCRP can further direct pharmacotherapeutic intervention aimed at lowering residual inflammatory risk.[103]

Summary

Lp(a) exhibits the most promise as a routinely used marker and is particularly relevant for middle-aged adults.[99] While promising in adjudicating risk, other forms of advanced lipid testing should be reserved for specific situations and should not be used for routine risk assessment. ApoB may be helpful in enhancing risk estimation in patients with dyslipidemia.[95] hsCRP has declined in popularity and is a relatively weak and nonspecific marker when compared with imaging—especially, CAC scoring.[104] Thus, hsCRP should be used occasionally—particularly, for further risk stratification in patients with metabolic risks, such as in metabolic syndrome.

ENDOCRINE SOCIETY'S 2020 LIPID MANAGEMENT GUIDELINE

The Endocrine Society's 2020 Guideline on Lipid Management in Patients with Endocrine Disorders recommends a 10-year risk estimation via the PCE. CAC is indicated for adjudicating statin therapy for borderline and intermediate-risk individuals with additional risk-enhancing factors and for whom the decision to initiate statin therapy as determined by the PCE score, is uncertain. If baseline CAC = 0, scoring should be repeated every 5 to 7 years (low-risk); 3 to 5 years (borderline-to-intermediate risk); or 3 years (high-risk or with concurrent DM) for patients. CAC scoring is considered the gold standard for assessing subclinical atherosclerosis. Statin therapy is not indicated for all individuals and is determined by a personalized assessment of risk factor burden. For adults with a personal history of ASCVD or family history of either ASCVD or elevated Lp(a), it is recommended that Lp(a) is measured to enhance short- and long-term risk discrimination and clarify the need to increase the pharmacologic intensity of LDL-C lowering. Lp(a) ≥50 mg/dL is associated with increased ASCVD risk. Further, the Endocrine Society does not endorse the routine measurement of advanced lipids, including apoB and hsCRP, for risk assessment. Lp(a) testing does not need to be repeated if it was previously measured in childhood or early adulthood.[67]

FUTURE DIRECTIONS
Calculators: Recalibrations and the Future of Hybrid Risk Calculators

Clinical risk assessment must reflect the most contemporaneous data. The PCE and SCORE should be updated, recalibrated, and validated with contemporary data of cohort studies with expanded representation of race/ethnicity, age, and specific (eg, low SES and comorbid chronic inflammatory) conditions. Future versions of already existing ASCVD risk calculators should also be updated with a hybrid risk calculation option incorporating CAC scoring. A recent CAC percentile calculator exhibits an expanded age range.[49] These innovations must continue, and clinical guidelines must be concomitant. More recently, a calculator which estimates the optimal age for incident CAC testing in young adults was derived.[105] Subsequent guidelines should incorporate this calculator into guideline recommendations.

Hybrid risk calculators are calculators which conflate the risk factors operationalized in traditional risk calculators and imaging, such as CAC scoring. The MESA CHD Risk Score is similar to the PCE[21] but includes additional risk factors (eg, CAC score, family history of MI, and whether the patient is currently taking a lipid-lowering medication)[106] in its 10-year assessment of CVD risk. Inclusion of CAC in MESA CHD risk scoring yielded a greater C-statistic (0.80 vs 0.75, $P < .0001$) and discrimination between events and nonevents.[106] As the risk score was derived from data obtained from the MESA Study,[63] the risk score addresses the impact of ethnicity in assessing risk; however, the MESA Study only included ages 45 to 84 years, thus, limiting the generalizability of the MESA CHD Risk Score to individuals within this range.[106] When compared with the Framingham Risk Study (FRS), MESA show a greater ability to predict the severity of CAD in the population and had a better performance in specific subgroups (diabetes, nondiabetes, smoking, male).[107]

Going forward, there needs to be a clarified indication for the routine use of the MESA CHD Risk Score (and the forthcoming MESA CVD Risk Score) in primary risk assessment. Additionally, the development of additional hybrid risk calculators should be encouraged, especially those which operationalize traditionally underrepresented risk factors in their risk estimate.

New and Innovative Uses of Coronary Artery Calcium

Imaging presents as the most efficacious subclinical atherosclerotic assessment and has exciting potential in early risk assessment and monitoring, especially in dyslipidemia. However, it lacks concise indication beyond that of an adjunctive role, despite its enhanced discrimination over traditional risk calculators (eg, Framingham risk score and Reynolds risk score).[108] Potential uses for CAC scoring have been conceptualized but are yet to be incorporated into guidelines (**Fig. 4**).[73]

Risk assessment in conditions like familial hypercholesterolemia could improve from this degree of personalization. It could enhance a benefit-versus-risk analysis of nonstatin pharmacologic interventions (eg, ezetimibe and PCSK9 inhibitors).[20] Additionally, it could be used to indicate benefit for statin initiation and augmentation in younger age groups. Future research will further elucidate the utility of broadened

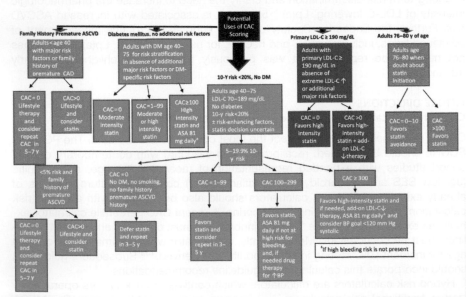

Fig. 4. Potential CAC scoring uses in the NLA Statement on CAC Scoring to Guide ASCVD Prevention. (*Adapted from* Orringer CE, Blaha MJ, Blankstein R, Budoff MJ, Goldberg RB, Gill EA, Maki KC, Mehta L, Jacobson TA. The National Lipid Association scientific statement on coronary artery calcium scoring to guide preventive strategies for ASCVD risk reduction. J Clin Lipidol. 2021 Jan-Feb;15(1):33-60.)

indications for CAC and provide the data necessary to construct risk calculators for specific high- or special-risk populations that could guide advanced preventive therapy choices.

Future of Cardiac Computed Tomographic Angiography

Further, a transition from CAC to CCTA for the assessment of subclinical atherosclerosis may be forthcoming. CCTA visualizes both calcified and noncalcified plaque through the use of intravenous (IV) contrast[79,109,110] and has shown increased prognostic value for major adverse coronary events (MACEs) than CAC in asymptomatic older (>62 y) individuals.[111] However, specific situations where CCTA may be favored over CAC testing are not yet delineated. New technologic advances continue to reduce the radiation dose associated with CCTA, and with emerging technologies such as dual-energy CCTA, IV contrast may one day be optional.

Future of Polygenic Risk Scoring

Additionally, there needs to be a focus on improving risk assessment in young people. Previously, there has been a large emphasis on age in the construction of traditional risk calculators.[112] While age is associated with the accumulation of risk factors,[113] the concept of heart and vascular age may be more appropriate in guiding treatment than chronologic age.[112] Personalized medicine should be emphasized. While CAC scoring can offer this, PRS may be a further progression toward personalized medicine.

PRS have recently emerged as an option for assessing the risk of developing complex traits,[112] including CVDs.[114,115] PRS approximates an individual's susceptibility to developing a complex trait, based on their genotype.[116] Estimates are derived from established associations of genotypic profiles with these traits, as made apparent through the data from genome-wide association studies (GWAS).[116] PRS has a suggested utility in cohorts with predetermined increased risk, especially, early in prognosis to assist in guiding preventive efforts or treatment.[117] However, the National Lipid Association (NLA) does not currently suggest the use of genetic testing in assessing CVD risk, citing a lack of concise clinical indication and formal guidelines, and stating that the use of PRS will only drastically affect the prognosis or treatment of dyslipidemia in select individuals with severe dyslipidemia.[82] The PRS presents itself as a potential CVD risk assessment that offers the unique ability of concise personalization from as early as birth.

CLINICS CARE POINTS

- When initially assessing ASCVD risk, traditional 10-year risk calculators such as the pooled cohort equations (PCE) and Systemic COronary Risk Evaluation 2 (SCORE2) should be used and then augmented with the appraisal of risk-enhancing factors (eg, family history).

- When using the PCE to assess the 10-year ASCVD risk in non-African American (AA) or non-White patients, the equation for non-White individuals should be used and results cautiously interpreted.

- If the indication for initiating statin or aspirin therapy is unclear in patients with borderline- or intermediate-risk, coronary artery calcium (CAC) should be used.

- To reassess the potential benefit of statin or aspirin therapy in primary prevention in patients with initial CAC = 0, CAC scanning should be repeated every 5 to 7 y for low-risk patients; every 3 to 5 y for borderline-to-intermediate-risk patients; and every 3 y for high-risk patients or those with diabetes; risk factors should be assessed at every visit.

- When assessing ASCVD risk in specific populations (eg, women, those with chronic inflammatory conditions or endocrine disorders, racial/ethnic minorities), which portend an increased risk of ASCVD due to factors under-represented in traditional risk calculators, an assessment of risk factors, risk-enhancing factors, and potentially CAC should be used to further arbitrate risk and benefit of preventive therapy.

- When assessing ASCVD risk in the young (<40 y) and elderly (>75 y), consideration of age, sex, and race/ethnicity-specific CAC percentiles are critical for driving nuanced discussion of the net benefit of preventive therapies.

- When considering advanced lipid testing to assess ASCVD risk, measuring lipoprotein(a) (Lp(a)) once has been shown to be the most helpful in further adjudicating risk, especially in women with hypercholesterolemia, those with strong family history, those of intermediate- or high-risk, and middle-aged adults.

ACKNOWLEDGMENTS

M. Blaha reports grants from the NIH, FDA, AHA, Amgen, Novo Nordisk, and Bayer. M. Blaha reports serving on Advisory Boards for Amgen, Novartis, Novo Nordisk, Bayer, Roche, Inozyme, 89Bio, Kaleido, VoxelCloud, Kowa, and emocha health.

DISCLOSURE

E. Goldsborough has no financial disclosures or competing interests to report. N. Osuji has no financial disclosures or competing interests to report.

REFERENCES

1. World Health Organization. Cardiovascular diseases. World Health Organization. Available at: https://www.who.int/health-topics/cardiovascular-diseases/#tab=tab_1. Accessed June 13, 2021.
2. Benjamin EJ, Muntner P, Alonso A, et al. Heart disease and stroke statistics— 2019 update: a report from the American Heart Association. Circulation 2019; 139(10). https://doi.org/10.1161/CIR.0000000000000659.
3. European Heart Network. European cardiovascular disease statistics. 2017. Available at: https://ehnheart.org/images/CVD-statistics-report-August-2017. pdf. Accessed December 15, 2021.
4. Roth GA, Mensah GA, Johnson CO, et al. Global burden of cardiovascular diseases and risk factors, 1990–2019. J Am Coll Cardiol 2020;76(25):2982–3021.
5. Roth GA, Nguyen G, Forouzanfar MH, et al. Estimates of global and regional premature cardiovascular mortality in 2025. Circulation 2015;132(13):1270–82.
6. Johnson NB, Hayes LD, Brown K, et al. CDC national health report: leading causes of morbidity and mortality and associated behavioral risk and protective factors—United States, 2005-2013. MMWR Suppl 2014;63:3–27.
7. Yusuf S, Hawken S, Ounpuu S, et al. Effect of potentially modifiable risk factors associated with myocardial infarction in 52 countries (the INTERHEART study): case-control study. Lancet 2004;364(9438):937–52.
8. Wickramasinghe M, Weaver JU. Lipid disorders in obesity. In: Weaver J, editor. Practical guide to obesity medicine. St. Louis, Missouri: Elsevier; 2018. p. 99–108.
9. Pekkanen J, Linn S, Heiss G, et al. Ten-year mortality from cardiovascular disease in relation to cholesterol level among men with and without preexisting cardiovascular disease. N Engl J Med 1990;322(24):1700–7.

10. Urbina EM, Daniels SR. Hyperlipidemia. In: Slap GB, editor. Adolescent medicine. Elsevier; 2008. p. 90–6.

11. Linton MRF, Yancey PG, Davies SS, et al. The role of lipids and lipoproteins in atherosclerosis. [Updated 2019 Jan 3]. In: Feingold KR, Anawalt B, Boyce A, et al, editors. Endotext. South Dartmouth (MA): MDText.com, Inc; 2000.

12. Michos ED, Blaha MJ, Martin SS, et al. Screening for atherosclerotic cardiovascular disease in asymptomatic individuals. In: Delemos J, Omland T, editors. Chronic coronary artery disease: a companion to Braunwald's heart disease. Philadelphia, PA: Elsevier; 2018. p. 459–78.

13. Arnett DK, Blumenthal RS, Albert MA, et al. 2019 ACC/AHA Guideline on the primary prevention of cardiovascular disease. J Am Coll Cardiol 2019;74(10): e177–232.

14. Cholesterol Treatment Trialists' (CTT) Collaborators. The effects of lowering LDL cholesterol with statin therapy in people at low risk of vascular disease: meta-analysis of individual data from 27 randomised trials. Lancet 2012;380(9841): 581–90.

15. Sandesara P, Bogart DB. Almost everyone over 50 should be put on a statin to reduce the risk of cardiovascular disease: a protagonist view. Mo Med 2013; 110(4):332–8.

16. 27th Bethesda Conference. Matching the intensity of risk factor management with the hazard for coronary disease events. September 14-15, 1995. J Am Coll Cardiol 1996;27(5):957–1047.

17. Califf RM, Armstrong PW, Carver JR, et al. 27th Bethesda Conference: matching the intensity of risk factor management with the hazard for coronary disease events. Task Force 5. Stratification of patients into high, medium and low risk subgroups for purposes of risk factor management. J Am Coll Cardiol 1996; 27(5):1007–19.

18. Pearson TA, McBride PE, Miller NH, et al. 27th Bethesda Conference: matching the intensity of risk factor management with the hazard for coronary disease events. Task Force 8. Organization of preventive cardiology service. J Am Coll Cardiol 1996;27(5):1039–47.

19. Mach F, Baigent C, Catapano AL, et al. 2019 ESC/EAS Guidelines for the management of dyslipidaemias: lipid modification to reduce cardiovascular risk. Eur Heart J 2020;41(1):111–88.

20. Grundy SM, Stone NJ, Bailey AL, et al. 2018 AHA/ACC/AACVPR/AAPA/ABC/ACPM/ADA/AGS/APhA/ASPC/NLA/PCNA Guideline on the management of blood cholesterol: executive summary. J Am Coll Cardiol 2019;73(24):3168–209.

21. Goff DC, Lloyd-Jones DM, Bennett G, et al. 2013 ACC/AHA Guideline on the assessment of cardiovascular risk. J Am Coll Cardiol 2014;63(25):2935–59.

22. European Association of Preventive Cardiology. About HeartScore. HeartScore. Available at: https://www.heartscore.org/el_CY/about-heartscore. Accessed December 15, 2021.

23. Conroy RM, Pyörälä K, Fitzgerald AP, et al. Estimation of ten-year risk of fatal cardiovascular disease in Europe: the SCORE project. Eur Heart J 2003; 24(11):987–1003.

24. Bostom AG, Gagnon DR, Cupples LA, et al. A prospective investigation of elevated lipoprotein (a) detected by electrophoresis and cardiovascular disease in women. The Framingham Heart Study. Circulation 1994;90(4):1688–95.

25. Bostom AG. Elevated plasma lipoprotein(a) and coronary heart disease in men aged 55 years and younger: a prospective study. JAMA 1996;276(7):544.

26. SCORE2 Working Group and ESC Cardiovascular Risk Collaboration, Hageman S, Pennells L, et al. SCORE2 risk prediction algorithms: new models to estimate 10-year risk of cardiovascular disease in Europe. Eur Heart J 2021; 42(25):2439–54.

27. Visseren FLJ, Mach F, Smulders YM, et al. 2021 ESC guidelines on cardiovascular disease prevention in clinical practice. Eur Heart J 2021;42(34):3227–337.

28. Ridker PM, Buring JE, Rifai N, et al. Development and validation of improved algorithms for the assessment of global cardiovascular risk in women: the reynolds risk score. JAMA 2007;297(6):611.

29. Ridker PM, Paynter NP, Rifai N, et al. C-reactive protein and parental history improve global cardiovascular risk prediction: the Reynolds Risk Score for men. Circulation 2008;118(22):2243–51, 4p following 2251.

30. Hippisley-Cox J, Coupland C, Vinogradova Y, et al. Derivation and validation of QRISK, a new cardiovascular disease risk score for the United Kingdom: prospective open cohort study. BMJ 2007;335(7611):136.

31. Hippisley-Cox J, Coupland C, Vinogradova Y, et al. Predicting cardiovascular risk in England and Wales: prospective derivation and validation of QRISK2. BMJ 2008;336(7659):1475–82.

32. Hippisley-Cox J, Coupland C, Brindle P. Development and validation of QRISK3 risk prediction algorithms to estimate future risk of cardiovascular disease: prospective cohort study. BMJ 2017;357:j2099.

33. SCORE2-OP Working Group and ESC Cardiovascular Risk Collaboration, de Vries TI, Cooney MT, et al. SCORE2-OP risk prediction algorithms: estimating incident cardiovascular event risk in older persons in four geographical risk regions. Eur Heart J 2021;42(25):2455–67.

34. Armitage J, Baigent C, Barnes E, et al. Efficacy and safety of statin therapy in older people: a meta-analysis of individual participant data from 28 randomised controlled trials. Lancet 2019;393(10170):407–15.

35. Newman CB, Blaha MJ, Boord JB, et al. Lipid management in patients with endocrine disorders: an Endocrine Society clinical practice guideline. J Clin Endocrinol Metab 2020;105(12):3613–82.

36. Tanz LJ, Stuart JJ, Williams PL, et al. Preterm delivery and maternal cardiovascular disease in young and middle-aged adult women. Circulation 2017;135(6): 578–89.

37. Garcia M, Mulvagh SL, Bairey Merz CN, et al. Cardiovascular disease in women: clinical perspectives. Circ Res 2016;118(8):1273–93.

38. Schultz WM, Kelli HM, Lisko JC, et al. Socioeconomic status and cardiovascular outcomes: challenges and interventions. Circulation 2018;137(20):2166–78.

39. Li R, Hou J, Tu R, et al. Associations of mixture of air pollutants with estimated 10-year atherosclerotic cardiovascular disease risk modified by socioeconomic status: the Henan Rural Cohort Study. Sci The Total Environ 2021; 793:148542.

40. Colantonio LD, Richman JS, Carson AP, et al. Performance of the atherosclerotic cardiovascular disease pooled cohort risk equations by social deprivation status. JAHA 2017;6(3). https://doi.org/10.1161/JAHA.117.005676.

41. Libby P, Ridker PM. Inflammation and atherothrombosis. J Am Coll Cardiol 2006; 48(9):A33–46.

42. Mason JC, Libby P. Cardiovascular disease in patients with chronic inflammation: mechanisms underlying premature cardiovascular events in rheumatologic conditions. Eur Heart J 2015;36(8):482–489c.

43. Hansen PR. Chronic inflammatory diseases and atherosclerotic cardiovascular disease: innocent bystanders or partners in crime? CPD 2018;24(3):281–90.

44. Rosenson RS, Hubbard D, Monda KL, et al. Excess risk for atherosclerotic cardiovascular outcomes among US adults with HIV in the current era. JAHA 2020; 9(1). https://doi.org/10.1161/JAHA.119.013744.

45. Feinstein MJ, Hsue PY, Benjamin LA, et al. Characteristics, prevention, and management of cardiovascular disease in people living with HIV: a scientific statement from the American Heart Association. Circulation 2019;140(2). https://doi.org/10.1161/CIR.0000000000000695.

46. American Heart Association, American Stroke Association. Facts: bridging the gap – CVD health disparities. Heart. Available at: https://www.heart.org/idc/groups/heart-public/@wcm/@hcm/@ml/documents/downloadable/ucm_429240.pdf. Accessed December 15, 2021.

47. Osei AD, Uddin SMI, Dzaye O, et al. Predictors of coronary artery calcium among 20-30-year-olds: The Coronary Artery Calcium Consortium. Atherosclerosis 2020;301:65–8.

48. Miedema MD, Dardari ZA, Nasir K, et al. Association of coronary artery calcium with long-term, cause-specific mortality among young adults. JAMA Netw Open 2019;2(7):e197440.

49. Javaid A, Mitchell JD, Villines TC. Predictors of coronary artery calcium and long-term risks of death, myocardial infarction, and stroke in young adults. JAHA 2021;10(22):e022513.

50. Patel J, Al Rifai M, Scheuner MT, et al. Basic vs more complex definitions of family history in the prediction of coronary heart disease: the Multi-Ethnic Study of Atherosclerosis. Mayo Clin Proc 2018;93(9):1213–23.

51. Lloyd-Jones DM, Nam B-H, D'Agostino RB, et al. Parental cardiovascular disease as a risk factor for cardiovascular disease in middle-aged adults: a prospective study of parents and offspring. JAMA 2004;291(18):2204–11.

52. Bachmann JM, Willis BL, Ayers CR, et al. Association between family history and coronary heart disease death across long-term follow-up in men: the Cooper Center Longitudinal Study. Circulation 2012;125(25):3092–8.

53. Mehta A, Virani SS, Ayers CR, et al. Lipoprotein(a) and family history predict cardiovascular disease risk. J Am Coll Cardiol 2020;76(7):781–93.

54. Patel J, Al Rifai M, Blaha MJ, et al. Coronary artery calcium improves risk assessment in adults with a family history of premature coronary heart disease: results from Multiethnic Study of Atherosclerosis. Circ Cardiovasc Imaging 2015;8(6):e003186.

55. Pandey AK, Pandey S, Blaha MJ, et al. Family history of coronary heart disease and markers of subclinical cardiovascular disease: where do we stand? Atherosclerosis 2013;228(2):285–94.

56. Shara NM, Desale S, Howard BV, et al. Modified pooled cohort atherosclerotic cardiovascular disease risk prediction equations in American Indians. J Nephrol Sci 2020;2(1):5–14.

57. Yadlowsky S, Hayward RA, Sussman JB, et al. Clinical implications of revised pooled cohort equations for estimating atherosclerotic cardiovascular disease risk. Ann Intern Med 2018;169(1):20.

58. Volgman AS, Palaniappan LS, Aggarwal NT, et al. Atherosclerotic cardiovascular disease in South Asians in the United States: epidemiology, risk factors, and treatments: a scientific statement from the American Heart Association. Circulation 2018;138(1). https://doi.org/10.1161/CIR.0000000000000580.

59. Lloyd-Jones DM, Braun LT, Ndumele CE, et al. Use of risk assessment tools to guide decision-making in the primary prevention of atherosclerotic cardiovascular disease: a special report from the American Heart Association and American College of Cardiology. Circulation 2019;139(25). https://doi.org/10.1161/CIR.0000000000000638.

60. Dalton JE, Perzynski AT, Zidar DA, et al. Accuracy of cardiovascular risk prediction varies by neighborhood socioeconomic position: a retrospective cohort study. Ann Intern Med 2017;167(7):456–64.

61. Feinstein MJ, Nance RM, Drozd DR, et al. Assessing and refining myocardial infarction risk estimation among patients with human immunodeficiency virus: a study by the Centers for AIDS Research Network of Integrated Clinical Systems. JAMA Cardiol 2017;2(2):155–62.

62. Ungprasert P, Matteson EL, Crowson CS. Reliability of cardiovascular risk calculators to estimate accurately the risk of cardiovascular disease in patients with sarcoidosis. Am J Cardiol 2017;120(5):868–73.

63. Agatston AS, Janowitz WR, Hildner FJ, et al. Quantification of coronary artery calcium using ultrafast computed tomography. J Am Coll Cardiol 1990;15(4):827–32.

64. Bild DE, Bluemke DA, Burke GL, et al. Multi-Ethnic Study of Atherosclerosis: objectives and design. Am J Epidemiol 2002;156(9):871–81.

65. Lackland DT, Elkind MSV, D'Agostino R, et al. Inclusion of stroke in cardiovascular risk prediction instruments: a statement for healthcare professionals from the American Heart Association/American Stroke Association. Stroke 2012;43(7):1998–2027.

66. Piepoli MF, Hoes AW, Agewall S, et al. 2016 European guidelines on cardiovascular disease prevention in clinical practice: the Sixth Joint Task Force of the European Society of Cardiology and other societies on cardiovascular disease prevention in clinical practice (constituted by representatives of 10 societies and by invited experts) developed with the special contribution of the European Association for Cardiovascular Prevention & Rehabilitation (EACPR). Eur Heart J 2016;37(29):2315–81.

67. Budoff MJ, Young R, Burke G, et al. Ten-year association of coronary artery calcium with atherosclerotic cardiovascular disease (ASCVD) events: the multi-ethnic study of atherosclerosis (MESA). Eur Heart J 2018;39(25):2401–8.

68. Martin SS, Blaha MJ, Blankstein R, et al. Dyslipidemia, coronary artery calcium, and incident atherosclerotic cardiovascular disease: implications for statin therapy from the Multi-Ethnic Study of Atherosclerosis. Circulation 2014;129(1):77–86.

69. Sandesara PB, Mehta A, O'Neal WT, et al. Clinical significance of zero coronary artery calcium in individuals with LDL cholesterol ≥190 mg/dL: The Multi-Ethnic Study of Atherosclerosis. Atherosclerosis 2020;292:224–9.

70. Greenland P, Blaha MJ, Budoff MJ, et al. Coronary calcium score and cardiovascular risk. J Am Coll Cardiol 2018;72(4):434–47.

71. Yeboah J, McClelland RL, Polonsky TS, et al. Comparison of novel risk markers for improvement in cardiovascular risk assessment in intermediate-risk individuals. JAMA 2012;308(8):788.

72. Peng AW, Mirbolouk M, Orimoloye OA, et al. Long-term all-cause and cause-specific mortality in asymptomatic patients with CAC ≥1,000: results from the CAC Consortium. JACC Cardiovasc Imaging 2020;13(1 Pt 1):83–93.

73. Orringer CE, Blaha MJ, Blankstein R, et al. The National Lipid Association scientific statement on coronary artery calcium scoring to guide preventive strategies for ASCVD risk reduction. J Clin Lipidol 2021;15(1):33–60.

74. Corrigendum to: "Lipid management in patients with endocrine disorders: an Endocrine Society clinical practice guideline. J Clin Endocrinol Metab 2021; 106(6):e2465.

75. Hecht H, Blaha MJ, Berman DS, et al. Clinical indications for coronary artery calcium scoring in asymptomatic patients: expert consensus statement from the Society of Cardiovascular Computed Tomography. J Cardiovasc Comput Tomogr 2017;11(2):157–68.

76. Anderson JL, Le VT, Min DB, et al. Comparison of three atherosclerotic cardiovascular disease risk scores with and without coronary calcium for predicting revascularization and major adverse coronary events in symptomatic patients undergoing positron emission tomography-stress testing. Am J Cardiol 2020; 125(3):341–8.

77. Lorenz MW, Markus HS, Bots ML, et al. Prediction of clinical cardiovascular events with carotid intima-media thickness: a systematic review and meta-analysis. Circulation 2007;115(4):459–67.

78. Mehta A, Rigdon J, Tattersall MC, et al. Association of carotid artery plaque with cardiovascular events and incident coronary artery calcium in individuals with absent coronary calcification: the MESA. Circ Cardiovasc Imaging 2021;14(4): e011701.

79. Divakaran S, Cheezum MK, Hulten EA, et al. Use of cardiac CT and calcium scoring for detecting coronary plaque: implications on prognosis and patient management. Br J Radiol 2015;88(1046):20140594.

80. Pellikka PA, Arruda-Olson A, Chaudhry FA, et al. Guidelines for performance, interpretation, and application of stress echocardiography in ischemic heart disease: from the American Society of Echocardiography. J Am Soc Echocardiogr 2020;33(1):1–41.e8.

81. Arbab-Zadeh A. Stress testing and non-invasive coronary angiography in patients with suspected coronary artery disease: time for a new paradigm. Heart Int 2012;7(1):e2.

82. Brown EE, Sturm AC, Cuchel M, et al. Genetic testing in dyslipidemia: A scientific statement from the National Lipid Association. J Clin Lipidol 2020. https://doi.org/10.1016/j.jacl.2020.04.011.

83. Burge MR, Eaton RP, Schade DS. The role of a coronary artery calcium scan in type 1 diabetes. Diabetes Technol Ther 2016;18(9):594–603.

84. Mortensen MB, Dzaye O, Steffensen FH, et al. Impact of plaque burden versus stenosis on ischemic events in patients with coronary atherosclerosis. J Am Coll Cardiol 2020;76(24):2803–13.

85. Cigna. Coronary calcium scan: should I have this test? Cigna. Available at: https://www.cigna.com/individuals-families/health-wellness/hw/medical-topics/coronary-calcium-scan-av2072. Accessed December 15, 2021.

86. Cleveland Clinic. Calcium-score screening heart scan. Cleveland Clinic. Available at: https://my.clevelandclinic.org/health/diagnostics/16824-calcium-score-screening-heart-scan. Accessed December 15, 2021.

87. Blaha MJ, Mortensen MB, Kianoush S, et al. Coronary Artery Calcium Scoring. JACC Cardiovascular Imaging 2017;10(8):923–37.

88. American College of Radiology. Radiation dose to adults from common imaging examinations. Available at: https://www.acr.org/-/media/ACR/Files/Radiology-

Safety/Radiation-Safety/Dose-Reference-Card.pdf. Accessed December 15, 2021.

89. United States Nuclear Regulatory Commission. Biological effects of radiation. Available at: https://www.nrc.gov/docs/ML0333/ML033390088.pdf. Accessed December 15, 2021.

90. Pradubpongsa P, Dhana N, Jongjarearnprasert K, et al. Adverse reactions to iodinated contrast media: prevalence, risk factors and outcome-the results of a 3-year period. Asian Pac J Allergy Immunol 2013;31(4):299–306.

91. Jacobson TA, Ito MK, Maki KC, et al. National lipid association recommendations for patient-centered management of dyslipidemia: part 1–full report. J Clin Lipidol 2015;9(2):129–69.

92. Davidson MH, Ballantyne CM, Jacobson TA, et al. Clinical utility of inflammatory markers and advanced lipoprotein testing: advice from an expert panel of lipid specialists. J Clin Lipidol 2011;5(5):338–67.

93. Feingold KR. Introduction to lipids and lipoproteins. In: Feingold KR, Anawalt B, Boyce A, et al, editors. Endotext. MDText.com, Inc; 2000. Available at: http://www.ncbi.nlm.nih.gov/books/NBK305896/. Accessed August 1, 2021.

94. Sniderman AD, Williams K, Contois JH, et al. A meta-analysis of low-density lipoprotein cholesterol, non-high-density lipoprotein cholesterol, and apolipoprotein B as markers of cardiovascular risk. Circ Cardiovasc Qual Outcomes 2011; 4(3):337–45.

95. Sniderman AD, Tremblay A, De Graaf J, et al. Phenotypes of hypertriglyceridemia caused by excess very-low-density lipoprotein. J Clin Lipidol 2012;6(5): 427–33.

96. Choi S. The potential role of biomarkers associated with ASCVD risk: risk-enhancing biomarkers. J Lipid Atheroscler 2019;8(2):173–82.

97. Cook NR, Mora S, Ridker PM. Lipoprotein(a) and cardiovascular risk prediction among women. J Am Coll Cardiol 2018;72(3):287–96.

98. Nordestgaard BG, Chapman MJ, Ray K, et al. Lipoprotein(a) as a cardiovascular risk factor: current status. Eur Heart J 2010;31(23):2844–53.

99. Patel AP, Wang M, Pirruccello JP, et al. Lp(a) (lipoprotein[a]) concentrations and incident atherosclerotic cardiovascular disease: new insights from a large national biobank. ATVB 2020. https://doi.org/10.1161/ATVBAHA.120.315291.

100. Mehta A, Vasquez N, Ayers CR, et al. Available at: https://pubmed.ncbi.nlm.nih.gov/35210030/.

101. Verweij SL, de Ronde MWJ, Verbeek R, et al. Elevated lipoprotein(a) levels are associated with coronary artery calcium scores in asymptomatic individuals with a family history of premature atherosclerotic cardiovascular disease. J Clin Lipidol 2018;12(3):597–603.e1.

102. Quispe R, Michos ED, Martin SS, et al. High-sensitivity C-reactive protein discordance with atherogenic lipid measures and incidence of atherosclerotic cardiovascular disease in primary prevention: the ARIC study. JAHA 2020;9(3). https://doi.org/10.1161/JAHA.119.013600.

103. Aday AW, Ridker PM. Targeting residual inflammatory risk: a shifting paradigm for atherosclerotic disease. Front Cardiovasc Med 2019;6:16.

104. Blaha MJ, Budoff MJ, DeFilippis AP, et al. Associations between C-reactive protein, coronary artery calcium, and cardiovascular events: implications for the JUPITER population from MESA, a population-based cohort study. Lancet 2011;378(9792):684–92.

105. Dzaye O, Razavi AC, Dardari ZA, et al. Available at: https://pubmed.ncbi.nlm.nih.gov/34649694/.

106. McClelland RL, Jorgensen NW, Budoff M, et al. 10-Year coronary heart disease risk prediction using coronary artery calcium and traditional risk factors. J Am Coll Cardiol 2015;66(15):1643–53.
107. Wang Y, Lv Q, Wu H, et al. Comparison of MESA of and Framingham risk scores in the prediction of coronary artery disease severity. Herz 2020;45(S1):139–44.
108. Zeb I, Budoff M. Coronary artery calcium screening: does it perform better than other cardiovascular risk stratification tools? Int J Mol Sci 2015;16(3):6606–20.
109. Miller JM, Rochitte CE, Dewey M, et al. Diagnostic performance of coronary angiography by 64-row CT. N Engl J Med 2008;359(22):2324–36.
110. Budoff MJ, Dowe D, Jollis JG, et al. Diagnostic performance of 64-multidetector row coronary computed tomographic angiography for evaluation of coronary artery stenosis in individuals without known coronary artery disease: results from the prospective multicenter ACCURACY (Assessment by Coronary Computed Tomographic Angiography of Individuals Undergoing Invasive Coronary Angiography) trial. J Am Coll Cardiol 2008;52(21):1724–32.
111. Han D, Hartaigh BÓ, Gransar H, et al. Incremental prognostic value of coronary computed tomography angiography over coronary calcium scoring for major adverse cardiac events in elderly asymptomatic individuals. Eur Heart J Cardiovasc Imaging 2018;19(6):675–83.
112. Martin SS, Abd TT, Jones SR, et al. 2013 ACC/AHA cholesterol treatment guideline. J Am Coll Cardiol 2014;63(24):2674–8.
113. Sniderman AD, Furberg CD. Age as a modifiable risk factor for cardiovascular disease. Lancet 2008;371(9623):1547–9.
114. Singh A. Complex Traits. In: Gellman MD, Turner JR, editors. Encyclopedia of behavioral medicine. New York: Springer; 2013. p. 478–9.
115. Abbate R, Sticchi E, Fatini C. Genetics of cardiovascular disease. Clin Cases Miner Bone Metab 2008;5(1):63–6.
116. Choi SW, Mak TS-H, O'Reilly PF. Tutorial: a guide to performing polygenic risk score analyses. Nat Protoc 2020;15(9):2759–72.
117. Lewis CM, Vassos E. Polygenic risk scores: from research tools to clinical instruments. Genome Med 2020;12(1):44.
118. Woodward M, Brindle P, Tunstall-Pedoe H, SIGN group on risk estimation. Adding social deprivation and family history to cardiovascular risk assessment: the ASSIGN score from the Scottish Heart Health Extended Cohort (SHHEC). Heart 2005;93(2):172–6.
119. Yang X, Li J, Hu D, et al. Predicting the 10-year risks of atherosclerotic cardiovascular disease in Chinese population: the China-PAR project (prediction for ASCVD risk in China). Circulation 2016;134(19):1430–40.
120. D'Agostino RB, Vasan RS, Pencina MJ, et al. General cardiovascular risk profile for use in primary care: The Framingham Heart Study. Circulation 2008;117(6):743–53.
121. Joint British Societies' consensus recommendations for the prevention of cardiovascular disease (JBS3). Heart 2014;100(Suppl 2):ii67, ii1.
122. Joint British Societies for the Prevention of Cardiovascular Disease. JBS3 report. JBS3Risk. Available at: http://www.jbs3risk.com/pages/report.htm. Accessed December 15, 2021.

Race and Modifiable Factors Influencing Cardiovascular Disease

Alvis Coleman Headen, BS[a,1],
Andrew Siaw-Asamoah, BA, MPhil[a,1],
Howard M. Julien, MD, MPH, ML[a,b,c,1,*]

KEYWORDS

- Hypertension • Hyperlipidemia • Race • Health care disparities

KEY POINTS

- Cardiovascular disease remains the leading cause of death in the United States with differences in cardiovascular disease mortality between Black and white Americans first manifesting in young and middle-aged adults.
- A modern approach to mitigating the impact of cardiovascular disease on Americans demands not only an understanding of modifiable conditions that contribute to its development but also a greater appreciation of the heterogeneous distribution of these conditions based on race.
- As race is a social construct, observed differences by race in modifiable risk factors that contribute to the development of cardiovascular disease demands further investigation into the numerous social and economic influences that underpin these findings.

INTRODUCTION

Cardiovascular disease remains the leading cause of death in the United States.[1] The disparate impact of race in influencing morbidity and mortality associated with cardiovascular disease has been well described.[2] The difference in cardiovascular disease mortality between Black and white Americans first manifests in young and middle-aged adults.[3]

Before any attempt to study the impact of race on cardiovascular disease, an appreciation for the construct of race is necessary to avoid pitfalls born of its unintended

This article originally appeared in *Medical Clinics*, Volume 106, Issue 2, March 2022.
[a] Perelman School of Medicine, University of Pennsylvania, Philadelphia, PA, USA; [b] Penn Cardiovascular Outcomes, Quality, and Evaluative Research Center; [c] Penn Cardiovascular Center for Health Equity and Social Justice
[1] Present address: Perelman Center for Advanced Medicine, 3400 Civic Center Boulevard, 2nd Floor East, Philadelphia, PA 19104.
* Corresponding author.
E-mail address: Howard.Julien@pennmedicine.upenn.edu

Clinics Collections 13 (2023) 91–99
https://doi.org/10.1016/j.ccol.2023.02.024
2352-7986/23/Published by Elsevier Inc.

application. Race has its origins between the sixteenth and eighteenth centuries as a folk idea in English language cultures[4]; it evolved to encompass the groups of North America by the seventeenth century and gained traction in the early eighteenth century in parallel with the rise of the transatlantic slave trade. The race-based classification of people persists as a vestige from this era with no discernible genetic basis.[5] Despite the absence of a discrete genetic underpinning, societies have, and continue to, use the classification to implicitly and explicitly allocate resources and treatment creating the foundation of racism in social institutions. Consequently, the use of race in scientific literature should indicate the presence of a complex interaction of mostly social, economic, and cultural influences along with some genetic factors that have been aggregated into one variable. Some of the social, economic, and cultural influences that influence the impact of race on cardiovascular disease owe their origins to institutional, personal/perceived, and internalized racism.[6]

Epidemiology of Hyperlipidemia in Black Americans

The Centers for Disease Control and Prevention has estimated that approximately 71 million or 33.5% of US adults older than 20 years have high low-density lipoprotein cholesterol (LDL-C), whereas only 48% of those people received treatment for it and only 33% of them had their LDL-C levels less than the goal level (controlled) when treated. Education is an important indicator for pathologic LDL-C values. In populations that had not completed high school, 41% had hyperlipidemia, whereas college graduates had prevalence of only 28.7%. In addition to education, self-described race has played a large role in hyperlipidemia prevalence. The prevalence of hyperlipidemia is highest in non-Hispanic whites at 34.5%, non- Hispanic Black Americans at 30.4%, and Mexican Americans at 27.7%. These numbers are likely an underestimate because Black Americans have one of the highest uninsured rates at 11.5% and are thus less likely to receive routine cardiovascular risk factor screening.[7] In addition to lower physical activity, alcohol consumption, and diet, perceived racism may play a role in dyslipidemia within Black communities. One study conducted in 2011 showed that endorsing behavioral coping responses to perceived racism predicted higher levels of LDL-C.[8] The relationship between stress and increased LDL-C levels was not associated with other stress response systems such as cortisol, norepinephrine, epinephrine, and interleukin-6.[8] This study implies that other forms of stress may also be associated with elevated LDL-C values.

Management of Hyperlipidemia in Black Americans

Treatment of hyperlipidemia aims to reduce the risk of atherosclerotic cardiovascular disease and resultant events through reduction of LDL-C levels. The foundation of therapy is nonpharmacologic lifestyle changes. Dietary changes including reducing saturated fat, cholesterol, and alcohol intake have been shown to lower lipid blood levels. Maintaining a healthy weight as well as increasing physical activity has been shown to yield similar results.[9,10] Pharmacologic treatments of hyperlipidemia typically include statins, which inhibit cholesterol synthesis in the liver leading to lower lipid levels circulating in the blood, and are a mainstay of therapy.[11–13] Second-line lipid-lowering agents include fibrates, bile acid resins, niacin, ezetimibe, and most recently, injectable proprotein convertase subtilisin/kexin type 9 (PCSK9) inhibitors.[14] Most frequently used are ezetimibe, which is indicated with statin intolerance, and PCSK9 inhibitors, indicated when LDL-C levels remain elevated despite receiving treatment with statins along with a history of atherosclerotic cardiovascular disease.[15] When compared with non-Hispanic white Americans, black Americans have a lower prevalence of hyperlipidemia but were less likely to be treated.

Black Americans were less likely to be aware of and have their LDL-C levels controlled upon receiving treatment than their white counterparts.[16,17] Among black patients, hyperlipidemia is less likely to be controlled and has been a main contributor to cardiovascular disease and death. Despite nationwide reductions in cardiovascular disease rates black Americans continue to suffer from cardiovascular disease at greater rates than other groups. Potential solutions lie in strengthening the patient-provider relationship. Black patients are less likely to be prescribed guideline-recommended statin therapy than their white counterparts.[18] Compounding this undertreatment is a lower propensity of Black patients to trust their clinician (82.3% vs 93.8%), to believe that statin therapy is safe (36.2% vs 57.3%) or believe that it is effective (70.0% vs 74.4%), when compared with whites.

In addition, dietary changes that result in reduction of consumption of saturated fats and transfats can help lower LDL-C levels. A move toward a more plant-based diet can help manifest these changes and has been shown to be effective at lowering LDL-C levels and consequently, incidence of cardiovascular events.[19] Finally, regular forms of exercise can lower LDL-C levels. These modifiable risk factors for dyslipidemia may be particularly hard to correct considering a lack of free exercise facilities and prevalence of food deserts in urban areas.[20]

Overview of hypertension

Hypertension, defined as sustained elevated systolic blood pressure (SBP) or diastolic blood pressure (DBP), is associated with adverse clinical end points such as target organ damage, heart disease, and end-stage renal disease.[21] Although the relationship between elevated blood pressure and the risk of cardiovascular disease is continuous, SBP and DBP thresholds have been used in clinical practice to help physicians identify and treat patients at risk.[21,22] Notably, different institutions use distinct cutoffs for the clinical definition of hypertension, allowing either SBP/DBP greater than or equal to 140/90 mm Hg[23] or SBP/DBP greater than or equal to 130/80 mmHg[21,24] to signal a need for blood pressure-lowering intervention.

To measure blood pressure, modern clinical settings have generally replaced the mercury sphygmomanometer with validated electronic upper-arm cuff devices or calibrated auscultatory devices, such as aneroid sphygmomanometers.[3]

Although calibrated measurement technologies can accurately measure blood pressure in the clinic, they struggle to identify some notable manifestations of hypertension, including white coat, masked, and nocturnal hypertension.[25] White coat hypertension, a short-term and reversible increase in blood pressure, either due to the clinical environment or the presence of an observer, is not thought to be associated with cardiovascular disease.[22,26] Masked hypertension, the clinical opposite of white coat hypertension, in which patients exhibit an increased daytime ambulatory blood pressure but a normal blood pressure in clinical settings can be more dangerous and potentially prevents proper diagnosis and treatment.[22,26] Nocturnal hypertension is defined as an elevated nocturnal blood pressure (mean nocturnal SBP/DBP $\geq$120/70 mm Hg) and, like masked hypertension, is associated with increased cardiovascular disease risk.[26,27] Although these clinical presentations can each frustrate epidemiologic efforts to quantify the burden of hypertension, the rates of masked and nocturnal hypertension suggest that the true prevalence of hypertension may be underestimated. Guidance from the International Society of Hypertension (ISH) recognizes the unique challenges that these subtypes present, offering out-of-office blood pressure measurement using ambulatory blood pressure monitoring (ABPM) as a more reproducible method of diagnosing high blood pressure in patients.[25]

Epidemiology of Hypertension in Black Patients

As in other industrialized nations, hypertension is very common in the United States, with an age-adjusted prevalence estimate of 45.4% for adults older than 18 years.[24] The prevalence of hypertension is higher in men than in women (51.0% vs 39.7%) and increases with age.[24] Blacks face the highest burden of hypertension among all the racial and ethnic groups in the United States.[28] During 2017 to 2018, 57.1% of non-Hispanic Black adults had hypertension after adjusting for age compared with 43.6% of non-Hispanic whites and 50.1% of Hispanics.[24] Other estimates suggest that Black Americans consistently experience more than 10% higher prevalence of hypertension than non-Hispanic whites and Mexican Americans since 2008.[9] Disparities in hypertension between black Americans and other racial groups extend beyond prevalence estimates. Evidence suggests that black Americans develop hypertension younger and have higher recorded blood pressures than their white counterparts,[29] and National Health and Nutrition Examination Survey (NHANES) data demonstrated that differences in blood pressure can be observed between white and black women before 10 years of age.[30] The gap further widens when investigating hypertension-related deaths, with Black Americans experiencing 3 times the association between SBP and stroke risk than whites do.[9] Black Americans can expect 4.2 times the rate of end-stage renal disease and 1.5 times the rate of heart disease mortality when compared with the general population in both cases.[30] Overall, as many as 49.6% of cardiovascular disease deaths in Black males were attributable to hypertension; only 14.4% of cardiovascular disease deaths were due to hypertension among their white counterparts.[30]

In addition to traditional risk factors for hypertension, including a sedentary lifestyle, high-salt diet, and family history, researchers have proposed that racism and discrimination are associated with cardiovascular diseases and hypertension. A study showed that Blacks in areas with greater structural racism were more likely to have experienced a heart attack in the past year.[31] A random effects meta-analysis model demonstrated that perceived racial discrimination was associated with a hypertension diagnosis.[32]

Another study found that for each unit increase of racism-related vigilance, a form of anticipatory stress, Blacks faced a 4% increase in the odds of high blood pressure.[33] After accounting for other social explainers such as socioeconomic status, researchers across multiple studies found that disparities between Black and white Americans persisted, suggesting that research into other risk factors, including racism, may be needed to fully understand the observed and persistent gap in hypertension prevalence.

Although the gap in the prevalence of hypertension and associated cardiovascular diseases between Black Americans and non-Blacks in the United States is large, it is likely an underestimation. In the Jackson Heart Study, researchers showed that when using ABPM to measure daytime blood pressure, 34% of patients thought to be normotensive in a clinical evaluation were found to be hypertensive; when using daytime, nighttime, and 24-hour blood pressure from ABPM, this percentage ballooned to 52%.[26] Further research demonstrated that Black Americans with masked hypertension diagnosed via ABPM were at greater risk of a future incident clinic hypertension diagnosis than normotensive Blacks, suggesting that masked hypertension may be an intermediate step between normal and clinically high blood pressure.[34] Together, these estimates suggest that the diagnostic sensitivity of in-clinic blood pressure measurements is low and may contribute to the observed health disparities between Black Americans and their non-Black peers.

Management of Hypertension in Black Patients

Although Black patients demonstrate a greater awareness of their hypertension status and were more likely to have it treated than whites or Hispanics,[9] some estimates show that as many as 40% of self-identifying hypertensive Black Americans were not receiving antihypertensive therapy.[30] In addition, Black Americans experienced lower rates of hypertension control, which is defined as previously elevated blood pressure brought within target ranges by blood pressure-lowering interventions such as pharmaceuticals, than whites.[35,36] These estimates suggest that both untreated and resistant hypertension play important roles in cardiovascular disease disparities experienced by Black Americans.

Common pharmacologic interventions include diuretics, calcium channel blockers (CCB), angiotensin-converting enzyme inhibitors (ACEI), angiotensin II receptor blockers (ARB), and β-blockers. Although each of these drugs can lower blood pressure in the general population, studies have shown that some drugs confer more modest reductions in blood pressure in Black Americans than in whites.[36] A meta-analysis of studies with ACEI monotherapy showed that the average Black patient had a final SBP/DBP blood pressure that was 4.6/2.8 mm Hg higher than that of white patients.[36] In addition, ACEI/ARB treatment has been demonstrated to be less effective in Black patients than other drug treatment classes.[23,36,37] Angioedema, an adverse drug effect of ACEI therapy, seems to occur as much as 3 times more often in black patients than non-Black patients,[38] but with a general population risk of ACEI-associated angioedema of less than 1%, it is unclear to what degree this difference should impact clinical decision making.[25,36] Interpreting these data with the knowledge that race is a social construct calls for additional research to determine the biological factors responsible for these differences. These findings have inspired differential recommendations for first-line therapy in Black versus non-Black populations; the Joint National Committee (JNC) 8 recommends ACEI or ARBs as options for initial antihypertension treatment in non-Blacks but drops these suggestions when considering Black patients.[23]

Differences in drug responses have sparked investigations into causal pathways of hypertension in Black Americans, such as increased dietary sodium sensitivity and low renin levels.[36] These theories imply that genetic differences can simultaneously explain increased rates of hypertension as well as reduced responses to therapy, but a genetic explanation of these observed and perceived differences has yet to be clearly identified. Studies that quantified ancestry using models that characterize genomic similarity suggest no association between West African ancestry and nocturnal hypertension or reduced hypertension control.[27,39] Importantly, studies have shown that known genetic factors for hypertension together explain less than 3% of observed individual differences[39]; other environmental factors, such as access to affordable health care and healthy food, likely play a larger role in the significant and persistent disparities faced by Black Americans over the past 20 years and beyond.

The emphasis on the effects of individual drugs also distracts from the well-established benefits of multidrug therapy in hypertension control. Monotherapy with ACEI and ARB treatment did not significantly increase odds of hypertension control in Black Americans,[37] but when combined with other treatments such as diuretics or CCB, they provided even stronger clinical benefits in blood pressure reduction than any drug individually.[23,25,30,35–37] It is estimated that if dosages for antihypertensives were increased on 1 of 3 visits with observed elevated blood pressure, hypertension control would increase from 45% to 66% in a single year.[40] Indeed, the Kaiser

Permanente Southern California health system, implementing strategies like treatment intensification to increase dosages and combine drugs, raised the rate of hypertension control among Black patients to more than 80%, simultaneously cutting the previous gap with whites by 50% and suggesting that hypertension control can be better achieved with team-based approaches to disease management and flexible treatment strategies rather than forms of genetic scapegoating.[26,41]

Behavioral interventions are a critical tool in combating hypertension. The Dietary Approaches to Stop Hypertension (DASH) diet, similar to the Mediterranean diet, has been shown to lower SBP by as much as 11 mm Hg, a reduction that mirrors the effects of some antihypertensive drugs.[29,35,42] In spite of these purported benefits, adherence to the DASH-type diet among hypertensive adults in the United States has steadily decreased over the past few decades, especially in Black American populations.[29,42] Challenges to adherence include DASH's limited integration with the cultural practices of Black communities as well as poor guidance on specific steps required for implementation, such as recipe modifications and grocery shopping.[42] Although diet and other individual changes, such as regular exercise, are known to reduce blood pressure in hypertensive patients, these challenges and others faced by Black Americans are influenced by community-level conditions, such as access to health care. Community outreach efforts such as barbershop engagement has had notable success in studies, with one project achieving a mean SBP reduction of 27.0 mm Hg from a baseline mean SBP of 152.8 mm Hg.[43]

SUMMARY

A modern approach to mitigating the impact of cardiovascular disease on Americans demands not only an understanding of modifiable conditions that contribute to its development but also a greater appreciation of the heterogeneous distribution of these conditions based on race. As race is not a biological construct, further research is needed to fully elucidate the mechanisms that contribute to these differences.

The consequences of the differential impact of modifiable risk factors on cardiovascular disease outcomes among Black Americans compared with white Americans cannot be understated. Because race is a social construct, observed differences by race in modifiable risk factors that contribute to the development of cardiovascular disease demands further investigation into the numerous social and economic influences that underpin these findings.

CLINICS CARE POINTS

- The prevalence of hyperlipidemia is highest in non-Hispanic whites at 34.5%, non- Hispanic Black Americans at 30.4%, and Mexican Americans at 27.7% though these data likely underestimate prevalence in Black Americans who have one of the highest uninsured rates in America.

- Black patients are less likely to be prescribed guideline-recommended statin therapy than their white counterparts.

- Blacks face the highest burden of hypertension among all the racial and ethnic groups in the United States.

- Black Americans develop hypertension younger and have higher recorded blood pressures than their white counterparts.

DISCLOSURE

The authors have nothing to disclose.

REFERENCES

1. Prevention. CfDCa. Underlying Cause of Death, 1999–2018. CDC WONDER Online Database. 2018.
2. Writing Group M, Mozaffarian D, Benjamin EJ, et al. American Heart Association Statistics C and Stroke Statistics S. Heart Disease and Stroke Statistics-2016 Update: A Report From the American Heart Association. Circulation 2016;133: e38–360.
3. Jolly S, Vittinghoff E, Chattopadhyay A, et al. Higher cardiovascular disease prevalence and mortality among younger blacks compared to whites. Am J Med 2010;123:811–8.
4. Smedley A, Smedley BD. Race as biology is fiction, racism as a social problem is real: Anthropological and historical perspectives on the social construction of race. Am Psychol 2005;60:16–26.
5. Ioannidis JPA, Powe NR, Yancy C. Recalibrating the Use of Race in Medical Research. JAMA 2021;325:623–4.
6. Wyatt SB, Williams DR, Calvin R, et al. Racism and cardiovascular disease in African Americans. Am J Med Sci 2003;325:315–31.
7. Artiga S. Changes in Health Coverage by Race and Ethnicity since the ACA, 2010-2018. 2020;2021. Available at: https://files.kff.org/attachment/Issue-Brief-Changes-in-Health-Coverage-by-Race-and-Ethnicity-since-the-ACA-2010-2018.pdf.
8. Mwendwa DT, Sims RC, Madhere S, et al. The influence of coping with perceived racism and stress on lipid levels in African Americans. J Natl Med Assoc 2011; 103:594–601.
9. Carnethon MR, Pu J, Howard G, et al, American Heart Association Council on E, Prevention, Council on Cardiovascular Disease in the Y, Council on C, Stroke N, Council on Clinical C, Council on Functional G, Translational B and Stroke C. Cardiovascular Health in African Americans: A Scientific Statement From the American Heart Association. Circulation 2017;136:e393–423.
10. Koutsari C, Karpe F, Humphreys SM, et al. Exercise prevents the accumulation of triglyceride-rich lipoproteins and their remnants seen when changing to a high-carbohydrate diet. Arterioscler Thromb Vasc Biol 2001;21:1520–5.
11. Stone NJ, Robinson JG, Lichtenstein AH, et al. Tomaselli GF and American College of Cardiology/American Heart Association Task Force on Practice G. 2013 ACC/AHA guideline on the treatment of blood cholesterol to reduce atherosclerotic cardiovascular risk in adults: a report of the American College of Cardiology/American Heart Association Task Force on Practice Guidelines. Circulation 2014;129:S1–45.
12. Cholesterol Treatment Trialists C, Mihaylova B, Emberson J, et al. The effects of lowering LDL cholesterol with statin therapy in people at low risk of vascular disease: meta-analysis of individual data from 27 randomised trials. Lancet 2012; 380:581–90.
13. Taylor F, Ward K, Moore TH, et al. Statins for the primary prevention of cardiovascular disease. Cochrane Database Syst Rev 2011;(1):CD004816.
14. Grundy SM, Stone NJ, Bailey AL, et al. 2018 AHA/ACC/AACVPR/AAPA/ABC/ACPM/ADA/AGS/APhA/ASPC/NLA/PCNA Guideline on the Management of Blood Cholesterol: A Report of the American College of Cardiology/American Heart

Association Task Force on Clinical Practice Guidelines. Circulation 2019;139: e1082–143.

15. Giugliano RP, Sabatine MS. Are PCSK9 Inhibitors the Next Breakthrough in the Cardiovascular Field? J Am Coll Cardiol 2015;65:2638–51.

16. Massing MW, Foley KA, Carter-Edwards L, et al. Disparities in lipid management for African Americans and Caucasians with coronary artery disease: a national cross-sectional study. BMC Cardiovasc Disord 2004;4:15.

17. Zweifler RM, McClure LA, Howard VJ, et al. Racial and geographic differences in prevalence, awareness, treatment and control of dyslipidemia: the reasons for geographic and racial differences in stroke (REGARDS) study. Neuroepidemiology 2011;37:39–44.

18. Nanna MG, Navar AM, Zakroysky P, et al. Association of patient perceptions of cardiovascular risk and beliefs on statin drugs with racial differences in statin use: insights from the patient and provider assessment of lipid management registry. JAMA Cardiol 2018;3:739–48.

19. Clifton PM. Diet, exercise and weight loss and dyslipidaemia. Pathology 2019;51: 222–6.

20. Kelli HM, Hammadah M, Ahmed H, et al. Association between living in food deserts and cardiovascular risk. Circ Cardiovasc Qual Outcomes 2017;10:e003532.

21. Whelton PK, Carey RM, Aronow WS, et al. 2017 ACC/AHA/AAPA/ABC/ACPM/ AGS/APhA/ASH/ASPC/NMA/PCNA Guideline for the Prevention, Detection, Evaluation, and Management of High Blood Pressure in Adults: A Report of the American College of Cardiology/American Heart Association Task Force on Clinical Practice Guidelines. Hypertension 2018;71:e13–115.

22. Staessen JA, Wang J, Bianchi G, et al. Essential hypertension. Lancet 2003;361: 1629–41.

23. James PA, Oparil S, Carter BL, et al. 2014 evidence-based guideline for the management of high blood pressure in adults: report from the panel members appointed to the Eighth Joint National Committee (JNC 8). JAMA 2014;311:507–20.

24. Ostchega Y, Fryar CD, Nwankwo T, et al. Hypertension Prevalence Among Adults Aged 18 and Over: United States, 2017-2018. NCHS Data Brief 2020;(364):1–8.

25. Unger T, Borghi C, Charchar F, et al. 2020 International Society of Hypertension Global Hypertension Practice Guidelines. Hypertension 2020;75:1334–57.

26. Muntner P, Abdalla M, Correa A, et al. Hypertension in blacks: unanswered questions and future directions for the JHS (Jackson Heart Study). Hypertension 2017; 69:761–9.

27. Booth JN III, Li M, Shimbo D, et al. West African Ancestry and Nocturnal Blood Pressure in African Americans: The Jackson Heart Study. Am J Hypertens 2018;31:706–14.

28. Kramer H, Han C, Post W, et al. Racial/ethnic differences in hypertension and hypertension treatment and control in the multi-ethnic study of atherosclerosis (MESA). Am J Hypertens 2004;17:963–70.

29. Go AS, Mozaffarian D, Roger VL, et al. American Heart Association Statistics C and Stroke Statistics S. Heart disease and stroke statistics–2013 update: a report from the American Heart Association. Circulation 2013;127:e6–245.

30. Ferdinand KC, Saunders E. Hypertension-related morbidity and mortality in African Americans–why we need to do better. J Clin Hypertens (Greenwich) 2006;8: 21–30.

31. Lukachko A, Hatzenbuehler ML, Keyes KM. Structural racism and myocardial infarction in the United States. Soc Sci Med 2014;103:42–50.

32. Dolezsar CM, McGrath JJ, Herzig AJM, et al. Perceived racial discrimination and hypertension: a comprehensive systematic review. Health Psychol 2014;33: 20–34.
33. Hicken MT, Lee H, Morenoff J, et al. Racial/ethnic disparities in hypertension prevalence: reconsidering the role of chronic stress. Am J Public Health 2014; 104:117–23.
34. Abdalla M, Booth JN 3rd, Seals SR, et al. Masked hypertension and incident clinic hypertension among blacks in the Jackson Heart Study. Hypertension 2016;68:220–6.
35. Ferdinand K, Batieste T, Fleurestil M. Contemporary and future concepts on hypertension in African Americans: COVID-19 and Beyond. J Natl Med Assoc 2020;112:315–23.
36. Helmer A, Slater N, Smithgall S. A Review of ACE Inhibitors and ARBs in black patients with hypertension. Ann Pharmacother 2018;52:1143–51.
37. Clemmer JS, Pruett WA, Lirette ST. Racial and sex differences in the response to first-line antihypertensive therapy. Front Cardiovasc Med 2020;7:608037.
38. Kostis JB, Kim HJ, Rusnak J, et al. Incidence and characteristics of angioedema associated with enalapril. Arch Intern Med 2005;165:1637–42.
39. Rao S, Segar MW, Bress AP, et al. Association of Genetic West African Ancestry, Blood Pressure Response to Therapy, and Cardiovascular Risk Among Self-Reported Black Individuals in the Systolic Blood Pressure Reduction Intervention Trial (SPRINT). JAMA Cardiol 2020;6(4):388–98.
40. Okonofua EC, Simpson KN, Jesri A, et al. Therapeutic inertia is an impediment to achieving the Healthy People 2010 blood pressure control goals. Hypertension 2006;47:345–51.
41. Bartolome RE, Chen A, Handler J, et al. Population care management and team-based approach to reduce racial disparities among African Americans/Blacks with Hypertension. Perm J 2016;20:53–9.
42. Scisney-Matlock M, Bosworth HB, Giger JN, et al. Strategies for implementing and sustaining therapeutic lifestyle changes as part of hypertension management in African Americans. Postgrad Med 2009;121:147–59.
43. Victor RG, Lynch K, Li N, et al. A cluster-randomized trial of blood-pressure reduction in black barbershops. N Engl J Med 2018;378:1291–301.

Cardiovascular Disease in Older Women

Essraa Bayoumi, MD[a], Pamela Karasik, MD[b],*

KEYWORDS

- Older women • Cardiovascular risk • CVD prevention and treatment

KEY POINTS

- Risk with aging, risk mitigation, better diagnosis, and treatment in women.
- Cardiovascular disease remains the most frequent cause of morbidity and mortality in women, despite recent advances in disease prevention, detection and treatment.
- Clinical presentation of cardiovascular disease can be variable and atypical in women, and clinicians need a high degree of sensitivity to make the diagnosis.
- Risk factors in women are in general similar to those in men, but do include non traditional clinical risks such as a history of auto immune disease, pregnancy related diabetes, and prior treatment of malignancy.
- Risk factor modification even in the older population can reduce future risk of cardiovascular events.

INTRODUCTION

Great strides have been made in the prevention, diagnosis, and treatment of cardiovascular disease (CVD) over the past 40 years. In the past decade, death attributable to coronary heart disease has declined by one-third.[1] Despite this, CVD, including cerebrovascular and atherosclerotic heart disease, remains the most frequent cause of death in women.[2,3] As women age, this burden of disease becomes an even greater threat to the quality and quantity of their lives.[2] In truth, the prevention of CVD starts early in life with adherence to a heart-healthy diet, regular exercise, avoidance of tobacco and excessive alcohol, and treatment of nonmodifiable risk factors, such as hypertension and hyperlipidemia. Mitigation of risk, however, is not age limited, and women at any age can adopt lifestyle changes and begin appropriate medical therapy that can have positive effects on future morbidity and mortality. The Framingham

This article originally appeared in *Clinics in Geriatric Medicine*, Volume 37, Issue 4, November 2022.

No Financial Disclosures, No COI for either author.

[a] Medstar Washington Hospital Center, Georgetown University, VA Medical Center, 110 Irving Street Northwest, Washington, DC 20422, USA; [b] Medical Service VA Medical Center, 50 Irving Street Northwest 4A 154, Washington, DC 20422, USA

* Corresponding author.

E-mail address: Pamela.karasik@va.gov

Heart Study showed that even those who are free from CVD at age 70 still have a 24% risk of developing coronary disease.[4] Women have often been underrepresented in clinical trials, in part because of the erroneous notion that women were not at the same risk as men for CVD. It was also not recognized until recently that women may have more atypical presentation of disease, sometimes leading to underdiagnosis of CVD, which resulted in increased mortalities. In this article, the authors review the current state of CVD in older women with a view toward modifying risk, improving diagnosis, and accessing treatment. Although not the subject of this article, the presence of noncoronary atherosclerotic diseases, such as peripheral arterial disease, abdominal aortic aneurysm, and carotid artery disease, is associated with a more than 20% risk of developing CVD.[5,6]

INCIDENCE AND RISK

According to the American Heart Association (AHA) heart disease and stroke statistics 2019 update,[1] the leading cause of death in the United States is heart disease, and if hypertension is included, 48% of American adults over the age of 20 has CVD.[2] In men and women over the age of 60, as many as 75% may have CVD, with the number going up as the population ages.[7] With that as the background, it is important to consider what risks exist for the development of CVD, what are unique to women, which are modifiable, and which are not. Although this focus is on the older woman, in assessing any individual's risk, one should start with a focused history, and for women, that should include an understanding of their early years. For example, women who have experienced complications during pregnancy, such as gestational diabetes and preeclampsia, carry an increased risk of future CVD. These are some of the gender-specific risks that are addressed first (**Fig. 1**).

PREGNANCY RELATED

According to the American College of Obstetrics and Gynecology, preeclampsia is defined as hypertension and proteinuria after 20 weeks' gestation in a previously normotensive patient. It affects 5% to 7% of all pregnancies worldwide and is a leading cause of both maternal and fetal death in the United States and worldwide.[8] Rates

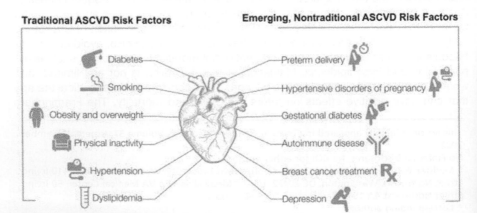

Fig. 1. Traditional versus new, emerging risk factors for CVD in women. ASCVD, atherosclerotic cardiovascular disease. (*From* Garcia M, Mulvagh SL, Merz CN, Buring JE, Manson JE. Cardiovascular Disease in Women: Clinical Perspectives. Circ Res. 2016;118(8):1273-1293. https://doi.org/10.1161/CIRCRESAHA.116.307547; with permission.)

of preeclampsia have increased 25% between 1987 and 2004 in the United States.[9] Although preeclampsia and CVD share many of the same risk factors, preeclampsia itself is also a risk factor for the development of CVD later in life, presenting a vicious cycle.[8] Preeclampsia occurs in 2 stages, including abnormal placentation in the first and early second trimester followed by a maternal syndrome defined as excess anti-angiogenic factors, which antagonize vascular endothelial growth factor, causing a reduction in levels and leading to local and systemic endothelial dysfunction, which ultimately result in hypertension, coagulation disorders, and proteinuria.[8] Although delivery cures the woman of preeclampsia, the endothelial dysfunction persists, leading to future atherosclerotic disease.[10] Several months and years after pregnancy, women with preeclampsia have been shown to have decreased endothelium-dependent dilation as well as increased sensitivity to angiotensin II.[10–12] Studies have shown up to a 3- to 4-fold increased risk of hypertension in women with preeclampsia.[10,13] A history of preeclampsia confers up to a 2-fold increase in death from CVD.[10] Those with early preeclampsia, defined as occurring before 34 weeks' gestation, have up to a 4- to 8-fold increase of death from CVD.[10,13–15] Prepregnancy risk factors, such as hypertension, diabetes, and obesity, lead to an increased risk of preeclampsia as well as CVD.[10] There is also evidence of elevated levels of C-reactive protein (CRP) up to 30 years after pregnancy in patients with subclinical insulin resistance, increasing the risk of CVD.[10,16] Pregnancy may be a stressor that either unmasks subclinical disease or injures the endothelium and increases inflammation, thereby predisposing to later CVD.[10,17]

In addition, those women who develop gestational diabetes have a 7-fold increased risk for developing diabetes type 2, which is a risk factor for CVD.[18–20] They also have a 2- to 4-fold increased risk for the development of CVD risk independent of the development for diabetes type 2.[18–20]

AUTOIMMUNE DISEASES

Systemic lupus erythematosus (SLE), rheumatoid arthritis, and systemic sclerosis are autoimmune diseases that disproportionately affect women, with SLE affecting woman at a ratio of 7:1.[21] One theory for the gender discrepancy is the role of estrogen in the development of disease.[22] Some of these syndromes are marked by increased inflammation that may lead to atherosclerosis.[23] The multiorgan involvement and subsequent therapies may result in the development of CVD. In SLE, hypertension secondary to renal involvement and steroid use, insulin insensitivity and obesity from corticosteroid use, thrombosis from antiphospholipid antibody, atherosclerosis from immune dysregulation and inflammation as well as valvular damage from Libman-Sacks endocarditis all contribute to the development of CVD.[24,25] Those with SLE also have a 2- to 10-fold increase in stroke and myocardial infarction as well as death compared with others of the same age.[24,26] One study found that those with SLE have elevated risks of CVD that are well beyond those captured by Framingham Scoring metrics.[24]

BREAST CANCER

According to the Centers for Disease Control and Prevention, breast cancer is the second most common cancer among women in the United States. Many who now survive owing to improved screening, surveillance, and treatment develop CVD from chemotherapy and radiation.[18] Studies have shown that women receiving radiation to the left breast developed coronary artery disease (CAD) at higher rates than those receiving radiation to the right breast.[18,27] Furthermore, the risk of CAD increased by 7.8% for every increase in Gray delivered.[18,27] Women may also develop valvular disease as well as cardiomyopathies from radiation.[18] Anthracycline-based chemotherapy is also implicated in the development of cardiomyopathies. Experts recommend surveillance for cardiomyopathy with an echocardiogram (ECHO) every 2 years for asymptomatic patients, and for valvular disease within 10 years of radiation and repeated in 5-year intervals. For CAD, they recommend noninvasive stress testing within 10 years of radiation and repeated in 5-year intervals.[28]

POLYCYSTIC OVARY SYNDROME

Polycystic ovary syndrome (PCOS) is defined by oligomenorrhea, infertility, acne, and hirsutism with polycystic ovaries. Although patients with PCOS have been shown to have a higher risk for other CVD risk factors, including hypertension, a negative lipid profile, obesity, and insulin resistance, it has not been shown to be an independent risk factor for CVD, especially in postmenopausal women.[29,30]

MENOPAUSE

Menopause is an inevitable transition that every woman who lives long enough will experience. Menopause confers an independent risk factor for CVD apart from the normal aging process.[31] The SWAN study demonstrated that within 1 year of the last menstrual period, total cholesterol, low-density lipoprotein (LDL), and apolipoprotein B levels all increased independent of ethnicity, weight, or age.[31] Early menopause has also been associated with increased risk for CVD, which has been postulated to be secondary to a drop in estrogen.[32] Large-scale trials (Women's Health Initiative and Heart and Estrogen-Progestin Replacement Study) looking at whether hormone replacement improved cardiovascular health in postmenopausal women failed to demonstrate a positive correlation.[32–34] This has led some to question whether early menopause confers an increased CVD risk or whether those with an increased risk for CVD have earlier menopause.[32] In either case, menopause and the age at which it occurs can lend important information regarding the possible risk of CVD in a woman.

TRADITIONAL RISK FACTORS

In addition to the gender-specific risk factors that all women should be asked about, traditional risk factors are common and require attention, especially as there are ample data that show women are underdiagnosed and undertreated.[35]

DIABETES

Approximately 13.4 million women in the United States have diabetes, and this appears to be a greater risk factor for the development of CVD in women as compared with men. In 1 study, women with diabetes type 2 had a higher adjusted hazard ratio (HR) of fatal CAD (HR = 14.74; 95% confidence interval [CI], 6.16–35.27) compared with men with diabetes (HR = 3.77; 95% CI, 2.52–5.65).[18,36] In another study, the relative risk for CVD in those with diabetes was 44% greater in women as compared with men.[18,37] The theory behind the gender discrepancy is that diabetes in women leads to greater hypercoagulability, dyslipidemia, and metabolic syndrome.[18]

SMOKING AND OBESITY

Although fewer adult women (15%) than men (19%) smoke, women over the age of 44 who smoke had a 25% increased risk for CVD compared with men.[18,38] Likewise, obesity has a greater impact on the development of CVD in women as compared with men, as demonstrated in the Framingham Heart Study, where the relative risk of CVD was increased by 64% in women, as opposed to 46% in men.[18,39]

HYPERLIPIDEMIA

Dyslipidemia confers the greatest risk for CVD compared with all other risk factors, which only becomes apparent after menopause even if levels are elevated before.[18] Statins are recommended for both men and women; however, the benefit of primary prevention in women is still unclear.[18] Despite the evidence for the benefit of statins, women continue to be prescribed these drugs less frequently than men for unknown reasons and demonstrate the need for physicians to be more vigilant in discovering and preventing CVD.[18]

HYPERTENSION

In women, hypertension develops on average 10 years later than men, as estrogen serves as an antihypertensive via vasodilation.[18] The incidence of hypertension is more in elderly women than elderly men.[18] Antihypertensive medications are recommended for a goal of systolic blood pressure less than 130 mm Hg.

Metabolic syndrome as defined by the National Cholesterol Education Program Adult Treatment Panel III is having 3 of the following 5 traits: elevated glucose, elevated blood pressure, low high-density lipoprotein (HDL), high triglycerides, and an increased waist circumference.[40] Although equally common in both men and women, African American and Mexican American women have twice the prevalence as compared with men.[41] The presence of metabolic syndrome is associated with a significant increase in the relative risk of developing CVD, as well as an increased mortality and thus requires early identification and aggressive treatment.[42] HIV is another disease that is associated with an increased risk for CVD because of a cascade of events that lead to increased inflammation and coagulation disorders. In addition, antiretrovirals have side effects similar to metabolic syndrome, including insulin resistance, dyslipidemia, and endothelial dysfunction.[43]

The foundation of preventing CVD begins with an assessment of the individual's personal risk for development of CVD. There are numerous tools available to the clinician to make that assessment. Perhaps the most well known is the Framingham Risk Score, first published in 1998, developed from the landmark Framingham Heart Study and last revised in 2008. This model incorporates well-known easily obtained information and laboratory test values and is gender specific. The variables include age, total cholesterol, smoking status, HDL cholesterol, and systolic blood pressure. The Reynolds Risk Score calculator is another simple system used to calculate CVD risk over 10 years. It adds CRP and family history to the algorithm, and it also shows how modifying these factors can reduce the risk of future CVD. The AHA recommends using a pooled risk assessment tool available at http://tools.acc.org/ASCVD-Risk-Estimator-plus, every three to five years.

The AHA guidelines for primary prevention of CVD aligns risk as follows, based on atherosclerotic risk factor estimators: low risk is less than 5%; borderline risk is 5% to less than 7.5%; intermediate risk is 7.5% to less than 20%; and greater than 20% is identified as being at high risk. These assessments should be used to engage the patient in discussions regarding risk-factor modification and mitigation. As clinicians, the goal is to match the intensity of the therapy with the absolute risk to the patient.

Once risk has been estimated, appropriate efforts should be made with a patient-centered approach, to lower the risk of development or progression of CVD. The

2019 American College of Cardiology (ACC)/AHA guidelines state that initial recommendations for risk reduction begin with following a diet high in vegetables, fruit, whole grains, and fish, along with reduction in saturated fats and cholesterol. Second, there is ample evidence to support encouragement of regular exercise and other types of physical activity, of at least 150 minutes per week. If the person is overweight or obese, then weight loss, especially if diabetic, is a critical nonpharmacologic intervention. Smoking cessation is an equally important recommendation, and it has been suggested that tobacco status should be treated as a vital sign.[1] Once these behavioral risk modifications have been initiated, if blood pressure and cholesterol remain uncontrolled (blood pressure >130/90 mm Hg and CVD risk >7.5%), then there is class 1a support for initiation of medical therapy. Current guidelines suggest that patients with CVD risk greater than 7.5% and less than 20% who choose to start medication should aim for a 30% reduction in LDL levels. In women at high risk (>20%), an early conversation about initiation of high-intensity statins is indicated. Patients with diabetes should be started on a moderate-intensity statin regardless of risk. For women with hypertension, despite adoption of appropriate lifestyle modification and CVD risk more than 10%, it is recommended in the ACC/AHA guidelines that treatment with blood pressure–lowering medication is indicated. Unfortunately, women have historically been undertreated with both antihypertensive and lipid-lowering medications. In 2010, it was reported that the proportion of women receiving lipid-lowering medication was 5.7% versus 7.3% in men.[44] Although aspirin use is supported by numerous randomized clinical trials for secondary prevention of myocardial infarction, its use in primary prevention in women remains controversial. It is not recommended that adults over the age of 70 take primary-prevention aspirin, as this group has an elevated bleeding risk. In response to several recent trials of primary-prevention low-dose aspirin in adults with high CVD risk, the use of 81-mg aspirin is now a class 2b recommendation.[45]

TESTING

For those patients who need diagnostic testing, either for symptoms or for enhanced risk stratification, there are numerous diagnostic strategies available. Some have better sensitivity and specificity in women than others, and there are pros and cons to all of them. Decisions regarding what testing or imaging to pursue will depend on the age of the patient, the desire to avoid ionizing radiation exposure, and the differential diagnosis under consideration. All patients regardless of gender should have a baseline 12-lead electrocardiogram (ECG) obtained at the time of initial evaluation. Although a full discussion of the ECG and CVD is beyond the scope of this article, the ECG is critical for guiding the next step in evaluating a patients' symptoms (after history and physical examination).

EXERCISE TREADMILL STRESS TEST

Exercise stress testing is the oldest and first-line diagnostic tool for the evaluation of ischemic heart disease. The ACC/AHA 2002 guidelines recommend exercise stress test with ECG as the initial noninvasive test for symptomatic, intermediate-risk women with a normal baseline ECG who are able to exercise.[46] ECG stress testing has excellent negative predictive value; however, positive results are less diagnostic in women. In 1 study, it was found that the positive predictive value in women as compared with men was 47% versus 77%, respectively.[47] There are gender differences in ST segment changes during exercise, which have been hypothesized to be due to more baseline ST-T segment changes in women, greater ST depressions, and estrogen, causing digitalis-like changes.[48,49] It has also been shown that postmenopausal women on estrogen replacement therapy have greater ST segment depressions than other women, thus affecting results.[50-52] Therefore, ST segment changes, although helpful for diagnostic purposes, have less prognostic value in regards to cardiovascular mortality in women.[49,52] In addition to informing about ischemic disease, exercise stress testing also gives prognostic information regarding functional capacity, chronotropic and blood pressure response, and heart rate recovery and thus remains a useful tool.[49,53]

ECHOCARDIOGRAM

Stress echocardiography is often used when there are baseline ECG changes, inability to exercise, and nondiagnostic ECG stress tests.[53] Adding imaging to stress testing results in increased sensitivity in the hands of experienced sonographers and cardiologists.[54] The level of sensitivity, however, has been shown to be different among men and women. In the Women's Ischemia Syndrome Evaluation study, dobutamine stress echo (DSE) was shown to have a sensitivity of about 40%.[55] One reason is that DSE has a lower sensitivity in identifying single-vessel disease, and women tend to have more single-vessel disease than men.[56] Nonetheless, stress ECHO still remains an excellent option for stress testing, given the lack of radiation, high negative predictive value, and ability to assess ventricular and valvular function.

MYOCARDIAL PERFUSION IMAGING

Like ECHO, myocardial perfusion imaging (MPI) with either single-photon emission computed tomography (SPECT) or PET, is another method of imaging used in stress testing that has a higher sensitivity than exercise stress test.[53] Despite breast attenuation lowering specificity of MPI with SPECT to 74% in women as compared with 94% in men, it still remains an important tool with a sensitivity of about 81%.[53] PET offers even more sensitivity and specificity even in obese patients.[53] PET also offers the ability to better detect severe multivessel disease that may be missed on SPECT because of balanced ischemia.[53] As with computed tomography (CT), MPI carries the risk of radiation and is important to consider in women when choosing a modality of stress imaging.

CARDIAC MRI

Cardiac MRI is the newest imaging technique in cardiology. It is used for its ability to combine high-quality images to evaluate both cardiac structure and function. It is also preferred for women in the premenopausal stage of life and is safe for pregnant women because of its lack of ionizing radiation.[55,57] Unfortunately, the available literature is lacking regarding female-specific reference values and diseases. Several publications have shown that women in general have smaller absolute and indexed right and left mass and volume.[58] There are also several disease states that primarily affect women and for which MRI functions as an important tool for diagnosis and prognostication for diseases like nonischemic heart failure and SLE.[58]

Another area for which cardiac MRI is an emerging and important diagnostic tool is diagnosing myocardial infarction with nonobstructive coronary artery disease. In a systematic review, it was found that in women presenting with a myocardial infarction, 43% had nonobstructive disease versus 24% of women who had obstructive coronary disease.[59] In those with elevated troponins, but nonobstructive disease, cardiac MRI was able to identify the cause in 74% to 87% of patients.[60,61] Diagnosis is important, as it informs prognosis.[61] Although the incidence of obstructive disease increases with age (approximately 48% of women between the ages of 55 and 64 years, 65% of women between the ages of 65 and 74 years, and 79% of women ≥75 years), women's diagnosis is often missed or delayed, leading to excess morbidity and mortality as compared with men.[62] Not only are women more likely to present with atypical features but also traditional methods of diagnosing CAD are oftentimes less sensitive in women.[62] In addition, many women have microvascular disease that will not be picked up with traditional stress testing and for which stress cardiac MRI can be useful.[58,62] Cardiac MRI demonstrated subendocardial hypoperfusion in women with nonobstructive disease presenting with symptoms.[63] The AHA recommends cardiac MRI in symptomatic women with intermediate risk of CAD and resting ST-segment abnormalities or inability to exercise.[54]

For women who require serial monitoring of cardiac function after cardiotoxic therapy, ECHO is the recommended modality. However, this can be problematic, as the ejection fraction (EF) estimation with transthoracic ECHO is reader dependent, and changes as small as 10% in ejection fraction may result in yearly cardiac evaluation after completion of therapy.[64] One study found that as compared with TTE, cardiac MRI was able to capture more patients with an EF less than 50%.[65] Furthermore, TTE may be difficult to do as frequently in women who have completed surgery because of pain.[58]

CARDIAC COMPUTED TOMOGRAPHY

Cardiac CT, both coronary artery calcium (CAC) and coronary CT angiography (CCTA), are noninvasive methods to detect CAD. In 2018, the ACC/AHA Cholesterol Guidelines suggested that "coronary artery calcium (CAC) testing may be considered in adults 40-75 years of age without diabetes mellitus and with LDL-C levels ≥70 mg/dl-189 mg/dl at a 10-year atherosclerotic cardiovascular disease (ASCVD) risk of ≥7.5% to <20% (i.e., intermediate risk group) if a decision about statin therapy is uncertain."[66,67] If CAC is ≥1, statin therapy is recommended especially in those ≥55 years of age.

For symptomatic, intermediate-risk patients, CCTA is often a good alternative for those with poor exercise capacity, baseline ECG abnormalities, or an intermediate-risk stress test.[53] In referring patients for these tests, be aware that a slower heart rate can help with obtaining better images, and patients should have normal renal function, as the test requires administration of contrast. Radiation, especially the cumulative risk, is a growing concern within medicine and specifically in cardiology. One study estimated that the absolute risk for cancer from 1 CCTA was 0.35% (1 in 284) for a 40-year-old woman, 0.22% (1 in 466) for a 60-year-old woman, and 0.075% (1 in 1338) for an 80-year-old woman.[67] One possible obstacle for CT imaging in women is the poor image quality of mid to distal segments of the coronaries because of smaller-caliber vessels.[68] In the ACCURACY (Assessment by Coronary Computed Tomographic Angiography of Individuals Undergoing Invasive Coronary Angiography) trial, CCTA was found to have a sensitivity of 90% and specificity of 88% in women and thus did not differ in its diagnostic accuracy between men and women, rendering it a great tool for the evaluation of ischemic heart disease in women.[69]

THERAPEUTICS

Improvements in clinical outcomes in women with CVD have lagged those metrics in men.[70] There are many reasons for this disturbing trend, which includes women underreporting their symptoms and not seeking necessary health care, health care providers underestimating a woman's risk of heart disease and misdiagnosing symptoms as noncardiac, and the lack of women in clinical trials. In fact, a recent report from AHA noted that women's awareness that CVD is the leading cause of death has declined over the decade from 2009 to 2019, especially among women of color and in younger women.[71,72]

In the United States, acute coronary syndrome (ACS) affects more than 250,000 women per year.[70] More women will present with non-ST elevation myocardial infarction than men and are more likely to have unusual manifestations of heart disease, such as spontaneous coronary artery dissection and Takatsubo cardiomyopathy.[70] Women are also older than men at the first presentation (71.8 years old as compared with men at 65 years of age).[70]

There are many reasons women have a poorer prognosis than men. In general, women present for evaluation of symptoms less often than men and with greater delay. Several studies have shown that women with ACS present up to 2 days later than men with similar symptoms. Symptoms of acute myocardial ischemia/infarction can be different in women as compared with men. The classic complaint of squeezing substernal chest pressure, radiating to the arm and jaw may be present, but women often will present with more "atypical" symptoms. These symptoms may include marked fatigue, shortness of breath, nausea, palpitations, anxiety, and dizziness. Women may have more frequent complaints of shoulder and arm pain as compared with men. The combination of unusual symptoms and delay in presentation for evaluation may contribute to the undertreatment of women.

There are no gender-specific guidelines for the treatment of ACS, and as such, women should receive the same guideline-directed therapy as men, as reflected in the AHA/ACC ACS guidelines. Lytic therapy is indicated for patients without timely access to percutaneous intervention, but women have a higher likelihood of complications. This higher likelihood of complications may be due in part to their higher frequency of comorbidities, including older age at presentation. Early studies of lytic-based reperfusion strategies showed that women had higher rates of bleeding complications, both peripheral and intracranial, as well as heart failure and shock. Subsequent trials of PCI showed improvement in outcomes for women as compared with lytic therapy.[73] In fact, several studies have confirmed that women with high-risk features in general fare better with an invasive strategy of percutaneous coronary intervention (PCI) for non-STEMI, as compared with a noninvasive strategy. In 2013, Stefanini and colleagues[74] performed a pooled analysis of 12 trials that included women, with a primary safety endpoint of death or myocardial infarction in patients who received drug-eluting stents (DES). When compared with bare metal stents and early-generation DES, women who received DES had better outcomes. Although they did not report on the outcomes in the male patients, the outcomes for women compare favorably with that reported for men who receive DES. Despite this and other similar reports, the AHA Scientific Statement on Acute Myocardial Infarction in women in 2016 still reports that women are less likely to receive appropriate intervention for ACS and are less likely to be discharged on evidence-based medication for established coronary disease.[70]

Early reviews of coronary artery bypass grafting (CABG) from the landmark CASS study (Coronary Artery Surgery Study) reported in 1982 showed marked difference in mortality between men and women. In men, operative mortality was 1.9%, and in women, operative mortality was 4.5%. In part, this was attributed to the smaller stature of women.[75] Two decades later, in a cohort study of more than 68,000 patients of which 15,000 were women, data again showed that women were older, were more often operated on urgently, and were less likely to receive arterial bypass grafts.[76]

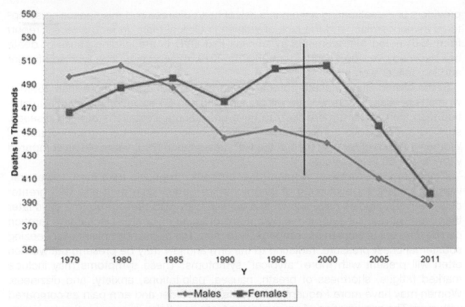

Fig. 2. CVD mortality trends for men and women in the United States from 1979 to 2011. *Reprinted with permission from* Mehta LS, Beckie TM, DeVon HA, et al. Acute Myocardial Infarction in Women: A Scientific Statement From the American Heart Association. Circulation. 2016;133(9):916-947. https://doi.org/10.1161/CIR.0000000000000351 ©2015 American Heart Association, Inc.

Others have reported that although women under 50 years of age may have higher adverse outcomes from CABG, the gender difference is reduced in older women as compared with men. Better use of arterial grafting and better attention to postoperative care may yield improved outcomes in women undergoing bypass surgery.[77]

SUMMARY

After decades of progress in the diagnosis, treatment, and prevention of CVD, women are starting to receive the attention they deserve (**Fig. 2**) Recognition of gender-specific risk factors in addition to traditional risks, variable symptom profiles, and improved outcomes with guideline-directed medical therapy are slowly improving the outlook for women's health and quality of life. Although much ground has been broken, there remains more work to be done to improve the lives of women with CVD.

CLINICS CARE POINTS

- Cardiovascular disease is the leading cause of death in women in the United States.

- Traditional risk factors portend a higher risk for the development of cardiovascular diseasein women as compared with men and thus should be aggressively prevented and treated.

- Pregnancy-related complications are common and carry an increased risk for the development of cardiovascular disease. Although traditional risk calculators do not include them in scoring, every clinician should be incorporating these elements of a patient's history into their medical decisions.

- Testing for ischemic disease is the same for men and women; however, the ordering provider should be aware of certain limitations that are unique to women and how this will impact the results and plan of care.

- There are no gender-specific guidelines or treatments, yet women continue to be underdiagnosed and undertreated, and efforts should be made to make sure therapies, including statins and PCI, are done appropriately and timely.

REFERENCES

1. Arnett DK, Blumenthal RS, Albert MA, et al. 2019 ACC/AHA guideline on the primary prevention of cardiovascular disease: executive summary: a report of the American College of Cardiology/American Heart Association Task Force on Clinical Practice Guidelines. J Am Coll Cardiol 2019;74(10):1376.
2. Mosca L, Appel LJ, Benjamin EJ, et al. Evidence-based guidelines for cardiovascular disease prevention in women. J Am Coll Cardiol 2004;43(5):900–21.
3. Benjamin EJ, Muntner P, et al. Heart disease and stroke statistics-2019 update. A report from the American Heart Association. Circulation 2019.
4. Lloyd-Jones DM, Larson MG, Beiser A, et al. Lifetime risk of developing coronary heart disease. Lancet 1999;353(9147):89.
5. Golomb BA, Dang TT, Criqui MH. Peripheral arterial disease: morbidity and mortality implications. Circulation 2006;114(7):688–99.
6. Kallikazaros I, Tsioufis C, Sideris S, et al. Carotid artery disease as a marker for the presence of severe coronary artery disease in patients evaluated for chest pain. Stroke 1999;30(5):1002–7.
7. Lloyd-Jones D, Adams R, Carnethon M, et al. Heart disease and stroke statistics–2009 update: a report from the American Heart Association Statistics Committee and Stroke Statistics Subcommittee. Circulation 2009;119(3):e21–181.
8. Rana S, Lemoine E, Granger JP, et al. Preeclampsia: pathophysiology, challenges, and perspectives. Circ Res 2019;124(7):1094–112.
9. Wallis AB, Saftlas AF, Hsia J, et al. Secular trends in the rates of preeclampsia, eclampsia, and gestational hypertension, United States, 1987-2004. Am J Hypertens 2008;21(5):521–6.
10. Powe CE, Levine RJ, Karumanchi SA. Preeclampsia, a disease of the maternal endothelium: the role of antiangiogenic factors and implications for later cardiovascular disease. Circulation 2011;123(24):2856–69.
11. Chambers JC, Fusi L, Malik IS, et al. Association of maternal endothelial dysfunction with preeclampsia. JAMA 2001;285(12):1607–12.
12. Saxena AR, Karumanchi SA, Brown NJ, et al. Increased sensitivity to angiotensin II is present postpartum in women with a history of hypertensive pregnancy. Hypertension 2010;55(5):1239–45.
13. Bellamy L, Casas JP, Hingorani AD, et al. Pre-eclampsia and risk of cardiovascular disease and cancer in later life: systematic review and meta-analysis. BMJ 2007;335(7627):974.
14. Ray JG, Vermeulen MJ, Schull MJ, et al. Cardiovascular health after maternal placental syndromes (CHAMPS): population-based retrospective cohort study. Lancet 2005;366(9499):1797–803.
15. Lykke JA, Langhoff-Roos J, Sibai BM, et al. Hypertensive pregnancy disorders and subsequent cardiovascular morbidity and type 2 diabetes mellitus in the mother. Hypertension 2009;53(6):944–51.

16. Hubel CA, Powers RW, Snaedal S, et al. C-reactive protein is elevated 30 years after eclamptic pregnancy. Hypertension 2008;51(6):1499–505.
17. Wolf M, Kettyle E, Sandler L, et al. Obesity and preeclampsia: the potential role of inflammation. Obstet Gynecol 2001;98(5 Pt 1):757–62.
18. Garcia M, Mulvagh SL, Merz CN, et al. Cardiovascular disease in women: clinical perspectives. Circ Res 2016;118(8):1273–93.
19. Bellamy L, Casas JP, Hingorani AD, et al. Type 2 diabetes mellitus after gestational diabetes: a systematic review and meta-analysis. Lancet 2009;373(9677): 1773–9.
20. Vrachnis N, Augoulea A, Iliodromiti Z, et al. Previous gestational diabetes mellitus and markers of cardiovascular risk. Int J Endocrinol 2012;2012:458610.
21. Chakravarty EF, Bush TM, Manzi S, et al. Prevalence of adult systemic lupus erythematosus in California and Pennsylvania in 2000: estimates obtained using hospitalization data. Arthritis Rheum 2007;56(6):2092–4.
22. Cunningham MA, Richard ML, Wirth JR, et al. Novel mechanism for estrogen receptor alpha modulation of murine lupus. J Autoimmun 2019;97:59–69.
23. Willerson J, Ridker P. Inflammation as a cardiovascular risk factor. Circulation 2004; 109. https://doi.org/10.1161/01.CIR.0000129535.04194.38Circulation. II-2–II-10.
24. Esdaile JM, Abrahamowicz M, Grodzicky T, et al. Traditional Framingham risk factors fail to fully account for accelerated atherosclerosis in systemic lupus erythematosus. Arthritis Rheum 2001;44(10):2331–7.
25. Casey KA, Smith MA, Sinibaldi D, et al. Modulation of cardiometabolic disease markers by type I interferon inhibition in systemic lupus erythematosus. Arthritis Rheumatol 2021;73(3):459–71.
26. Yazdany J, Pooley N, Langham J, et al. Systemic lupus erythematosus; stroke and myocardial infarction risk: a systematic review and meta-analysis RMD. Open 2020;6:e001247.
27. Darby SC, Ewertz M, McGale P, et al. Risk of ischemic heart disease in women after radiotherapy for breast cancer. N Engl J Med 2013;368:987–98.
28. Lancellotti P, Nkomo VT, Badano LP, et al. Expert consensus for multi-modality imaging evaluation of cardiovascular complications of radiotherapy in adults: a report from the European Association of Cardiovascular Imaging and the American Society of Echocardiography. J Am Soc Echocardiogr 2013;26:1013–32.
29. Schmidt J, Landin-Wilhelmsen K, Brännström M, et al. Cardiovascular disease and risk factors in PCOS women of postmenopausal age: a 21-year controlled follow-up study. J Clin Endocrinol Metab 2011;96(12):3794–803.
30. Wild S, et al. Cardiovascular disease in women with polycystic ovary syndrome at long-term follow-up: a retrospective cohort study. Clin Endocrinol 2000;52: 595±600.
31. Matthews K, Crawford SL, Chae CU, et al. Are changes in cardiovascular disease risk factors in midlife women due to chronological aging or to the menopausal transition? J Am Coll Cardiol 2009;54(25):2366–73.
32. Kok H, van Asselt KM, van der Schouw YT, et al. Heart disease risk determines menopausal age rather than the reverse. J Am Coll Cardiol 2006;47(10):1976–83.
33. Hulley S, Grady D, Bush T, et al. Randomized trial of estrogen plus progestin for secondary prevention of coronary heart disease in postmenopausal women. Heart and Estrogen/Progestin Replacement Study (HERS) Research Group. JAMA 1998;280:605–13. 10.
34. Rossouw JE, Anderson GL, Prentice RL, et al. Risks and benefits of estrogen plus progestin in healthy postmenopausal women: principal results from the Women's Health Initiative randomized controlled trial. JAMA 2002;288(3):321–33.

35. Wengner N. Women and coronary heart disease: a century after Herrick; understudied, underdiagnosed, and undertreated. Circulation 2011;124:A612.
36. Juutilainen A, Kortelainen S, Lehto S, et al. Gender difference in the impact of type 2 diabetes on coronary heart disease risk. Diabetes Care 2004;27: 2898–904.
37. Huxley R, Barzi F, Woodward M. Excess risk of fatal coronary heart disease associated with diabetes in men and women: meta-analysis of 37 prospective cohort studies. Bmj 2006;332:73–8.
38. Huxley RR, Woodward M. Cigarette smoking as a risk factor for coronary heart disease in women compared with men: a systematic review and meta-analysis of prospective cohort studies. Lancet 2011;378:1297–305.
39. Wilson PW, D'Agostino RB, Sullivan L, et al. Overweight and obesity as determinants of cardiovascular risk: the Framingham experience. Arch Intern Med 2002; 162:1867–72.
40. Executive summary of the third report of the National Cholesterol Education Program (NCEP) expert panel on detection, evaluation, and treatment of high blood cholesterol in adults (Adult Treatment Panel III). JAMA 2001;285:2486–97.
41. Ford ES, Giles WH, Dietz WH, et al. Prevalence of the metabolic syndrome among US adults: findings from the third National Health and Nutrition Examination Survey. JAMA 2002;287:356–9.
42. Wilson PW, D'Agostino RB, Parise H, et al. Metabolic syndrome as a precursor of cardiovascular disease and type 2 diabetes mellitus. Circulation 2005;112(20): 3066–72.
43. Vachiat A, McCutcheon K, Tsabedze N, et al. HIV and ischemic heart disease. J Am Coll Cardiol 2017;69(1):73–82.
44. Koopman C, Vaartjes I, Heintjes, et al. Persisting gender differences and attenuating age differences in cardiovascular drug use for prevention and treatment of coronary heart disease, 1998-2010. Eur Heart J 2013;34:3198–205.
45. McNeil JJ, Woods RL, Tonkin AM, et al. Effect of aspirin on cardiovascular events and bleeding in the healthy elderly. N Engl J Med 2018;379:16.
46. Gibbons RJ, Balady GJ, Bricker JT, et al. Smith SCACC/AHA 2002 guideline update for exercise testing: summary article: a report of the American College of Cardiology/American Heart Association Task Force on Practice guidelines (committee to update the 1997 exercise testing guidelines). Circulation 2002;106: 1883–92.
47. Barolsky SM, Gilbert CA, Faruqui A, et al. Differences in electrocardiographic response to exercise of women and men: a non-Bayesian factor. Circulation 1979;60:1021–7.
48. Kohli P, Gulati M. Exercise stress testing in women: going back to the basics. Circulation 2010;122(24):2570–80.
49. Weiner DA, Ryan TJ, McCabe CH, et al. Exercise stress testing: correlations among history of angina, ST-segment response and prevalence of coronary-artery disease in the Coronary Artery Surgery Study (CASS). N Engl J Med 1979;301:230–5.
50. Morise AP, Beto R. The specificity of exercise electrocardiography in women grouped by estrogen status. Int J Cardiol 1997;60:55–65.
51. Henzlova MJ, Croft LB, Diamond JA. Effect of hormone replacement therapy on the electrocardiographic response to exercise. J Nucl Cardiol 2002;9(4):385–7.
52. Gulati M, Pandey DK, Arnsdorf MF, et al. Exercise capacity and the risk of death in women: the St James Women Take Heart Project. Circulation 2003;108:1554–9.

53. Mieres JH, Gulati M, Bairey Merz N, et al, American Heart Association Cardiac Imaging Committee of the Council on Clinical Cardiology; Cardiovascular Imaging and Intervention Committee of the Council on Cardiovascular Radiology and Intervention. Role of noninvasive testing in the clinical evaluation of women with suspected ischemic heart disease: a consensus statement from the American Heart Association. Circulation 2014;130(4):350–79 [Erratum in: Circulation. 2014;130(4):e86].

54. Picano E, Lattanzi F, Orlandini A, et al. Stress echocardiography and the human factor: the importance of being expert. J Am Coll Cardiol 1991;17(3):666–9.

55. Expert Panel on MRS, Kanal E, Barkovich AJ, et al. ACR guidance document on MR safe practices: 2013. J Magn Reson Imaging 2013;37:501–30, 183.

56. Lewis JF, Lin L, McGorray S, et al. Dobutamine stress echocardiography in women with chest pain. Pilot phase data from the National Heart, Lung and Blood Institute Women's Ischemia Syndrome Evaluation (WISE). J Am Coll Cardiol 1999; 33(6):1462–8.

57. Ray JG, Vermeulen MJ, Bharatha A, et al. Association between MRI exposure during pregnancy and fetal and childhood outcomes. JAMA 2016;316:952–61.

58. Bucciarelli-Ducci C, Ostenfeld E, Baldassarre LA, et al. Cardiovascular disease in women: insights from magnetic resonance imaging. J Cardiovasc Magn Reson 2020;22:71.

59. Pasupathy S, Air T, Dreyer RP, et al. Systematic review of patients presenting with suspected myocardial infarction and nonobstructive coronary arteries. Circulation 2015;131:861–70.

60. Pathik B, Raman B, Mohd Amin NH, et al. Troponin-positive chest pain with unobstructed coronary arteries: incremental diagnostic value of cardiovascular magnetic resonance imaging. Eur Heart J Cardiovasc Imaging 2016;17(10):1146–52.

61. Dastidar AG, Baritussio A, De Garate E, et al. Prognostic role of CMR and conventional risk factors in myocardial infarction with nonobstructed coronary arteries. JACC Cardiovasc Imaging 2019;12(10):1973–82.

62. Bairey Merz CN, Shaw LJ, Reis SE, et al, WISE Investigators. Insights from the NHLBI-Sponsored Women's Ischemia Syndrome Evaluation (WISE) Study: part II: gender differences in presentation, diagnosis, and outcome with regard to gender-based pathophysiology of atherosclerosis and macrovascular and microvascular coronary disease. J Am Coll Cardiol 2006;47(3 Suppl):S21–9.

63. Panting JR, Gatehouse PD, Yang GZ, et al. Abnormal subendocardial perfusion in cardiac syndrome X detected by cardiovascular magnetic resonance imaging. N Engl J Med 2002;346:1948–53.

64. Mackey JR, Clemons M, Côté MA, et al. Cardiac management during adjuvant trastuzumab therapy: recommendations of the Canadian Trastuzumab Working Group. Curr Oncol 2008;15(1):24–35.

65. Armstrong GT, Plana JC, Zhang N, et al. Screening adult survivors of childhood cancer for cardiomyopathy: comparison of echocardiography and cardiac magnetic resonance imaging. J Clin Oncol 2012;30(23):2876–84.

66. Grundy SM, Stone NJ, Bailey AL, et al. 2018 AHA/ACC/AACVPR/AAPA/ABC/ACPM/ADA/AGS/APhA/ASPC/NLA guideline on the management of blood cholesterol: a report of the American College of Cardiology/American Heart Association Task Force on Practice guidelines. J Am Coll Cardiol 2019;73(24):3234–7.

67. Einstein AJ, Henzlova MJ, Rajagopalan S. Estimating risk of cancer associated with radiation exposure from 64-slice computed tomography coronary angiography. JAMA 2007;298(3):317–23.

68. Pampolano M. Imaging of heart disease in women: an updated review. ACC 2018.
69. Tsang JC, Min JK, Lin FY, et al. Sex comparison of diagnostic accuracy of 64-multidetector row coronary computed tomographic angiography: results from the multicenter ACCURACY trial. J Cardiovasc Comput Tomogr 2012;6:246–51.
70. Mehta LS, Beckie TM, DeVon HA, et al. Acute myocardial infarction in women. Circulation 2016;133:916–47.
71. Cushman M, Shay CM, Howard VJ, et al. Ten-year differences in women's awareness related to coronary heart disease: results of the 2019 American Heart Association National Survey. Circulation 2020;142:e1–10.
72. Mozaffarian D, Benjamin EJ, Go AS, et al. Heart disease and stroke statistics—2015 update. A report from the American Heart Association. Circulation 2015; 131(4):e29–322.
73. Boersma E, the PCAT Group. Does time matter? A pooled analysis of randomized clinical trials comparing primary PCI and in hospital fibrinolysis in acute myocardial infarction patients. Eur Heart J 2006;27:779–88.
74. Stefanini GG, Baber U, Windecker S, et al. Safety and efficacy of drug-eluting stents in women: a patient-level pooled analysis of randomised trials. Lancet 2013;382:1879–88.
75. Fisher L, Kennedy J, Davis K, et al. Association of sex, physical size, and operative mortality after CABG in the Coronary Artery Surgery Study (CASS). J Thorac Cardiovasc Surg 1982;84:334–41.
76. Guru V, Fremes S, Tu J. Time-related mortality for women after CABG surgery: a population-based study. J Thorac Cardiovasc Surg 2004;127:1158–65.
77. Nicolini F, Vezzani A, Fortuna D, et al. Gender differences in outcomes following isolated coronary artery bypass grafting: long-term results. J Thorac Cardiothorac Surg 2016;11:144.

Drug Interactions

What Are Important Drug Interactions for the Most Commonly Used Medications in Preventive Cardiology?

Aziz Hammoud, MD[a], Michael D. Shapiro, DO, MCR[a,b,c,*]

KEYWORDS

- Drug interactions • Preventive cardiology • Statins

KEY POINTS

- Drug interactions are a major concern in preventive cardiology because of the widespread use of statins.
- Clinically significant statin interactions are predictable and preventable with an understanding of statin pharmacokinetics and how they differ from statin to statin.
- Novel lipid-lowering therapies, such as proprotein convertase subtilisin/kexin type 9 inhibition with monoclonal antibodies or small interfering RNAs, have favorable drug interaction profiles.

INTRODUCTION

Drug interactions are defined as 2 or more substances that interact in such a way that the effectiveness or toxicity of 1 or more substance is modified. Many interactions are theoretic or clinically trivial; however, some may have serious or life-threatening consequences.[1] They are estimated to cause approximately 2.8% of all hospitalizations annually in the United States, representing more than 245,000 hospitalizations and costing the health care system $1.3 billion.[2] Moreover, the actual incidence of hospitalization secondary to clinically significant drug interactions is likely to be underestimated because medication-related issues are reported more commonly as adverse

This article originally appeared in *Medical Clinics*, Volume 106, Issue 2, March 2022.
[a] Section on Cardiovascular Medicine, Department of Medicine, Wake Forest University School of Medicine, Winston-Salem, NC, USA; [b] Section on Cardiovascular Medicine, Department of Internal Medicine, Wake Forest University School of Medicine, Winston-Salem, NC, USA; [c] Center for Prevention of Cardiovascular Disease, Medical Center Boulevard, Winston Salem, NC 27157, USA
* Corresponding author. Section on Cardiovascular Medicine, Department of Internal Medicine, Wake Forest University School of Medicine, Winston-Salem, NC.
E-mail address: mdshapir@wakehealth.edu

Clinics Collections 13 (2023) 117–127
https://doi.org/10.1016/j.ccol.2023.02.025
2352-7986/23/

drug reactions and often confounded by complex underlying disease states.[3] The aging population, high prevalence of chronic diseases, and polypharmacy are some factors closely associated with potential drug interactions.[4]

Several types of drug interactions exist: drug-drug, drug-food, drug-supplement, and drug-patient.[5] Drug-drug interactions—the focus of this review—can be pharmacokinetic or pharmacodynamic in nature. Pharmacokinetics involve the effects of one drug on the absorption, distribution, metabolism, or excretion of another drug, which can result in changes in serum drug concentrations and clinical response.[6] Pharmacokinetic drug interactions frequently involve isoenzymes of the hepatic cytochrome P450 (CYP) system and membrane transporters, such as organic anion transporting polypeptides (OATPs) and P-glycoprotein (P-gp), also known as multidrug resistance-associated protein (MRP) 1. Pharmacodynamics are related to the pharmacologic activity of the interacting drugs, and the outcome is an amplification or decrease in the therapeutic effects or side-effects of a specific drug in an additive, a synergistic, or an antagonistic fashion.[3]

Clinically significant drug interactions usually are preventable. To optimize patient safety, providers should understand the mechanisms, magnitude, and potential consequences of any given drug interaction. This article provides an overview of important drug interactions for commonly used medications in preventive cardiology, with an emphasis on clinically important drug-drug interactions involving conventional lipid-lowering agents.

DISCUSSION
Statin Pharmacology

One in 4 Americans greater than 40 years of age takes a statin to reduce the risk of atherosclerotic cardiovascular disease (ASCVD).[7] Statins reduce hepatic cholesterol synthesis by competitively blocking 3-hydroxy-3-methylglutaryl coenzyme A reductase, thereby leading to increased cell surface low-density lipoprotein (LDL) receptor expression and clearance of LDL-cholesterol (LDL-C) from the bloodstream.[8] The most effective statins produce a mean reduction in LDL-C of 55% to 60% at the maximum dosage.[7] They also may exhibit non–lipid-related pleiotropic effects, including improved endothelial function, atherosclerotic plaque stabilization, anti-inflammatory, immunomodulatory, and antithrombotic effects.[9] They reduce morbidity and mortality in individuals with ASCVD and thus are a mainstay of therapy for these individuals. The 2018 American Heart Association/American College of Cardiology Guideline on the Management of Blood Cholesterol also recommends statins for individuals with diabetes mellitus, individuals with LDL-C greater than or equal to 190 mg/dL, and adults in primary prevention with an estimated 10-year ASCVD risk greater than or equal to 7.5%.[10]

Statin toxicity or intolerance presents most commonly as statin-associated muscle symptoms (SAMs)—muscle aches or pains reported during statin therapy but not necessarily caused by the statin. The incidence of SAMs is 10% to 15% of patients in observational studies, as high as 30% according to clinic data, and 1.5% to 5% in randomized controlled trials, which likely is an underestimation because most studies exclude patients with a history of statin intolerance.[8] Myopathy, defined as unexplained muscle pain or weakness accompanied by increases in creatine kinase above 10 times the upper limit of normal, is the hallmark adverse effect of statins; however, it is rare, occurring in less than 1 in 1000 patients treated with maximum recommended doses and with an even lower risk at lower doses. Approximately 1 in 10,000 patients experience rhabdomyolysis, a severe form of myopathy leading to acute renal failure because of myoglobinuria. Prompt cessation of therapy usually reverses statin myopathy, whose mechanism remains unknown. Hepatotoxicity is also associated with statins in approximately 1% of patients, usually in the form of an asymptomatic and temporary transaminitis without histopathologic changes and inconsistent with true liver injury. Monitoring transaminases is not useful in preventing clinically significant statin hepatotoxicity, which occurs in approximately 0.001% of patients.[7]

The metabolic pathway of statins is summarized in **Fig. 1**. Statin pharmacokinetics are highly dependent on membrane transporters that can be broadly classified into uptake and efflux transporters. Uptake transporters belong to the solute-linked carrier (SLC) superfamily and are responsible for the movement of substrates into cells.[6] In contrast, efflux transporters belong to the adenosine triphosphate–binding cassette (ABC) superfamily and are responsible for the movement of substrates out of cells. Statins enter portal circulation through enterocytes by both passive and active transport via OATP1B3 and OATP1A2.[11] P-gp, breast cancer resistance protein (BCRP), and MRP2 also are expressed on the apical membrane of enterocytes and modulate statin absorption. Enterocyte CYP isoenzymes may metabolize some statins before they are absorbed. OATP1B1 and OATP1B3 are expressed on the basolateral membrane of hepatocytes and are involved in hepatic uptake of statins. In the liver, statins undergo phase I oxidation (mediated by CYP isoenzymes) and phase II glucuronidation (mediated by uridine 5'-diphospho-glucuronosyltransferases [UGT]). The main pathway of elimination is biliary excretion mediated by P-gp, BCRP, and MRP2 expressed on the bile canalicular membrane.

The pharmacokinetic properties of statins are complex, variable from statin to statin, and central in understanding statin interactions (**Table 1**). Except for simvastatin and lovastatin, which are given as prodrugs, all statins are administered in the active hydroxyl acid form.[6] Systemic bioavailability for all statins is considered low, ranging from less than 5% for simvastatin and lovastatin to 51% for pitavastatin. All statins except pravastatin and rosuvastatin are considered lipophilic, and most statins

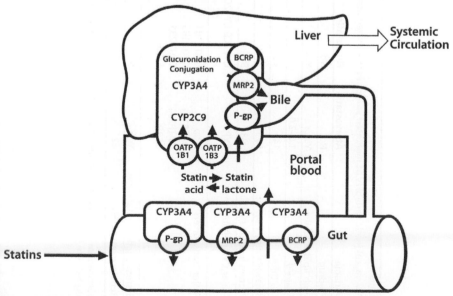

Fig. 1. Metabolic pathway of statins. (*Adapted from* Neuvonen et al.[13])

Table 1
Pharmacokinetic variables of marketed statins in the United States

Variable	Atorvastatin	Fluvastatin	Lovastatin	Pitavastatin	Pravastatin	Rosuvastatin	Simvastatin
Prodrug	No	No	Yes	No	No	No	Yes
High lipid solubility	Yes	Yes	Yes	Yes	No	No	Yes
T_{max} (h)	1.0–2.0	<1.0	2.0–4.0	1.0	1.0–1.5	3.0–5.0	4.0
$T_{1/2}$ (h)	14	<3	2	12	2	19	2
Bioavailability (%)	14	24	<5	51	17	20	<5
Protein binding (%)	>98	98	>95	99	50	88	95
Major CYP metabolism	CYP3A4	CYP2C9 CYP2C8	CYP3A4	CYP2C9 CYP2C8 (minor)	None	CYP2C9 (minor)	CYP3A4
Major transporters	P-gp OATP1B1 OATP2B1 BCRP	OATP1B1 OATP1B3 OATP2B1 BCRP	P-gp OATP1B1 BCRP	P-gp OATP1B1 OATP1B3 OATP2B1 BCRP	OATP1B1 OATP1B3 OATP2B1 BCRP	OATP1B1 OATP1B3 OAT2B1 BCRP NTCP	P-gp OATP1B1
Systemic active metabolites	Yes[2]	No	Yes[4]	No	No	Minimal	Yes[3]
Renal excretion (%)	<2	<6	10	15	20	10	13

Abbreviations: T_{max}, amount of time that a drug is present at the maximum concentration in serum; NTCP, sodium–taurocholate cotransporting polypeptide; $T_{1/2}$, drug half-life.[6]

consequently are highly protein bound. Lipophilic statins require a greater degree of metabolism to convert the statin into water-soluble salts and conjugates that are eliminated from the body. Simvastatin and lovastatin undergo significant CYP3A4 metabolism, and atorvastatin undergoes a lesser amount as one of its minor metabolic pathways. In contrast, fluvastatin, pitavastatin, and rosuvastatin undergo significant CYP2C9 metabolism. Pravastatin is the only statin that does not undergo CYP metabolism. The overall dependence of statin metabolites on renal elimination is modest, with pravastatin the highest at 20% and atorvastatin the lowest at less than 2%.[12]

Clinically Significant Statin-Drug Interactions

Drugs that inhibit the CYP3A4 enzyme can interfere with the metabolism of simvastatin, lovastatin, and, to a lesser extent, atorvastatin. The principal drugs that inhibit CYP3A4 are the azole antifungals ketoconazole and itraconazole (but not fluconazole); the macrolide antibiotics clarithromycin and erythromycin (but not azithromycin); the human immunodeficiency virus protease inhibitors; the antiarrhythmics amiodarone and dronedarone; and the non-dihydropyridine calcium channel blockers diltiazem and verapamil (no effect on atorvastatin).[13,14] Current Food and Drug Administration (FDA) labeling advises that the dose of simvastatin not exceed 10 mg daily and the dose of lovastatin not exceed 20 mg daily when coprescribed with diltiazem or verapamil in adults (**Table 2**).[3] Similarly, the FDA-approved product labeling for amlodipine, a substrate of CYP3A4, indicates that there may be an increased risk of muscle-related toxicity when combined with simvastatin and recommends a dose limit of 20 mg daily when coprescribed. Furthermore, FDA labeling recommends a dose limit of simvastatin, 20 mg daily, and of lovastatin, 40 mg daily, when coprescribed with amiodarone and a dose limit of simvastatin, 10 mg daily, and lovastatin, 20 mg daily, when coprescribed with dronedarone.[3]

Some drugs that inhibit CYP2C9 are azole antifungals, omeprazole, cimetidine, and tolbutamide. Although these drugs theoretically may interact with fluvastatin, few clinically important fluvastatin interactions have been reported. The most significant fluvastatin interaction occurs with fluconazole, and prescribing information for fluvastatin advises a dose limit of 20 mg daily when used with fluconazole. This caution does not extend to pitavastatin, which also relies on CYP2C9 metabolism. CYP2C9 plays an important role in the metabolism of warfarin, a vitamin K antagonist and commonly used oral anticoagulant, yet it has no clinically significant interactions with statins.[3] Until more definitive data are available, the international normalized ratio (INR) should be monitored more closely after the initiation of a statin or any change in statin dose.

Some foods and supplements also have been associated with clinically significant statin interactions. For instance, grapefruit products contain bergamottin, a natural furanocoumarin, which can inhibit intestinal CYP3A4 and increase systemic statin exposure in a dose-dependent manner that increases with the concentration and volume of grapefruit consumed.[6] According to FDA labeling, grapefruit juice should be avoided with lovastatin, and excessive consumption of grapefruit juice (>1 L/d) should be avoided with simvastatin and atorvastatin. Alternatively, any of the statins that are not metabolized by CYP3A4 may be safely used with grapefruit products. St. John's wort, a common supplement for depression, induces CYP3A4 and P-gp.[15] It decreases the metabolism of simvastatin and possibly atorvastatin but not the others in the class.[6] Health care providers also should be aware of red yeast rice extract, a popular cholesterol-lowering supplement. Red rice yeast contains varying amounts of monacolin K, which structurally is identical to lovastatin. Thus, patients on statins should be advised to avoid red yeast rice products.

Table 2
Clinically significant statin-drug interactions and recommended dose limits

Drug	Atorvastatin	Fluvastatin	Lovastatin	Pitavastatin	Pravastatin	Rosuvastatin	Simvastatin
Amiodarone			40 mg/d				20 mg/d
Amlodipine			20 mg/d				20 mg/d
Colchicine	Caution	Caution	Caution	Caution	Caution	Caution	Caution
Conivaptan	Avoid	Avoid	Avoid	Avoid	Avoid	Avoid	Avoid
Calcineurin inhibitors	10 mg/d	40 mg/d	Avoid	Avoid	20 mg/d	5 mg/d	Avoid
mTOR inhibitors	10 mg/d	40 mg/d	Avoid	Avoid	20 mg/d	5 mg/d	Avoid
Diltiazem			20 mg/d				10 mg/d
Dronedarone			10 mg/d				10 mg/d
Gemfibrozil	Avoid	Avoid	Avoid	Avoid	Avoid	Avoid	Avoid
Ranolazine			20 mg/d				20 mg/d
Ticagrelor			40 mg/d				40 mg/d
Verapamil			20 mg/d				10 mg/d
Warfarin	Monitor INR more closely after initiation of a statin or change in statin dose.						
Ketoconazole			Avoid				Avoid
Fluconazole		20 mg/d					
Posaconazole			Avoid				Avoid
Itraconazole	20 mg/d						
Clarithromycin	20 mg/d						
Erythromycin				1 mg/d			
Danazol			Avoid				Avoid
Digoxin	Coadministration is reasonable, if clinically indicated.						
Niacin	Limit dose of niacin to 1 g/d						
Bempedoic acid					40 mg/d		20 mg/d
Atazanavir + ritonavir			Avoid			10 mg/d	Avoid

Darunavir + ritonavir	20 mg/d		Avoid
Fosamprenavir + ritonavir	20 mg/d		Avoid
Lopinavir + ritonavir	Caution		Avoid
Nelfinavir	40 mg/d	10 mg/d	Avoid
Tipranavir + ritonavir	Avoid		Avoid
Saquinavir + ritonavir	20 mg/d		Avoid

Dose limits derived from FDA labels. Empty cells represent the absence of conclusive data on clinically significant interactions. Cells with numbers represent the dose limit based on drug labeling. "Avoid" indicates that the combination is contraindicated. Caution indicates that the combination may be considered with close monitoring.

Statins commonly are coprescribed with immunosuppressants, especially among heart transplant recipients. Current guidelines strongly recommend initiation of statins within 1 week to 2 weeks of heart transplantation, irrespective of lipid profiles, because statins have been associated with a reduction in mortality, hemodynamically significant rejection episodes, and incidence of coronary vasculopathy.[16,17] Calcineurin inhibitors, such as cyclosporine and tacrolimus, are metabolized extensively by hepatic and intestinal CYP3A4, both inhibitors and substrates of P-gp, and inhibitors of OATP1B1 and OATP1B3.[13] As a result, calcineurin inhibitors are predisposed to potential pharmacokinetic interactions with all statins. Additionally, numerous cases of rhabdomyolysis have occurred with concomitant use of cyclosporine and various statins, except for fluvastatin.[13] Similarly, sirolimus and everolimus have extensive hepatic and intestinal metabolism by CYP3A4 and P-gp. Few data exist, however, on the interactions between mammalian target of rapamycin inhibitors and statins (mTOR). Combination therapy of any of these immunosuppressants with lovastatin, simvastatin, or pitavastatin potentially is harmful and should be avoided. Daily doses of fluvastatin, pravastatin, rosuvastatin, and atorvastatin should be limited to 40 mg, 20 mg, 5 mg, and 10 mg daily, respectively, when combined with calcineurin inhibitors or mTOR inhibitors.[3]

Drug Interactions with Other Lipid-lowering Therapies

Coadministration of statins with a fibrate may be warranted for treatment of severe hypertriglyceridemia or complex dyslipidemias.[3] In the United States, gemfibrozil, fenofibrate, and fenofibric acid are the only fibrates approved for clinical use. Both statins and fibrates have been independently associated with a risk of muscle-related toxicity, and the statin-fibrate combination therapy increases this risk.[18,19] Gemfibrozil, but not fenofibrate, adversely affects the pharmacokinetics of most statins due to several mechanisms, including inhibition of OATP1B1-mediated hepatic uptake, CYP2C8 metabolism, and glucuronidation and subsequent lactonization by UGT1A1 and UGT1A3 enzymes.[20,21] Gemfibrozil and its glucuronide metabolite also are substrates of CYP3A4. The net result of these interactions is a higher concentration of active, open acid statins in the systemic circulation and a greater risk of adverse effects. Thus, the combination of any statin and gemfibrozil should be avoided. When statin-fibrate combination therapy is indicated, fenofibrate is preferred.[3]

Other LDL-C–lowering agents that may be coadministered with statins are ezetimibe and bempedoic acid. Initially approved in the United States in 2002, ezetimibe inhibits absorption of cholesterol in the small intestine by targeting the sterol transporter, Niemann-Pick C1-Like 1.[22] It is metabolized primarily in the small intestine and liver via glucuronide conjugation (phase II reaction) with subsequent biliary and renal excretion.[23] Ezetimibe and statins can be used together without significant concern for adverse interactions; however, the current FDA labeling warns of increased risk of myopathy and cholelithiasis when combining ezetimibe and fibrates. In February 2020, the FDA approved bempedoic acid for treatment of adults with heterozygous familial hypercholesteremia or established ASCVD who require additional lowering of LDL-C.[24] Bempedoic acid lowers LDL-C by inhibiting adenosine triphosphate citrate lyase, a key enzyme in the cholesterol biosynthesis pathway that acts upstream of 3-hydroxy-3-methylglutaryl coenzyme A reductase.[25] It is a prodrug that requires activation by the enzyme very-long-chain acyl–coenzyme A synthetase 1, which is present in the liver but absent in most peripheral tissue, including muscle. Bempedoic acid and its metabolite are converted by UGT2B7 to glucuronide conjugates that are inactive.[24] Concurrent use of bempedoic acid with greater than 20 mg of simvastatin or 40 mg of pravastatin increases the risk of myopathies and should be avoided, according to the FDA label. Additionally, a combination of statins or bempedoic acid with ezetimibe may offer synergistic lipid-lowering activity compared with monotherapy because of their complementary mechanisms of actions that couple inhibition of hepatic cholesterol synthesis and inhibition intestinal cholesterol absorption.[26–28]

There is little concern for drug interactions among novel lipid-lowering therapies targeting proprotein convertase subtilisin/kexin type 9 (PCSK9), an enzyme that binds LDL receptors, leading to their degradation and subsequently higher plasma LDL-C levels, given their novel mechanisms of action. Evolocumab and alirocumab are FDA-approved fully human monoclonal antibodies that inhibit plasma PCSK9. Although statins stimulate PCSK9 through an increased release of sterol regulatory element-binding protein 2, the percent of LDL-C reduction with PCSK9monoclonal antibodies is independent of statin use.[29,30] An alternative approach to antagonizing PCSK9leverages small interfering RNAs that prevent intracellular translation of PCSK9 messenger RNA to protein. Inclisiran, a long-acting, synthetic, small interfering RNA directed against PCSK9 messenger RNA conjugated to triantennary *N*-acetylgalactosamine carbohydrates, which bind liver-expressed asialoglycoprotein receptors with high affinity, is associated with LDL-C reduction that rivals the therapeutic monoclonal antibodies.[31] Inclisiran was approved by the European Commission in December 2020, for the treatment of adults with primary hypercholesteremia or mixed dyslipidemia and currently is awaiting regulatory approval in the United States.

Principles of Drug Interaction Avoidance

Health care providers should be aware of serious drug interactions and tailor drug combinations to avoid them. General strategies for reducing the risk of drug-drug interactions include minimizing the number of drugs prescribed, re-evaluating therapy on a regular basis, considering nonpharmacologic options when possible, monitoring for signs and symptoms of toxicity and/or effectiveness, and adjusting drug doses or administration times, when indicated.[1] Software within the electronic health record that detects and alerts providers of potential drug interactions lowers the risk of some drug interactions at the cost of alert fatigue.[32] Additionally, medication review and reconciliation by a pharmacist may reduce the risk of clinically significant drug interactions.

SUMMARY

Many of the most common drug interactions within preventive cardiology involve statins. These interactions often are predictable by understanding the pharmacokinetics of this class of medications. The variation in their pharmacokinetics allows providers to tailor drug combinations to avoid clinically significant interactions. Although statins will continue to be the backbone of lipid-lowering therapy for primary and secondary ASCVD prevention, novel lipid-lowering agents may offer more favorable drug interaction profiles.

CLINICS CARE POINTS

- Statins are the primary lipid-lowering therapy but have several drug interactions dictated by their metabolism.

- The pharmacokinetics of statins differ from statin to statin, so drug combinations can be tailored in such a way to avoid clinically significant interactions.

- Simvastatin and lovastatin have the most documented drug interactions because of their CYP3A4 metabolism.
- Providers should screen patients for possible drug-food and drug-supplement interactions with statins.
- Drug interaction screening using the electronic health record and pharmacists may help prevent clinically significant drug interactions.
- Novel lipid-lowering therapies often have favorable drug interaction profiles.

DISCLOSURE

A. Hammoud has nothing to disclose. M.D. Shapiro reports scientific advisory activities with Amgen, Esperion, and Novartis.

REFERENCES

1. Carpenter M, Berry H, Pelletier AL. Clinically Relevant Drug-Drug Interactions in Primary Care. Am Fam Physician 2019;99(9):558–64.
2. Nikolic B, Jankovic S, Stojanov O, et al. Prevalence and predictors of potential drug-drug interactions. Cent Eur J Med 2014;9:348–56.
3. Wiggins BS, Saseen JJ, Page RL 2nd, et al. Recommendations for Management of Clinically Significant Drug-Drug Interactions With Statins and Select Agents Used in Patients With Cardiovascular Disease: A Scientific Statement From the American Heart Association. Circulation 2016;134(21):e468–95.
4. Sánchez-fidalgo S, Guzmán-ramos MI, Galván-banqueri M, et al. Prevalence of drug interactions in elderly patients with multimorbidity in primary care. Int J Clin Pharm 2017;39(2):343–53.
5. Mallet L, Spinewine A, Huang A. The challenge of managing drug interactions in elderly people. Lancet 2007;370(9582):185–91.
6. Kellick KA, Bottorff M, Toth PP. The National Lipid Association's Safety Task F. A clinician's guide to statin drug-drug interactions. J Clin Lipidol 2014;8(3 Suppl): S30–46.
7. Newman CB, Preiss D, Tobert JA, et al. Statin Safety and Associated Adverse Events: A Scientific Statement From the American Heart Association. Arterioscler Thromb Vasc Biol 2019;39(2):e38–81.
8. Ward NC, Watts GF, Eckel RH. Statin Toxicity. Circ Res 2019;124(2):328–50.
9. Kavalipati N, Shah J, Ramakrishan A, et al. Pleiotropic effects of statins. Indian J Endocrinol Metab 2015;19(5):554–62.
10. Arnett DK, Blumenthal RS, Albert MA, et al. 2019 ACC/AHA Guideline on the Primary Prevention of Cardiovascular Disease: Executive Summary: A Report of the American College of Cardiology/American Heart Association Task Force on Clinical Practice Guidelines. Circulation 2019;140(11):e563–95.
11. Whirl-Carrillo M, Huddart R, Gong L, et al. An evidence-based framework for evaluating pharmacogenomics knowledge for personalized medicine. Clin Pharmacol Ther 2021;110(3):563–72.
12. Ballantyne C. Clinical Lipidology: A Companion to Braunwald's Heart Disease. 2014. Available at: https://www.elsevier.com/books/clinical-lipidology-a-companion-to-braunwalds-heart-disease/ballantyne/978-0-323-28786-9.
13. Neuvonen PJ, Niemi M, Backman JT. Drug interactions with lipid-lowering drugs: Mechanisms and clinical relevance. Clin Pharmacol Ther 2006;80(6):565–81.

14. Bellosta S, Corsini A. Statin drug interactions and related adverse reactions. Expert Opin Drug Saf 2012;11(6):933–46.
15. Holtzman CW, Wiggins BS, Spinler SA. Role of P-glycoprotein in statin drug interactions. Pharmacotherapy 2006;26(11):1601–7.
16. Costanzo MR, Dipchand A, Starling R, et al. The International Society of Heart and Lung Transplantation Guidelines for the care of heart transplant recipients. J Heart Lung Transplant 2010;29(8):914–56.
17. Vallakati A, Reddy S, Dunlap ME, et al. Impact of Statin Use After Heart Transplantation. Circ Heart Fail 2016;9(10):e003265.
18. Farnier M. Safety review of combination drugs for hyperlipidemia. Expert Opin Drug Saf 2011;10(3):363–71.
19. Graham DJ, Staffa JA, Shatin D, et al. Incidence of hospitalized rhabdomyolysis in patients treated with lipid-lowering drugs. Jama 2004;292(21):2585–90.
20. Shitara Y, Hirano M, Sato H, et al. Gemfibrozil and its glucuronide inhibit the organic anion transporting polypeptide 2 (OATP2/OATP1B1:SLC21A6)-mediated hepatic uptake and CYP2C8-mediated metabolism of cerivastatin: analysis of the mechanism of the clinically relevant drug-drug interaction between cerivastatin and gemfibrozil. J Pharmacol Exp Ther 2004;311(1):228–36.
21. Prueksaritanont T, Tang C, Qiu Y, et al. Effects of fibrates on metabolism of statins in human hepatocytes. Drug Metab Dispos 2002;30(11):1280–7.
22. Jia L, Betters JL, Yu L. Niemann-pick C1-like 1 (NPC1L1) protein in intestinal and hepatic cholesterol transport. Annu Rev Physiol 2011;73:239–59.
23. Kosoglou T, Statkevich P, Johnson-Levonas AO, et al. Ezetimibe: a review of its metabolism, pharmacokinetics and drug interactions. Clin Pharmacokinet 2005;44(5):467–94.
24. Nguyen D, Du N, Sulaica EM, et al. Bempedoic Acid: A New Drug for an Old Problem. Ann Pharmacother 2021;55(2):246–51.
25. Ray KK, Bays HE, Catapano AL, et al. Safety and Efficacy of Bempedoic Acid to Reduce LDL Cholesterol. N Engl J Med 2019;380(11):1022–32.
26. Gagné C, Gaudet D, Bruckert E. Efficacy and safety of ezetimibe coadministered with atorvastatin or simvastatin in patients with homozygous familial hypercholesterolemia. Circulation 2002;105(21):2469–75.
27. Kerzner B, Corbelli J, Sharp S, et al. Efficacy and safety of ezetimibe coadministered with lovastatin in primary hypercholesterolemia. Am J Cardiol 2003;91(4):418–24.
28. Khan SU, Michos ED. Bempedoic acid and ezetimibe - better together. Eur J Prev Cardiol 2020;27(6):590–2.
29. Mayne J, Dewpura T, Raymond A, et al. Plasma PCSK9 levels are significantly modified by statins and fibrates in humans. Lipids Health Dis 2008;7(1):22.
30. Robinson JG, Nedergaard BS, Rogers WJ, et al. Effect of evolocumab or ezetimibe added to moderate- or high-intensity statin therapy on LDL-C lowering in patients with hypercholesterolemia: the LAPLACE-2 randomized clinical trial. Jama 2014;311(18):1870–82.
31. German CA, Shapiro MD. Small Interfering RNA Therapeutic Inclisiran: A New Approach to Targeting PCSK9. BioDrugs 2020;34(1):1–9.
32. Yeh ML, Chang YJ, Wang PY, et al. Physicians' responses to computerized drug-drug interaction alerts for outpatients. Comput Methods Programs Biomed 2013;111(1):17–25.

Heart-Healthy Diets and the Cardiometabolic Jackpot

Cameron K. Ormiston, BS, Ashley Rosander, BS,
Pam R. Taub, MD*

KEYWORDS

- Plant-based diet • Cardiovascular disease • Nutrition • Cultural competency
- Obesity

KEY POINTS

- The key elements of a heart-healthy diet are a variety of vegetables, fruits, whole grains, low-fat or fat-free dairy, plant-based protein sources, and unsaturated oils. Saturated fats, red meat, and added sugars should be reduced and replaced by healthier alternatives.
- The "cardiometabolic jackpot" involves supplementing nutritional intervention with lifestyle changes, such as exercise or time-restricted eating (having a daily eating window of 8–10 hours), maximizing the benefits of healthy eating.
- Among popular diets currently available, the Mediterranean diet and Ornish diet have the strongest evidence supporting their clinical use.
- A patient's sociocultural and socioeconomic context must be considered when implementing dietary or lifestyle interventions. This includes cultural food practices, affordable and accessible foods, and cultural values or expectations.

 Video content accompanies this article at http://www.medical.theclinics.com.

INTRODUCTION

The increasing rate of cardiovascular disease (CVD) is intricately linked with diet and lifestyle, although health care providers are often poorly educated on evidence-based lifestyle interventions. Given both medical students and physicians report receiving inadequate training in nutrition education and more than 25% of primary care visits are nutrition-related, the need to address this knowledge gap is becoming increasingly important.[1,2]

This article originally appeared in *Medical Clinics*, Volume 106, Issue 2, March 2022.
Division of Cardiovascular Medicine, UC San Diego, 9500 Gilman Drive MC 7411, La Jolla, San Diego, CA 92037-7411, USA
* Corresponding author. Division of Cardiovascular Medicine, University of California San Diego, 9300 Campus Point Drive, Mail Code #7414, La Jolla, CA 92037.
E-mail address: ptaub@health.ucsd.edu

Clinics Collections 13 (2023) 129–141
https://doi.org/10.1016/j.ccol.2023.02.026

Unfortunately, foods high in sodium, saturated fat (SF), added sugar, and processed foods are on the rise because of globalization, convenience, affordability, and widespread popularity and marketing. Consequently, US CVD rates have increased by 25% since 1990 and greater than 66% of Americans are overweight or obese.[3,4] Obesity is a gateway to chronic disease conditions, such as metabolic syndrome, hyperlipidemia, type 2 diabetes (T2D), and hypertension, which all confer increased risk of CVD. Moreover, obesity disproportionately impacts ethnic and racial minorities, with African American and Hispanic/Latino adults having double the risk of developing obesity compared to White Americans.[5] These disparities are due to inequitable access to economic, educational, and health resources, where racial and ethnic minorities experience significantly greater socioeconomic, structural, and environmental barriers to health.[6]

To address the increase of CVD and obesity, the American Heart Association (AHA) issued diet guidelines arguing for the increased consumption of fruits, vegetables, fish, and fiber, and the cutting down on foods that are processed and/or high in sodium, cholesterol, and SF.[7] This review focuses on the key elements of a heart-healthy diet, popular diets and their strengths and limitations, the cardiometabolic jackpot, and special considerations for nutritional counseling.

DISCUSSION: HEART-HEALTHY DIET GUIDELINES

A diet focused on nutrient-rich foods from a variety of natural sources is the foundation of health optimization and CVD risk reduction, reducing myocardial infarction (MI) risk by 17% to 23%.[8] A healthy diet includes a moderate consumption of a variety of colorful vegetables, legumes, fruits, whole grains, low-fat or fat-free dairy, plant-based protein sources, and unsaturated oils (**Table 1**). SF and added sugars should be less than 10% of one's total daily caloric intake, and sodium consumption should be < 2300 mg/d[7] Alarmingly, people who acquire ≥25% of their calories from sugar have double the risk of CVD mortality compared with those who have sugar comprising less than 10%

Table 1 Best foods to consume and avoid		
Consume Most of the Time	**Consume Occasionally**	**Avoid**
Whole fruits and raw vegetables (citrus fruits, apples, pears, and berries; allium, carrots, c ruciferous, and leafy greens)	Roasted/salted nuts	Highly processed foods
Fish and lean meats (salmon, poultry)	Moderate alcohol consumption	Foods with added sugars
Legumes	Fruit and vegetable juices can be high in calories and sugar, but low in fiber	Artificial sweeteners
Raw nuts		High sodium foods
Low sodium and no added sugar options		Excess alcohol
Fortified foods (eg, whole-grain cereals)		Oils or fats that are solid at room temperature (coconut oil, margarine)
Foods that fit the Mediterranean or other plant-based diets		

of their diet (P = .004).[9] Although advertised as sugar-free and healthier, diet soda is associated with increased risk of metabolic syndrome and T2D, possibly because of artificial sweeteners increasing the risk of insulin resistance due to the pancreas equating the sweeteners as glucose, triggering an insulin response.[10] Also, every 1000 mg of dietary sodium intake is linked to a 6% increase in CVD risk.[11]

Legumes, plant-based proteins, and fish are excellent protein sources and preferable to red meat because chronic red meat consumption increases the risk of adverse cardiovascular events and mortality.[12] Legumes and plant-based sources are nutritious and cardioprotective substitutes for meat-based protein sources. In fact, having 1 daily serving of legumes (130 g) significantly decreases low-density lipoprotein (LDL) levels compared with no legume consumption.[13] Legumes are high in antioxidants, fiber, and nutrients, very low in SF, and are cholesterol free.[14] Legume protein content is on par with red meat, containing 20% to 45% protein, whereas lean red meat contains 26% to 27%.[15] Legumes can also play a key role in preventing CVD, cancers, and other degenerative diseases, with Bazzano and colleagues[16] showing legume consumption significantly decreases the incidence of coronary heart disease (CHD) (P = .002) and CVD (P = .02). Furthermore, Kelemen and colleagues[17] showed replacing animal proteins with plant-based proteins can decrease CHD events by 30% (P = .02). When comparing legume consumption $\geq$4 times per week to <1 time per week, eating legumes lowered CHD and CVD risk by 22% and 11%, respectively.[16] Legumes can also aid in weight loss, with 1 daily serving of legumes significantly decreasing body weight compared with diets without legumes, even when adhering to noncaloric restriction diets (P = .03).[18] One concern of having solely plant-based protein sources, however, is the risk of becoming deficient in essential micronutrients, such as vitamin B12, which can be prevented through supplementation.[19]

Fruit and vegetables are essential, universal components of a heart-healthy diet. Total fruit and vegetable consumption has an inverse relationship with CVD, CHD, and stroke incidence.[20] Three to 4 daily servings of fruits and vegetables (375–500 g) can significantly reduce all-cause mortality and improve cardiovascular health. Among fruits, citrus, apples, pears, and berries exhibit the most cardiovascular benefits; allium, carrots, cruciferous, and leafy greens are the most beneficial among vegetables.[20] Fruits and vegetables have a benefits threshold, however, with CVD risk and mortality being inversely related to combined fruit and vegetable consumption until 800 g/d, after which no benefits are observed.[21] Raw vegetables are more strongly associated with lower mortality, cancer, and CVD risk than cooked vegetables, possibly because of degradation and loss of nutrients during the cooking process.[21]

Substituting high-glycemic carbohydrates and refined grains with complex and low-glycemic carbohydrates can reduce all-cause mortality, CVD, and cancer risk.[22,23] In fact, 1 to 2 daily servings (16–32 g) of whole grains and fibrous foods, which contain phytonutrients and germ layers that are absent in refined grains, decreases CVD risk by 10% to 20%.[22] Current AHA guidelines suggest eating 6 servings of grain per day ($\geq$3 of which should be whole grain).[24]

Comparing fiber types, viscous fiber (fruits, beans, oats) and cereal grains are more cardioprotective than insoluble fiber (whole wheat). Although high-glycemic foods' exacerbation of CVD risk is well known, the benefits of low-glycemic foods have come under recent scrutiny. For example, Sacks and colleagues[25] showed low-glycemic foods had minimal effects on insulin sensitivity, blood pressure (BP), triglyceride, and cholesterol levels. Fiber content is therefore a more reliable measure of cardiovascular benefits.[26]

Dietary fats are generally classified as unsaturated, saturated, or trans fats. Higher consumption of trans fats is positively correlated with lipid risk factors for CVD, raising

CHD risk and mortality by 21% and 28%, respectively.[27] Trans fats and SF should be substituted with unsaturated fat (polyunsaturated is preferred), complex carbohydrates/whole grains, and protein. Meta-analyses show every 5% of energy from SF replaced with an isocaloric amount of polyunsaturated fats can reduce CHD events and risk by 10% and 27%, respectively.[23,28] Moreover, decreasing SF consumption can improve lipid profiles.[29] Fish, particularly fatty fish like salmon, are excellent sources of protein and omega-3 polyunsaturated fatty acids, significantly lowering BP and mortality.[30] In the Diet and Reinfarction trial (n = 2033), higher fish consumption was linked to a 29% reduction in total mortality and 32% reduction in CHD mortality compared with increased intake of grains or decreased total fat.[31] In addition, replacing SF with whole grains can reduce CHD risk by 6%.[32]

Although typically high in SF, dairy products can have a positive impact on CVD risk or diabetes, regardless of fat content. The PURE study (n = 135,335) showed greater than 2 daily servings of dairy is inversely correlated with mortality, major CVD, and stroke when compared with no dairy consumption.[33] Compared with unsaturated fat, however, dairy fat significantly increases LDL and total cholesterol levels ($P > .05$).[34] Current literature and guidelines therefore suggest limiting SF intake and replacing it with polyunsaturated fats and complex carbohydrates.

CURRENT EVIDENCE ON POPULAR DIETS

Several diets have recently emerged as popular in the health care field and mainstream media. Each diet's key components, current evidence, and utility for cardiovascular risk reduction are discussed below (**Table 2**).

Mediterranean Diet

Named for its regional and historical roots, the Mediterranean diet (MD) consists of high consumption of whole grains and cereal, legumes, fruits, and vegetables as well as moderate consumption of dairy products and alcohol. It is also characterized by low consumption of meat and meat products, although fish is often a source of protein.[35]

The MD has some of the strongest evidence for CVD prevention.[29] Many trials and critical reviews have validated the health effects of this diet, showing that it reduces CHD, ischemic stroke, and total CVD.[35–37] In fact, MD adherence is associated with a 40% CVD risk reduction.[38] In the Lyon Diet Heart study (n = 423), post-MI participants who were randomized to the MD group experienced protective effects of the lifestyle change even 4 years after the MI and had significantly lower incidence of recurrent MI compared with the Western diet group ($P = 0.0001$).[39] In addition, the degree of MD adherence has been shown to have an inverse relationship with total mortality, and cardiovascular and MI incidence and mortality.[40]

As a result of strong evidence supporting this dietary lifestyle, major societies recommend the MD to address multiple comorbidities, including hyperlipidemia (recommended by AHA), T2D (recommended by ADA), and obesity (recommended by the American Association of Clinical Endocrinology).[29]

Ornish Diet

The Ornish diet is vegetarian and consists of 10% fat, complex carbohydrates, and whole foods while discouraging simple sugars.[41]

The LIFESTYLE Heart Trial (n = 35) examined the difference in coronary atherosclerosis progression and cardiac event incidence in a control group versus an "Ornish" intensive lifestyle change, which includes dietary intervention, aerobic exercise, stress

Table 2
Key components of the Mediterranean, Ornish, Pritikin, ketogenic, and paleolithic diet

Diet	Components of Diet	Key Studies	Long-Term Adherence
Mediterranean	High consumption: whole-grains and cereal, legumes, fruits, and vegetables Moderate consumption: dairy products and alcohol. Low consumption: meat and meat products	Lyon Diet Heart study (n = 204 control, n = 219 experimental)[39] PREDIMED study (n = 7447)[51]	Lyon Diet Heart study: most intervention patients were still closely adhering to the Mediterranean diet several years after randomization PREDIMED: Mediterranean diet group adherence scores were significantly higher than the control group 6 y after study completion (P < .0001); patients maintained sufficient adherence to the Mediterranean diet after 6 y
Ornish	Vegetarian, 10% fat, complex carbohydrates, and whole foods. Discourages simple sugars	LIFESTYLE Heart Trial (n = 35)[41]	LIFESTYLE Heart Trial: 100% compliance after 5 y
Pritikin	Whole foods, whole-grains, fruits, vegetables, and lean meats, such as fish and poultry. Low fat	"Effect of short-term Pritikin diet therapy on the metabolic syndrome" (n = 67)[52]	80% of patients reported dietary compliance after 5 y; however, more trials are needed[52,53]
Ketogenic	Low consumption of carbohydrates and a high ingestion of fats, including saturated fats	"Effect of a plant-based, low-fat diet vs an animal-based, ketogenic diet on ad libitum energy intake" (n = 20)[47]	Unlikely to be sustained beyond 1–2 y[54]
Paleolithic	Meat, fruits, vegetables. No dairy or grains	"Effects of a short-term intervention with a paleolithic diet in healthy volunteers" (n = 14)[49]	80% compliance in 29 male patients with ischemic heart disease after 12 wk[55] Trials still needed for long-term assessment

management coaching, smoking cessation, and psychosocial support groups. After 5 years, the Ornish group experienced coronary atherosclerosis regression, whereas the control group experienced progression and more cardiac event incidence.[41] In a 1-year randomized trial of 4 popular diets in which diet was the only intervention, the Ornish diet (n = 40) exhibited an ~10% reduction in the high-density lipoprotein (HDL)/LDL ratio and reduced body weight, insulin, total cholesterol/HDL ratio, and inflammation.[42]

Pritikin Diet

The Pritikin diet consists of whole foods, whole grains, fruits, vegetables, and lean meats, such as fish and poultry.[43] This diet limits calorically dense, high-fat foods, which leads to a reduced total caloric and cholesterol intake.[43] Therefore, the Pritikin diet is used as a low-fat diet to promote weight loss and overall cardiovascular health.

Ketogenic Diet

Although this diet has proven to be popular for weight loss in the past decade, there are precautions that patients should take note of before starting this diet.

The ketogenic diet consists of a very low consumption of carbohydrates and a high ingestion of fats, including SF.[44] In cancer treatment, the ketogenic diet can sensitize cancer cells to treatment by creating an unfavorable metabolic environment.[45] This diet has also exhibited both positive and negative effects on the gut microbiota.[46]

In a randomized controlled trial (n = 20) in which the ketogenic diet was tested against a low-fat plant-based diet, the ketogenic diet resulted in significantly more caloric intake ($P < .0001$).[47] Although the ketogenic diet may lead to short-term weight loss, it also raises LDL-cholesterol and can lead to hyperlipidemia, which has long-term cardiovascular consequences.[44]

Paleolithic Diet

The paleolithic, or "paleo" diet, has been controversially advertised by non–health experts as a "cure-all" for various diseases. This diet stems from the idea that modern life is not in tune with our ancestral human metabolism and people should only eat what cave people ate. This means meat, fruits, and vegetables, but no farm-born foods, such as grains and dairy products.[48]

In individuals with ischemic heart disease, the paleo diet decreased waist circumference (WC) and increased sensitivity to glucose.[48] In a 3-week pilot study (n = 14), paleo diet adherence significantly decreased body weight ($P < .001$), WC ($P = .001$), and systolic blood pressure (SBP; $P = .03$).[49] However, it should be noted that calcium consumption significantly decreased compared with prestudy consumption levels.

Some of the validity of the paleo diet stems from its focus on whole foods, leading to the benefits of avoiding the processed and artificial foods that plague the western menu. High glucose-containing foods found on the market today are avoided altogether, helping combat insulin resistance.[48] Although there is convincing evidence for short-term use of the paleo diet, long-term trials with varying patient populations are still needed.[50]

THE CARDIOMETABOLIC JACKPOT

A lifestyle-based approach using exercise and one's circadian rhythm can maximize the benefits of a heart-healthy diet (Video 1). Compared with diet-alone (D) and exercise-alone (E) interventions, exercise plus diet (E + D) produces the most changes in body composition.[56] In a study on 1-year D, E, and E + D interventions, the E + D arm exhibited significantly greater reductions in weight ($P_{D + E \text{ vs } D}$ = 0.03; $P_{D + E \text{ vs } E}$ < 0.0001), percent body fat ($P_{D + E \text{ vs } D}$ = 0.005; $P_{D + E \text{ vs } E}$ < 0.0001), and WC ($P_{D + E \text{ vs } D}$ = 0.004; $P_{D + E \text{ vs } E}$ < 0.0001).[57] Moreover, resistance training reduces more fat mass compared with endurance training and retains fat free mass.[56]

Time-restricted eating (TRE) is when one constricts all their caloric intake to a daily 8- to 10-hour eating window. A consistent feeding-fasting cycle facilitates circadian alignment, promoting metabolic and physiologic homeostasis.[58] This is crucial, as erratic or prolonged eating patterns increase the risk of CVD, insulin resistance, and obesity.[58] TRE has been shown to be effective in patients who are overweight/obese and in patients with metabolic syndrome, reducing insulin resistance, oxidative stress, WC, body fat %, and improving HbA_{1c}, BP, LDL, and non-HDL-cholesterol.[58] Moreover, TRE is more effective and easier to sustain than calorie counting or restriction.[59]

Early findings on combining TRE and exercise are promising. Comparing a 16:8 alternating TRE schedule with non-TRE while performing resistance training, Moro and colleagues[60] reported similar increases in muscle mass in both groups. However, the TRE group showed a greater reduction in fat mass and total body mass (P = .04), and improvements in glucose, HDL, and triglycerides.

SPECIAL CONSIDERATIONS
Low Socioeconomic Status

Even though plant-based diets are the most beneficial to cardiovascular health, they are not always accessible to everyone, particularly communities of low socioeconomic status (SES), which are disproportionately comprised of racial/ethnic minorities. Patients of low SES often cite food costs and a lack of knowledge about measuring or incorporating foods into their diet as significant barriers to prescribed diets.[61] Clinicians should therefore discuss with their patients the socioeconomic (eg, low-income, family responsibilities) or geographic barriers (eg, food deserts) they may face and tailor clinical guidance accordingly. For example, legumes, poultry, oils, nuts, milk, eggs, and whole-grain cereals are foods with ideal ratios of nutrition to price (**Fig. 1**).[62]

The use of smartphone applications to promote physical activity, health access, and community engagement has also shown promise in decreasing CVD disparities for minority populations.[63] Improving health literacy, physician and patient nutritional education, and access to resources and affordable foods is imperative to ameliorating barriers to health.

Cultural Competency

Given greater than 50% of the US population will be composed of individuals from different cultural backgrounds by 2050, practitioner knowledge of cultural food practices is essential to personalizing care to the patient.[64] Foods can have different roles and impacts on health across different cultures. For example, white rice is often cautioned against in some diets but holds symbolic and physical significance in some cultures; rice is a staple of many East Asian diets and is seen as vital and healthful. Moreover, clinicians should be aware of their patient's sociocultural role. For example, women with T2D may place the needs of others over their own and may not make family meals diabetes-friendly due to cultural expectations.[65]

Culture can also guide how one views foods and their nutritional quality. In traditional Chinese medicine, foods can be classified as "hot" or "cold," and one must eat a balance of hot and cold foods to maintain internal harmony or health.[61] Navajo

Proteins

Canned and frozen legumes, poultry, nuts, and eggs have good nutrition to price ratios.

Fats

Olive oil, roasted nuts with no salt added, low-fat dairy options.

Fruits & Vegetables

Canned or frozen options. Choose no salt or sugar added.

Carbohydrates

Rice (brown preferred), white potatoes, whole grain/whole wheat cereal (low sugar).

Dairy

Low-fat or fat-free milk, yogurt, and cheese.

Beverages

Substitute sugar sweetened beverages with water or milk.

Fig. 1. Heart-healthy diet on a budget. A guide for more affordable healthy food options.

tribes also have binary food classifications, categorizing them as "strong" or "filler" foods. Strong foods (eg, mutton, stew) promote health and are therapeutic and essential parts of religious ceremonies. Filler foods (eg. cheese, refined flour, and canned meat) are eaten daily.[61] Prescribed diets that suggest decreasing or discontinuing the consumption of these culturally valued foods may conflict with food practices and lifestyles. Practitioners should be mindful of possible conflicts between dietary counseling and the patient's sociocultural needs and adapt the care plan to those needs.

Patients with Hypertension

Combining reduced sodium intake (2-g restriction) with the Dietary Approaches to Stop Hypertension (DASH) diet, which focuses on low SF and cholesterol, lots of fruits and vegetables, and low-fat dairy, can be effective for patients with hypertension, significantly lowering SBP compared with the control diet ($P < .001$).[66] Furthermore, the low-sodium DASH diet has greater benefits for patients with higher baseline SBP, yielding a −11-mm Hg reduction in those with ≥150 mm Hg baseline SBP and −4 mm Hg in those with less than 130 mm Hg baseline SBP.[66] The DASH diet can be an effective alternative to pharmacotherapy for patients with hypertension or can delay the need for antihypertensives for patients at risk for hypertension.[67]

The DASH diet can also reduce inflammation and LDL-cholesterol.[68] For patients not at risk for hyperkalemia, increasing dietary potassium intake can also decrease BP and has the largest effect for those with higher baseline BP.[29]

Patients with Diabetes

Managing and preventing T2D involves much of the same guidelines described above. The American Diabetes Association has also suggested restricting carbohydrate intake to ~40% of total calories and focusing on whole grains, fruits, vegetables, and low-fat milk as one's carbohydrate sources. In addition, refined grains and foods with added sugar should be replaced by complex carbohydrate and low-glycemic alternatives. Sugar-sweetened beverage consumption should also be reduced, as each daily serving confers a 20% increase in T2D risk.[29] Trans fats can also increase T2D risk, and replacing 2% of trans fat consumption with polyunsaturated fats can reduce risk by 40%.[69] Lifestyle changes, such as increasing physical activity, should also be encouraged.

SUMMARY

To address the increase of CVD and obesity, clinicians should promote increased consumption of fruits, vegetables, fish, and foods high in fiber, and decreased consumption of foods that are processed and/or high in sugar, sodium, cholesterol, and SF. Combining a heart-healthy diet with synergistic lifestyle modification strategies, such as increased physical activity or TRE, can further optimize health, improving health outcomes. Special considerations should be made for patients of diverse backgrounds, patients of low SES, and patients with hypertension or diabetes, tailoring the diet intervention to their unique needs.

CLINICS CARE POINTS

- The Mediterranean diet and Ornish diet have the strongest evidence showing their effectiveness in lowering cardiovascular disease risk and mortality.
- Clinicians should be aware of other diets to educate their patients to follow them safely. For example, the ketogenic diet can easily be misconstrued and potentially lead to negative cardiovascular outcomes.
- Plant-based diets may run the risk of vitamin B12 deficiency because it is typically found in animal products. Supplementation may be necessary.
- To maximize the benefits of a healthy diet, lifestyle therapies, such as exercise, should also be implemented.
- Socioeconomic status and geographic region can be barriers to a patient's ability to adhere to dietary intervention, and clinicians should be aware of the barriers their patients face while giving nutritional advice.

DISCLOSURES

PRT: Amgen (consultant), Novo-Nordisk (consultant), Sanofi (consultant), Boehringer-Ingelheim (consultant), Epirium Bio (shareholder), Esperion therapeutics (consultant). CKO and AR have no disclosures to report. No funding was received in the writing of this manuscript.

SUPPLEMENTARY DATA

Supplementary data related to this article can be found online at https://doi.org/10.1016/j.mcna.2021.11.001.

REFERENCES

1. Kolasa KM, Rickett K. Barriers to providing nutrition counseling cited by physicians: a survey of primary care practitioners. Nutr Clin Pract 2010;25(5):502–9.

2. Devries S, Freeman AM. Nutrition education for cardiologists: the time has come. Curr Cardiol Rep 2017;19(9):77.

3. Products - data briefs - number 360 - February 2020. 2020. Available at: https://www.cdc.gov/nchs/products/databriefs/db360.htm. Accessed January 11, 2021.

4. Roth GA, Forouzanfar MH, Moran AE, et al. Demographic and epidemiologic drivers of global cardiovascular mortality. N Engl J Med 2015;372(14):1333–41.

5. Wang L, Southerland J, Wang K, et al. Ethnic differences in risk factors for obesity among adults in California, the United States. J Obes 2017;2017:2427483.

6. Petersen R, Pan L, Blanck HM. Racial and ethnic disparities in adult obesity in the United States: CDC's tracking to inform state and local action. Prev Chronic Dis 2019;16:E46.

7. The American Heart Association diet and lifestyle recommendations. Available at: https://www.heart.org/en/healthy-living/healthy-eating/eat-smart/nutrition-basics/aha-diet-and-lifestyle-recommendations. Accessed April 29, 2021.

8. Hansen-Krone IJ, Enga KF, Njølstad I, et al. Heart healthy diet and risk of myocardial infarction and venous thromboembolism. Thromb Haemost 2017;108(09): 554–60.

9. Yang Q, Zhang Z, Gregg EW, et al. Added sugar intake and cardiovascular diseases mortality among US adults. JAMA Intern Med 2014;174(4):516–24.

10. Mathur K, Agrawal RK, Nagpure S, et al. Effect of artificial sweeteners on insulin resistance among type-2 diabetes mellitus patients. J Family Med Prim Care 2020;9(1):69.

11. Wang Y-J, Yeh T-L, Shih M-C, et al. Dietary sodium intake and risk of cardiovascular disease: a systematic review and dose-response meta-analysis. Nutrients 2020;12(10). https://doi.org/10.3390/nu12102934.

12. Al-Shaar L, Satija A, Wang DD, et al. Red meat intake and risk of coronary heart disease among US men: prospective cohort study. BMJ 2020;371. https://doi.org/10.1136/bmj.m4141.

13. Ha V, Sievenpiper JL, de Souza RJ, et al. Effect of dietary pulse intake on established therapeutic lipid targets for cardiovascular risk reduction: a systematic review and meta-analysis of randomized controlled trials. CMAJ 2014;186(8): E252–62.

14. Polak R, Phillips EM, Campbell A. Legumes: health benefits and culinary approaches to increase intake. Clin Diabetes 2015;33(4):198.

15. Maphosa Y, Jideani VA. The role of legumes in human nutrition. Functional food - improve health through adequate food. Published online 2017. Available at: https://www.google.com/books/edition/Functional_Food/-vyPDwAAQBAJ?hl=en&gbpv=0.

16. Bazzano LA, He J, Ogden LG, et al. Legume consumption and risk of coronary heart disease in US men and women: NHANES I Epidemiologic Follow-up Study. Arch Intern Med 2001;161(21):2573–8.

17. Kelemen LE, Kushi LH, Jacobs DR, et al. Associations of dietary protein with disease and mortality in a prospective study of postmenopausal women. Am J Epidemiol 2005;161(3). https://doi.org/10.1093/aje/kwi038.

18. Kim SJ, de Souza RJ, Choo VL, et al. Effects of dietary pulse consumption on body weight: a systematic review and meta-analysis of randomized controlled trials. Am J Clin Nutr 2016;103(5). https://doi.org/10.3945/ajcn.115.124677.

19. Pawlak R, Parrott SJ, Raj S, et al. How prevalent is vitamin B(12) deficiency among vegetarians? Nutr Rev 2013;71(2):110–7.

20. Zurbau A, Au-Yeung F, Blanco Mejia S, et al. Relation of different fruit and vegetable sources with incident cardiovascular outcomes: a systematic review and

meta-analysis of prospective cohort studies. J Am Heart Assoc 2020;9(19). https://doi.org/10.1161/JAHA.120.017728.

21. Miller V, Mente A, Dehghan M, et al. Fruit, vegetable, and legume intake, and cardiovascular disease and deaths in 18 countries (PURE): a prospective cohort study. Lancet 2017;390(10107):2037–49.

22. Temple NJ. Fat, sugar, whole grains and heart disease: 50 years of confusion. Nutrients 2018;10(1). https://doi.org/10.3390/nu10010039.

23. Li Y, Hruby A, Bernstein AM, et al. Saturated fats compared with unsaturated fats and sources of carbohydrates in relation to risk of coronary heart disease: a prospective cohort study. J Am Coll Cardiol 2015;66(14). https://doi.org/10.1016/j.jacc.2015.07.055.

24. Suggested servings from each food group. Available at: https://www.heart.org/en/healthy-living/healthy-eating/eat-smart/nutrition-basics/suggested-servings-from-each-food-group. Accessed April 5, 2021.

25. Sacks FM, Carey VJ, Anderson CAM, et al. Effects of high vs low glycemic index of dietary carbohydrate on cardiovascular disease risk factors and insulin sensitivity: the OmniCarb randomized clinical trial. JAMA 2014;312(23):2531–41.

26. Reynolds A, Mann J, Cummings J, et al. Carbohydrate quality and human health: a series of systematic reviews and meta-analyses. Lancet 2019;393(10170): 434–45.

27. Sacks FM, Lichtenstein AH, Wu JHY, et al. Dietary fats and cardiovascular disease: a presidential advisory from the American Heart Association. Circulation 2017;136(3). https://doi.org/10.1161/CIR.0000000000000510.

28. Mozaffarian D, Micha R, Wallace S. Effects on coronary heart disease of increasing polyunsaturated fat in place of saturated fat: a systematic review and meta-analysis of randomized controlled trials. PLoS Med 2010;7(3). https://doi.org/10.1371/journal.pmed.1000252.

29. Pallazola VA, Davis DM, Whelton SP, et al. A clinician's guide to healthy eating for cardiovascular disease prevention. Mayo Clin Proc Innov Qual Outcomes 2019; 3(3):251–67.

30. Naini AE, Keyvandarian N, Mortazavi M, et al. Effect of omega-3 fatty acids on blood pressure and serum lipids in continuous ambulatory peritoneal dialysis patients. Am J Pharmacogenomics 2015;4(3):135–41.

31. Burr ML, Fehily AM, Gilbert JF, et al. Effects of changes in fat, fish, and fibre intakes on death and myocardial reinfarction: diet and reinfarction trial (DART). Lancet 1989;2(8666):757–61.

32. Zong G, Li Y, Wanders AJ, et al. Intake of individual saturated fatty acids and risk of coronary heart disease in US men and women: two prospective longitudinal cohort studies. BMJ 2016;355. https://doi.org/10.1136/bmj.i5796.

33. Dehghan M, Mente A, Rangarajan S, et al. Association of dairy intake with cardiovascular disease and mortality in 21 countries from five continents (PURE): a prospective cohort study. Lancet 2018;392(10161). https://doi.org/10.1016/S0140-6736(18)31812-9.

34. Engel S, Tholstrup T. Butter increased total and LDL cholesterol compared with olive oil but resulted in higher HDL cholesterol compared with a habitual diet. Am J Clin Nutr 2015;102(2):309–15.

35. Martínez-González MA, Gea A, Ruiz-Canela M. The Mediterranean diet and cardiovascular health. Circ Res 2019;124(5):779–98.

36. Buil-Cosiales P, Toledo E, Salas-Salvadó J, et al. Association between dietary fibre intake and fruit, vegetable or whole-grain consumption and the risk of

CVD: results from the PREvención con DIeta MEDiterránea (PREDIMED) trial. Br J Nutr 2016;116(3):534–46.

37. Hayes J, Benson G. What the latest evidence tells us about fat and cardiovascular health. Diabetes Spectr 2016;29(3):171–5.
38. Grosso G, Marventano S, Yang J, et al. A comprehensive meta-analysis on evidence of Mediterranean diet and cardiovascular disease: are individual components equal? Crit Rev Food Sci Nutr 2017;57(15):3218–32.
39. de Lorgeril Michel, Patricia Salen, Jean-Louis Martin, et al. Mediterranean diet, traditional risk factors, and the rate of cardiovascular complications after myocardial infarction. Circulation 1999;99(6):779–85.
40. Tognon G, Lissner L, Sæbye D, et al. The Mediterranean diet in relation to mortality and CVD: a Danish cohort study. Br J Nutr 2014;111(1):151–9.
41. Ornish D, Scherwitz LW, Billings JH, et al. Intensive lifestyle changes for reversal of coronary heart disease. JAMA 1998;280(23):2001–7.
42. Dansinger ML, Gleason JA, Griffith JL, et al. Comparison of the Atkins, Ornish, Weight Watchers, and Zone diets for weight loss and heart disease risk reduction: a randomized trial. JAMA 2005;293(1):43–53.
43. Li Z, Heber D. The Pritikin diet. JAMA 2020;323(11):1104.
44. Hartman AL, Vining EPG. Clinical aspects of the ketogenic diet. Epilepsia 2007; 48(1):31–42.
45. Weber DD, Aminzadeh-Gohari S, Tulipan J, et al. Ketogenic diet in the treatment of cancer - where do we stand? Mol Metab 2020;33:102–21.
46. Paoli A, Mancin L, Bianco A, et al. Ketogenic diet and microbiota: friends or enemies? Genes 2019;10(7). https://doi.org/10.3390/genes10070534.
47. Hall KD, Guo J, Courville AB, et al. Effect of a plant-based, low-fat diet versus an animal-based, ketogenic diet on ad libitum energy intake. Nat Med 2021;27(2): 344–53.
48. Lindeberg S, Jönsson T, Granfeldt Y, et al. A Palaeolithic diet improves glucose tolerance more than a Mediterranean-like diet in individuals with ischaemic heart disease. Diabetologia 2007;50(9):1795–807.
49. Osterdahl M, Kocturk T, Koochek A, et al. Effects of a short-term intervention with a paleolithic diet in healthy volunteers. Eur J Clin Nutr 2008;62(5):682–5.
50. Andrikopoulos S. The Paleo diet and diabetes. Med J Aust 2016;205(4):151–2.
51. Estruch R, Ros E, Salas-Salvadó J, et al. Primary prevention of cardiovascular disease with a Mediterranean diet supplemented with extra-virgin olive oil or nuts. N Engl J Med 2018;378(25):e34.
52. Sullivan S, Samuel S. Effect of short-term Pritikin diet therapy on the metabolic syndrome. J Cardiometab Syndr 2006;1(5):308–12.
53. Barnard R, Guzy P, Rosenberg J, et al. Effects of an intensive exercise and nutrition program on patients with coronary artery disease: five-year follow-up. Eur J Cardiovasc Prev Rehabil 1983;3(3):183–94.
54. Masood W, Annamaraju P, Uppaluri KR. Ketogenic diet. In: StatPearls. Treasure Island, Florida: StatPearls Publishing; 2020.
55. Rydhög B, Granfeldt Y, Frassetto L, et al. Assessing compliance with Paleolithic diet by calculating Paleolithic diet fraction as the fraction of intake from Paleolithic food groups. Clin Nutr Exp 2019;25:29–35.
56. Clark JE. Diet, exercise or diet with exercise: comparing the effectiveness of treatment options for weight-loss and changes in fitness for adults (18-65 years old) who are overfat, or obese; systematic review and meta-analysis. J Diabetes Metab Disord 2015;14:31.

57. Foster-Schubert KE, Alfano CM, Duggan CR, et al. Effect of diet and exercise, alone or combined, on weight and body composition in overweight-to-obese postmenopausal women. Obesity 2012;20(8):1628–38.
58. Wilkinson MJ, Manoogian ENC, Zadourian A, et al. Ten-hour time-restricted eating reduces weight, blood pressure, and atherogenic lipids in patients with metabolic syndrome. Cell Metab 2020;31(1):92–104.e5.
59. O'Connor SG, Boyd P, Bailey CP, et al. Perspective: time-restricted eating compared with caloric restriction: potential facilitators and barriers of long-term weight loss maintenance. Adv Nutr 2021. https://doi.org/10.1093/advances/nmaa168.
60. Moro T, Tinsley G, Bianco A, et al. Effects of eight weeks of time-restricted feeding (16/8) on basal metabolism, maximal strength, body composition, inflammation, and cardiovascular risk factors in resistance-trained males. J Transl Med 2016;14(1). https://doi.org/10.1186/s12967-016-1044-0.
61. Tripp-Reimer T, Choi E, Kelley LS, et al. Cultural barriers to care: inverting the problem. Diabetes Spectr 2001;14(1):13–22.
62. Darmon N, Drewnowski A. Contribution of food prices and diet cost to socioeconomic disparities in diet quality and health: a systematic review and analysis. Nutr Rev 2015;73(10):643–60.
63. Ceasar JN, Claudel SE, Andrews MR, et al. Community engagement in the development of an mhealth-enabled physical activity and cardiovascular health intervention (Step It Up): Pilot Focus Group Study. JMIR Form Res 2019;3(1):e10944.
64. Colby S, Ortman JM, Others. Projections of the size and composition of the US population: 2014 to 2060. 2015. Available at: https://mronline.org/wp-content/uploads/2019/08/p25-1143.pdf. Accessed March 3, 2021.
65. Chesla CA, Kwan CML, Chun KM, et al. Gender differences in factors related to diabetes management in Chinese American immigrants. West J Nurs Res 2014;36(9):1074–90.
66. Juraschek SP, Miller ER 3rd, Weaver CM, et al. Effects of sodium reduction and the DASH diet in relation to baseline blood pressure. J Am Coll Cardiol 2017;70(23):2841–8.
67. Appel LJ, Moore TJ, Obarzanek E, et al. A clinical trial of the effects of dietary patterns on blood pressure. DASH Collaborative Research Group. N Engl J Med 1997;336(16):1117–24.
68. Hodson L, Harnden KE, Roberts R, et al. Does the DASH diet lower blood pressure by altering peripheral vascular function? J Hum Hypertens 2010;24(5):312–9.
69. Rice Bradley BH. Dietary fat and risk for type 2 diabetes: a review of recent research. Curr Nutr Rep 2018;7(4):214.

The Role of Physical Activity and Exercise in Preventive Cardiology

Paul D. Thompson, MD[a,b,*]

KEYWORDS

- Physical activity • Exercise • Exercise training • Coronary disease
- Atherosclerotic risk factors • Angina • Claudication

KEY POINTS

- Increased physical activity is associated with an approximately 50% reduction in cardiac events between the least and most active individuals.
- Exercise rarely cures a markedly abnormal cardiac risk factor but is excellent adjunctive treatment of dyslipidemia, hypertension, glucose intolerance, and increased body weight.
- Exercise-based cardiac rehabilitation should be recommended to essentially all patients after a myocardial infarction, valve or bypass surgery, or the diagnosis of heart failure.
- Walking is an effective treatment of claudication in patients without critical limb ischemia.

INTRODUCTION

My preventive clinical cardiology career started in 1978 after training in cardiology/ preventive cardiology at the Stanford Heart Disease Prevention Program. I am not sure if other preventive cardiology training programs existed at that time, but I was attracted to the Stanford program because the faculty included Peter Wood, PhD and William Haskell, PhD. Dr Wood was the first to report that endurance athletes had markedly higher high-density lipoprotein (HDL) cholesterol levels[1]; Dr Haskell was a premier exercise physiologist. They were joined during my second year by Ralph Paffenbarger, MD, DrPH, principal investigator of the San Francisco Long-shoreman[2] and subsequent Harvard Alumni[3] studies, both showing that more physically active individuals had fewer cardiovascular events. It was a different time. The drug treatment of hyperlipidemia consisted of clofibrate, bile acid sequestrants, and niacin. The drug treatment of diabetes consisted of insulin and sulfonylureas. I had never heard of coronary angioplasty until Andreas Gruentzig lectured at Stanford in 1977 during my fellowship. I was terribly skeptical of the procedure, but one of my co-fellows, John Simpson, MD, was enthralled with the concept and visited Gruentzig

This article originally appeared in *Medical Clinics*, Volume 106, Issue 2, March 2022.
[a] Emeritus, Hartford Hospital, 80 Seymour Street Hartford, Hartford, CT 06070, USA;
[b] University of Connecticut
* Hartford Hospital, 80 Seymour Street Hartford, CT 06070.
E-mail address: Paul.thompson@hhchealth.org

in Switzerland. John returned convinced that he could invent a better catheter and with co-fellow Ned Roberts, MD launched an incredibly successful business career by inventing the Simpson/Roberts angioplasty catheter. In contrast to such inventions, exercise and physical activity (PA) have been advocated by expert clinicians since antiquity. Herodicus (480–? BC) was a Greek physician and martial arts teacher who integrated exercise and medicine.[4] Knowledge of exercise medicine has also advanced. There are more and better designed epidemiologic studies supporting the value of PA, and there is a better understanding of the basic science mechanisms by which exercise reduces atherosclerotic vascular disease (ASCVD) risk, but PA remains underutilized as a therapeutic modality. I last reviewed the role of exercise in cardiology in 2001.[5] The present article updates the previous report and reviews the value of exercise for preventing and treating ASCVD disease with an emphasis on what clinicians should know and do about exercise and PA.

PHYSICAL ACTIVITY, EXERCISE, AND CARDIORESPIRATORY FITNESS

Physical activity (PA) refers to any voluntary, bodily movement that burns calories. *Exercise* is PA "with a purpose" including to increase muscular strength, endurance, physical performance, or health. *Cardiorespiratory fitness* (CRF) is a measurement of the exercise performance capacity of the cardiovascular system. CRF is determined using exercises requiring large muscle groups such as treadmill walking or running, stationary cycling, or the time to walk or run a fixed distance. CRF is an indirect measurement of maximal oxygen uptake (VO_{2max}) or the maximal ability to consume oxygen during a specific exercise task. VO_{2max} is the product of maximal cardiac output (heart rate [HR] x stroke volume [SV]) and the maximal arterial-venous oxygen difference (A-VO2 Δ).[6] Because HR is largely age determined and the A-VO2 Δ varies relatively little among individuals, CRF is an indirect measurement of maximum SV. CRF increases with habitual PA and with exercise training, so it is often used as a measure of PA; this is an attractive approach because CRF is less variable than measurements of PA by self-report, but CRF is not a direct measure of PA. Other factors such as genetics and innate exercise capacity also affect CRF. I refer to this innate exercise capacity as the "hardiness factor" or the fact that some individuals are innately hardier and have increased CRF. And remember that increased CRF indicates an increased SV. CRF is one of the best predictors of reduced ASCVD risk and increased survival; this is attributed to PA in many studies, but it is important to acknowledge that this enhanced prognosis may be due to the hardiness factor and the larger stroke volume. Similar to the Timex watch commercial from the 1970s, subjects with increased CRF have a larger SV and a heart that can "take a licking and keep on ticking."

PHYSICAL ACTIVITY AND DECREASED ATHEROSCLEROTIC VASCULAR DISEASE RISK

PA is *associated* with decreased ACVD risk but has never been subjected to testing in healthy people to the most stringent form of medical evidence, the randomized, controlled clinical trial (RCCT). I was part of a group that performed what I think is the first comprehensive review of epidemiologic studies examining the relationship between PA and coronary artery disease (CAD).[7] We concluded that PA was inversely and causally related to a reduction in CAD and that CAD was approximately 50% lower in the highest versus the lowest physical activity groups. That study was initiated by Ken Powell, MD, a career-long, physical activity researcher at the Centers for Disease Control. I had published several early studies on sudden cardiac death (SCD) during vigorous exercise.[8,9] Dr Powell invited me to the Centers for Disease Control to debate Henry Solomon, MD the author of the book, *The Exercise Myth*.[10] Dr

Solomon proposed that the danger of acute cardiac events during exercise outweighed its benefits, that people should exercise less vigorously, and that exercise did little to prevent CAD. This was a highly controversial topic when his book was published in 1984, given that interest in marathons and endurance exercise was exploding at the time. Indeed, there was a California pathologist, Dr Thomas Bassler, who had an incredible number of publications, composed almost entirely of letters to the editor, maintaining that running a marathon, a 42 km foot race, guaranteed protection against cardiac events, the so-called "Bassler Hypothesis."[11] My approach to the Solomon debate was to acknowledge that cardiac events did occur during exercise, since I had written about them,[8,9] but to emphasize that the benefits of physical activity outweighed the risk.

At that time there had never been, and likely there never will be, an RCCT comparing physical activity and sedentary behavior in previously healthy adults. Such a trial would require large numbers of subjects and would need to follow those subjects for a prolonged time. The number of subjects would need to be "huge," because the cardiac event rate in healthy subjects over a reasonable study duration would be low and also because there would be cross-overs from the PA group to the sedentary group and vice versa. At that time there had also never been, nor will there likely be, an RCCT of smoking versus nonsmoking, but Dr Luther L. Terry had already issued the first Surgeon General's report on smoking and health in 1964. Dr Terry determined that smoking caused adverse health outcomes by examining the relationship between smoking and health and epidemiologic characteristics. These included the strength of the relationship, its consistency study to study, whether it was appropriately sequenced meaning that smoking proceeded the disease and not the reverse, if there was a biological gradient in which more packs-per-day produced more disease, whether the relationship was biologically probable, and whether the relationship was coherent with all the facts.[12] These 5 criteria have since been criticized,[12] but I used them and a similar approach to the evidence in my debate with Dr Solomon. Dr Powell liked this approach and enlisted me and 2 of his colleagues to use epidemiologic data to conclude that PA reduces CAD.[7]

There have been multiple studies using more sophisticated techniques including meta-analysis since our publication.[13] These studies confirm that the risk of CAD is approximately 50% lower between the most and least active subjects. These studies also show that the greatest decrease in CVD is associated with increasing from the lowest to the next lowest PA cohort; this suggests that reductions in CAD events require only modest increases in physical activity. The lowest rate of CAD events is seen in the most active subjects, but the biggest decrease in CAD events occurs with only modest increases in PA[13]; this is partly because large portions of the population engage in no physical activity so that the population benefit is greatest with small increases in PA. These studies also show that CRF is a better predictor of CAD outcomes than PA, likely because CRF can be measured more accurately than the self-reported PA assessed in most trials but also because CRF measures the "hardiness factor" mentioned earlier.

HOW DOES PHYSICAL ACTIVITY REDUCE CORONARY ARTERY DISEASE EVENTS?

Exercise likely reduces CAD risk by multiple mechanisms. An analysis of subjects in the Women's Health Study demonstrated that compared with women self-reporting less than 200 kcal/wk of PA, the risk of CVD decreased 27%, 32%, and 41% as PA increased to 200 to 599, 600 to 1499, and greater than or equal to 1500 kcal/wk.[14] Known risk factors (listed later) explained 59% of the CVD reduction. Inflammatory/

hemostatic factors contributed the most, 32.6%, to the reduction, whereas blood pressure (−27.1%), total cholesterol (C), low-density lipoprotein cholesterol (LDL-C), HDL-C (−19.1%), lipoprotein (a) and apolipoproteins A-1 and B-100 (−15.5%), body mass index (−10.1%), and hemoglobin a1c/diabetes (−8.9%) contributed less. Why these risk factors add up to greater than 100% is unclear.

Many other exercise effects likely contribute. Exercise training lowers HR and increases parasympathetic or vagal tone. Every 10 beat per minute decrease in HR is associated with a 7% decrease in CHD and an 18% decrease in SCD.[15] Parasympathetic tone itself reduces cardiovascular risk. Exercise training in dogs increases HR variability, a marker of parasympathetic tone, and reduces the incidence of ischemia-induced ventricular fibrillation.[16] Exercise training increases coronary artery vasodilatory capacity and may increase coronary artery diameter. Runners who completed the Western States 100 miles run did not have larger coronary artery cross-sectional area at rest but did have markedly larger cross-sectional areas of their left anterior descending and circumflex coronary arteries after nitroglycerin administration.[17] Acetylcholine (ACH) produces vasoconstriction in atherosclerotic coronary arteries. Only 4 weeks of exercise training reduces this ACH vasoconstriction in patients with CAD.[18] The autopsy of Clarence DeMar, winner of 7 Boston Marathons, as reported by Currens and Paul Dudley White, the famous Boston cardiologist, showed extensive coronary atherosclerosis but large residual coronary lumens because of the coronaries' overall diameters.[19]

EXERCISE EFFECTS ON ATHEROSCLEROTIC VASCULAR DISEASE RISK FACTORS

Exercise affects multiple ASCVD risk factors, but exercise alone rarely cures clinically abnormal risk factors so should generally be viewed as adjunctive therapy. Exercise helps to control body weight and helps to prevent weight gain after weight loss but seems most useful for weight loss when combined with dietary caloric restriction.[20] Caloric expenditure during locomotive exercise is determined by the distance traveled and the body weight moved. The speed of locomotion matters because humans become less energy efficient with increased locomotive speed, but speed is less important than distance traveled and the grade of any elevation. Overweight individuals risk orthopedic injury with activities such as running. We recommend brisk walking to patients, rather than other exercises such as cycling or swimming, because the increased body weight of heavy individuals requires more caloric expenditure over the same distance than for a lighter person. I tell patients they can use their weight to "make lemonade out of their lemon."

Exercise can improve serum lipids. HDL cholesterol levels are 50% higher in endurance athletes, whereas triglycerides (TG) and LDL-C are approximately 50% and 10% lower, respectively.[21] Lipoprotein lipase activity (LPLA)[22] and intravenous fat clearance[23] are also higher in endurance athletes. Free fatty acids are a key energy source during endurance exercise. Using several marathons in Newport, RI as the laboratory, we demonstrated that exercise acutely reduces TGs and increases HDL-C[24,25] by increasing LPLA[25] and the clearance of intravenously administered fat.[25]

We postulated that decreased intramuscular fat from endurance exercise increases LPLA, which removes TGs from very low-density lipoproteins (VLDL).[21] The excess cholesterol on the VLDL surface that remains after TG removal is transferred to HDL by core lipid transport protein where it is esterified to increase HDL-C.[21] LDL-C is only slightly lower in endurance athletes possibly due to the expanded plasma volume that accompanies exercise training. Distance runners running 10 miles daily increased their LDL-C 10% within 2 days of exercise cessation[26] and decreased their plasma volume 5%,[27] suggesting that the expended plasma volume from training dilutes LDL-C. However, the newly available angiopoietin-like-3 (ANGPL3) monoclonal antibody, evinacumab, reduces LDL-C even in individuals lacking LDL receptors.[28] ANGPL3 inhibits LPLA, so increased LPLA from ANGPL3 inhibition suggests that the increased LPLA with acute exercise and exercise training may also contribute to lower LDL-C levels in very active subjects.

There is controversy about the role of HDL-C as a CVD risk factor because 2 trials of niacin therapy, which increases HDL-C, failed to demonstrate benefit, but in both instances, niacin was added to statin therapy. LDL-C levels at baseline in the AIM-HIGH[29] and the HPS-THRIVE[30] trials averaged only 72 and 63 mg/dL, making it difficult for niacin to demonstrate an effect. Other studies before statins were available, including the Coronary Drug Project using niacin[31] and the VA HDL Intervention Trial using gemfibrozil[32] did show reductions in CVD events and support the concept that HDL modification is important. Nevertheless, HDL-C remains the most predictive CAD lipid risk factor in many epidemiologic studies, so its increase with exercise is probably valuable.

I have focused on the effect of exercise on blood lipid because this was the focus of our National Institutes of Health–supported research for 11 years, but exercise also reduces systolic blood pressure[33] and improves insulin sensitivity[34] as well as many other risk factors.

Many of exercise's effects on risk factors are acute effects of recent exercise. TGs decrease within 24 hours of an exercise session.[35] Exercise acutely reduces systolic, and in some studies diastolic, blood pressure[36] likely from vasodilatation, and this reduction persists for up to 9 hours after exercise.[36] The average reduction in systolic blood pressure (SBP) and diastolic blood pressure (DBP) in subjects with prehypertension can be approximately 6 and 4 mm Hg, respectively, compared with the subjects' control session,[36] suggesting that the acute exercise effect is at least as powerful as some antihypertensive medicines.

Indeed, we have speculated that some of the risk factor effects attributed to exercise training are a cumulative effect of recent exercise. Exercise training increases fitness, which allows more exertion per session, which produces a larger acute effect when measured in fit subjects. At any rate, the observation that exercise produces an acute exercise effect argues for daily or at least frequent exercise to achieve the most beneficial effect on risk factors.

Despite the beneficial effect of exercise on CVD risk factors, it is important to recognize that exercise alone rarely normalized significantly abnormal risk factors. Patients need to know this because many delay effective drugs for long periods and are discouraged when their exercise efforts are insufficient.

EXERCISE-BASED CARDIAC REHABILITATION

Medicare approves exercise-based cardiac rehabilitation for patients after acute myocardial infarction, coronary revascularization, and valve surgery and for patients with angina pectoris and heart failure. The data are most robust for patients with CAD. A meta-analysis of 63 randomized control trials of exercise-based cardiac rehabilitation included 47 with mortality outcomes. These 47 studies followed 12, 455 patients for more than or equal to 6 months. Exercise-based rehab significantly reduced cardiac mortality in patients with CAD by 26% and hospital admissions by 18%.[37] Total mortality, MI, and revascularization were not significantly different between the rehab and control groups, although an earlier meta-analysis of 36 randomized trials including 6,111 patients post-MI found a 36% reduction in cardiac deaths, a 26%

reduction in total mortality, and a 47% reduction in reinfarction.[38] At least 2 observational studies of cardiac rehab including 846 and 3,975 patients after coronary artery bypass graft surgery (CABG) reported risk reductions of 46% and 40%.[38] Neither study was an RCCT, but both used propensity matching to try to adjust for selection bias. There are insufficient data to evaluate the effect of exercised-based rehab on patients after valve surgery, but the few available studies are supportive.

Exercise Training for Heart Failure

A meta-analysis of cardiac rehab in patients with heart failure and reduced ejection fraction (HFrEF) found that those randomized to rehab had a 45% reduction in mortality and a 28% reduction in death or hospital admission.[39] Medicare approval of rehab for HFrEF is largely based on HF-ACTION or the Heart Failure: A Controlled Trial Investigating Outcomes of Exercise Training, which randomized 2331 patients with HFrEF to exercise training or standard therapy.[40] All-cause mortality and hospitalization was reduced by 11% ($P = .03$) after adjustment for the prespecified baseline confounders of atrial fibrillation/flutter, psychological depression, ejection fraction, and exercise capacity. The secondary combined endpoint of cardiovascular mortality or HF hospitalizations was also reduced by 9% ($P = .03$) after adjustment for baseline variables. The investigators did nearly everything possible to keep the exercise-assigned patients actually exercising, including providing home exercise cycles or treadmills, but the increase in VO_{2max} in the training group was only 4%; this suggests that many of the exercise training participants did very little exercise training and that the benefits in patients with HFrEF could be significantly greater if patients would exercise.

Exercise Training for Angina Pectoris

Classic stable angina has essentially disappeared from modern cardiology because of β-blocker therapy, angioplasty, and CABG. Exercise-based therapy was an extremely useful therapy for stable angina and remains an underutilized adjunctive treatment for those patients who are not candidates for revascularization or who have symptoms despite medicines and revascularization. William Heberden, the English physician who first described angina, stated that he knew a patient who sawed wood for half an hour daily and was "nearly cured."[6] Medical historians think that Heberden was knowledgeable about the disease and the effects of exercise training because he was both physician and patient.

At least 2 factors contribute to the reduction in angina with exercise training.[6] HR is the primary determinant of myocardial oxygen demand. Exercise training reduces the HR response to any exercise workload so that after exercise training the patient can perform more exercise work before the onset of symptoms. Exercise training also improves abnormal endothelial function. Normal coronary arteries vasodilate with exercise, but atherosclerosis injures the endothelium so that the normal coronary vasodilatory response to exercise either does not occur or the arteries vasoconstrict. Reducing this exercise-induced vasoconstriction increases coronary blood flow and exercise capacity; this should not be interpreted as indicating that exercise is a replacement for modern medical therapy but that exercise training is valuable as adjunctive treatment of patients with angina who are not candidates for revascularization, refuse operative intervention, or have angina due to minor vessel disease.

Exercise Training for Claudication

Exercise training is an excellent treatment of claudication and has Medicare approval for this indication. Exercise training can produce remarkable increases in walking tolerance in patients who adhere to the program. An analysis of 25 RCCTs comparing walking exercise versus control found that the average increase in walking distance was 180 m.[41] Improvement in walking distance is greatest when walking is used as the exercise modality, patients walk to their maximal pain tolerance, and walking is pursued for greater than 6 months.[42] Another meta-analysis including stent revascularization found the greatest improvement with combined exercise and revascularization than with either therapy alone.[43] Patients need to know that the benefits of exercise on walking distance disappear with inactivity.

CLINICS CARE POINTS

The clinical implications of this review are as follows:

1. Clinicians should ask patients if they are physically active and for the specifics of the patient's activity program. Some have recommended that exercise be considered a vital sign for patient visits.[44] Many patients think that if the doctor does not ask it cannot be important.

2. Clinicians should know the 2018 Physical Activity Guidelines for Americans in order to advise patients to achieve at least the minimal recommended activity.[45] These guidelines recommend the following: move more/sit less, accumulate 150 to 300 min/wk of moderately vigorous exercise such as brisk walking or 75 to 150 min/wk of vigorous exercise such as jogging plus 2 resistance exercise sessions weekly to maintain muscle strength.

3. Exercise alone rarely normalizes a seriously abnormal cardiac risk factor, but exercise training is excellent adjunctive therapy for many cardiac risk factors including abnormal lipids, hypertension, excess body weight, and diabetes.

4. Clinician should be involved in advocating for physically active lifestyles in their community. Such advocating could be for walking paths, bicycle lanes, facility access, and other environmental engineering changes that enhance the population's ability to exercise. Jerry Morris, the British epidemiologist who led physical activity and outcomes studies of London bus drivers and conductors, called exercise "The best bargain in public health."[46] Clinicians should do what they can to make this bargain easily available to the public.

5. Clinicians should do their best to remove barriers from exercise participation; this includes not recommending exercise stress tests before starting a gradually progressive exercise program unless there are worrisome clinical symptoms. Exercise stress tests have long been known to predict angina and not SCD or acute MI (AMI). Positive exercise stress tests require ischemia from a significant coronary stenosis, whereas exercise-related SCD and AMI are usually produced by disruption of a previously nonobstructive lesion. Patients should be advised to promptly report new symptoms to the clinician but otherwise most patients can start exercise programs without undue risk.

6. All patients after AMI, valve or bypass surgery, or the diagnosis of HF should be referred to cardiac rehab. Utilization of cardiac rehabilitation is woefully low in the United States, and one of the biggest determinants as to whether or not a patient attends rehab is whether or not their clinician recommended it.

7. All patients with claudication in the absence of critical limb ischemia should be referred to a supervised exercise training program or advised to start a walking program on their own. Because maximal benefit is obtained when patients walk to maximal pain, I often recommend that patients buy a "cane chair" on the Internet so that they can walk to maximum pain, deploy the tripod cane chair, sit down to recover, and then walk again without having to find some other place to sit.

REFERENCES

1. Wood PD, Haskell W, Klein H, et al. The distribution of plasma lipoproteins in middle-aged male runners. Metabolism 1976;25:1249–57.

2. Paffenbarger RS, Laughlin ME, Gima AS, et al. Work activity of longshoremen as related to death from coronary heart disease and stroke. N Engl J Med 1970;282: 1109–14.

3. Paffenbarger RS, Hyde RT, Wing AL, et al. Physical activity, all-cause mortality, and longevity of college alumni. N Engl J Med 1986;314:605–13.

4. Thompson PD. D. Bruce Dill Historical lecture. Historical concepts of the athlete's heart. Med Sci Sports Exerc 2004;36:363.

5. Thompson PD, Moyna N. The therapeutic role of exercise in contemporary cardiology Cardiovascular Reviews & Reports. Cardiovasc Rev Rep 2001;22:279–80, 22:279-280, 282-284, 2001. 282-284.

6. Thompson D. Exercise Prescription and Proscription for Patients With Coronary Artery Disease. Circulation 2005;112:2354–63.

7. Powell KE, Thompson PD, Caspersen CJ, et al. Physical activity and the incidence of coronary heart disease. Annu Rev Public Health 1987;8:253–87.

8. Thompson PD, Stern MP, Williams P, et al. Death during jogging or running. A study of 18 cases. JAMA 1979;242:1265–7.

9. Thompson PD, Funk EJ, Carleton RA, et al. Incidence of death during jogging in Rhode Island from 1975 through 1980. JAMA 1982;247:2535–8.

10. Solomon HA. The exercise Myth. 1984. Harcourt Brace Jovanovich; 1984.

11. Bassler TJ. Coronary-artery disease in marathon runners. N Engl J Med 1980; 302:57–8.

12. Burch PR. The surgeon general's "epidemiologic criteria for causality." A critique. J Chronic Dis 1983;36:821–36.

13. Eijsvogels TM, Molossi S, Lee DC, et al. Exercise at the Extremes: The Amount of Exercise to Reduce Cardiovascular Events. J Am Coll Cardiol 2016;67:316–29.

14. Mora S, Cook N, Buring JE, et al. Physical activity and reduced risk of cardiovascular events: potential mediating mechanisms. Circulation 2007;116:2110–8.

15. Aune D, Sen A, o'Hartaigh B, et al. Resting heart rate and the risk of cardiovascular disease, total cancer, and all-cause mortality - A systematic review and dose-response meta-analysis of prospective studies. Nutr Metab Cardiovasc Dis 2017;27:504–17.

16. Hull SS, Vanoli E, Adamson PB, et al. Exercise training confers anticipatory protection from sudden death during acute myocardial ischemia. Circulation 1994; 89:548–52.

17. Haskell WL, Sims C, Myll J, et al. Coronary artery size and dilating capacity in ultradistance runners. Circulation 1993;87:1076–82.

18. Hambrecht R, Wolf A, Gielen S, et al. Effect of exercise on coronary endothelial function in patients with coronary artery disease. N Engl J Med 2000;342:454–60.

19. CURRENS JH, WHITE PD. Half a century of running. Clinical, physiologic and autopsy findings in the case of Clarence DeMar ("Mr. Marathon"). N Engl J Med 1961;265:988–93.

20. Donnelly JE, Blair SN, Jakicic JM, et al. American College of Sports Medicine Position Stand. Appropriate physical activity intervention strategies for weight loss and prevention of weight regain for adults. Med Sci Sports Exerc 2009;41: 459–71.

21. Thompson PD. What do muscles have to do with lipoproteins? Circulation 1990; 81:1428–30.

22. Herbert PN, Bernier DN, Cullinane EM, et al. High-density lipoprotein metabolism in runners and sedentary men. JAMA 2021;252:1034–7.

23. Sady SP, Cullinane EM, Saritelli A, et al. Elevated high-density lipoprotein cholesterol in endurance athletes is related to enhanced plasma triglyceride clearance. Metabolism 1988;37:568–72.

24. Thompson PD, Cullinane E, Henderson LO, et al. Acute effects of prolonged exercise on serum lipids. Metabolism 1980;29:662–5.

25. Sady SP, Thompson PD, Cullinane EM, et al. Prolonged exercise augments plasma triglyceride clearance. JAMA 1986;256:2552–5.

26. Thompson PD, Cullinane EM, Eshleman R, et al. The effects of caloric restriction or exercise cessation on the serum lipid and lipoprotein concentrations of endurance athletes. Metabolism 1984;33:943–50.

27. Cullinane EM, Sady SP, Vadeboncoeur L, et al. Cardiac size and VO2max do not decrease after short-term exercise cessation. Med Sci Sports Exerc 1986;18: 420–4.

28. Raal FJ, Rosenson RS, Reeskamp LF, et al. Evinacumab for homozygous familial hypercholesterolemia. N Engl J Med 2020;383:711–20.

29. AIM-HIGH Investigators, Boden WE, Probstfield JL, et al. Niacin in patients with low HDL cholesterol levels receiving intensive statin therapy. N Engl J Med 2011;365:2255–67.

30. HPS2-THRIVE Collaborative Group, Landray MJ, Haynes R, et al. Effects of extended-release niacin with laropiprant in high-risk patients. N Engl J Med 2014;371:203–12.

31. Canner PL, Berge KG, Wenger NK, et al. Fifteen year mortality in Coronary Drug Project patients: long-term benefit with niacin. J Am Coll Cardiol 1986;8:1245–55.

32. Rubins HB, Robins SJ. Conclusions from the VA-HIT study. Am J Cardiol 2000;86: 543–4.

33. Boutcher YN, Boutcher SH. Exercise intensity and hypertension: what's new? J Hum Hypertens 2017;31:157–64.

34. Goodyear LJ, Kahn BB. Exercise, glucose transport, and insulin sensitivity. Annu Rev Med 1998;49:235–61.

35. Cullinane E, Siconolfi S, Saritelli A, et al. Acute decrease in serum triglycerides with exercise: is there a threshold for an exercise effect? Metabolism 1982;31: 844–7.

36. Ash GI, Taylor BA, Thompson PD, et al. The antihypertensive effects of aerobic versus isometric handgrip resistance exercise. J Hypertens 2017;35:291–9.

37. Anderson L, Oldridge N, Thompson DR, et al. Exercise-based cardiac rehabilitation for coronary heart disease: cochrane systematic review and meta-analysis. J Am Coll Cardiol 2016;67:1–12.

38. McMahon SR, Ades PA, Thompson PD. The role of cardiac rehabilitation in patients with heart disease. Trends Cardiovasc Med 2017;27:420–5.

39. Piepoli MF, Davos C, Francis DP, et al, ExTraMATCH Collaborative. Exercise training meta-analysis of trials in patients with chronic heart failure (ExTra-MATCH). BMJ 2004;328:189.

40. O'Connor CM, Whellan DJ, Lee KL, et al. Efficacy and safety of exercise training in patients with chronic heart failure: HF-ACTION randomized controlled trial. JAMA 2009;301:1439–50.

41. McDermott MM. Exercise training for intermittent claudication. J Vasc Surg 2017; 66:1612–20.

42. Gardner AW, Poehlman ET. Exercise rehabilitation programs for the treatment of claudication pain. A meta-analysis. JAMA 1995;274:975–80.

43. Saratzis A, Paraskevopoulos I, Patel S, et al. Supervised exercise therapy and revascularization for intermittent claudication: network meta-analysis of randomized controlled trials. JACC Cardiovasc Interv 2019;12:1125–36.
44. Golightly YM, Allen KD, Ambrose KR, et al. Physical activity as a vital sign: a systematic review. Prev Chronic Dis 2017;14:E123.
45. Piercy KL, Troiano RP, Ballard RM, et al. The physical activity guidelines for Americans. JAMA 2018;320:2020–8.
46. Morris JN. Exercise in the prevention of coronary heart disease: today's best buy in public health. Med Sci Sports Exerc 1994;26:807–14.

Management of Coronary Artery Disease

Eric Francis Sulava, MD[a], Jeffery Chad Johnson, MD[b],*

KEYWORDS

- Coronary artery bypass grafting (CABG) • Heart team • Hybrid revascularization
- Minimally invasive CABG

KEY POINTS

- Surgical revascularization coronary artery bypass grafting (CABG) continues to be the preferred treatment of most patients with multivessel and left main coronary artery disease (CAD).
- The heart team approach is recommended when evaluating patients with CAD who may be candidates for surgical revascularization; this ensures the patient is considered individually and all factors are taken into account to develop the best, tailored treatment strategy.
- Use of arterial conduits, when available and appropriate, is preferred to venous grafts with internal thoracic artery conduits being superior to radial artery conduits.
- Minimally invasive and hybrid surgical/percutaneous revascularization strategies are being used more often and present additional options for some patients.
- Off-pump CABG presents an alternative revascularization treatment of some patients who are not good candidates for traditional CABG due to technical considerations (eg, heavily calcified aorta that cannot be cross-clamped).

BACKGROUND

Heart disease is the number one cause of death in the United States and is responsible for more than 650,000 deaths annually. Coronary heart disease results in more than 800,000 myocardial infarctions per year and is responsible for 13% of all deaths.[1] Although there has been a recent decrease in both the overall number and rate of deaths in recent years, it remains a significant economic and health burden. Moreover, with the population aging it is likely to remain a significant cause of death and morbidity.

This article originally appeared in *Cardiac Electrophysiology Clinics*, Volume 13, Issue 1, March 2021.

[a] Department of Emergency Medicine, Naval Medical Readiness & Training Center Portsmouth, 620 John Paul Jones Circle, Portsmouth, VA 23708, USA; [b] Department of Surgery, Division of Cardiothoracic Surgery, Naval Medical Readiness & Training Center Portsmouth, 620 John Paul Jones Circle, Portsmouth, VA 23708, USA
* Corresponding author.
E-mail address: jchadjohnson@gmail.com

Surgical therapy for ischemic heart disease was first performed in the 1960s and coronary artery bypass grafting (CABG) techniques have been continually refined since that time.[2,3] In the 1970s, percutaneous coronary intervention (PCI) was introduced and has advanced from angioplasty, to the deployment of bare metal stents, and to modern drug eluting stents.[4–6] These 2 procedures comprise the mainstays of procedural treatment of coronary artery disease (CAD) today. A comprehensive examination the of medical, percutaneous, and surgical treatment of CAD in all settings is extremely far reaching. For this reason, this review outlines the surgical management of CAD, primarily in the stable setting. Patient presentation, evaluation, surgical indications, and surgical treatment are also examined.

PATIENT EVALUATION AND OVERVIEW

CAD is a pathologic process that leads to inadequate blood supply to the myocardium secondary to atherosclerotic plaque accumulation in the epicardial coronary arteries. This chronic and progressive disease can have dynamic and seemingly unpredictable transitions. There are long, clinically silent periods of plaque accumulation that lead to acute decompensation following plaque rupture. This widespread variation of clinical presentation can be conveniently organized into the disease classification of acute coronary syndrome (ACS) or stable ischemic heart disease (SIHD).[7]

ACS is defined as an abrupt reduction in coronary blood flow or a mismatch in myocardial oxygen supply and demand.[8] The 3 presentations of ACS are unstable angina, acute non-ST elevation myocardial infarction, and acute ST elevation myocardial infarction.[9] SIHD, also referred to as chronic coronary syndrome, encompasses stable anginal pain syndromes (chronic angina) and new-onset, low-risk chest pain. Differentiation will initially be largely history based, following a reassuring initial workup of nondiagnostic electrocardiogram (ECG), negative cardiac biomarkers, and exclusion of secondary causes of chest pain.[10]

DETERMINATION OF PRETEST RISK

Once the initial clinical evaluation suggests SIHD, the probability of SIHD must be determined before recommending further testing. When the probability is low, testing is usually not warranted because of the higher likelihood of a false-positive test. The same is true for high probability of SIHD, with noninvasive testing being unable to completely exclude underlying disease.

The 2012 American College of Cardiology Foundation (ACCF)/American Heart Association (AHA) Guidelines on SIHD reference combined tables based on data from the Coronary Artery Surgery Study (CASS), Diamond-Forrester model, and the Duke Databank for Cardiovascular Disease. These models determine pretest probability of SIHD by using multiple clinical and demographic factors. Intermediate ranges from 20% to 70% pretest probability of SIHD. There are limitations for these risk calculations, including risk overestimation for low-risk SIHD in patients, inappropriately excluding patients older than 70 years, and performing less well in the female population.[11]

APPROACH TO TESTING

Several factors influence the choice of additional diagnostic testing for patients with suspected CAD. In addition to calculating pretest probability, the clinician must consider the patient's ability to exercise, body habitus, cardiac medications, and resting ECG abnormalities that might affect interpretation of test results. Further testing is delineated by the method of stressing (exercise or pharmacologic) and the method to identify and measure ischemia (ECG, echocardiography, PET, single-photon emission computed tomography [SPECT], or MRI).[10] Functional, or stress testing, to detect inducible ischemia has been the "gold standard" and is the most common noninvasive test used to diagnose SIHD.

EXERCISE VERSUS PHARMACOLOGIC TESTING

In the testing environment, induced ischemia depends on the severity of stress imposed and the severity of the pathologic flow disturbance. Submaximal exercise or incomplete pharmacologic vasodilation can fail to produce ischemia, and therefore coronary stenoses less than 70% are often undetected by functional testing.[11] Exercise testing is generally preferred because it often can provide a higher physiologic stress than would be achieved by pharmacologic testing, while eliciting the prognostic indicator of exercise capacity.[11,12]

TESTING MODALITIES
Exercise Electrocardiography

The exercise ECG has been the cornerstone of diagnostic testing of patients with SIHD for several decades, although recent research calls its utility into question. The 2012 ACCF/AHA Guidelines on SIHD recommend starting with exercise ECG without imaging for intermediate-risk patients who can exercise and have an interpretable ECG.

There are limitations to this modality. Research has shown that exercise ECG has inferior performance compared with diagnostic imaging tests and has limited power to rule in/out obstructive CAD.[13] The addition of coronary computed tomography angiography (CCTA) or functional imaging clarifies the diagnosis, enables the targeting of preventive therapies and interventions, and potentially reduces the risk of myocardial infarction. The 2019 European Society of Cardiology (ESC) Guidelines for the Diagnosis and Management of Chronic Coronary Syndromes removed the recommendation for exercise ECG to be used as the initial test to establish a diagnosis of stable CAD.[7]

Functional Noninvasive Testing

Some cardiologists prefer to add imaging to the initial exercise evaluation. Noninvasive functional tests detect ischemia by wall motion abnormalities on stress cardiac magnetic resonance (CMR), stress echocardiography, or perfusion changes by SPECT or PET. These are highly accurate for the detection of high-grade, flow-limiting coronary stenosis when compared with coronary angiography and fractional flow reserve (FFR).[13] However, lower grade coronary atherosclerosis can remain undetected by functional testing.[7]

Stress Echocardiography

Echocardiography is a reliable noninvasive test that can detect evidence of myocardial ischemia or infarction. It can reveal new or worsening regional wall motion abnormalities (RWMA) and changes in global left ventricular (LV) function during or immediately following pharmacologically induced stress. Severe ischemia produces RWMA that can be visualized within seconds of coronary artery occlusion occurring before the onset of ECG changes or symptoms.[14,15] In several meta-analyses, the diagnostic sensitivity ranged from 70% to 85% for exercise and 85% to 90% for pharmacologic stress echocardiography, with specificity ranging from 77% to 89% and 79% to 90%, respectively.[16–18]

Nuclear Myocardial Perfusion Imaging

Nuclear myocardial perfusion imaging (MPI), using SPECT or PET, uses a radioactive tracer to identify myocardial tissue uptake using pharmacologic or exercise-induced stress. Sensitivity is similar between stress echocardiography and SPECT, with the caveat that SPECT provides better quality images in the obese population.[10] PET, which is less widely available, has increased sensitivity over traditional SPECT with values of 90% and 85%, respectively.[19] In the special population of patients with a known diagnosis of CAD, nuclear MPI and CMR have the ability to identify myocardium with reversible ischemia that may be amenable to revascularization.[11]

Stress Cardiac Magnetic Resonance

CMR has the ability to provide information on cardiac structure, function, and myocardial perfusion.[7,20] Unfortunately, CMR is more difficult to obtain, given the lack of widespread expertise, increased scan times, and compatibility issues with medical implants. CMR incorporates gadolinium contrast, which is contraindicated in patients with renal dysfunction. The 2012 ACCF/AHA Guideline on SIHD states that CMR is reasonable for patients with intermediate to high pretest probability of IHD who are incapable of moderate physical function and for patients with known SIHD who have an uninterpretable ECG. The 2019 ESC Guidelines also allow for CMR in patients with inconclusive echocardiographic testing.[7,11]

Coronary Computed Tomography Angiography

CCTA is a noninvasive alternative to stress testing that provides anatomic instead of functional information. This multislice imaging technique allows for noninvasive visualization of anatomic CAD with high-resolution images, similar to invasive coronary angiography. Its advantage over functional testing is the ability to identify nonobstructive CAD conditions.[10] Noting its tendency to overestimate the severity of coronary lesions in the presence of heavy coronary calcification, the strength of CCTA is its near-perfect negative predictive value.[11]

Coronary Angiography

Invasive coronary angiography (ICA) remains the "gold-standard" testing modality for the diagnosis of CAD. ICA defines coronary anatomy, the presence of coronary intraluminal obstruction, and the extent of coronary and collateral blood flow. ICA is recommended for initial testing only in patients who have survived sudden cardiac death, had a life-threatening ventricular arrythmia, or developed signs of heart failure. ICA is more routinely used for further diagnostic evaluation following a high-risk or inconclusive initial workup with noninvasive cardiac testing.[11]

The most commonly used nomenclature for defining coronary anatomy was developed for CASS. The extent of disease is defined as 1-vessel, 2-vessel, 3-vessel, or left main disease, with a significant stenosis being generally greater than 70% diameter occlusion. Unprotected left main CAD is considered significantly stenotic at greater than 50% diameter occlusion.[11] For lesions with intermediate severity stenoses, FFR can measure the pressure proximal and distal to stenotic lesions and determine proportional decrease of flow across a stenosis to assist in differentiation. Values less than 0.80 are associated with provocable ischemia and significant coronary artery stenosis.[11,21]

MEDICAL TREATMENT OPTIONS

Goals of SIHD treatment are to diminish disease progression, limit complications, and reduce ischemic symptoms. Medical providers must address risk modification and determine guideline-directed medical therapy (GDMT). Risk modification includes life-style changes such as dietary modification, weight reduction, smoking cessation, frequent exercise, and management of stress and depression. GDMT includes therapies that slow down the atherosclerotic disease, decrease future events of myocardial infarction, and attempts to eliminate angina. Medications used to decrease mortality include antiplatelet agents, β-blockers, renin-angiotensin-aldosterone blockers and lipid-lowering drugs. Medications for symptom control include nitrates, β-blockers, calcium channel blockers, and sodium channel blockers.[11] A summary of the ACCF/AHA approach to GDMT is included in **Table 1**. Medical therapy alone is inferior revascularization with regard to survival.

SURGICAL AND INTERVENTIONAL TREATMENT OPTIONS

The decision to treat CAD with PCI versus CABG is, from a procedural standpoint, one of the most critical decisions that can affect patient outcome. Timing and presentation will initially drive the choice of procedure. In patients with an acute presentation, restoration of coronary blood flow is the most important consideration. Such patients are typically treated with PCI initially to expeditiously restore myocardial blood flow, with CABG being reserved for salvage of failed intervention or those with unfavorable anatomy for PCI in such situations.

For patients with stable CAD a thoughtful, guidelines-based approach developed jointly by cardiologists and cardiac surgeons is followed. These guidelines were published by the ACC, AHA, the American Association for Thoracic Surgery, the Society of Thoracic Surgeons (STS), the Preventive Cardiovascular Nurses Association, and the Society for Cardiac Angiography and Interventions for the treatment of SIHD in 2014 and for CABG in 2011.[22,23] They were updated in 2016 to include dual antiplatelet therapy recommendations.[24] These guidelines provide an evidence-based framework to direct patient-tailored coronary revascularization strategies. Surgical management remains the best choice of treatment of patients with significant multivessel and unprotected left main CAD who are able to undergo CABG. Central concepts of the guidelines important for cardiac surgeons in the management of CAD are summarized in **Fig. 1**.

Heart Team Approach

Multidisciplinary evaluation of stable patients with cardiovascular disease, including significant CAD, allows for tailored evidence-based treatment of individual patients.[25] The heart team typically consists of an interventional cardiologist, a noninterventional cardiologist, and cardiac surgeon who review the patient's coronary disease pattern and complexity, technical feasibility of PCI and CABG, overall patient health and condition, STS risk estimate, and any other factors that might affect patient outcome. The recommendations of the heart team are discussed with the patient, and an informed treatment decision can then be made.

This approach can lead to a different recommended procedural treatment of CAD than that recommended by the original treating interventional cardiologist alone in up to 30% of multivessel CAD cases according to one retrospective study.[26] Although randomized controlled trial data are not currently available to assess impact on outcome, this approach nonetheless carries the highest level of recommendation (LOR 1) in the ACC/AHA guidelines.[22]

Table 1
Overview of guideline-directed medical therapy in stable ischemic heart disease

Modification	Intervention	Indication	Explanation
Lipid management Moderate- to high-potency statin	Atorvastatin, 40–80 mg/d Rosuvastatin, 20–40 mg/d	With, or at high risk for, CVD. High potency for age <75 y, if tolerated. Moderate potency preferred for >75 y	LDL-C goal of ≤70 mg/dL
Lipid-lowering medication	Ezetimibe, 10 mg	If LDL-C is not at goal with maximum statin therapy. Primary therapy for patients who cannot tolerate statins.	LDL-C goal of ≤70 mg/dL
PCSK9 inhibitor	Evolucumab or alirocumab SQ	Not at goal with statin–ezetimibe combination therapy.	Not routinely used due to high cost and mode of delivery
Blood pressure management SIHD goal of <130/80	β-Blocker (not atenolol), ACE inhibitors, or ARBs	First-line therapy for SIHD	β-blockers have additional benefit in patients with reduced EF following MI
	Dihydropyridine CCBs	Second-line therapy: BP not at goal and angina is present	With angina: β-blockers and CCB are preferred
	Dihydropyridine CCBs, thiazide diuretics, MRAs	Second-line therapy: BP not at goal and angina is absent	DM initial antihypertension treatment: combination of an ACE-I with a CCB or thiazide-/thiazide-like diuretic
Diabetes management Goal HbA1c level of <7%	SGLT2 inhibitor or GLP-1 agonist	SGLT2 inhibitors have been shown to reduce cardiovascular events. GLP-1 agonist reduces ischemic events in patients with SIHD	SGLT2 inhibitors (empagliflozin, canagliflozin) increase loss of glucose through urinary tract. GLP-1 agonists (liraglutide, semaglutide) promote insulin secretion

Category	Intervention	Recommendation	Target/Indication	Comment
Behavior modification	Physical activity	30–60 min of moderate aerobic activity on 5–7 d/wk	Patients with, or at risk for, CVD	Regular exercise reduces heart disease mortality, improves functional capacity, and can decrease angina
	Weight management	BMI $\leq$35 kg/m^2		Risk of CVD, cardiovascular morbidity/mortality, is higher in overweight/obese patients
	Social historical factors	Tobacco and alcohol cessation		Smoking increases CVD mortality by 50%. Relationship between alcohol consumption and CVD, with probable harm beyond 2 drinks per day
Thrombotic risk management	Antiplatelet therapy	Aspirin, 75–162 mg/d	Used indefinitely (in the absence of contraindications) in patients with SIHD	Platelet aggregation is a key element of the thrombotic response to plaque disruption
		Clopidogrel, 75 mg/d	Can be used when aspirin is contraindicated	Can be used in patients with a history of GI bleeds

Abbreviations: ACEI, angiotensin-converting enzyme inhibitor; ARB, angiotensin-receptor blocker; BMI, body mass index; BP, blood pressure; CCB, calcium channel blocker; CVD, cardiovascular disease; DM, diabetes mellitus; EF, ejection fraction; GI, gastrointestinal; GLP-1, glucagon-like peptide 1; HbA1c, hemoglobin A1c; LDL-C, low-density lipoprotein cholesterol; MI, myocardial infarction; MRAs, mineralocorticoid receptor antagonists; PCSK9, proprotein convertase subtilisin/kexin type 9; SGLT2, sodium-glucose cotransporter-2; SIHD, stable ischemic heart disease.

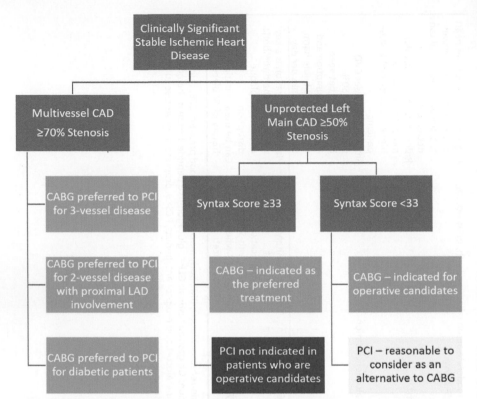

Fig. 1. Condensed summary of recommendations for surgical treatment of coronary artery disease and percutaneous treatment alternatives according to AHA/ACC/STS/AATS/PCNA/SCAI guidelines. Level of recommendation (LOR) is indicated by color: Green—LOR 1, yellow—LOR 2a/2b, red—LOR 3.

Unprotected Left Main Coronary Artery Disease

For patients with significant left main CAD, CABG is the preferred therapy to improve survival for patients who are surgical candidates. For patients with anatomically complex stenosis (SYNTAX score ≥33), CABG is superior to PCI for major adverse cardiac or cerebrovascular events (MACCE).[27] Patients with low to moderate anatomic complexity stenosis (SYNTAX score <33) and for whom the risk of adverse surgical outcomes is high, can be considered for PCI as an alternative to CABG without an increase in mortality.[28]

Multivessel Coronary Artery Disease

Patients with clinically significant multivessel CAD, defined as greater than or equal to 70% stenosis in 3 coronary arteries or in 2 coronary arteries with one being the proximal left anterior descending (LAD), should be considered for CABG as the preferred method of revascularization.[29] The left internal thoracic artery (LITA), if available, should be used to revascularize the LAD. Patients with significant stenoses in 2 coronary arteries with extensive ischemia, patients with mild to moderate LV dysfunction and multivessel CAD, and patients with isolated proximal LAD stenosis and extensive ischemia are also candidates to be considered for CABG to improve survival.[22]

Among patients with multivessel CAD, multiple arterial grafting is preferred to single arterial grafting and is associated with a lower all-cause mortality when compared with single arterial grafting CABG or PCI.[30,31]

Diabetic Patients

Patients with diabetes mellitus with clinically significant multivessel or unprotected left main CAD should preferentially receive CABG over PCI if they are suitable surgical candidates.[32] Multiple arterial grafting, including bilateral internal thoracic artery (BITA), can be considered with wound complication risk being mitigated to an acceptable level if ITA grafts are skeletonized.[33–35]

Conduit Selection

When planning surgical revascularization, it is critical to consider the type and amount of conduit available for use. The conduit type and source can affect long-term patency and clinical outcome. Likewise, when limited conduit is available, innovative configurations to achieve the most complete and highest quality revascularization should be considered. There is recent evidence to suggest that the use of multiple arterial grafting lowers all-cause mortality in multivessel and left main CAD, and liberal use of arterial grafts should be considered when available.[30] **Fig. 2** provides a summary of preferred conduits for use in CABG.

Internal thoracic artery

The right and left internal thoracic arteries are the best performing conduits over time, provided they are prepared appropriately and their target vessels are selected well. The LITA is the conduit of choice for the LAD. The right internal thoracic artery (RITA) can be used to revascularize the right coronary system, the distal circumflex coronary system, and the LAD. There is no difference in long-term patency between RITA and LITA grafts to equivalent targets, with both exhibiting greater than 90% patency at 10 years for appropriately chosen targets.[36] An important consideration when using the RITA to revascularize the right coronary circulation is to ensure there is a high-grade (>70%) stenosis proximal to the target when grafting the main RCA, use a free RITA graft, or use the RITA to graft more distal right coronary targets to

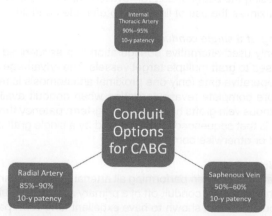

Fig. 2. Simplified summary of options for coronary revascularization conduits, including long-term patency rates for each.

prevent competitive flow and graft failure.[37,38] Both internal thoracic arteries can be prepared as in situ pedicled, skeletonized, or as free grafts.

There is an important caveat when preparing BITA grafts. The pedicled BITA technique is associated with a higher incidence of sternal wound complications than the skeletonized BITA technique. This effect may be magnified in the presence of diabetes and may affect single ITA grafting as well.[33–35] These are considerations that should be taken into account when considering a BITA technique in diabetic patients. Diabetic patients seem to benefit the most as a group from long-term mortality reduction when BITA revascularization is the chosen revascularization strategy. However, long-term mortality is similar between skeletonized and pedicled BITA grafts, although late MACCE may be higher among surgeons who perform the technique less often.[39]

Radial artery

The second most durable conduit available for use in CABG is the radial artery. Careful selection of eligible patients is required, including an Allen test to ensure adequate arterial circulation remains for the hand. The 10-year patency exceeds 85%, which is intermediate between ITA grafts and venous grafts.

Saphenous vein

The most commonly used conduit in CABG is the saphenous vein graft, typically in combination with the LITA. It is chosen for its ready availability, abundance, and caliber. However, these grafts are more prone to occlusion. The 1-month occlusion rate is greater than 10% and the 10-year patency rate is 50% to 60%.[40–42] Recent data on "no-touch" vein harvesting techniques seem to show a significant reduction in early occlusion and may improve long-term patency rates.[43]

Alternative conduits

Although surgical revascularization can usually be accomplished with the aforementioned conduit options, others have been described. These include the right gastroepiploic artery, lesser saphenous vein, and cryopreserved vein. These are not first-line or widely used options and are generally only entertained when none of other options are available.

Conduit Configurations

In addition to choosing the best conduit for revascularization, different configurations can be used to maximize the use of limited or preferable conduits.

Sequenced grafting of a single conduit

The most commonly used alternative configuration is a sequenced graft, wherein a single conduit is used to graft multiple target vessels. The advantage of this technique is that it reduces operative time (only one proximal anastomosis is required per graft) and enables a more complete revascularization when conduit availability is limited. Sequenced saphenous vein grafts have higher long-term patency than single grafts.[41] The disadvantage is that sequenced targets served by a single graft are jeopardized if inflow is occluded or otherwise compromised.

Composite conduit grafting

Another option that is used when performing all arterial or majority arterial revascularization is to branch one arterial conduit off of a primary arterial conduit as a composite graft. This technique has been shown to have excellent long-term patency when performed by surgeons experienced with this approach.[44,45] The disadvantage of branched grafting is that it is technically challenging with a learning curve and can jeopardize multiple vascular territories; it is particularly devastating if such a complication were to affect an LITA graft to the LAD territory.

COMBINED THERAPY

Combining PCI with DES and CABG to achieve LITA to LAD grafting and effectively treat multivessel CAD has attracted great interest in recent years. The concept behind this hybrid approach is to achieve the most complete and high-quality revascularization possible when all targets may not be suitable for grafting. Likewise, this strategy opens the possibility to use minimally invasive CABG techniques for LITA to LAD grafting and to complete treatment of other significant stenoses with PCI.

One randomized controlled trial that compared hybrid CABG/PCI with CABG found no difference in mortality or MACCE at 5 years; however, this was not powered to definitively prove equivalence.[46] Other retrospective studies have likewise suggested no difference in outcome between these 2 treatment strategies.[47] For selected patients this option is reasonable to consider.

TREATMENT FAILURE AND COMPLICATIONS

Although CABG is considered the superior treatment option for multivessel and left main CAD in appropriately selected patients, treatment failure necessitating repeat revascularization does occur; this can often be addressed by PCI, although there is occasionally a role for redo CABG. Approximately 2% of contemporary CABG procedures in the United States are redo operations.[48]

Perioperative mortality is increased in redo CABG compared with primary CABG, although long-term survival is similar.[48,49] The procedure should be performed at centers with a higher volume of redo cardiac surgery. The usual indication for redo CABG is primary graft failure leading to LAD territory ischemia. If the LITA is available, it should be used in these situations; otherwise, the best available remaining conduit should be chosen for grafting. In non-LAD bypass situations, decisions are made on an individual case basis with the Heart Team.

Preoperative preparation for redo CABG should be thorough. In addition to the usual diagnostic studies that are obtained to define progressive or recurrent disease, adjunct studies should be obtained. At a minimum, a contrasted CT of the chest should be performed to assess patient anatomy as well as patency and location of prior grafts. Surgeons should also identify and confirm the presence of the conduit they plan to use for revascularization.

INNOVATIVE APPROACHES AND NEW DEVELOPMENTS

Innovative surgical approaches have been developed for surgical revascularization as well. Hybrid revascularization was discussed earlier, but minimally invasive and off-pump techniques expand the surgeon's armamentarium to treat CAD as well.

Off-Pump Coronary Artery Bypass Grafting

The ability to perform surgical revascularization without having to cannulate, cross-clamp, or place a patient on cardiopulmonary bypass is advantageous for select patients. Debate regarding equivalence or superiority of CABG versus off-pump CABG (OPCAB) is robust. Three large randomized controlled trials have been performed over the past 2 decades, all with 5-year follow-up.[50–54] The ROOBY trial found that OPCAB had a higher 5-year mortality and lower graft patency.[53] The CORNARY and GOPCABE trials showed no difference in MACCE or mortality between OPCAB and traditional CABG.[52,54]

Others have argued that high-volume surgeons at high-volume centers can achieve OPCAB outcomes comparable to traditional CABG.[55,56] An important takeaway for OPCAB techniques is that they can be appropriate for the treatment of certain subgroups of patients, such as those with aortic disease that prevents cross-clamp application.

Minimally Invasive Approaches

Minimally invasive direct coronary artery bypass (MIDCAB) refers to a variation of OPCAB that uses a technique typically involving a small thoracotomy and off-pump LITA to LAD bypass grafting. This procedure has been refined in recent years to use robotic technology and revascularization of additional territories is possible. The benefits of this approach include less pain, shorter length of stay, and less scarring. The technique is superior in outcome compared with PCI with regard to long-term mortality and need for revascularization.[57] MIDCAB can be combined with PCI in a hybrid approach to allow for complete revascularization with the benefit of an LITA to LAD graft as well.

EVALUATION OF OUTCOME AND LONG-TERM RECOMMENDATIONS

Patients are typically discharged from the care of their CT surgeon after a postoperative visit if there are no complications. They will, however, require cardiology/medical follow-up and testing as indicated. Optimal GDMT is very important in the postoperative setting for best results. Full recommendations can be found in the 2015 AHA statement on postoperative therapy.[58] When symptoms of progressive or recurrent CAD occur, diagnostic evaluation using coronary catheterization is usually indicated.

SUMMARY

Surgical management of CAD has been refined over almost 6 decades and is the standard of care for coronary revascularization among patients with multivessel or unprotected left main CAD. The goal of surgical therapy is complete revascularization, and using arterial conduits, specifically the LITA to LAD, is advocated. Minimally invasive, OPCAB, and hybrid procedures may benefit subsets of patients for whom traditional CABG is not advised or who have conditions that are more suited to these techniques. Optimizing long-term outcomes depends on diligent medical follow-up and adherence to optimal postoperative medical therapy.

CLINICS CARE POINTS

- Surgical treatment of coronary artery disease is most safely done in an elective setting; therefore, screening at-risk patients to identify them prior to acute presentation is critical.

- A learning curve exists for off-pump and multi-arterial grafting techniques; surgeons should achieve proficiency in these techniques before they employ them in practice in order to ensure the best possible outcomes.- Failure to initiate and maintain medical therapy after surgical intervention will result in inferior long-term outcomes; therefore, it is imperative to ensure postoperative medical therapy (i.e., beta blockers, statins, and aspirin) is prescribed and medical follow up is ensured.

DISCLOSURE

The authors have nothing to disclose.

REFERENCES

1. Underlying cause of death 1999-2019. Centers for Disease Control and Prevention, National Center for Health Statistics. Available at: http://wonder.cdc.gov/ucd-icd10.html. Accessed 31 August 2021.
2. Kolesov VI, Potashov LV. [Surgery of coronary arteries]. Eksp Khir Anesteziol 1965;10(2):3–8. Operatsii na venechnykh arteriiakh serdtsa.
3. Kolesov VI. [Initial experience in the treatment of stenocardia by the formation of coronary-systemic vascular anastomoses]. Kardiologiia 1967;7(4):20–5. Pervyi opyt lecheniia stenokardii nalozheniem venechno-sistemnykh sosudistykh soust'ev.
4. Gruntzig A. Transluminal dilatation of coronary-artery stenosis. Lancet 1978; 1(8058):263.
5. Sigwart U, Puel J, Mirkovitch V, et al. Intravascular stents to prevent occlusion and restenosis after transluminal angioplasty. N Engl J Med 1987;316(12):701–6.
6. Sousa JE, Costa MA, Abizaid A, et al. Lack of neointimal proliferation after implantation of sirolimus-coated stents in human coronary arteries: a quantitative coronary angiography and three-dimensional intravascular ultrasound study. Circulation 2001;103(2):192–5.
7. Knuuti J, Wijns W, Saraste A, et al. 2019 ESC Guidelines for the diagnosis and management of chronic coronary syndromes. Eur Heart J 2020;41(3):407–77.
8. Anderson JL, Morrow DA. Acute Myocardial Infarction. N Engl J Med 2017; 376(21):2053–64.
9. Amsterdam EA, Wenger NK, Brindis RG, et al. 2014 AHA/ACC Guideline for the Management of Patients with Non-ST-Elevation Acute Coronary Syndromes: a report of the American College of Cardiology/American Heart Association Task Force on Practice Guidelines. J Am Coll Cardiol 2014;64(24):e139–228.
10. Katz D, Gavin MC. Stable Ischemic Heart Disease. Ann Intern Med 2019;171(3): ITC17–32.
11. Fihn SD, Gardin JM, Abrams J, et al. 2012 ACCF/AHA/ACP/AATS/PCNA/SCAI/STS Guideline for the diagnosis and management of patients with stable ischemic heart disease: a report of the American College of Cardiology Foundation/American Heart Association Task Force on Practice Guidelines, and the American College of Physicians, American Association for Thoracic Surgery, Preventive Cardiovascular Nurses Association, Society for Cardiovascular Angiography and Interventions, and Society of Thoracic Surgeons. J Am Coll Cardiol 2012;60(24):e44–164.
12. Myers J, Prakash M, Froelicher V, et al. Exercise capacity and mortality among men referred for exercise testing. N Engl J Med 2002;346(11):793–801.
13. Knuuti J, Ballo H, Juarez-Orozco LE, et al. The performance of non-invasive tests to rule-in and rule-out significant coronary artery stenosis in patients with stable angina: a meta-analysis focused on post-test disease probability. Eur Heart J 2018;39(35):3322–30.
14. Wohlgelernter D, Cleman M, Highman HA, et al. Regional myocardial dysfunction during coronary angioplasty: evaluation by two-dimensional echocardiography and 12 lead electrocardiography. J Am Coll Cardiol 1986;7(6):1245–54.
15. Hauser AM, Gangadharan V, Ramos RG, et al. Sequence of mechanical, electro-cardiographic and clinical effects of repeated coronary artery occlusion in human

beings: echocardiographic observations during coronary angioplasty. J Am Coll Cardiol 1985;5(2 Pt 1):193–7.

16. Fleischmann KE, Hunink MG, Kuntz KM, et al. Exercise echocardiography or exercise SPECT imaging? A meta-analysis of diagnostic test performance. JAMA 1998;280(10):913–20.

17. Imran MB, Palinkas A, Picano E. Head-to-head comparison of dipyridamole echocardiography and stress perfusion scintigraphy for the detection of coronary artery disease: a meta-analysis. Comparison between stress echo and scintigraphy. Int J Cardiovasc Imaging 2003;19(1):23–8.

18. Picano E, Molinaro S, Pasanisi E. The diagnostic accuracy of pharmacological stress echocardiography for the assessment of coronary artery disease: a meta-analysis. Cardiovasc Ultrasound 2008;6:30.

19. Mc Ardle BA, Dowsley TF, deKemp RA, et al. Does rubidium-82 PET have superior accuracy to SPECT perfusion imaging for the diagnosis of obstructive coronary disease?: A systematic review and meta-analysis. J Am Coll Cardiol 2012; 60(18):1828–37.

20. Tarantini G, Cacciavillani L, Corbetti F, et al. Duration of ischemia is a major determinant of transmurality and severe microvascular obstruction after primary angioplasty: a study performed with contrast-enhanced magnetic resonance. J Am Coll Cardiol 2005;46(7):1229–35.

21. Pijls NH, De Bruyne B, Peels K, et al. Measurement of fractional flow reserve to assess the functional severity of coronary-artery stenoses. N Engl J Med 1996; 334(26):1703–8.

22. Fihn SD, Blankenship JC, Alexander KP, et al. 2014 ACC/AHA/AATS/PCNA/SCAI/STS focused update of the guideline for the diagnosis and management of patients with stable ischemic heart disease: a report of the American College of Cardiology/American Heart Association Task Force on Practice Guidelines, and the American Association for Thoracic Surgery, Preventive Cardiovascular Nurses Association, Society for Cardiovascular Angiography and Interventions, and Society of Thoracic Surgeons. J Am Coll Cardiol 2014;64(18):1929–49.

23. Hillis LD, Smith PK, Anderson JL, et al. 2011 ACCF/AHA Guideline for Coronary Artery Bypass Graft Surgery. A report of the American College of Cardiology Foundation/American Heart Association Task Force on Practice Guidelines. Developed in collaboration with the American Association for Thoracic Surgery, Society of Cardiovascular Anesthesiologists, and Society of Thoracic Surgeons. J Am Coll Cardiol 2011;58(24):e123–210.

24. Levine GN, Bates ER, Bittl JA, et al. 2016 ACC/AHA Guideline Focused Update on Duration of Dual Antiplatelet Therapy in Patients With Coronary Artery Disease: A Report of the American College of Cardiology/American Heart Association Task Force on Clinical Practice Guidelines. J Am Coll Cardiol 2016;68(10):1082–115.

25. Holmes DR Jr, Rich JB, Zoghbi WA, et al. The heart team of cardiovascular care. J Am Coll Cardiol 2013;61(9):903–7.

26. Tsang MB, Schwalm JD, Gandhi S, et al. Comparison of heart team vs interventional cardiologist recommendations for the treatment of patients with multivessel coronary artery disease. JAMA Netw Open 2020;3(8):e2012749.

27. Serruys PW, Morice MC, Kappetein AP, et al. Percutaneous coronary intervention versus coronary-artery bypass grafting for severe coronary artery disease. N Engl J Med 2009;360(10):961–72.

28. Stone GW, Sabik JF, Serruys PW, et al. Everolimus-Eluting Stents or Bypass Surgery for Left Main Coronary Artery Disease. N Engl J Med 2016;375(23):2223–35.

29. Head SJ, Milojevic M, Daemen J, et al. Mortality after coronary artery bypass grafting versus percutaneous coronary intervention with stenting for coronary artery disease: a pooled analysis of individual patient data. Lancet 2018; 391(10124):939–48.
30. Davierwala PM, Gao C, Thuijs D, et al. Single or multiple arterial bypass graft surgery vs. percutaneous coronary intervention in patients with three-vessel or left main coronary artery disease. Eur Heart J 2021. https://doi.org/10.1093/eurheartj/ehab537.
31. Rocha RV, Tam DY, Karkhanis R, et al. Multiple arterial grafting is associated with better outcomes for coronary artery bypass grafting patients. Circ 2018;138(19): 2081–90.
32. Esper RB, Farkouh ME, Ribeiro EE, et al. SYNTAX Score in patients with diabetes undergoing coronary revascularization in the FREEDOM trial. J Am Coll Cardiol 2018;72(23 Pt A):2826–37.
33. Peterson MD, Borger MA, Rao V, et al. Skeletonization of bilateral internal thoracic artery grafts lowers the risk of sternal infection in patients with diabetes. J Thorac Cardiovasc Surg 2003;126(5):1314–9.
34. Sa MP, Ferraz PE, Escobar RR, et al. Skeletonized versus pedicled internal thoracic artery and risk of sternal wound infection after coronary bypass surgery: meta-analysis and meta-regression of 4817 patients. Interact Cardiovasc Thorac Surg 2013;16(6):849–57.
35. Ding WJ, Ji Q, Shi YQ, et al. Incidence of deep sternal wound infection in diabetic patients undergoing off-pump skeletonized internal thoracic artery grafting. Cardiology 2016;133(2):111–8.
36. Tatoulis J, Buxton BF, Fuller JA. The right internal thoracic artery: the forgotten conduit–5,766 patients and 991 angiograms. Ann Thorac Surg 2011;92(1):9–15 [discussion 15-17].
37. Tatoulis J, Buxton BF, Fuller JA. Results of 1,454 free right internal thoracic artery-to-coronary artery grafts. Ann Thorac Surg 1997;64(5):1263–8 [discussion: 1268-1269].
38. Sabik JF 3rd, Stockins A, Nowicki ER, et al. Does location of the second internal thoracic artery graft influence outcome of coronary artery bypass grafting? Circulation 2008;118(14 Suppl):S210–5.
39. Gaudino M, Audisio K, Rahouma M, et al. Comparison of long-term clinical outcomes of skeletonized vs pedicled internal thoracic artery harvesting techniques in the arterial revascularization trial. JAMA Cardiol 2021. https://doi.org/10.1001/jamacardio.2021.3866.
40. Sabik JF 3rd, Lytle BW, Blackstone EH, et al. Comparison of saphenous vein and internal thoracic artery graft patency by coronary system. Ann Thorac Surg 2005; 79(2):544–51 [discussion: 544-551].
41. Vural KM, Sener E, Tasdemir O. Long-term patency of sequential and individual saphenous vein coronary bypass grafts. Eur J Cardiothorac Surg 2001;19(2): 140–4.
42. Goldman S, Zadina K, Moritz T, et al. Long-term patency of saphenous vein and left internal mammary artery grafts after coronary artery bypass surgery: results from a Department of Veterans Affairs Cooperative Study. J Am Coll Cardiol 2004;44(11):2149–56.
43. Tian M, Wang X, Sun H, et al. No-touch versus conventional vein harvesting techniques at 12 months after coronary artery bypass grafting surgery: multicenter randomized, controlled trial. Circulation 2021. https://doi.org/10.1161/CIRCULATIONAHA.121.055525.

44. Kim KB, Hwang HY, Hahn S, et al. A randomized comparison of the Saphenous Vein Versus Right Internal Thoracic Artery as a Y-Composite Graft (SAVE RITA) trial: one-year angiographic results and mid-term clinical outcomes. J Thorac Cardiovasc Surg 2014;148(3):901–7 [discussion: 907-908].
45. Kim MS, Hwang HY, Kim JS, et al. Saphenous vein versus right internal thoracic artery as a Y-composite graft: five-year angiographic and clinical results of a randomized trial. J Thorac Cardiovasc Surg 2018;156(4):1424–33.e1.
46. Ganyukov V, Kochergin N, Shilov A, et al. Randomized clinical trial of surgical vs. percutaneous vs. hybrid revascularization in multivessel coronary artery disease: residual myocardial ischemia and clinical outcomes at one year-hybrid coronary REvascularization Versus Stenting or Surgery (HREVS). J Interv Cardiol 2020; 2020:5458064. https://doi.org/10.1155/2020/5458064.
47. Basman C, Hemli JM, Kim MC, et al. Long-term survival in triple-vessel disease: Hybrid coronary revascularization compared to contemporary revascularization methods. J Card Surg 2020;35(10):2710–8.
48. Elbadawi A, Hamed M, Elgendy IY, et al. Outcomes of Reoperative Coronary Artery Bypass Graft Surgery in the United States. J Am Heart Assoc 2020;9(15): e016282.
49. Gallo M, Trivedi JR, Monreal G, et al. Risk factors and outcomes in redo coronary artery Bypass Grafting. Heart Lung Circ 2020;29(3):384–9.
50. Shroyer AL, Grover FL, Hattler B, et al. On-pump versus off-pump coronary-artery bypass surgery. N Engl J Med 2009;361(19):1827–37.
51. Lamy A, Devereaux PJ, Prabhakaran D, et al. Effects of off-pump and on-pump coronary-artery bypass grafting at 1 year. N Engl J Med 2013;368(13):1179–88.
52. Lamy A, Devereaux PJ, Prabhakaran D, et al. Five-year outcomes after off-pump or on-pump coronary-artery bypass grafting. N Engl J Med 2016;375(24): 2359–68.
53. Shroyer AL, Hattler B, Wagner TH, et al. Five-year outcomes after on-pump and off-pump coronary-artery bypass. N Engl J Med 2017;377(7):623–32.
54. Diegeler A, Borgermann J, Kappert U, et al. Five-Year Outcome After Off-Pump or On-Pump Coronary Artery Bypass Grafting in Elderly Patients. Circulation 2019; 139(16):1865–71.
55. Polomsky M, He X, O'Brien SM, et al. Outcomes of off-pump versus on-pump coronary artery bypass grafting: Impact of preoperative risk. J Thorac Cardiovasc Surg 2013;145(5):1193–8.
56. Taggart DP, Gaudino MF, Gerry S, et al. Ten-year outcomes after off-pump versus on-pump coronary artery bypass grafting: Insights from the Arterial Revascularization Trial. J Thorac Cardiovasc Surg 2021;162(2):591–9.e8.
57. Benedetto U, Raja SG, Soliman RF, et al. Minimally invasive direct coronary artery bypass improves late survival compared with drug-eluting stents in isolated proximal left anterior descending artery disease: a 10-year follow-up, single-center, propensity score analysis. J Thorac Cardiovasc Surg 2014;148(4):1316–22.
58. Kulik A, Ruel M, Jneid H, et al. Secondary prevention after coronary artery bypass graft surgery: a scientific statement from the American Heart Association. Circ 2015;131(10):927–64.

Approach to the Patient with a Murmur

John Landefeld, MD, MS*, Melody Tran-Reina, MD,
Mark Henderson, MD, MACP

KEYWORDS

- Cardiac auscultation • Valvular heart disease • Murmurs • Physical examination

KEY POINTS

- The cardiac examination consists of auscultation, visualization, palpation, and special maneuvers, all of which can reveal abnormalities suggestive of valvular heart disease.
- Likelihood ratios, calculated from the sensitivity and specificity of a physical finding (or test result), are useful to adjust one's clinical impression or likelihood of a given diagnosis, providing practical information regarding the need for further evaluation or management.
- The most robust likelihood ratios for the cardiac examination pertain to systolic murmurs, the primary focus of this review.

 Video content accompanies this article at http://www.medical.theclinics.com.

INTRODUCTION

As average life expectancy approaches 80 years in the United States, and exceeds 80 years in many other wealthy countries, the prevalence of valvular heart disease is growing, impacting patient quality of life, functional status, and mortality. Recently, advances in valve replacement and repair for patients with valvular heart disease have led to improvements in outcomes for patients with conditions such as mitral regurgitation and aortic stenosis.[1] The identification of patients who might benefit from these and other treatments often depends on a clinician's ability to evaluate for valvular pathologies through the physical examination. Murmurs are initially classified according to their timing in the cardiac cycle, specifically, systolic or diastolic. As they are most common, systolic murmurs will be the focus of this article. Diastolic murmurs generally indicate important underlying valvular pathology, but there is less

This article originally appeared in *Medical Clinics*, Volume 106, Issue 3, May 2022.
Department of Internal Medicine, UC Davis School of Medicine, 4150 V Street, Suite 2400, Sacramento, CA 95817, USA
* Corresponding author.
E-mail address: jclandefeld@ucdavis.edu

Clinics Collections 13 (2023) 169–180
https://doi.org/10.1016/j.ccol.2023.02.009

evidence supporting the diagnostic utility of the accompanying physical examination findings.

Likelihood Ratios

Interpreting the physical examination findings for valvular heart disease requires a basic understanding of likelihood ratios. Likelihood ratios serve to define the relative utility of a given physical examination maneuver (or test result) and can be applied in clinical scenarios to determine the likelihood that a patient has (or does not have) a particular valvular pathology.

Likelihood ratios are a function of test sensitivity and specificity. A *positive likelihood ratio* (+LR) can be calculated as follows:

$$+LR = \frac{Sensitivity}{1 - Specificity}$$

A + LR can also be articulated as:*

$$+LR = \frac{The\ probability\ that\ a\ person\ with\ Condition\ A'\ tested\ ^{2}\ positive\ for\ Condition\ A}{The\ probability\ that\ a\ person\ without\ Condition\ A'\ tested'\ positive\ for\ Condition\ A}$$

$$ie. + LR = \frac{The\ probability\ of\ a\ true\ positive}{The\ probability\ of\ a\ false\ positive}$$

A *negative likelihood ratio* can be calculated as follows:

$$-LR = \frac{1 - Sensitivity}{Specificity}$$

A −LR can also be read as:

$$-LR = \frac{The\ probability\ that\ a\ person\ \textbf{with}\ Condition A\ tested\ negative\ for\ Condition A}{The\ probability\ that\ a\ person\ \textbf{without}\ Condition A\ tested\ negative\ for\ Condition A}$$

$$ie. - LR = \frac{The\ probability\ of\ a\ false\ negative}{The\ probability\ of\ a\ true\ negative}$$

An LR close to 1 means that the test result or clinical finding does not appreciably change the likelihood of disease. A +LR informs the clinician how much a positive test result (or the presence of a given clinical finding) changes the probability of a disease. A −LR suggests how much a negative test result (or the absence of a given clinical finding) changes the probability of a disease. In this review, we include physical examination findings with LRs greater than 5 or less than 0.2, because such findings sufficiently impact post-test probabilities as to be clinically useful.

Clinicians can apply physical examination findings with a known likelihood ratio to their pretest probability of disease by using a Fagan nomogram, to thus arrive at a post-test probability (**Fig. 1**).[2] The post-test probability informs further diagnostic and therapeutic planning.

---

* In the case of a physical exam finding, 'tested' refers to the probability that a person with Condition A has a particular characteristic physical exam finding associated with Condition A.

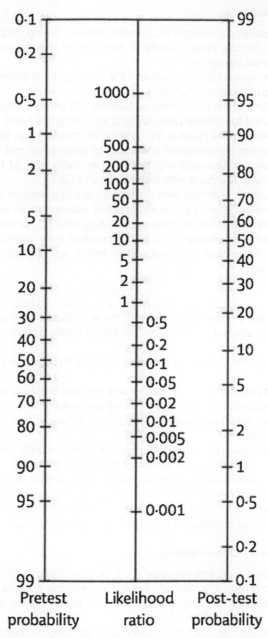

Fig. 1. Fagan nomogram. (*Adapted from* Fagan TJ. Nomogram for Bayes's theorem. N Engl J Med Jul 31, 1975; 293(5):257.)

AUSCULTATION IN VALVULAR HEART DISEASE

Auscultation of the heart in a patient with suspected valvular heart disease centers around 4 core components: timing, intensity, onomatopoeia, and location. A precise description of murmurs is fundamental to identifying valvular pathology and informing appropriate next steps.

Timing in the Cardiac Cycle

The first step in classifying a murmur is to characterize its timing. Murmurs may occur in either part of the cardiac cycle (systole or diastole), or in some instances, may be continuous throughout the cycle.

Systolic murmurs, which occur in between the closing of the atrioventricular valves (S1) and the closing of the semilunar valves (S2), are the most common. Diastolic murmurs occur at any time in the longer interval between S2 and S1. One can first identify S1 and S2 by palpating the carotid pulse while auscultating the heart. The heart sound that nearly coincides with the pulse is S1. Systolic murmurs, by far the most common murmurs, should further be described according to when in systole they occur.[3]

Early systolic murmurs: Murmurs with indistinct or obliterated S1 but distinct S2.

Midsystolic murmurs: Murmurs with distinct S1 *and* S2.

Late systolic murmurs: Murmurs with distinct S1 but indistinct or obliterated S2.

Holosystolic murmurs: Murmurs with indistinct or obliterated S1 *and* S2.

Diastolic murmurs tend to occur either immediately after S2, in mid-diastole, or late in diastole (also termed "presystolic"). Early murmurs may obscure S2 and mid-diastolic murmurs (eg, mitral stenosis) often follow an opening *snap* (more on *onomatopoeia* below).

Murmur Intensity

Once the timing of the murmur is established, the examiner should describe its intensity. By convention, intensity is categorized into 6 levels according to the Levine grading system.

Grade 1: Murmurs only audible by listening carefully through the stethoscope for a period of time.

Grade 2: Murmurs audible as soon as the stethoscope is placed on the chest wall.

Grade 3: Murmurs which are loud with the stethoscope but without a palpable thrill.

Grade 4: Murmurs which are loud, still require a stethoscope to be heard, and are associated with a thrill.

Grade 5: Murmurs which are very loud, associated with a thrill, but only require the edge of the stethoscope to contact the chest in order to be heard.

Grade 6: An unusually loud murmur, associated with a thrill, and audible with the stethoscope even when the stethoscope is just off the surface of the chest wall.

The intensity of a murmur alone is not particularly predictive of the underlying cause, but may be useful when considered in context with other findings.

Nature of the Sounds—Onomatopoeia

After determining the timing and intensity of the murmur, the clinician should describe the nature of the murmur. Phonetically imitating aloud the sounds auscultated is a practical way to differentiate various murmurs and to accurately communicate the findings to colleagues and learners.[4]

The clinician should mimic the sound while demonstrating its relationship to the first and second heart sounds. For instance, the high-pitched murmur of mitral regurgitation might be described as "lubHoooooooodub," with "lub" indicating mitral valve closure, "Hoooooooo" indicating the regurgitant flow across the mitral valve, and "dub" indicating aortic valve closure. The murmur of aortic stenosis is often described as "harsh," owing to the combination of both high-pitched and low-pitched sounds. The clinician may hear a guttural "lub gRRRrrr dub" murmur with aortic stenosis. An aortic murmur that has a "blowing" nature is less likely to be severe aortic stenosis (−LR 0.1).[5]

Mitral valve prolapse is a common pathology accompanied by a "midsystolic click" that sounds similar to a "*k*" sound. Regurgitant flow across the mitral valve may develop over time. The combined sound of mitral valve prolapse and mitral regurgitation may be described as "lub...kHoooooooodub."

Sound intensity may also be indicated with onomatopoeia. For example, the early diastolic high frequency blowing decrescendo murmur of aortic regurgitation may obscure S2 and be indicated as "Lub... PEWWww....". If this murmur is grade 3 intensity or louder, the patient likely has moderate to severe aortic regurgitation (+LR 8.2). The absence of the characteristic diastolic murmur is strong evidence against the existence of moderate to severe aortic regurgitation (−LR 0.1).

The low-pitched murmur of mitral stenosis begins in mid-diastole, occasionally after a snap (the sound of the stenotic leaflets opening). It may sound like "up bu duprrrrRR-Rup," with "up" being S1 (which may be louder than normal), "bu" being S2, and "dup" being the opening snap. The rumble may eclipse the beginning of S1.

Location on Chest Wall (Broad or Small Apical-base, Broad Apical, LLSB, Apical Only, Base Only)

The distribution of sound on the chest wall is helpful in differentiating systolic murmurs. The *third left parasternal space* overlies both the aortic and mitral valves and is thus used as a landmark to help classify systolic murmurs into 1 of 6 possible patterns (**Fig. 2**). The primary determinant of a murmur's radiation is *not* necessarily the direction of blood flow, but rather how the abnormal blood flow generates vibrations in the ventricles and/or great arteries, which are also transmitted because of adjacent bony vibration. Vibrations of the ventricles and lower ribs will generate sound *below* the third left parasternal space, and vibrations of the great arteries, sternum, and clavicles will generate sound *above* the third left parasternal space.

The location on the chest wall helps to identify whether murmurs are characteristic for certain valvular pathologies. Increased aortic valve velocity (suggestive of aortic stenosis) results in a broad apical-base pattern (+LR 9.7) on the chest wall. A broad apical pattern increases the probability of mitral regurgitation (+LR 6.8), whereas the left lower sternal pattern increases the probability of tricuspid regurgitation (+LR 8.4).[6]

The diastolic murmur of aortic regurgitation is often heard most prominently at the left sternal border (and occasionally at the right sternal border). The diastolic murmur of pulmonic regurgitation is typically loudest at the left sternal border at the second intercostal space.

All 4 components of auscultation—timing, intensity, onomatopoeia, and location— should be interpreted in relation to one another with their associated likelihood ratios (**Table 1**).

Visualization and Palpation in Valvular Heart Disease

Direct observation of the patient's undraped chest and neck may help determine the etiology of a murmur. Visualization and/or palpation of the cardiac apex may also be helpful; normally there is a single apical impulse per cardiac cycle. A double apical impulse may suggest left ventricular (LV) hypertrophy (+LR 5.6). A hyperkinetic apical impulse may be seen in mitral regurgitation (+LR 11.2). On the other hand, the *absence* of an enlarged apical impulse decreases the probability of moderate to severe aortic regurgitation (−LR 0.1).

With severe tricuspid regurgitation, the right ventricle becomes dilated and occupies the cardiac apex. In systole, the apex may be seen to move inward, and a simultaneous outward motion may be seen at the left or right lower sternal border signifying the increased flow into the dilated right atrium. This visual finding is known

ABOVE AND BELOW THIRD LEFT PARASTERNAL SPACE

Broad apical-base pattern
Murmur extends at least
from the first right parasternal
space to fourth intercostal
space at MCL; may have
diminished intensity at LLSB

Small apical-base pattern
Murmur oriented obliquely
but does not meet criteria
of broad apical-base pattern

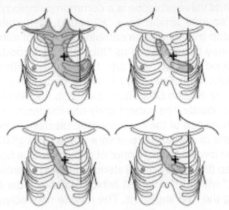

ENTIRELY BELOW THIRD LEFT PARASTERNAL SPACE

Left lower sternal pattern
Murmur along left sternal
edge; may extend to MCL

Broad apical pattern
Murmur in fourth or fifth intercostal
space, or both, and extends at
least from MCL to anterior
axillary line; may extend to
sternum

Isolated apical pattern
Murmur near MCL, fourth or fifth
intercostal space, confined to
diameter of stethoscope

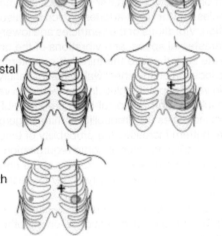

ENTIRELY ABOVE THIRD LEFT PARASTERNAL SPACE

Isolated base pattern
Murmur centered at second
intercostal space or
higher; may radiate to neck
or along clavicles

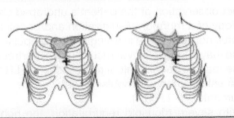

Fig. 2. Location on the chest wall of 6 systolic murmur patterns. (*Reproduced with permission from* Evidence-Based Physical Diagnosis, 4th Ed., Steven McGee, Fig 43.1 Six systolic murmur patterns. Copyright Elsevier 20.)

Table 1
Clinically useful examination findings, as determined by likelihood ratios (+LR > 5, −LR < 0.2)

Finding	Sensitivity (%)	Specificity (%)	Likelihood Ratio if Finding is	
			Present	Absent
Characteristic Systolic Murmur				
Mild tricuspid regurgitation or worse (*LubSHSHSHSHdub in a left-lower sternal pattern*)	23	98	**14.6**	0.8
Mild or worse aortic stenosis (*Lub GRRRR dub in a broad apical-base pattern or small apical-base pattern*)	90	85	**5.9**	**0.1**
Mild or worse mitral regurgitation (*LubSHSHSHSHdub in a broad apical pattern*)	56–75	89–93	**5.4**	0.4
Mitral valve prolapse (*Lub...kSHSHSHdub with midsystolic click in broad apical pattern*)	55	96	**12.1**	0.5
"Blowing" sound throughout aortic flow murmur for significant aortic stenosis	4	67	**0.1**	1.4
Characteristic Diastolic Murmur				
Mild or worse aortic regurgitation (*early diastolic high-frequency decrescendo murmur along lower sternal border*)	54–87	75–98	**9.9**	0.3
Detecting pulmonary regurgitation (*diastolic decrescendo murmur in 2nd intercostal space at left upper sternal border*)	15	99	**17.4**	NS
Intensity of S1 and S2				
S2 inaudible for increased aortic valve peak velocity in aortic stenosis			**12.7**	
Maneuvers				
Louder during inspiration (for TR)	78–95	87–97	**7.8**	0.2
Louder with Valsalva strain for HCM	70	95	**14**	0.3
Louder with squat-to-stand (for HCM)	95	84	6	**0.1**
Softer with stand-to-squat (for HCM)	88–95	84–97	**7.6**	**0.1**
Softer with passive leg elevation (for HCM)	90	90	9	**0.1**

(continued on next page)

Table 1
(continued)

Finding	Sensitivity (%)	Specificity (%)	Likelihood Ratio if Finding is	
			Present	Absent
Visualization and Palpation				
Hyperkinetic apical movement (for detecting MR)	74	93	11.2	0.3
Double apical movement (for LVH)	57	90	5.6	0.5
Right ventricular rock (for TR)	5	100	31.4	NS
Pulsatile liver (for TR)	12–30	92–99	6.5	NS
C-V wave (for TR)	37	97	10.9	0.7

Abbreviation: HCM, hypertrophic cardiomyopathy; LVH, left ventricular hypertrophy; MR, mitral regurgitation; TR, tricuspid regurgitation.

as the right ventricular rock (+LR 31.4). A pulsatile liver may also be palpated with severe tricuspid regurgitation (+LR 6.5).[7]

The jugular veins may demonstrate prominent outward pulsations or giant (fused) "c-v" waves in severe tricuspid regurgitation. The x-descent is obliterated and the "v" wave, representing right atrial filling, increases when the regurgitant jet crosses the tricuspid valve from the right ventricle. This finding, also known by the eponym Lancisi sign, can be seen in Video 1 in the online version of this text. It is important to differentiate the jugular venous pulsation from the carotid pulse; bounding carotid arteries may be seen in severe aortic regurgitation.

Patients with aortic regurgitation generate a large stroke volume followed by rapid diastolic emptying of aortic blood into the left ventricle, causing the arterial pulse wave to both rise and collapse abruptly. This is known as water-hammer pulses or Corrigan pulse. The same physiology produces fascinating pulsations throughout the body and has generated many eponyms such as Quincke pulse (capillary pulsations in the nail bed), de Musset sign (bobbing of the head), Müller sign (pulsation of the uvula), and Landolfi sign (pulsatile constriction of the iris, seen in Video 2 in the online version of this text). Although interesting, such findings do not offer particular diagnostic value in terms of likelihood ratios. However, widened pulse pressure (>80 mm Hg) or low diastolic pressure (<50 mm Hg) strongly suggest underlying aortic regurgitation (+LR 10.9 and +LR 19.3, respectively).[8]

By applying these findings on visualization and observation to the findings heard on auscultation, the clinician can further hone the differential diagnosis for a given murmur.

Maneuvers in Valvular Heart Disease

Special maneuvers that change venous return and afterload, can aid the clinician in differentiating the cause of a systolic murmur.

With inspiration, intrathoracic pressure decreases, increasing the volume of blood entering the right-sided chambers from the vena cava, while decreasing return to the left side of the heart. This elevated right-sided volume causes increased flow across the tricuspid and pulmonic valves. A murmur that increases or varies in intensity with inspiration suggests a murmur across the tricuspid or pulmonic valve.

Maneuvers that affect venous return are useful in evaluating suspected hypertrophic cardiomyopathy (HCM), in which the characteristic harsh midsystolic murmur is influenced by the degree of LV outflow tract obstruction by the anterior mitral valve leaflet and the hypertrophic interventricular septum. With the Valsalva maneuver or changing from squatting-to-standing, venous return to the right side of the heart decreases and the LV cavity size diminishes, which aggravates the degree of outflow tract obstruction and thus *increases* the intensity of the murmur (+LR 14 for Valsalva). On the other hand, standing-to-squatting or passive leg elevation both increase venous return, which enlarges the LV cavity size and causes the murmur intensity to decrease (+LR 9 for passive leg elevation). The absence of this characteristic response decreases the probability of HCM (−LR 0.1). Although the greatest risk of sudden death from HCM occurs in patients younger than 30 years, the average age at diagnosis of the condition is increasing (currently at over 50 years).[9] This increasing age likely reflects increased provider awareness and greater use of sensitive imaging modalities. Some of the maneuvers described earlier may be more challenging to conduct in physically limited or frail patients, but the Valsalva maneuver can usually be performed regardless of the patient's functional status.

Proper technique in performing maneuvers such as the Valsalva maneuver is key to eliciting the findings for which you can apply likelihood ratios to aid clinical decisions.

The Valsalva maneuver involves expiration against a closed airway for at least 20 seconds. As described by Valsalva, this was accomplished by breathing against a pinched nose and closed mouth. However, this approach can increase pressure in the Eustachian tubes, causing discomfort. Alternatively, breathing out against a closed glottis is a modified technique that may be more tolerable to patients. Patients should be instructed to strain their abdominal muscles as if to rapidly breath out, but to close their mouth and their airway in the back of their throat. To assess whether Valsalva is being performed correctly, the clinician should observe for distended neck veins or facial flushing, and palpate the patient's contracted abdominal muscles. The examiner should listen for a change in the murmur after a 20-second Valsalva strain.

Functional or Innocent Murmurs

Systolic murmurs may be present but without associated valvular pathology by echocardiography. Such murmurs, termed "functional" or "innocent" murmurs based on lack of structural heart disease, are quite common, although their prevalence varies with age. In young adults, the vast majority of systolic murmurs are functional. Although the peak incidence of functional murmurs is around age 3 to 4 years, studies suggest that 86% to 100% of younger adults with a systolic murmur will have a normal echocardiogram. Echocardiograms of elderly patients with systolic murmurs are often normal, although the percentage ranges widely (from 44% to 100%, depending on the study).

Functional murmurs tend to be of lower intensity (usually 2/6 or lower on the Levine grading scale), in early systole or midsystole, and are frequently loudest near the left upper sternal border. Functional murmurs are particularly common in children, and pediatricians have described the "7 S's" as key findings suggestive of a functional murmur: sensitive (the murmur changes in intensity with bodily position or respiration), short duration (not holosystolic), single (no clicks or gallops), small (the location is limited or nonradiating), soft (low volume), sweet (not harsh or coarse), and systolic.[10] However, because other pathologic murmurs can also have these characteristics, functional murmurs are defined by the *absence* of other abnormal findings. This includes normal jugular veins, normal apical impulse, normal pulses, no cardiopulmonary symptoms attributable to a pathologic murmur, and a decrease in intensity of the murmur with standing or the Valsalva maneuver.

When a patient has an examination consistent with a functional murmur, the likelihood ratio of the patient having a normal echocardiogram is 4.7. Although not particularly compelling compared with other likelihood ratios discussed in this article, depending on the pretest probability for valvular disease, a clinician could reasonably defer echocardiography in such a patient in accordance with principles of high-value care. It is important to note, however, that functional murmurs may be associated with other high cardiac output disease states (anemia, thyrotoxicosis) that may not present with echocardiographic abnormalities, but may still merit evaluation and treatment.

Putting It Together

After a comprehensive cardiac examination, the clinician can integrate findings to arrive at a differential diagnosis for the murmur in question. This may include the particular valve involved, the direction of flow, and the severity of disease. The flow chart in **Fig. 3** demonstrates one such approach to arriving at likelihood ratios based on these clinical examination results.

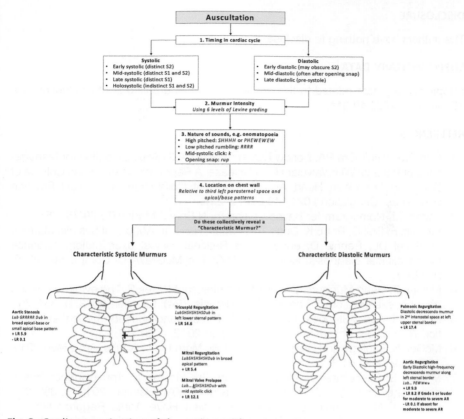

Fig. 3. Cardiac examination of the patient with a murmur.

CLINICS CARE POINTS

- A systematic approach to the cardiac examination can help determine the cause of a murmur.
- Auscultation forms the crux of the physical examination for patients with murmurs; visualization, palpation, and special maneuvers are useful adjuncts.
- The physical examination is most useful for systolic murmurs, although certain findings strongly suggest aortic regurgitation as the cause of a diastolic murmur.
- Findings with strong likelihood ratios (+LR > 5 or −LR < 0.2) should be applied to the pretest probability to ascertain a post-test probability to inform further evaluation.

SUMMARY

In this article, we presented an exam-based approach to narrowing the differential diagnoses for systolic and diastolic murmurs. The systematic examination of the patient, considering timing, intensity, onomatopoeia, and location of the murmur, as well as visualization, palpation, and special maneuvers, can meaningfully impact the clinician's interpretation of a murmur. Applying likelihood ratios for these findings to the pretest or prior probability of disease allows a prudent, timely, and thoughtful additional diagnostic workup and, in some instances, therapeutic intervention.

DISCLOSURE

The authors have nothing to disclose.

SUPPLEMENTARY DATA

Supplementary data related to this article can be found online at https://doi.org/10.1016/j.mcna.2021.12.011.

REFERENCES

1. Otto CM, Nishimura RA, Bonow RO, et al. 2020 ACC/AHA Guideline for Management of Patients With Valvular Heart Disease: A Report of the American College of Cardiology/American Heart Association Joint Committee on Clinical Practice Guidelines. Circulation 2021;143(5):e72–227.
2. Fagan TJ. Nomogram for Bayes's theorem. N Engl J Med 1975;293(5):257.
3. Etchells E, Bell C, Robb K. Does This Patient Have an Abnormal Systolic Murmur. In: Simel DL, Rennie D, editors. The Rational clinical examination: evidence based clinical diagnosis. New York, (NY): The McGraw-Hill Companies; 2009. p. 433–7.
4. McGee S. Heart Murmurs: General Principles. In: McGee S. The evidence-based physical examination. 3rd edition. Philadelphia, (PA): Elsevier; 2012. p. 351–70.
5. McGee S. Aortic Stenosis. In: McGee S. The evidence-based physical examination. 3rd edition. Philadelphia, (PA): Elsevier; 2012. p. 373–8.
6. McGee S. Etiology and Diagnosis of Systolic Murmurs in Adults. Am J Med 2010; 123(10):913–21.e1.
7. McGee S. Miscellaneous Heart Murmurs. In: McGee S. The evidence-based physical examination. 3rd edition. Philadelphia, (PA): Elsevier; 2012. p. 388–99.
8. Choudhry NK, Etchells EE. Does This Patient Have Aortic Regurgitation. In: Simel DL, Rennie D, editors. The Rational clinical examination: evidence based clinical diagnosis. New York, NY: The McGraw-Hill Companies; 2009. p. 419–27.
9. Canepa M, Fumagalli C, Tini G, et al. Temporal Trend of Age at Diagnosis in Hypertrophic Cardiomyopathy: An Analysis of the International Sarcomeric Human Cardiomyopathy Registry. Circ Heart Fail 2020;13(9):e007230.
10. Bronzetti G, Corzani A. The seven "S" murmurs: an alliteration about innocent murmurs in cardiac auscultation. Clin Pediatr (Phila) 2010;49(7):713.

Medical Management of Peripheral Artery Disease

Tara A. Holder, MD[a], J. Antonio Gutierrez, MD, MHS[b],
Aaron W. Aday, MD, MSc[a,c,*]

KEYWORDS

- Peripheral artery disease • Statins • Smoking cessation • Antiplatelet therapy
- Antithrombotic therapy

KEY POINTS

- Peripheral artery disease is a progressive atherosclerotic disease that remains underappreciated and poorly optimized.
- The target low-density lipoprotein cholesterol for this patient population is <70 mg/dL (1.8 mmol/L).
- Lipid-lowering therapy improves both cardiovascular and limb outcomes in peripheral artery disease.
- Angiotensin-converting enzyme inhibitors and aldosterone receptor antagonists remain the only antihypertensive therapies with a mortality benefit in peripheral artery disease.
- Aspirin plus low-dose rivaroxaban (2.5 mg twice daily) should be considered in high-risk patients with peripheral artery disease, such as those with a prior history of lower extremity revascularization or with atherosclerosis in other vascular territories.

INTRODUCTION

Lower extremity peripheral artery disease (PAD) is a malignant form of atherosclerosis associated with a heightened risk of cardiovascular morbidity and mortality.[1] Many patients with PAD have additional comorbidities, such as diabetes mellitus or atherosclerosis in additional vascular beds, further amplifying this risk.[2] Much of the medical

This article originally appeared in *Surgical Clinics*, Volume 102, Issue 3, June 2022.
Funding: This work was supported by NIH K23 HL151871 (Dr Aday).
[a] Division of Cardiovascular Medicine, Vanderbilt University Medical Center, 2220 Pierce Avenue, 383 PRB, Nashville, TN 37232-0021, USA; [b] Division of Cardiology, Department of Medicine, Duke University Medical Center, DUMC 3330, Durham, NC 27710, USA; [c] Vanderbilt Translational and Clinical Cardiovascular Research Center, Division of Cardiovascular Medicine, Vanderbilt University Medical Center, Nashville, TN, USA
* Corresponding author. Vanderbilt University Medical Center, 2525 West End Avenue Suite 300, Nashville, TN 37203.
E-mail address: aaron.w.aday@vumc.org
Twitter: @TaraHolder17 (T.A.H.); @JAGutierrezMD (J.A.G.); @AaronAdayMD (A.W.A.)

Clinics Collections 13 (2023) 181–196
https://doi.org/10.1016/j.ccol.2023.02.015

management of PAD overlaps with secondary prevention of coronary artery disease (CAD) and cerebrovascular disease. In the last 2 decades, greater attention to PAD has led to the development of novel therapies that decrease adverse cardiovascular and limb events in this patient population. This review focuses on the components of optimal medical management of patients with PAD.

SMOKING CESSATION

Tobacco use is strongly associated with cardiovascular disease and remains an important risk factor for the development and progression of PAD.[3] Ongoing smoking is associated with an increased risk of chronic limb-threatening ischemia (CLTI), need for revascularization and amputation, and major adverse cardiovascular events (MACE).[4,5] Observational data from patients with PAD who successfully stop smoking demonstrate improved outcomes,[6] making smoking cessation a primary target for clinicians.

Current smoking cessation strategies consist of both counseling and pharmacologic intervention with nicotine replacement therapy (NRT), bupropion, or varenicline. A previous study randomizing patients with PAD to either intensive counseling intervention or minimal intervention showed that patients in the intensive intervention group were more likely to achieve smoking abstinence at 6 months compared with the minimal intervention group (21.3% vs 6.8%, $P = .023$).[7] However, long-term abstinence often requires medical therapy (Table 1).

Bupropion is a norepinephrine and dopamine reuptake inhibitor. When used alone or in addition to nicotine replacement, bupropion leads to higher rates of smoking cessation at 12 months compared with placebo or NRT alone.[8] Varenicline is a partial agonist of α-4 and β-2 nicotinic acetylcholine receptors and remains the most effective smoking cessation aid. Randomized controlled trial data demonstrate that varenicline is more effective than placebo (odds ratio [OR], 3.61; 95% confidence interval [CI], 3.07–4.24), bupropion (OR, 1.68; 95% CI, 1.46–1.93) and nicotine patch (OR, 1.75; 95% CI, 1.52–2.01) at improving 12-week smoking abstinence rates.[9] Importantly, varenicline does not lead to an increase risk of neuropsychiatric side effects.[9]

Recommendations

Current professional guidelines recommend that all patients using tobacco should be advised to quit.[10] For patients that are willing to quit, shared decision-making can be used to determine the best pharmacologic treatment option with either NRT, bupropion, or varenicline.[11] Varenicline, either alone or in combination with NRT, is recommended as the first-line treatment in patients with cardiovascular disease. Based on availability of tobacco cessation programs and patient preference, counseling or group therapy may also be used.[11]

LIPID-LOWERING THERAPY

Dyslipidemia is an important modifiable risk factor in the development of cardiovascular disease and atherosclerosis. Atherogenic dyslipidemia, which is characterized by elevated concentrations of total cholesterol and low levels of high-density lipoprotein cholesterol, is a strong risk factor for PAD development.[12] In contrast with CAD, data demonstrating a link between low-density lipoprotein cholesterol (LDL-C) and incident PAD are sparse. Nonetheless, recent studies have shown a consistent benefit in lipid reduction to decrease MACE, as well as limb outcomes in patients with PAD.

Table 1
Pharmacologic treatment options for smoking cessation

Pharmaceutical	Dosing Strengths	Dosing	OTC	Evidence	Precautions	Side Effects	Dose Adjustments
Short-acting agents							
Nicotine gum	2 mg[a] 4 mg[b]	1 pc, q1–2 h × 6 wk 1 pc, q2–4 h × 3 wk 1 pc, q4–8 h × 3 wk Max: 24 pc/d	Yes	RCT[53]	None	Jaw pain, sleep disturbance, vivid dreams, oral irritation	None[c]
Nicotine lozenge	2 mg[a] 4 mg[b]	1 pc, q1–2 h × 6 wk 1 pc, q2–4 h × 3 wk 1 pc, q4–8 h × 3 wk Max: 20 pc/d	Yes	RCT[53]	None	Jaw pain, sleep disturbance, vivid dreams, oral irritation	None[c]
Nicotine inhaler	10 mg/cartridge	6–16 cartridges/d × 3–6 wk Reduce dose × 6–12 wk Max: 16 cartridges/d	No	RCT[54,55]	None	Headache, oral irritation, nasal discomfort, dyspepsia	None[c]
Nicotine intranasal spray	10 mg/mL (1 spray = 0.5 mg) (2 spray = 1 dose) (1 spray/nostril)	1–2 dose/h (1 spray/ nostril) No more than 5 doses (10 sprays) per hour Max: 40 mg/d (80 spray) or 3 mo treatment	No	ND	None	Headache, oral irritation, nasal discomfort, dyspepsia	None[c]
Long-acting agents							
Nicotine patch	14 mg (≤10 cig/d) 21 mg (>10 cig/d)	14 mg/d × 6 wk 7 mg/d × 2 wk 21 mg/d × 6 wk 14 mg/d × 2 wk 7 mg/d × 2 wk	No	RCT[56]	None	Local skin irritation, headaches, insomnia	None[c]
Bupropion	150 mg	150 mg/d × 3 d followed by 150 mg bid × 7–	No	RCT[8]	Seizure disorder, SI, use of MAOIs,	Insomnia, agitation, constipation	None[c]

(continued on next page)

Table 1
(continued)

Pharmaceutical	Dosing Strengths	Dosing	OTC	Evidence	Precautions	Side Effects	Dose Adjustments
		12 wk Max: 300 mg/d			simultaneous cessation of EtoH or Benzos		
Varenicline	0.5 mg	0.5 mg/d × 3 d 0.5 mg bid × 4–7 d 1.0 mg bid × 11 wk Max: 2.0 mg/d	No	RCT[9]	*Black box warning for neuropsychiatric events removed in 2016[57]	Nausea, vivid dreams	CrCl <30 mL/min Initial: 0.5 mg/d Max: 0.5 mg bid

Abbreviations: benzos, benzodiazepines; bid, twice daily; cig, cigarettes; CrCl, creatinine clearance; EtOH, alcohol; MAOi, monoamine oxidase inhibitors; ND, no data; OTC, over-the-counter; pc, piece; RCT, randomized controlled trial; SI, suicidal ideation.

Consider adjustments in moderate to severe renal/hepatic impairment.

[a] Smoke first cigarette after 30 minutes of waking.

[b] Smoke first cigarette within 30 minutes of waking.

[c] None provided on manufacturer labeling.

Statin Therapy

Although many patients with PAD participated in the landmark statin trials, PAD-specific outcome data are limited. In the Heart Protection Study, 20,536 high-risk patients with stable vascular disease, of whom 6748 had PAD, were randomized to either simvastatin or placebo. Simvastatin not only decreased the risk of all-cause mortality, but also led to a 16% relative decrease in the rate of first peripheral vascular event, irrespective of baseline LDL-C levels.[13] There was no decrease in amputations with simvastatin compared with placebo.

Observational studies have helped solidify the role of statins in improving PAD outcomes. The international Reduction of Atherothrombosis for Continued Health Registry, which included 5861 patients with symptomatic PAD, demonstrated that statin use was associated with a reduction in adverse limb events compared with those not taking statins (hazard ratio [HR] 0.82; 95% CI, 0.72–0.92, P = .01).[14] Among 155,647 patients with newly diagnosed PAD in the Veterans Affairs health system, statins, particularly high-intensity statin therapy, significantly decreased the rates of lower extremity amputation compared with antiplatelet therapy alone (HR, 0.67; 95% CI, 0.61–0.74).[15]

Ezetimibe

The Improved Reduction of Outcomes: Vytorin Efficacy International Trial (n = 18,144) examined the addition of ezetimibe, which inhibits absorption of cholesterol from the intestine, to simvastatin in patients with recent acute coronary syndrome. Within the trial, 1005 participants had a prior history of PAD. The addition of ezetimibe further decreased LDL-C by approximately 24% along with a reduction in MACE (HR, 0.94; 95% CI, 0.89–0.99; P = .016).[16] Limb events were not reported in this study.

PCSK9 inhibition

More recently, inhibitors of protein convertase subtilisin kexin type 9 (PCSK9) have been shown to not only decrease LDL-C concentrations in patients on statin therapy, but also to decrease the risk cardiovascular and limb events. The Further Cardiovascular Outcomes Research with PCSK9 Inhibition in Subjects with Elevated Risk trial randomized 27,564 patients with known atherosclerotic disease already on a statin to either evolocumab, a PCSK9 inhibitor, or placebo. In a subgroup analysis of 3642 patients with PAD, evolocumab led to a greater decrease in MACE (HR, 0.73; 95% CI, 0.59–0.91; P = .0040).[17] Although evolocumab led to a decrease in major adverse limb events in the overall study population, this decrease did not reach statistical significance in the PAD subgroup. In the ODYSSEY Outcomes trial, treatment with the PCSK9 inhibitor alirocumab did demonstrate a statistically significant reduction in a composite of CLTI, lower extremity amputation, or revascularization (HR, 0.69; 95% CI, 0.54–0.89; P = .004).[18]

Recommendations

The US guidelines recommend that all patients with PAD be treated with high-intensity statin therapy for a goal LDL-C decrease of 50% or greater,[19] whereas the European guidelines recommend a target LDL-C of less than 70 mg/dL.[20] High-intensity statin options include atorvastatin 40 to 80 mg/d or rosuvastatin 20 to 40 mg/d. In patients with PAD who do not achieve their target LDL-C on statin therapy alone, additional lipid-lowering therapy with ezetimibe or a PCSK9 inhibitor should be used.[19]

HYPERTENSION

Hypertension is associated with a doubling in the risk of death from stroke, heart disease, or other vascular disease.[21] Current professional guidelines recommend a target blood pressure less than 130/80 mm Hg in patients with cardiovascular disease, including PAD.[22] There remain few studies guiding target blood pressure or specific hypertensive therapeutic choices in patients with PAD. The subgroup analysis of the Appropriate Blood Pressure Control in Diabetes study examined patients with diabetes and PAD (ankle-brachial index [ABI] of <0.90) who were randomized to moderate blood pressure control (placebo, no intended change in diastolic blood pressure) or intensive blood pressure control (enalapril or nisoldipine, target decrease in diastolic blood pressure of 10 mm Hg). The intensive treatment group had a larger reduction in cardiovascular events compared with moderate treatment.[23] The Heart Outcomes Prevention Evaluation trial (n = 4051) randomized patients with vascular disease or diabetes, of whom 44% had PAD, to ramipril 10 mg/d or placebo. Overall, ramipril significantly decreased the risk of MACE in the PAD subgroup.[24] Other clinical trials have found similar reductions in MACE for patients with PAD treated with either angiotensin-converting enzyme inhibitors or angiotensin receptor blockers.[25,26]

There has long been concern that intensive blood pressure control may contribute to adverse limb outcomes in patients with PAD owing to worsened limb perfusion. Among 2699 participants with PAD in the INternational VErapamil-SR/Trandolapril Study, there was a J-shaped relationship between systolic blood pressure and a composite of all-cause death, myocardial infarction, or stroke.[27] Excess risk occurred with a systolic blood pressure of less than 135 mm Hg, suggesting that these patients might require different blood pressure targets. Similarly, the Antihypertensive and Lipid-Lowering Treatment to Prevent Heart Attack Trial (n = 33,357) found that patients with a systolic blood pressure of less than 120 mm Hg or greater than 160 mm Hg were at greater risk of PAD-related outcomes.[28] In contrast, recent data from the Examining the Use of Ticagrelor in Peripheral Artery Disease (EUCLID) trial showed that every 10 mm Hg decrease in systolic blood pressure of 125 mm Hg or less was associated with an increased risk of MACE (HR, 1.19; 95% CI, 1.09–1.31; $P<.001$) but no increased risk of adverse limb events (HR, 1.02%; 95%, 0.84–1.23; $P = .824$).[29] Additional work is needed to better understand the link between PAD and hypertension.

Recommendations

In patients with PAD, the American College of Cardiology/American Heart Association PAD guidelines recommend targeting a blood pressure of less than 130/80 mm Hg.[10] Angiotensin-converting enzyme inhibitors of angiotensin receptor blockers are the only antihypertensive medications with a mortality benefit in the PAD population and should remain the first-line therapies in this population. Current data suggest that intensive blood pressure control in patients with PAD, particularly those with more advanced PAD, may worsen limb symptoms, thus necessitating a more liberal target in select groups. PAD-specific blood pressure targets have yet to be defined.

ANTIPLATELET AND ANTITHROMBOTIC THERAPY
Antiplatelet Therapy

Antiplatelet and antithrombotic therapy remain key components of primary and secondary prevention of cardiovascular disease. Although antiplatelet therapy has historically been used to treat a wide range of atherosclerotic diseases, data supporting the use of these drugs in PAD, particularly in terms of decreasing adverse limb outcomes, are inconsistent. More recently, a combination of antiplatelet and antithrombotic therapy has shown significant benefits among patients with PAD, and these drug regimens represent a paradigm shift in PAD management (**Table 2**).

Table 2
Antiplatelet and antithrombotic trials in patients with PAD

Trial	POPADAD[31]	Aspirin for Asymptomatic Atherosclerosis Trialists[32]	CAPRIE[33]	CHARISMA[36]	EUCLID[34]	TRA 2°P-TIMI 50[35]
			Antiplatelet therapy			
Intervention	Aspirin 100 mg/d vs placebo	Aspirin 100 mg/d vs placebo	Aspirin 325 mg/d vs clopidogrel 75 mg/d	Clopidogrel 75 mg/d plus either aspirin 75–162 mg/d or placebo	Ticagrelor 90 mg twice daily vs clopidogrel 75 mg/d	Vorapaxar 2.5 mg/d vs placebo
Study population	1276 patients with diabetes and an ABI of ≤0.99	3350 patients with an ABI of ≤0.95	19,185 total 6452 patients with intermittent claudication and either an ABI of ≤0.85 or prior revascularization/amputation	15,603 total 3096 patients with intermittent claudication and either an ABI of ≤0.85 or prior revascularization/amputation	13,885 patients with and ABI of ≤0.85 or prior revascularization	26,449 total 3787 patients with an ABI of ≤0.85 or prior revascularization
MACE outcomes	Vascular death, MI, stroke: HR, 0.98; 95% CI, 0.76–1.26	Fatal or nonfatal MI, stroke, or revascularization: HR, 1.03; 95% CI, 0.84–1.27	Vascular death, MI, or ischemic stroke in PAD subgroup: HR, 0.76; 95% CI, 0.64–0.91	CV death, MI, or stroke: HR, 0.85; 95% CI, 0.66–1.08	CV death, MI, or stroke: HR, 1.02; 95% CI, 0.92–1.13	CV death, MI, stroke: HR, 0.94; 95% CI, 0.78–1.14
MALE outcomes	Major amputation: 2% vs 2%	None reported	None reported	None reported	Hospitalization for ALI: HR, 1.03; 95% CI, 0.79–1.33 Lower limb revascularization: HR, 0.95; 95% CI, 0.90–1.05	Hospitalization for ALI: HR, 0.58; 95% CI, 0.39–0.86 Lower limb revascularization: HR, 0.84; 95% CI, 0.73–0.97

Antithrombotic therapy

Trial	WAVE[38]	COMPASS[40]	VOYAGER PAD[42]
Intervention	Warfarin with an INR goal of 2.0–3.0 plus antiplatelet monotherapy vs antiplatelet monotherapy alone	Rivaroxaban 2.5 mg twice daily plus aspirin 100 mg/d, rivaroxaban 5 mg twice daily plus placebo, or aspirin 100 mg/d plus placebo	Rivaroxaban 2.5 mg twice daily plus aspirin 100 mg/d vs aspirin plus placebo
Study population	2161 patients with symptomatic PAD or carotid/subclavian stenosis	27,395
7470 patients with symptomatic PAD or carotid stenosis	6564 patients with PAD and recent lower extremity revascularization
MACE outcomes	CV death, MI, stroke: RR, 0.92; 95% CI, 0.73–1.16	CV death, MI or stroke:	

ASA + rivaroxaban vs ASA + placebo: HR, 0.72; 95% CI, 0.57–0.90; *P* = .0047Primary outcome MACE + MALE: HR, 0.85; 95% CI, 0.76–0.96   MALE outcomesRevascularization: 3.3% vs 3.7%; *P* = .64

Amputation: 0.7% vs 1.1%; *P* = .37MALE: HR, 0.54; 95% CI, 0.35–0.82; *P* = .0037ALI: HR, 0.67; 95% CI, 0.55–0.82*Abbreviations:* ABI, ankle-brachial index; ALI, acute limb ischemia; CAPRIE, Clopidogrel versus Aspirin in Patients at Risk of Ischaemic Events; CHARISMA, Clopidogrel for High Atherothrombotic Risk and Ischemic Stabilization, Management, and Avoidance; COMPASS, Cardiovascular Outcomes for People Using Anticoagulation Strategies; CV, cardiovascular; INR, international normalized ratio; MALE, major adverse limb event; MI, myocardial infarction; POPADAD, Progression of Arterial Disease and Diabetes; RR, relative risk; VOYAGER PAD, Vascular Outcomes Study of ASA Along with Rivaroxaban in Endovascular or Surgical Limb Revascularization for PAD; WAVE, Warfarin Antiplatelet Vascular Evaluation.

Aspirin

Aspirin is a cyclooxygenase-1 inhibitor that inhibits the effect of thromboxane A2, thus inhibiting platelet aggregation. The ATT Collaboration meta-analysis showed that patients with symptomatic PAD on antiplatelet therapy had a 22% reduction in MACE. Although this analysis used various aspirin doses and other antithrombotic therapies, this marks the earliest clinical evidence supporting antiplatelet therapy in PAD.[30]

More recent studies have shown a less consistent benefit of aspirin therapy. The Prevention of Progression of Arterial Disease and Diabetes trial (n = 1276) assessed the efficacy of aspirin 100 mg versus placebo in patients with diabetes and PAD. The study found no difference between groups in cardiovascular end points (18.2% vs 18.3%), nor was there a difference in lower extremity amputation.[31] The Aspirin for Asymptomatic Atherosclerosis Trial (n = 3350) examined aspirin 100 mg versus placebo in patients with PAD (ABI of $\leq$0.95), and once again found no difference in cardiovascular end points or improvement in intermittent claudication.[32]

Clopidogrel

Clopidogrel is a prodrug, metabolized by the liver, that irreversibly binds and inactivates the platelet receptor, $P2Y_{12}$. The Clopidogrel versus Aspirin in Patients at Risk of Ischaemic Events (CAPRIE) trial (n = 19,185) randomized patients with symptomatic atherosclerotic disease to clopidogrel 75 mg/d versus aspirin 325 mg/d. In the PAD subgroup (n = 6452), clopidogrel decreased MACE (relative risk reduction 23.8%; 95% CI, 8.9–36.2; P = .0028) compared with aspirin with similar bleeding rates.[33]

Ticagrelor

The EUCLID trial sought to build on the results of CAPRIE. Ticagrelor is also an inhibitor of the $P2Y_{12}$ platelet receptor but, unlike clopidogrel, is not a prodrug and does not require activation by the body. In this study, 13,885 patients with symptomatic PAD (ABI of <0.80 or prior revascularization) were randomized to either ticagrelor 90 mg or clopidogrel 75 mg/d. The primary end point of MACE was similar between groups (HR, 1.02; 95% CI, 0.92–1.13; P = .65) with no differences observed in the rates of acute limb ischemia (ALI) or lower limb revascularization.[34]

Vorapaxar

Vorapaxar is a novel antiplatelet drug that inhibits platelet aggregation by the irreversible inhibition of protease-activated receptor-1. In TRA 2°P-TIMI 50, 20,170 patients with stable atherosclerotic vascular disease (myocardial infarction, stroke, or symptomatic PAD) were randomized to vorapaxar 2.5 mg/d or placebo. Among the subgroup with PAD (n = 3787), there was no significant reduction in MACE with vorapaxar therapy (HR, 0.94; 95% CI, 0.78–1.14; P = .53), although there was a decrease in hospitalization for ALI (HR, 0.58; 95% CI, 0.39–0.86; P = .006) and peripheral artery revascularization (HR, 0.84; 95% CI, 0.73–0.97; P = .017). This came at the cost of increased bleeding with vorapaxar (HR, 1.62; 95% CI, 1.21–2.18; P = .001), which has in part limited the use of this drug.[35]

Dual antiplatelet therapy

The Clopidogrel for High Atherothrombotic Risk and Ischemic Stabilization, Management, and Avoidance trial (n = 15,603) evaluated the effect of low-dose aspirin plus clopidogrel versus aspirin plus placebo in individuals with stable cardiovascular disease or multiple risk factors. In subgroup analyses (n = 3096) of patients with symptomatic (92%) and asymptomatic PAD (8%), there was similarly no decrease in MACE with dual antiplatelet therapy (DAPT) compared with aspirin (HR, 0.85; 95% CI, 0.66–

1.08; $P = .18$).[36] Similar results were seen in the Clopidogrel and Acetylsalicylic Acid in Bypass Surgery trial in PAD patients undergoing unilateral surgical bypass grafting. Although there was no benefit to DAPT in decreasing mortality, the trial did suggest a benefit in decreasing prosthetic graft occlusions.[37]

Antithrombotic Therapy

Vitamin K antagonism

Until recently, data on antithrombotic therapy in PAD were largely limited to the Warfarin Antiplatelet Vascular Evaluation trial. In this study, 2161 patients with PAD were randomized to warfarin (international normalized ratio of 2–3) plus aspirin versus aspirin alone.[38] There was no significant reduction in MACE (relative risk, 0.92; 95% CI, 0.73–1.16; $P = .48$) with warfarin, although there was a significant increase in life-threatening bleeding (relative risk, 3.41; 95% CI, 1.84–6.35; $P<.001$). Accordingly, professional guidelines do not support the use of warfarin in treating PAD.[10]

Factor Xa inhibition

After the development of numerous oral factor Xa inhibitors, several trials has assessed their efficacy in reducing atherosclerotic events in conjunction with anti-platelet therapy. In the Cardiovascular Outcomes for People Using Anticoagulation Strategies (COMPASS) trial, 27,396 patients with stable CAD, PAD, or carotid disease were randomized to 1 of 3 drug regimens: the factor Xa inhibitor rivaroxaban 5 mg twice daily plus placebo, rivaroxaban 2.5 mg twice daily plus aspirin, or aspirin mono-therapy plus placebo. The trial was terminated early after a mean follow-up period of 23 months owing to the decrease in MACE in the rivaroxaban plus aspirin versus the aspirin monotherapy group (HR, 0.76; 95% CI, 0.66–0.86; $P<.001$).[39]

The PAD subanalysis of COMPASS (n = 7470) included 4129 with symptomatic lower extremity PAD, 1422 patients with CAD and an ABI of less than 0.90, and 1919 patients with CAD and carotid disease. The combination of rivaroxaban plus aspirin compared with aspirin monotherapy showed significantly decreased rates of MACE (HR, 0.72; 95% CI, 0.57–0.90; $P = .0047$) and major adverse limb event (HR, 0.54; 95% CI, 0.35–0.82; $P = .0037$).[40] Similarly, this regimen led to decreases in ALI (HR, 0.56; 95% CI, 0.32–0.99; $P = .04$), vascular amputations (HR, 0.40; 95% CI, 0.20–0.79; $P = .007$), and peripheral vascular interventions (HR, 0.76; 95% CI, 0.60–0.97; $P = .03$).[40,41] Major bleeding was more common with the combination of low-dose rivaroxaban and aspirin (3.1% vs 1.9%, $P = .009$), but there was no increased risk in intracranial hemorrhage.[40]

To further evaluate the role of factor Xa inhibition in patients with PAD, the Vascular Outcomes Study of ASA Along with Rivaroxaban in Endovascular or Surgical Limb Revascularization for PAD (VOYAGER PAD) trial randomized 6564 patients with PAD who had undergone recent revascularization to rivaroxaban 2.5 mg twice daily plus aspirin versus aspirin alone. The addition of rivaroxaban led to a decrease in the primary outcome of MACE, ALI, or major amputation (HR, 0.85; 95% CI, 0.76–0.96; $P = .009$). The benefit for rivaroxaban was similar for endovascular and surgical revascularization and for revascularization for CLTI and non-CLTI. Bleeding risk was modestly increased (5.94% vs 4.06%; HR, 1.42; 95% CI, 1.10–1.84; $P = .007$) with no differences in life-threatening and intracranial hemorrhage.[42]

Antiplatelet and Antithrombotic Recommendations

The use of antiplatelet and antithrombotic in patients with PAD is based on multiple considerations including additional comorbidities, such as diabetes, the presence of polyvascular atherosclerotic disease, prior arterial revascularization, indications for therapeutic anticoagulation (eg, atrial fibrillation or venous thromboembolism), and other conditions that may further increase one's bleeding risk. This is an evolving field that is, not fully addressed in current professional guidelines. Our typical approach is as follows.

- For PAD without polyvascular disease or other risk factors, such as diabetes or prior revascularization, use single antiplatelet therapy. Data suggest clopidogrel is more effective than aspirin.[33] Ticagrelor is a reasonable alternative to clopidogrel, particularly in poor metabolizers of clopidogrel.[34]
- In patients with symptomatic PAD and polyvascular disease, use aspirin plus low-dose rivaroxaban 2.5 mg twice daily.[40]
- After revascularization, DAPT to decrease in-stent thrombosis remains common practice, although data within a PAD population are limited.[43] Recent trial data support the use of aspirin plus low-dose rivaroxaban 2.5 mg twice daily after revascularization.[42] Additional studies are needed to compare DAPT to aspirin plus low-dose rivaroxaban after lower extremity percutaneous revascularization.
- In patients with lower extremity PAD but no attributable symptoms and no history of symptomatic atherosclerosis in other arterial beds, defer antiplatelet therapy.

OTHER THERAPIES
Cilostazol

Cilostazol is a selective inhibitor of phosphodiesterase III with antiplatelet, antithrombotic, and vasodilating properties. A meta-analysis (n = 2702) examining patients with stable, moderate to severe claudication from 8 randomized controlled trials found an increase in maximum walking distance by 50% and pain-free walking distance by 67% with cilostazol therapy.[44] Another meta-analysis (n = 1258) then compared cilostazol with placebo resulting in an improved maximum walking distance (50.7% vs 24.3%, P = .001) and pain-free walking distance (67.8% vs 42.6%, P = .0001).[45] Cilostazol is contraindicated in patients with heart failure owing to concerns of increased ventricular arrhythmias. Side effects of gastrointestinal intolerance, dizziness, and headaches may limit its use.[46,47]

Pentoxifylline

Pentoxifylline is a theophylline derivative initially studied to improve claudication symptoms. A randomized controlled trial comparing cilostazol, pentoxifylline, and placebo in patients with moderate to severe claudication found no difference in walking distance between pentoxifylline and placebo.[48] Current guidelines do not recommend the use of pentoxifylline for intermittent claudication.[10]

Recommendations

Cilostazol remains the only drug that has demonstrated efficacy in improving claudication symptoms with benefits seen 4 weeks after initiation, and guidelines recommend its use to improve walking distance and claudication symptoms.[10,45,49]

FUTURE DIRECTIONS

Given the results of COMPASS and VOYAGER PAD, we will likely have additional data for other factor Xa inhibitors as well as novel antithrombotic agents in the near future. There is ongoing work on new therapies to improve walking distance and claudication metrics. A pilot study of daily cocoa supplementation, which contains flavanols that may promote vascular growth and function, demonstrated improved walking distance and increased calf muscle perfusion on biopsy.[50,51] Anti-inflammatory drugs are also being explored as modulators of the proinflammatory pathways involved in the development and progression of atherosclerosis.[52] A small study exploring the effect of canakinumab, an interleukin 1β antagonist, in patients with PAD demonstrated improved pain free walking distance as early as 3 months after treatment.[51] We hopefully will have more cardiovascular outcome trial data, including limb events, of anti-inflammatory therapies in the coming years.

SUMMARY

The medical management options for PAD has improved markedly over the last 2 decades. In addition to standard risk modification therapies, advances have been made in improving lipid therapy with the addition of ezetimibe and PCSK9 inhibitors. More recently, this complex patient population has finally established an antiplatelet and antithrombic regimen that improves both MACE and major adverse limb event outcomes. We hope that the recent attention to PAD and limb outcomes leads to the development of novel therapies for this high risk patient population. Regardless, undertreatment remains a critical issue for patients with PAD, and an emphasis on both patient and provider awareness remains paramount.

CLINICS CARE POINTS

- Smoking cessation remains paramount in PAD, and varenicline should be used as a first-line therapy to help patients attain and maintain cessation.
- Statin therapy in PAD remains underused despite a lower risk of mortality and limb-related events regardless of baseline LDL-C levels. High-intensity statins are recommend in individuals with PAD.
- Angiotensin-converting enzyme inhibitors or angiotensin receptor blockers are first-line antihypertensive therapies in patients with PAD.
- A regimen of low-dose rivaroxaban 2.5 mg twice daily plus aspirin has both mortality and limb-related benefits in stable patients with PAD patients and following lower extremity revascularization.
- Cilostazol remains the only PAD therapy to improve walking distance and claudication symptoms.

DISCLOSURE

Dr Aday reports receiving consulting fees from OptumCare. Dr J. A. Gutierrez discloses the following relationships: research support from the Veterans Health Administration Career Development Award; consulting from Janssen Pharmaceuticals and Amgen Inc.

REFERENCES

1. Criqui MH, Aboyans V. Epidemiology of peripheral artery disease. Circ Res 2015; 116(9):1509–26.
2. Gutierrez JA, Aday AW, Patel MR, et al. Polyvascular disease: reappraisal of the current clinical landscape. Circ Cardiovasc Interv 2019;12(12):e007385.
3. Willigendael EM, Teijink JA, Bartelink ML, et al. Influence of smoking on incidence and prevalence of peripheral arterial disease. J Vasc Surg 2004;40(6):1158–65.

4. Willigendael EM, Teijink JA, Bartelink ML, et al. Smoking and the patency of lower extremity bypass grafts: a meta-analysis. J Vasc Surg 2005;42(1):67–74.
5. Armstrong EJ, Wu J, Singh GD, et al. Smoking cessation is associated with decreased mortality and improved amputation-free survival among patients with symptomatic peripheral artery disease. J Vasc Surg 2014;60(6):1565–71.
6. Faulkner KW, House AK, Castleden WM. The effect of cessation of smoking on the accumulative survival rates of patients with symptomatic peripheral vascular disease. Med J Aust 1983;1(5):217–9.
7. Hennrikus D, Joseph AM, Lando HA, et al. Effectiveness of a smoking cessation program for peripheral artery disease patients: a randomized controlled trial. J Am Coll Cardiol 2010;56(25):2105–12.
8. Jorenby DE, Leischow SJ, Nides MA, et al. A controlled trial of sustained-release bupropion, a nicotine patch, or both for smoking cessation. N Engl J Med 1999; 340(9):685–91.
9. Anthenelli RM, Benowitz NL, West R, et al. Neuropsychiatric safety and efficacy of varenicline, bupropion, and nicotine patch in smokers with and without psychiatric disorders (EAGLES): a double-blind, randomised, placebo-controlled clinical trial. Lancet 2016;387(10037):2507–20.
10. Gerhard-Herman MD, Gornik HL, Barrett C, et al. 2016 AHA/ACC guideline on the management of patients with lower extremity peripheral artery disease: executive summary: a report of the American College of Cardiology/American Heart Association Task Force on Clinical Practice Guidelines. Circulation 2017;135(12): e686–725.
11. Barua RS, Rigotti NA, Benowitz NL, et al. 2018 ACC expert consensus decision pathway on tobacco cessation treatment: a report of the American College of Cardiology Task Force on Clinical Expert Consensus Documents. J Am Coll Cardiol 2018;72(25):3332–65.
12. Aday AW, Everett BM. Dyslipidemia profiles in patients with peripheral artery disease. Curr Cardiol Rep 2019;21(6):42.
13. Heart Protection Study Collaborative G. Randomized trial of the effects of cholesterol-lowering with simvastatin on peripheral vascular and other major vascular outcomes in 20,536 people with peripheral arterial disease and other high-risk conditions. J Vasc Surg 2007;45(4):645–54, discussion 653-644.
14. Kumbhani DJ, Steg PG, Cannon CP, et al. Statin therapy and long-term adverse limb outcomes in patients with peripheral artery disease: insights from the REACH registry. Eur Heart J 2014;35(41):2864–72.
15. Arya S, Khakharia A, Binney ZO, et al. Association of statin dose with amputation and survival in patients with peripheral artery disease. Circulation 2018;137(14): 1435–46.
16. Cannon CP, Blazing MA, Giugliano RP, et al. Ezetimibe added to statin therapy after acute coronary syndromes. N Engl J Med 2015;372(25):2387–97.
17. Bonaca MP, Nault P, Giugliano RP, et al. Low-density lipoprotein cholesterol lowering with evolocumab and outcomes in patients with peripheral artery disease: insights from the FOURIER trial (further cardiovascular outcomes research with PCSK9 inhibition in Subjects with elevated risk). Circulation 2018;137(4): 338–50.
18. Schwartz GG, Steg PG, Szarek M, et al. Peripheral artery disease and venous thromboembolic events after acute coronary syndrome. Circulation 2020; 141(20):1608–17.
19. Grundy SM, Stone NJ, Bailey AL, et al. 2018 AHA/ACC/AACVPR/AAPA/ABC/ ACPM/ADA/AGS/APhA/ASPC/NLA/PCNA guideline on the management of blood

cholesterol: a report of the American College of Cardiology/American Heart Association Task Force on Clinical Practice Guidelines. J Am Coll Cardiol 2019;73(24): e285–350.

20. Aboyans V, Ricco JB, Bartelink MEL, et al. 2017 ESC guidelines on the diagnosis and treatment of peripheral arterial diseases, in collaboration with the European Society for Vascular Surgery (ESVS): document covering atherosclerotic disease of extracranial carotid and vertebral, mesenteric, renal, upper and lower extremity arteries endorsed by: the European Stroke Organization (ESO)The Task Force for the Diagnosis and Treatment of Peripheral Arterial Diseases of the European Society of Cardiology (ESC) and of the European Society for Vascular Surgery (ESVS). Eur Heart J 2018;39(9):763–816.

21. Lewington S, Clarke R, Qizilbash N, et al. Age-specific relevance of usual blood pressure to vascular mortality: a meta-analysis of individual data for one million adults in 61 prospective studies. Lancet 2002;360(9349):1903–13.

22. Whelton PK, Carey RM, Aronow WS, et al. 2017 ACC/AHA/AAPA/ABC/ACPM/ AGS/APhA/ASH/ASPC/NMA/PCNA guideline for the prevention, detection, evaluation, and management of high blood pressure in adults: a report of the American College of Cardiology/American Heart Association Task Force on Clinical Practice Guidelines. J Am Coll Cardiol 2018;71(19):e127–248.

23. Mehler PS, Coll JR, Estacio R, et al. Intensive blood pressure control reduces the risk of cardiovascular events in patients with peripheral arterial disease and type 2 diabetes. Circulation 2003;107(5):753–6.

24. Ostergren J, Sleight P, Dagenais G, et al. Impact of ramipril in patients with evidence of clinical or subclinical peripheral arterial disease. Eur Heart J 2004;25(1): 17–24.

25. Fox KM, Investigators EUtOrocewPiscAd. Efficacy of perindopril in reduction of cardiovascular events among patients with stable coronary artery disease: randomised, double-blind, placebo-controlled, multicentre trial (the EUROPA study). Lancet 2003;362(9386):782–8.

26. Investigators O, Yusuf S, Teo KK, et al. Telmisartan, ramipril, or both in patients at high risk for vascular events. N Engl J Med 2008;358(15):1547–59.

27. Bavry AA, Anderson RD, Gong Y, et al. Outcomes Among hypertensive patients with concomitant peripheral and coronary artery disease: findings from the INternational VErapamil-SR/Trandolapril STudy. Hypertension 2010;55(1):48–53.

28. Officers A, Coordinators for the ACRGTA, Lipid-Lowering Treatment to Prevent Heart Attack T. Major outcomes in high-risk hypertensive patients randomized to angiotensin-converting enzyme inhibitor or calcium channel blocker vs diuretic: the Antihypertensive and Lipid-Lowering Treatment to Prevent Heart Attack Trial (ALLHAT). JAMA 2002;288(23):2981–97.

29. Fudim M, Hopley CW, Huang Z, et al. Association of hypertension and arterial blood pressure on limb and cardiovascular outcomes in symptomatic peripheral artery disease: the EUCLID trial. Circ Cardiovasc Qual Outcomes 2020;13(9): e006512.

30. Antithrombotic Trialists C. Collaborative meta-analysis of randomised trials of antiplatelet therapy for prevention of death, myocardial infarction, and stroke in high risk patients. BMJ 2002;324(7329):71–86.

31. Belch J, MacCuish A, Campbell I, et al. The prevention of progression of arterial disease and diabetes (POPADAD) trial: factorial randomised placebo controlled trial of aspirin and antioxidants in patients with diabetes and asymptomatic peripheral arterial disease. BMJ 2008;337:a1840.

32. Fowkes FG, Price JF, Stewart MC, et al. Aspirin for prevention of cardiovascular events in a general population screened for a low ankle brachial index: a randomized controlled trial. JAMA 2010;303(9):841–8.

33. Committee CS. A randomised, blinded, trial of clopidogrel versus aspirin in patients at risk of ischaemic events (CAPRIE). CAPRIE Steering Committee. Lancet 1996;348(9038):1329–39.

34. Hiatt WR, Fowkes FG, Heizer G, et al. Ticagrelor versus clopidogrel in symptomatic peripheral artery disease. N Engl J Med 2017;376(1):32–40.

35. Bonaca MP, Scirica BM, Creager MA, et al. Vorapaxar in patients with peripheral artery disease: results from TRA2{degrees}P-TIMI 50. Circulation 2013;127(14): 1522–9, 1529.e1521-1526.

36. Cacoub PP, Bhatt DL, Steg PG, et al. Patients with peripheral arterial disease in the CHARISMA trial. Eur Heart J 2009;30(2):192–201.

37. Belch JJ, Dormandy J, Committee CW, et al. Results of the randomized, placebo-controlled clopidogrel and acetylsalicylic acid in bypass surgery for peripheral arterial disease (CASPAR) trial. J Vasc Surg 2010;52(4):825–33, 833.e821-822.

38. Warfarin Antiplatelet Vascular Evaluation Trial I, Anand S, Yusuf S, et al. Oral anticoagulant and antiplatelet therapy and peripheral arterial disease. N Engl J Med 2007;357(3):217–27.

39. Eikelboom JW, Connolly SJ, Bosch J, et al. Rivaroxaban with or without aspirin in stable cardiovascular disease. N Engl J Med 2017;377(14):1319–30.

40. Anand SS, Bosch J, Eikelboom JW, et al. Rivaroxaban with or without aspirin in patients with stable peripheral or carotid artery disease: an international, randomised, double-blind, placebo-controlled trial. Lancet 2018;391(10117):219–29.

41. Anand SS, Caron F, Eikelboom JW, et al. Major adverse limb events and mortality in patients with peripheral artery disease. J Am Coll Cardiol 2018;71(20): 2306–15.

42. Bonaca MP, Bauersachs RM, Anand SS, et al. Rivaroxaban in peripheral artery disease after revascularization. N Engl J Med 2020;382(21):1994–2004.

43. Aday AW, Gutierrez JA. Antiplatelet therapy following peripheral arterial interventions: the choice is yours. Circ Cardiovasc Interv 2020;13(8):e009727.

44. Thompson PD, Zimet R, Forbes WP, et al. Meta-analysis of results from eight randomized, placebo-controlled trials on the effect of cilostazol on patients with intermittent claudication. Am J Cardiol 2002;90(12):1314–9.

45. Pande RL, Hiatt WR, Zhang P, et al. A pooled analysis of the durability and predictors of treatment response of cilostazol in patients with intermittent claudication. Vasc Med 2010;15(3):181–8.

46. Regensteiner JG, Ware JE Jr, McCarthy WJ, et al. Effect of cilostazol on treadmill walking, community-based walking ability, and health-related quality of life in patients with intermittent claudication due to peripheral arterial disease: meta-analysis of six randomized controlled trials. J Am Geriatr Soc 2002;50(12): 1939–46.

47. Lee C, Nelson PR. Effect of cilostazol prescribed in a pragmatic treatment program for intermittent claudication. Vasc Endovascular Surg 2014;48(3):224–9.

48. Dawson DL, Cutler BS, Hiatt WR, et al. A comparison of cilostazol and pentoxifylline for treating intermittent claudication. Am J Med 2000;109(7):523–30.

49. Beebe HG, Dawson DL, Cutler BS, et al. A new pharmacological treatment for intermittent claudication: results of a randomized, multicenter trial. Arch Intern Med 1999;159(17):2041–50.

50. McDermott MM, Criqui MH, Domanchuk K, et al. Cocoa to improve walking performance in older people with peripheral artery disease: the COCOA-PAD pilot randomized clinical trial. Circ Res 2020;126(5):589–99.

51. Russell KS, Yates DP, Kramer CM, et al. A randomized, placebo-controlled trial of canakinumab in patients with peripheral artery disease. Vasc Med 2019;24(5): 414–21.

52. Camara Planek MI, Silver AJ, Volgman AS, et al. Exploratory review of the role of statins, colchicine, and aspirin for the prevention of radiation-associated cardiovascular disease and mortality. J Am Heart Assoc 2020;9(2):e014668.

53. Hartmann-Boyce J, Chepkin SC, Ye W, et al. Nicotine replacement therapy versus control for smoking cessation. Cochrane Database Syst Rev 2018;5:CD000146.

54. Bolliger CT, Zellweger JP, Danielsson T, et al. Smoking reduction with oral nicotine inhalers: double blind, randomised clinical trial of efficacy and safety. BMJ 2000; 321(7257):329–33.

55. Croghan IT, Hurt RD, Dakhil SR, et al. Randomized comparison of a nicotine inhaler and bupropion for smoking cessation and relapse prevention. Mayo Clin Proc 2007;82(2):186–95.

56. Fiore MC, Smith SS, Jorenby DE, et al. The effectiveness of the nicotine patch for smoking cessation. A meta-analysis. JAMA 1994;271(24):1940–7.

57. Mohammadi D. Black-box warnings could be removed from varenicline. Lancet Respir Med 2016;4(11):861.

The Effects of Testosterone Treatment on Cardiovascular Health

Channa N. Jayasena, MA, PhD, MRCP, FRCPath[a],*,
Carmen Lok Tung Ho, BSc[a], Shalender Bhasin, MB, BS[b]

KEYWORDS

- Testosterone • Hypogonadism • Cardiovascular • Hypertension • Diabetes

KEY POINTS

- Testosterone has complex, direct effects on myocardial function.
- Some studies have observed minor reductions in total cholesterol and HDL cholesterol during testosterone replacement therapy.
- Clinical trials evidence on the cardiovascular safety of testosterone therapy is contradictory, owing to design, and/or lack of statistical power.

INTRODUCTION

The prescription rates for testosterone products have risen markedly over the last 20 years, due to multiple factors, including heighted awareness about TRT because of direct-to-consumer pharmaceutical marketing, media coverage, and increased off-label use of testosterone for middle-aged and older men with age-related conditions, such as obesity and type 2 diabetes mellitus. However, the cardiovascular safety of long-term TRT remains unknown because of insufficient RCT data and conflicting evidence from epidemiologic, pharmacovigilance, and retrospective studies and small trials. This has affected prescribing behavior among clinicians, leading to disparities in the treatment of men with hypogonadism. This article will provide a critical summary of the available evidence of the cardiovascular effects and safety of TRT. Areas of controversy and gaps in our current evidence are highlighted along with a synthesis of the available evidence.

This article originally appeared in *Endocrinology and Metabolism Clinics*, Volume 51, Issue 1, June 2022.
[a] Section of Endocrinology and Investigative Medicine, Imperial College London, W12 0HS, UK;
[b] Boston Claude D. Pepper Older Americans Independence Center, Research Program in Men's Health: Aging and Metabolism, Brigham and Women's Hospital, Harvard Medical School, 221 Longwood Avenue, Boston, MA 02115, USA
* Corresponding author.
E-mail address: c.jayasena@imperial.ac.uk

PHYSIOLOGIC EFFECTS OF TESTOSTERONE ON CARDIOVASCULAR HEALTH

Testosterone exerts several diverse effects on cardiovascular physiology; some of these physiologic effects may increase the risk of cardiovascular events while others may reduce cardiovascular risk. Androgen receptors (ARs) are located in cardiac myocytes, vascular smooth muscle, and vascular endothelial cells.[1-4]

Testosterone exerts some potentially beneficial effects on the cardiovascular system. Testosterone is a potent vasodilator; it inhibits L-type calcium channels, resulting in coronary vasodilatation and increased coronary blood flow.[5,6] DHT is more potent than testosterone in mediating these nongenomic effects on vascular smooth muscle relaxation. Testosterone improves endothelial function, reduces vascular reactivity,[7] and shortens QTc interval.[8] Furthermore, testosterone administration decreases whole body, subcutaneous, and intraabdominal fat.[9,10]

In mice, orchiectomy increases sarcoplasmic reticulum (SR) calcium load within ventricular myocytes and the expression of SERCA-2a which is implicated in the preservation of ventricular function after myocardial infarction.[11] Testosterone supplementation was associated with left ventricle dysfunction in orchiectomised mice. Testosterone administration by downregulating SERCA-2a expression causes reduced SR calcium accumulation[11] thereby attenuating the cardiac inotropic response.[12]

Several physiologic effects of testosterone could potentially increase the risk of cardiovascular events. As discussed later, testosterone administration reduces plasma HDL cholesterol depending on the administered dose, the route of administration.[13,14] Testosterone induces platelet aggregation by stimulating thromboxane A2[15] and promotes sodium and water retention,[16] which can contribute to edema formation and worsen preexisting heart failure. In preclinical models, testosterone promotes smooth muscle proliferation[17] and increases the expression of vascular cell adhesion molecule.[18] Testosterone increases hematocrit[19] by stimulating iron-dependent erythropoiesis by suppressing hepcidin,[20,21] increasing erythropoietin,[22] and by direct effects on the bone marrow to increase the numbers of erythropoietic progenitors. Older men experience greater increments in hematocrit than younger men.[23]

Testosterone administration increases the levels of prothrombotic as well as antithrombotic factors. It does not significantly affect myocardial infarct size in preclinical models of myocardial infarction.[24] Testosterone has been shown to retard atherosclerosis in some preclinical models[25] but not in others,[26] and induce myocardial hypertrophy in some mouse strains,[4,24] but not in others.

EFFECTS OF TESTOSTERONE ON BLOOD PRESSURE

Blood pressure is higher in men when compared with women.[27-29] Testosterone may play a role in the sex differences in BP, which only appears in boys and girls after puberty.[30] Orchiectomy or administration of the AR antagonist, flutamide, attenuates the development of salt-induced hypertension has been observed in the male rats.[31] However, the 5-alpha-reductase inhibitor, finasteride, does not affect the onset of hypertension, suggesting that testosterone's conversion to DHT may not be implicated in the development of hypertension in this model.[30] Female rats treated with testosterone during the neonatal period, develop higher blood pressures than control animals.[31] Furthermore, women with elevated androgens due to virilising tumors or polycystic ovarian syndrome (PCOS) have higher BP when compared with age-matched women without PCOS.[30] AR signaling increases the activity of the renin angiotensin aldosterone (RAA) system; male rats have higher plasma renin activity versus females, and castration reduces plasma renin activity in male rats.[30]

Testosterone exposure also increases renal angiotensinogen mRNA.[25] Testosterone administration is associated with transient sodium and water retention in men and women in the first few weeks after starting testosterone treatment and some men, especially older men, with hypogonadism experience edema during TRT.[32] However, clinical data suggest that the effects of testosterone on BP are complex; hypogonadal men have been observed to have higher systolic blood pressures than eugonadal men.[33] Although most testosterone studies have not reported an increase in BP during testosterone treatment,[32,34] recent studies of oral testosterone undecanoate that performed standardized measurements of blood pressure during the clinic visits as well as ambulatory blood pressure measurement found that the BP more than 24 hours was higher following 120 and 180 days of treatment with oral testosterone undecanoate than at baseline; the effects on diastolic BP more than 24 h were less than for the systolic BP.[35–37] The US Food and Drug Administration has required a boxed warning on oral testosterone undecanoate labeling stating that the drug can cause blood pressure to rise.[38]

EFFECTS OF TESTOSTERONE ON SERUM LIPID PARAMETERS

In epidemiologic studies, low testosterone levels are generally associated with a proatherogenic lipid profile and higher HDL cholesterol[39–42]; some studies have also reported a negative association between circulating testosterone and VLDL cholesterol.[43] Testosterone levels are positively associated with smaller or less atherogenic VLDL particles[44] and higher testosterone levels have also been associated with a lower apoB to apo A-1 ratio.[45]

The intervention studies generally have reported modest reductions in total and high-density lipoprotein (HDL) cholesterol during TRT[32,34,46,47] in men with hypogonadism; 2 of these studies reported significant reductions in low-density lipoprotein (LDL) cholesterol in hypogonadal men with T2DM.[34,46] However, some RCTs have failed to observe any significant changes in total, LDL or HDL cholesterol during treatment with transdermal testosterone.[48–52] Nonaromatizable oral androgens suppress HDL cholesterol substantially more than transdermal or injectable testosterone esters. Testosterone-induced suppression of HDL cholesterol is associated with the upregulation of hepatic triacylglycerol lipase, changes in HDL proteome, and suppression of apolipoprotein A1,[53] but does not seem to reduce the cholesterol efflux capacity of HDL particles. TRT seems to have no significant effect on serum triglyceride levels. In summary, overall, TRT is generally associated with a modest reduction in total cholesterol and HDL cholesterol without a concomitant reduction in LDL cholesterol.

EFFECTS OF TESTOSTERONE ON VENOUS THROMBOEMBOLISM

Testosterone stimulates erythropoiesis by multiple mechanisms[20,21] and increases haematocrit.[19] Erythrocytosis is the most frequent adverse event associated with TRT in randomized trials.[54] However, there is a paucity of high-quality evidence of an association between testosterone replacement therapy and venous thromboembolism (VTE) in men with hypogonadism.[21,55] To date, no RCTs of TRT administration have captured significant numbers of events to accurately determine VTE risk in men with hypogonadism. A case-control study reported an increased risk of VTE in the first 6 months following commencement of testosterone treatment.[56] Recently, the IBM MarketScan Commercial Claims and Encounter Database and the Medicare Supplemental Database was used to compare VTE events within 39,622 men during 1, 3, and 6 months before TRT commencement versus 1, 3, and 6 months after starting TRT.[57] This study suggested that men with hypogonadism have a twofold increased risk of

VTE within the 6 months following TRT commencement. However, the number of confirmed VTE events in RCTs has been exceedingly small. Most of the reported VTE events in published case reports have occurred in men with preexisting hypercoagulable condition.[58] It is prudent to consider VTE risk and counsel men with hypogonadism appropriately when considering TRT.

EFFECTS OF TESTOSTERONE ON GLUCOSE INTOLERANCE AND TYPE 2 DIABETES

In epidemiologic studies, low total testosterone levels are associated with increased visceral fat volume,[59] serum glucose concentration,[60] and increased risk of type 2 diabetes mellitus (T2DM) both cross-sectionally and longitudinally.[61] The association of free testosterone and T2DM has been inconsistent; some studies have reported a weak association[62] while others have failed to find any relation.[63] The lack of a strong correlation between free testosterone and T2DM suggests that SHBG may be the primary determinant of the observed relation between total testosterone levels and T2DM. Indeed, circulating SHBG level is an independent predictor of incident T2DM even after adjustment for free or total testosterone levels. Polymorphisms of the SHBG gene that are associated with low SHBG levels are associated with increased risk of T2DM.[64]

In Mendelian randomization studies, higher genetically determined testosterone levels are associated with the risk of T2DM in a sexually dimorphic manner; in men, higher genetically determined testosterone levels are associated with lower risk of T2DM, but in women, higher genetically determined testosterone levels are associated with increased risk of T2DM.[65]

The effects of testosterone on insulin sensitivity have been inconsistent across studies. In general studies of men in whom severe testosterone deficiency was induced rapidly by acute withdrawal of testosterone replacement therapy in men known to have hypogonadism[66] develop insulin resistance. Similarly, men receiving with prostate who receive androgen deprivation therapy are at increased risk of developing impaired glucose tolerance, insulin resistance, and T2DM.[67–69] The worsening of insulin sensitivity associated with the development of severe testosterone deficiency may be related in part to loss of skeletal muscle mass, increase in whole body and visceral fat mass, and to the effects of testosterone on lipid oxidation and mitochondrial function.[70] Dhindsa and colleagues performed euglycaemic hyperinsulinaemia clamp studies showing that 3 weeks of testosterone administration have no detectable effects on insulin sensitivity or other glucose parameters in men with type 2 diabetes; however, 24 weeks of testosterone administration were associated with significant changes in body composition and improvement in insulin sensitivity.[71] Changes in insulin sensitivity was accompanied by reductions in circulating free fatty acids (FFAs)[71] and increased adipose expression of insulin signaling markers such as insulin receptor β subunit, insulin reception substrate (IRS) 1, protein kinase B (AKT-2), and glucose transporter types 4 (GLUT-4).

However, well-controlled randomized trials of testosterone treatment that recruited men with mild testosterone deficiency or with low normal testosterone levels have failed to find consistent improvements in insulin sensitivity with testosterone treatment. For example, in the testosterone trials (TTrials),[72] testosterone treatment of older men with low testosterone levels and one or more symptoms of testosterone deficiency was associated with a small reduction in insulin but not glucose levels and only a small change in HOMA-IR. In another study, 2 years of testosterone treatment in elderly men with low or low normal testosterone levels did not improve carbohydrate tolerance, insulin secretion, insulin action, glucose effectiveness, hepatic insulin clearance, or the pattern of postprandial glucose metabolism.[73] Another placebo-controlled randomized trial also found no significant improvement in insulin sensitivity after 3 years of testosterone treatment relative to placebo in middle-aged and older men with low or low normal testosterone levels.[74]

The clinical effects of testosterone on diabetes risk and diabetes prevention are covered in detail by Yeap & Wittert elsewhere in this issue. In the T4DM Trial, testosterone treatment administered in combination with a lifestyle intervention for 2 years of men, 50 to 74 years, with impaired glucose tolerance or newly diagnosed type 2 diabetes, but without symptomatic testosterone deficiency, reduced the proportion of randomized men with type 2 diabetes beyond the effects of the lifestyle intervention.[75] However, the study participants in this large well-conducted trial were not hypogonadal. In the TIMES2 trial,[34] testosterone treatment did not consistently improve hemoglobin A_{1c} in hypogonadal men with T2DM or metabolic syndrome. Thus, in spite of strong association of low testosterone levels with increased risk of T2DM in epidemiologic studies, randomized intervention trials in hypogonadal men have not provided clear evidence of improvement in glycemic control, prevention of progression from prediabetes to diabetes, or diabetes remission.

THE EFFECTS OF TESTOSTERONE TREATMENT ON THE RISK OF MAJOR ADVERSE CARDIOVASCULAR EVENTS
Epidemiologic Studies

The relation of testosterone levels and coronary artery disease in cross-sectional and prospective cohort studies has been inconsistent. Some cross-sectional studies have shown low levels of testosterone to be associated with increased risk for coronary artery disease,[76] while others have shown no association.[77] The relationship between serum testosterone levels and the incidence of cardiovascular events also has been inconsistent in prospective epidemiologic studies.

Epidemiologic studies have found a consistent negative association between circulating testosterone concentrations and common carotid artery intima-media thickness, a measure of subclinical atherosclerosis. For example, in the Rotterdam study, the men in the lowest quartile of testosterone levels had greater progression of intima-media thickness than men in highest quartile of testosterone levels.[78] However, the same study did not identify a significant difference in the rates of change in coronary artery calcium between the group administered with testosterone or placebo.[78]

The relation of testosterone and mortality has been heterogeneous across studies. A meta-analysis by Corona and colleagues reported an association of low testosterone levels with increased risk of cardiovascular disease. Furthermore, study participants with the lowest testosterone levels seemed to have the highest overall mortality and cardiovascular mortality.[79] Another meta-analysis of 11 randomized trials by Araujo and colleagues found that in aggregate, lower testosterone levels were associated with higher risk of all-cause mortality, especially cardiovascular mortality.[80] Epidemiologic studies can only show association but cannot prove causality; reverse causality cannot be excluded. It is possible that testosterone is a marker of health, and those who are higher risk of dying have lower testosterone levels. Ruige and colleagues found that higher testosterone levels were associated with a lower risk for cardiovascular events in men more than 70 years of age but not in men who were younger than this age group.[77]

Pharmacovigilance Studies and Retrospective Analyses of Electronic Medical Records

The pharmacovigilance studies and retrospective analyses of electronic medical records have yielded inconsistent results because of their inherent limitations. In a retrospective analysis of male veterans who underwent angiography and had low testosterone concentrations, Vigen and colleagues observed that TRT was associated with an increased risk of the composite cardiovascular outcome of myocardial infarction, stroke, and death when (hazard ratio, HR = 1.29)[81] relative to no TRT. Finkle used an insurance database and found an increased risk of nonfatal myocardial infarction during the 90 days following initial prescription for TRT when compared with the period before commencing TRT (relative risk (RR) = 1.36).[82] However, another retrospective study of men with low testosterone concluded that TRT was associated with reduced all-cause mortality when compared with no TRT (HR = 0.61).[83] Muraleedharan and colleagues retrospectively concluded that low serum testosterone may predict increased all-cause mortality in 581 men with type 2 diabetes (HR 2.3).[84] Furthermore, Boden and colleagues conducted a post hoc analysis of the AIM-HIGH trial of men with metabolic syndrome and low baseline levels of HDL cholesterol. The 643 out of 2118 men with levels of serum testosterone less than 300 ng/dL had a higher risk of the primary composite outcome (coronary heart disease, death, MI, stroke, hospitalization for acute coronary syndrome, or coronary or cerebral revascularization) when compared with the normal testosterone group (HR 1.23).[85] Taken collectively, observational studies provide little consensus on TRT safety, and have each been used to substantiate claims TRT either reduces or increases the risk of MACE outcomes.

These pharmacovigilance and retrospective studies suffer from many limitations, including heterogeneous study populations and differences in treatment indications, treatment regimens and duration, and on-treatment testosterone levels, and in other aspects of study design. These studies used variable definitions of cardiovascular outcomes that were often not prespecified, and the ascertainment methods varied across studies. They also suffered from a potential for residual confounding in that the patients assigned to testosterone therapy differed from comparators in baseline cardiovascular risk factors. Due to the inherent limitations and inconsistency of findings, these pharmacovigilance and retrospective analyses do not permit strong inferences about the relation between testosterone therapy and mortality and cardiovascular outcomes.

Randomized Controlled Trials

The testosterone replacement for older men with sarcopenia (TOM) randomized controlled trial was designed to investigate functional mobility following TRT in 209 men with hypogonadism and frailty.[32] However, the study was stopped early by its data and safety monitoring board due to an unexpected increase in cardiovascular events within the TRT versus the placebo arm, albeit with small absolute number of events (23 vs 5, respectively). However, the cardiovascular events were not prespecified nor adjudicated prospectively. The number of major adverse cardiovascular events (MACEs) was small. Subsequent RCTs have often excluded men with the increased baseline cardiovascular risk, so it is unsurprising that the number of MACE has been small in most trials. Several meta-analyses have examined the association between testosterone replacement and cardiovascular events, major cardiovascular events, and death in RCTs and overall, these meta-analyses have not shown a statistically significant association between testosterone and cardiovascular events, major cardiovascular events, or deaths.[23,86–88] These meta-analyses are limited by the heterogeneity of randomized trials included in these analyses with respect to eligibility criteria, testosterone dose and formulation, and intervention durations. The variable quality of adverse event recording in clinical trials has been well-documented, and was particularly apparent in these trials, which reported a very low frequency of all adverse events as well cardiovascular events. The small size of

Table 1	
Key points of the biological plausibility: effects of testosterone on cardiovascular physiology	
Potential Cardiovascular Risks	**Potential Cardiovascular Benefits**
• Increase in hematocrit[19] • Suppression of HDL cholesterol[34] • Platelet aggregation[15] • Sodium retention • Smooth muscle proliferation[17] • Increased VCAM expression	• Vasodilator effect which increases coronary and penile blood flow[6] • Decreased whole body and visceral fat[59] • Improves vascular reactivity[5,7] • Shortens QTc interval[8]

many trials and the inclusion of pilot studies with very small sample sizes was another constraint. Cardiovascular outcomes were not prespecified, they were often defined post hoc, and were of varying clinical significance. The major cardiovascular events were not adjudicated, not specified prospectively, and the total number of major cardiovascular events was too small to draw strong inferences. None of the trials has been large enough or long enough to determine the effects of testosterone treatment on MACE.

Two randomized trials—the Cardiovascular Trial of the TTrials[32] and the Testosterone Effects on Atherosclerosis in Aging Men (The TEAAM Trial)[78] determined the effects of testosterone treatment relative to placebo on the rate of atherogenesis progression. The rate of atherosclerosis progressed assessed using the common carotid artery -intima-media thickness or the coronary calcium scores did not differ between testosterone-treated and placebo-treated men in either of the 2 trials. However, in the Cardiovascular Trial of the TTrials,[32] testosterone treatment was associated with greater increase in the volume of noncalcified plaque in the coronary arteries, assessed using computed tomography angiography, compared with placebo.

An extensive review by the FDA concluded that *"the studies...have significant limitations that weaken their evidentiary value for confirming a causal relationship between testosterone and adverse cardiovascular outcomes."* Nevertheless, the US Food and Drug Administration (FDA) directed the pharmaceutical companies to include in the label warning about the potential cardiovascular risks of TRT.[89] The European Medicines Agency also found no conclusive link between testosterone treatment and cardiovascular risk. Fortunately, 2 ongoing studies are aiming to close the evidence gap. The National Institute for Health Research (NIHR) TestES (Testosterone Effects and Safety) consortium is currently collating individual patient data (IPD) and adverse events from published RCTs to analyze the risks of subtypes of MACE within men with hypogonadism treated with TRT when compared with placebo (https://www.imperial.ac.uk/metabolism-digestion-reproduction/research/diabetes-endocrinology-metabolism/endocrinology-and-investigative-medicine/nihr-testosterone/). Furthermore, the Phase 4, randomized placebo-controlled trial (The TRAVERSE Trial) is recruiting approximately 6000 men aged 45 to 80 years with either preexisting cardiovascular disease or at least 3 cardiovascular risk factors, with the primary objective of comparing the effect of TRT versus placebo on the incidence of MACE.

SUMMARY

Overall, TRT exerts multiple physiologic effects, both positive and negative, on cardiovascular health (**Table 1**). Finally, there are insufficient RCT data to determine whether TRT increases MACE risk. Studies are underway to clarify this important question. The Endocrine Society's testosterone treatment guideline recommends avoiding testosterone treatment in hypogonadal men who incurred a MACE in the preceding 6 months and in men with a known hypercoagulable condition, such as a mutation on antithrombin 3, protein C or protein S. Testosterone treatment of hypogonadal men with increased risk of cardiovascular events requires consideration and counseling of the potential risks versus benefits of testosterone replacement therapy.

CLINICS CARE POINTS

- Testosterone replacement therapy for young men with classical hypogonadism due to known diseases of the testis, pituitary, or the hypothalamus is associated with low frequency of adverse events.
- The long-term cardiovascular safety of testosterone replacement therapy remains uncertain.
- Testosterone treatment of older men with age-related decline in testosterone levels is not currently approved by the US Food and Drug Administration. The long-term benefits, as well as long term risks of testosterone treatment in older men with age related decline in testosterone levels, remain unknown.
- Testosterone treatment should be avoided in men with hypogonadism who have suffered a major adverse cardiovascular event in the preceding 6 months or who suffer from a hypercoagulable state.
- Testosterone treatment of hypogonadal men with increased risk of cardiovascular events requires consideration and counseling of the potential risks versus benefits of testosterone replacement therapy.

DISCLOSURE

Dr C.N. Jayasena is funded by an NIHR Post-Doctoral Fellowship and NIHR Health Technology Assessment Grant. Dr S. Bhasin reports receiving research grants from the National Institute on Aging, the National Institute of Child Health and Human Development, the National Institute of Nursing Research, the Patient-Centered Outcomes Research Institute (PCORI), AbbVie, Transition Therapeutics, and Metro International Biotechnology and has an equity interest in FPT, LLC. These grants are managed by the Brigham and Women's Hospital. These conflicts are overseen and managed in accordance with the policies of the Office of Industry Interactions, Massachusetts General Brigham Healthcare System, Boston MA.

REFERENCES

1. Yeh S, Tsai M-Y, Xu Q, et al. Generation and Characterization of Androgen Receptor Knockout (ARKO) Mice: An in vivo Model for the Study of Androgen Functions in Selective Tissues. Proc Natl Acad Sci U S A 2002;99(21):13498–503. Available at: https://www.jstor.org/stable/3073435.
2. Yu I, Lin H, Liu N, et al. Neuronal androgen receptor regulates insulin sensitivity via suppression of hypothalamic NF-κB—Mediated PTP1B Expression. Diabetes 2013;62(2):411–23. Available at: https://www.ncbi.nlm.nih.gov/pubmed/23139353.
3. Huang C, Lee SO, Chang E, et al. Androgen receptor (AR) in cardiovascular diseases. J Endocrinol 2016;229(1):R1–16.
4. Marsh JD, Lehmann MH, Ritchie RH, et al. Androgen Receptors Mediate Hypertrophy in Cardiac Myocytes. Circulation 1998;98(3):256–61. Available at: http://circ.ahajournals.org/cgi/content/abstract/98/3/256.

5. Herring MJ, Oskui PM, Hale SL, et al. Testosterone and the cardiovascular system: a comprehensive review of the basic science literature. J Am Heart Assoc 2013;2(4):e000271. Available at: https://onlinelibrary.wiley.com/doi/abs/10.1161/JAHA.113.000271.

6. Scragg JL, Jones RD, Channer KS, et al. Testosterone is a potent inhibitor of L-type Ca 2+ channels. Biochem Biophys Res Commun 2004;318(2):503–6.

7. Empen K, Lorbeer R, Dörr M, et al. Association of testosterone levels with endothelial function in men: results from a population-based study. Arterioscler Thromb Vasc Biol 2012;32(2):481–6. Available at: http://ovidsp.ovid.com/ovidweb.cgi?T=JS&NEWS=n&CSC=Y&PAGE=fulltext&D=ovft&AN=00043605-201202000-00041.

8. Schwartz JB, Volterrani M, Caminiti G, et al. Effects of testosterone on the Q-T Interval in older men and older women with chronic heart failure. Int J Androl 2011; 34(5pt2):e415–21. Available at: https://api.istex.fr/ark:/67375/WNG-XMWPBTD2-M/fulltext.pdf.

9. Bhasin S. Effects of Testosterone Administration on Fat Distribution, Insulin Sensitivity, and Atherosclerosis Progression. Clin Infect Dis 2003;37(Supplement-2): S142–9. Available at: https://api.istex.fr/ark:/67375/HXZ-8KZGKG2P-D/fulltext.pdf.

10. Bhasin S, Parker RA, Sattler F, et al. Effects of testosterone supplementation on whole body and regional fat mass and distribution in human immunodeficiency virus-infected men with abdominal obesity. J Clin Endocrinol Metab 2007;92(3): 1049–57.

11. Ribeiro Júnior RF, Ronconi KS, Jesus ICG, et al. Testosterone deficiency prevents left ventricular contractility dysfunction after myocardial infarction. Mol Cell Endocrinol 2018;460:14–23.

12. Fernandes AA, Ribeiro RF, de Moura VGC, et al. SERCA-2a is involved in the right ventricular function following myocardial infarction in rats. Life Sci (1973) 2015; 124:24–30.

13. Bagatell CJ, Knopp RH, Vale WW, et al. Physiologic testosterone levels in normal men suppress high-density lipoprotein cholesterol levels. Ann Intern Med 1992; 116(12):967–73. Available at: https://www.ncbi.nlm.nih.gov/pubmed/1586105.

14. Bagatell CJ, Bremner WJ. Androgen and progestagen effects on plasma lipids. Prog Cardiovasc Dis 1995;38(3):255–71.

15. Ajayi AAL, Mathur R, Halushka PV. Testosterone increases human platelet thromboxane A2 receptor density and aggregation responses. Circulation 1995;91(11): 2742–7. Available at: http://circ.ahajournals.org/cgi/content/abstract/91/11/2742.

16. Johannsson G, Gibney J, Wolthers T, et al. Independent and combined effects of testosterone and growth hormone on extracellular water in hypopituitary men. J Clin Endocrinol Metab 2005;90(7):3989–94.

17. Fujimoto R, Morimoto I, Morita E, et al. Androgen receptors, 5 alpha-reductase activity and androgen-dependent proliferation of vascular smooth muscle cells. J Steroid Biochem Mol Biol 1994;50(3):169–74.

18. Death AK, McGrath KCY, Sader MA, et al. Dihydrotestosterone promotes vascular cell adhesion molecule-1 expression in male human endothelial cells via a nuclear factor-κb-dependent pathway. Endocrinology (Philadelphia) 2004; 145(4):1889–97.

19. Bhasin S, Brito J, Cunningham G, et al. Testosterone therapy in men with hypogonadism: an endocrine society clinical practice guideline. J Clin Endocrinol Metab 2018;103(5):1715–44. Available at: http://ovidsp.ovid.com/ovidweb.cgi?

T=JS&NEWS=n&CSC=Y&PAGE=fulltext&D=ovft&AN=00004678-201805000-00001.

20. Ohlander SJ, Varghese B, Pastuszak AW. Erythrocytosis following testosterone therapy. Sex Med Rev 2018;6(1):77–85.

21. Sharma R, Oni OA, Chen G, et al. Association Between Testosterone Replacement Therapy and the Incidence of DVT and pulmonary embolism: a retrospective cohort study of the veterans administration database. Chest 2016;150(3): 563–71. Available at: https://www.ncbi.nlm.nih.gov/pubmed/27179907.

22. Bachman E, Travison TG, Basaria S, et al. Testosterone induces erythrocytosis via increased erythropoietin and suppressed hepcidin: evidence for a new erythropoietin/hemoglobin set point. J Gerontol A Biol Sci Med Sci 2014;69(6):725–35. Available at: https://www.ncbi.nlm.nih.gov/pubmed/24158761.

23. Haddad RM, Kennedy CC, Caples SM, et al. Testosterone and cardiovascular risk in men: a systematic review and meta-analysis of randomized placebo-controlled trials. Mayo Clin Proc 2007;82(1):29–39. Available at: https://www.ncbi.nlm.nih.gov/pubmed/17285783.

24. Nahrendorf M, Frantz S, Neubauer S, et al. Effect of testosterone on post-myocardial infarction remodeling and function. Cardiovasc Res 2003;57(2): 370–8. Available at: https://www.ncbi.nlm.nih.gov/pubmed/12566109.

25. Nathan L, Shi W, Dinh H, et al. Testosterone Inhibits Early Atherogenesis by Conversion to Estradiol: Critical Role of Aromatase. Proc Natl Acad Sci U S A 2001; 98(6):3589–93. Available at: https://www.jstor.org/stable/3055279.

26. Bhasin S, Herbst K. Testosterone and atherosclerosis progression in men. Diabetes care 2003;26(6):1929–31. Available at: https://www.ncbi.nlm.nih.gov/pubmed/12766137.

27. Ganten U, Schröder G, Witt M, et al. Sexual dimorphism of blood pressure in spontaneously hypertensive rats: effects of anti-androgen treatment. J Hypertens 1989;7(9):721–6. Available at: http://ovidsp.ovid.com/ovidweb.cgi?T=JS&NEWS=n&CSC=Y&PAGE=fulltext&D=ovft&AN=00004872-198909000-00005.

28. Crofton J, Ota M, Share L. Role of vasopressin, the renin—angiotensin system and sex in Dahl salt-sensitive hypertension. J Hypertens 1993;11(10):1031–8. Available at: http://ovidsp.ovid.com/ovidweb.cgi?T=JS&NEWS=n&CSC=Y&PAGE=fulltext&D=ovft&AN=00004872-199310000-00005.

29. Chen Y, Meng Q. Sexual dimorphism of blood pressure in spontaneously hypertensive rats is androgen dependent. Life Sci (1973) 1991;48(1):85–96.

30. Reckelhoff JF. Gender Differences in the Regulation of Blood Pressure. Hypertension 2001;37(5):1199–208. Available at: http://hyper.ahajournals.org/cgi/content/abstract/37/5/1199.

31. Rowland NE, Fregly MJ. Role of gonadal hormones in hypertension in the dahl salt-sensitive rat. Clin Exp Hypertens (1993) 1992;A14(3):367–75. Available at: http://www.tandfonline.com/doi/abs/10.3109/10641969209036195.

32. Basaria S, Coviello AD, Travison TG, et al. Adverse Events Associated with Testosterone Administration. N Engl J Med 2010;363(2):109–22.

33. Rezanezhad B, Borgquist R, Willenheimer R, et al. The association between serum testosterone and risk factors for atherosclerosis. Curr Urol 2019;13(2): 101–6. Available at: https://www.karger.com/Article/FullText/499285.

34. Jones TH, Arver S, Behre HM, et al. Testosterone replacement in hypogonadal men with type 2 diabetes and/or metabolic syndrome (the TIMES2 Study). Diabetes care 2011;34(4):828–37. Available at: https://www.narcis.nl/publication/RecordID/oai:pure.atira.dk:publications%2Faae47901-c35f-4e3c-a15d-f7c3c9a599a8.

35. Swerdloff RS, Wang C, White WB, et al. A new oral testosterone undecanoate formulation restores testosterone to normal concentrations in hypogonadal men. J Clin Endocrinol Metab 2020;105(8):2515–31. Available at: http://ovidsp. ovid.com/ovidweb.cgi?T=JS&NEWS=n&CSC=Y&PAGE=fulltext&D=ovft&AN= 00004678-202008000-00003.

36. Gittelman M, Jaffe JS, Kaminetsky JC. Safety of a new subcutaneous testosterone enanthate auto-injector: results of a 26-week study. J Sex Med 2019; 16(11):1741–8.

37. White WB, Bernstein JS, Rittmaster R, et al. Effects of the oral testosterone undecanoate Kyzatrex™ on ambulatory blood pressure in hypogonadal men. J Clin Hypertens (Greenwich) 2021;23(7):1420–30. Available at: https://onlinelibrary. wiley.com/doi/abs/10.1111/jch.14297.

38. Aschenbrenner D. First oral testosterone product now available. Am J Nurs 2019; 119(8):22–3. Available at: http://ovidsp.ovid.com/ovidweb.cgi?T=JS&NEWS=n& CSC=Y&PAGE=fulltext&D=ovft&AN=00000446-201908000-00022.

39. Haffner SM, Mykkänen L, Valdez RA, et al. Relationship of sex hormones to lipids and lipoproteins in nondiabetic men. J Clin Endocrinol Metab 1993;77(6):1610–5.

40. Agledahl I, Skjærpe P, Hansen J, et al. Low serum testosterone in men is inversely associated with non-fasting serum triglycerides: The Tromsø study. Nutr Metab Cardiovasc Dis 2007;18(4):256–62. Available at: https://www.clinicalkey.es/ playcontent/1-s2.0-S0939475307000348.

41. Mäkinen JI, Perheentupa A, Irjala K, et al. Endogenous testosterone and serum lipids in middle-aged men. Atherosclerosis 2007;197(2):688–93. Available at: https://www.clinicalkey.es/playcontent/1-s2.0-S0021915007003401.

42. Zmuda JM, Cauley JA, Kriska A, et al. Longitudinal relation between endogenous testosterone and cardiovascular disease risk factors in middle-aged men: a 13-year follow-up of former multiple risk factor intervention trial participants. Am J Epidemiol 1997;146(8):609–17. Available at: https://www.ncbi.nlm.nih.gov/ pubmed/9345114.

43. Khaw KT, Barrett-Connor E. Endogenous sex hormones, high density lipoprotein cholesterol, and other lipoprotein fractions in men. Arterioscler Thromb Vasc Biol 1991;11(3):489–94. Available at: http://atvb.ahajournals.org/cgi/content/abstract/ 11/3/489.

44. Vaidya D, Dobs A, Gapstur SM, et al. The association of endogenous sex hormones with lipoprotein subfraction profile in the Multi-Ethnic Study of Atherosclerosis. Metab Clin Exp 2008;57(6):782–90. Available at: https://www.clinicalkey.es/ playcontent/1-s2.0-S0026049508000528.

45. Ohlsson C, Barrett-Connor E, Bhasin S, et al. High serum testosterone is associated with reduced risk of cardiovascular events in elderly men. The MrOS (Osteoporotic Fractures in Men) study in Sweden. J Am Coll Cardiol 2011;58(16): 1674–81. Available at: https://www.ncbi.nlm.nih.gov/pubmed/21982312.

46. Gianatti EJ, Hoermann R, Lam Q, et al. Effect of testosterone treatment on cardiac biomarkers in a randomized controlled trial of men with type 2 diabetes. Clin Endocrinol (Oxford) 2016;84(1):55–62. Available at: https://api.istex.fr/ark:/67375/ WNG-GPF8HBTD-R/fulltext.pdf.

47. Emmelot-Vonk MH, Verhaar HJJ, Nakhai Pour HR, et al. Effect of testosterone supplementation on functional mobility, cognition, and other parameters in older men : a randomized controlled trial. JAMA 2008;299(1):39–52.

48. Groti K, Žuran I, Antonič B, et al. The impact of testosterone replacement therapy on glycemic control, vascular function, and components of the metabolic syndrome in obese hypogonadal men with type 2 diabetes. The aging male 2018;

21(3):158–69. Available at: http://www.tandfonline.com/doi/abs/10.1080/13685538.2018.1468429.

49. Aversa A, Bruzziches R, Francomano D, et al. Effects of testosterone undecanoate on cardiovascular risk factors and atherosclerosis in middle-aged men with late-onset hypogonadism and metabolic syndrome: results from a 24-month, randomized, double-blind, placebo-controlled study. J Sex Med 2010;7(10): 3495–503.

50. Svartberg J, Agledahl I, Figenschau Y, et al. Testosterone treatment in elderly men with subnormal testosterone levels improves body composition and BMD in the hip. Int J Impot Res 2008;20(4):378–87.

51. Paduch DA, Polzer PK, Ni X, et al. Testosterone replacement in androgen-deficient men with ejaculatory dysfunction: a randomized controlled trial. J Clin Endocrinol Metab 2015;100(8):2956–62.

52. Kenny AM, Kleppinger A, Annis K, et al. Effects of Transdermal Testosterone on Bone and Muscle in Older Men with Low Bioavailable Testosterone Levels, Low Bone Mass, and Physical Frailty. J Am Geriatr Soc 2010;58(6):1134–43. Available at: https://api.istex.fr/ark:/67375/WNG-7SR5DCSQ-4/fulltext.pdf.

53. Rubinow KB, Tang C, Hoofnagle AN, et al. Acute sex steroid withdrawal increases cholesterol efflux capacity and HDL-associated clusterin in men. Steroids 2012; 77(5):454–60.

54. Ponce OJ, Spencer-Bonilla G, Alvarez-Villalobos N, et al. The efficacy and adverse events of testosterone replacement therapy in hypogonadal men: a systematic review and meta-analysis of randomized, placebo-controlled trials. J Clin Endocrinol Metab 2018;103(5):1745–54. Available at: http://ovidsp.ovid.com/ovidweb.cgi?T=JS&NEWS=n&CSC=Y&PAGE=fulltext&D=ovft&AN=00004678-201805000-00002.

55. Baillargeon J, Urban RJ, Morgentaler A, et al. Risk of Venous Thromboembolism in Men Receiving Testosterone Therapy. Mayo Clin Proc 2015;90(8):1038–45. Available at: https://www.clinicalkey.es/playcontent/1-s2.0-S0025619615004280.

56. Martinez C, Suissa S, Rietbrock S, et al. Testosterone treatment and risk of venous thromboembolism: population based case-control study. BMJ 2016; 355:i5968.

57. Walker RF, Zakai NA, MacLehose RF, et al. Association of testosterone therapy with risk of venous thromboembolism among men with and without hypogonadism. JAMA Intern Med 2020;180(2):190–7.

58. Glueck CJ, Prince M, Patel N, et al. Thrombophilia in 67 patients with thrombotic events after starting testosterone therapy. Clin Appl Thromb Hemostat 2016; 22(6):548–53. Available at: https://journals.sagepub.com/doi/full/10.1177/1076029615619486.

59. Fui MNT, Dupuis P, Grossmann M. Lowered testosterone in male obesity: Mechanisms, morbidity and management. Asian J Androl 2014;16(2):223–31. Available at: https://www.ncbi.nlm.nih.gov/pubmed/24407187.

60. MI EP. Low testosterone level increases fasting blood glucose level in adult males. Universa Medicina 2015;31(3):200–7. Available at: https://explore.openaire.eu/search/publication?articleId=dedup_wf_001:2129979ed51a29513d18ad3f426cecea.

61. Menéndez E, Valdés S, Botas P, et al. Glucose tolerance and plasma testosterone concentrations in men. Results of the Asturias Study. Endocrinol Nutr 2011;58(1): 3–8. Available at: https://www.ncbi.nlm.nih.gov/pubmed/21215713.

62. Haffner SM, Karhapaa P, Mykkanen L, et al. Insulin resistance, body fat distribution, and sex hormones in men. Diabetes 1994;43(2):212–9. Available at: http://diabetes.diabetesjournals.org/content/43/2/212.abstract.

63. Abate N, Haffner SM, Garg A, et al. Sex steroid hormones, upper body obesity, and insulin resistance. J Clin Endocrinol Metab 2002;87(10):4522–7.

64. Quan L, Wang L, Wang J, et al. Association between sex hormone binding globulin gene polymorphism and type 2 diabetes mellitus. Int J Clin Exp Pathol 2019; 12(9):3514–20. Available at: https://www.ncbi.nlm.nih.gov/pubmed/31934198.

65. Ruth KS, Day FR, Tyrrell J, et al. Using human genetics to understand the disease impacts of testosterone in men and women. Nat Med 2020;26(2):252–8. Available at: https://www.ncbi.nlm.nih.gov/pubmed/32042192.

66. Yialamas MA, Dwyer AA, Hanley E, et al. Acute Sex Steroid Withdrawal Reduces Insulin Sensitivity in Healthy Men with Idiopathic Hypogonadotropic Hypogonadism. J Clin Endocrinol Metab 2007;92(11):4254–9.

67. Smith MR, Lee H, Nathan DM. Insulin sensitivity during combined androgen blockade for prostate cancer. J Clin Endocrinol Metab 2006;91(4):1305–8.

68. Keating NL, O'Malley AJ, Smith MR. Diabetes and cardiovascular disease during androgen deprivation therapy for prostate cancer. J Clin Oncol 2006;24(27): 4448–56. Available at: http://jco.ascopubs.org/content/24/27/4448.abstract.

69. Keating NL, Liu P, O'Malley AJ, et al. Androgen-deprivation therapy and diabetes control among diabetic men with prostate cancer. Eur Urol 2013;65(4):816–24. Available at: https://www.clinicalkey.es/playcontent/1-s2.0-S0302283813001358.

70. Pitteloud N, Mootha VK, Hayes FJ, et al. Relationship Between Testosterone Levels, Insulin Sensitivity, and Mitochondrial Function in Men. Diabetes care 2005;28(7):1636–42. Available at: http://care.diabetesjournals.org/content/28/7/1636.abstract.

71. Dhindsa S, Ghanim H, Batra M, et al. Insulin resistance and inflammation in hypogonadotropic hypogonadism and their reduction after testosterone replacement in men with type 2 diabetes. Diabetes care 2016;39(1):82–91. Available at: https://www.ncbi.nlm.nih.gov/pubmed/26622051.

72. Mohler ER, Ellenberg SS, Lewis CE, et al. The Effect of Testosterone on Cardiovascular Biomarkers in the Testosterone Trials. J Clin Endocrinol Metab 2018; 103(2):681–8. Available at: https://www.ncbi.nlm.nih.gov/pubmed/29253154.

73. Basu R, Dalla Man C, Rizza RA, et al. Effect of 2 years of testosterone replacement on insulin secretion, insulin action, glucose effectiveness, hepatic insulin clearance, and postprandial glucose turnover in elderly men. Diabetes care 2007;30(8):1972–8. Available at: http://care.diabetesjournals.org/content/30/8/1972.abstract.

74. Huang G, Pencina KM, Li Z, et al. Long-term testosterone administration on insulin sensitivity in older men with low or low-normal testosterone levels. J Clin Endocrinol Metab 2018;103(4):1678–85. Available at: http://ovidsp.ovid.com/ovidweb.cgi?T=JS&NEWS=n&CSC=Y&PAGE=fulltext&D=ovft&AN=00004678-201804000-00052.

75. Wittert G, Bracken K, Robledo KP, et al. Testosterone treatment to prevent or revert type 2 diabetes in men enrolled in a lifestyle programme (T4DM): a randomised, double-blind, placebo-controlled, 2-year, phase 3b trial. Lancet Diabetes Endocrinol 2021;9(1):32–45.

76. Rosano GMC, Leonardo F, Pagnotta P, et al. Acute anti-ischemic effect of testosterone in men with coronary artery disease. Circulation 1999;99(13):1666–70. Available at: http://circ.ahajournals.org/cgi/content/abstract/99/13/1666.

77. Ruige JB, Mahmoud AM, De Bacquer D, et al. Endogenous testosterone and cardiovascular disease in healthy men: a meta-analysis. Heart 2011;97(11):870–5.
78. Basaria S, Harman SM, Travison TG, et al. Effects of testosterone administration for 3 years on subclinical atherosclerosis progression in older men with low or low-normal testosterone levels: a randomized clinical trial. JAMA 2015;314(6): 570–81.
79. Corona G, Rastrelli G, Monami M, et al. Hypogonadism as a risk factor for cardiovascular mortality in men: a meta-analytic study. Eur J Endocrinol 2011;165(5): 687–701.
80. Araujo AB, Dixon JM, Suarez EA, et al. Clinical review: endogenous testosterone and mortality in men: a systematic review and meta-analysis. J Clin Endocrinol Metab 2011;96(10):3007–19. Available at: https://www.ncbi.nlm.nih.gov/pubmed/21816776.
81. Vigen R, O'Donnell CI, Barón AE, et al. Association of testosterone therapy with mortality, myocardial infarction, and stroke in men with low testosterone levels. JAMA 2013;310(17):1829–36.
82. Finkle WD, Greenland S, Ridgeway GK, et al. Increased risk of non-fatal myocardial infarction following testosterone therapy prescription in men. PLoS One 2014; 9(1):e85805. Available at: https://www.ncbi.nlm.nih.gov/pubmed/24489673.
83. Shores MM, Smith NL, Forsberg CW, et al. Testosterone Treatment and Mortality in Men with Low Testosterone Levels. J Clin Endocrinol Metab 2012;97(6):2050–8.
84. Muraleedharan V, Marsh H, Kapoor D, et al. Testosterone deficiency is associated with increased risk of mortality and testosterone replacement improves survival in men with type 2 diabetes. Eur J Endocrinol 2013;169(6):725–33.
85. Boden WE, Miller MG, McBride R, et al. Testosterone concentrations and risk of cardiovascular events in androgen-deficient men with atherosclerotic cardiovascular disease. Am Heart J 2020;224:65–76.
86. Nguyen PL, Je Y, Schutz FAB, et al. Association of androgen deprivation therapy with cardiovascular death in patients with prostate cancer: a meta-analysis of randomized trials. JAMA 2011;306(21):2359–66.
87. Calof OM, Singh AB, Lee ML, et al. Adverse events associated with testosterone replacement in middle-aged and older men: a meta-analysis of randomized, placebo-controlled trials. J Gerontol A Biol Sci Med Sci 2005;60(11):1451–7. Available at: https://api.istex.fr/ark:/67375/HXZ-TVW8H35J-6/fulltext.pdf.
88. Fernández-Balsells MM, Murad MH, Lane M, et al. Adverse effects of testosterone therapy in adult men: a systematic review and meta-analysis. J Clin Endocrinol Metab 2010;95(6):2560–75.
89. US Food and Drug Administration. FDA cautions about using testosterone products for low testosterone due to aging; requires labeling change to inform of possible increased risk of heart attack and stroke with use. FDA Drug Safety Communication. January 31, 2014.

Obstructive Sleep Apnea and Cardiovascular Disease

Joseph A. Diamond, MD*, Haisam Ismail, MD

KEYWORDS

- Obstructive sleep apnea • Hypertension • Atrial fibrillation
- Premature ventricular contractions • Ventricular tachycardia • Nondipper
- Polysomnography

KEY POINTS

- Obstructive sleep apnea (OSA) is due to repetitive interruptions of ventilation each lasting for more than 10 seconds during sleep as a result of upper airway obstruction and resulting in increased respiratory effort.
- Normally, there is a 10% to 20% decrease in sleep blood pressure (BP) compared with wake BP (dip) on 24-hour ambulatory BP monitoring; however, individuals with OSA typically have an absent dip or paradoxic increase (reverse dip) in sleep period BP.
- The definitive diagnosis of OSA is made by polysomnography, a sleep study that may be performed in a sleep laboratory or at home.
- Clinical trials demonstrate modest reduction of BP with continuous positive airway pressure (CPAP).
- Treatment of OSA with CPAP is necessary for proper management of atrial fibrillation and maintenance sinus rhythm.

INTRODUCTION AND BACKGROUND

Obstructive sleep apnea (OSA) presents as repetitive interruptions of ventilation each lasting for more than 10 seconds during sleep as a result of upper airway obstruction and resulting in increased respiratory effort.[1] This is in contradistinction to central sleep apnea in which there is a loss of ventilatory drive, with a greater than 10-second pause in ventilation, but with no associated increase in respiratory effort. In this article, we explore the relationship between OSA and cardiovascular disease. Observational studies have associated OSA with hypertension often resistant to medication, coronary heart disease, cardiac arrhythmia (particularly atrial fibrillation), and heart failure.

This article originally appeared in *Clinics in Geriatric Medicine*, Volume 37, Issue 3, August 2022.
Department of Cardiology, Long Island Jewish Hospital, Northwell Health, 270-05 76th Avenue Room 2008, New Hyde Park, NY 11040, USA
* Corresponding author.
E-mail address: jdiamond@northwell.edu

PREVALENCE OF OBSTRUCTIVE SLEEP APNEA

OSA is a common worldwide problem. Population-based studies suggest the prevalence of OSA to be 3% to 7% for adult men and 2% to 5% for adult women in the general population, although higher in different population subsets, such as overweight or obese people and older individuals.[2] In a meta-analysis of 17 studies, Benjafield and colleagues[3] estimated that 936 million adult men and women aged 30 to 69 years worldwide have mild to severe OSA, with the highest prevalence exceeding 50% in some locations. Men are 3 times more likely than women to have OSA, and the prevalence increases with age, particularly in those older than 60 years. Patients with OSA are often obese and have an increased prevalence of other cardiovascular risk factors, such as hypertension and type 2 diabetes mellitus. Approximately 50% of patients with OSA have high blood pressure (BP), and up to 30% of hypertensive individuals may have OSA. Although OSA is associated with obesity, significant sleep-disordered breathing is more likely to be the sole cause of elevated BP in relatively lean versus obese individuals. Even minimal degree of sleep-disordered breathing can increase BP and may contribute to hypertension in 5% of hypertensive individuals.[4,5] The association between OSA and hypertension appears to be particularly prominent in patients with resistant hypertension. In one study, OSA was found in 71% of individuals with resistant hypertension, compared with 38% of individuals with controlled systemic hypertension.[6]

PATHOPHYSIOLOGY OF CARDIOVASCULAR DISEASE WITH OBSTRUCTIVE SLEEP APNEA

It is not clear if OSA causes cardiovascular disease or is only associated with cardiac disease, because the 2 conditions share independent risk factors, such as age and obesity. Intermittent hypoxia from OSA causes changes in oxygen concentration, carbon dioxide concentration, and blood pH, resulting in an increase in catecholamine production. Catecholamine production may be further enhanced in response to chronic sleep deprivation. Furthermore, carotid chemoreceptors are stimulated producing a vasomotor center reflex, which with increased catecholamines results in an increase in total peripheral resistance. The cyclic ventilatory pattern of sleep apnea also causes tachycardia and increased venous return, leading to an increase in cardiac output. The combination of increased total peripheral resistance and cardiac output promotes hypertension. The increase in catecholamines and heart rate contributes to tachyarrhythmias and heart failure. In addition to sympathetic excitation, intermittent hypoxia promotes inflammation, oxidative stress, and metabolic dysregulation, all of which promote atherosclerosis, myocardial ischemia, cerebrovascular ischemia, left ventricular hypertrophy, and heart failure.[7]

CLINICAL PRESENTATION OF OBSTRUCTIVE SLEEP APNEA WITH CARDIOVASCULAR DISEASE

Early recognition of the symptoms and signs of OSA is important to initiate treatment before the development of significant cardiovascular disease. Clinical features suggestive of OSA include witnessed gasping during sleep, morning headaches, excessive daytime somnolence, loud snoring, and neck circumference greater than 16 inches (40.6 cm).[8] Screening questionnaires for OSA, such as the Berlin Questionnaire, STOP- Bang Questionnaire, or the Epworth Sleepiness Scale may be helpful, but have varying degrees of accuracy. Features of the physical examination suggestive of OSA include large neck circumference, high body mass index, posterior chin position (retrognathia), reduced distance and increased angles from the chin to the thyroid cartilage, narrow oropharyngeal opening (pharyngeal crowding), macroglossia, chronic nasal or sinus congestion (eg, by trans-illumination), and a deviated nasal septum. Twenty-four–hour ambulatory BP monitoring may be done to assess for changes in the pattern of BP. Normally, there is a 10% to 20% decrease in sleep BP compared with wake BP (dip). Individuals with OSA typically have an absent dip or paradoxic increase (reverse dip) in sleep period BP (**Fig. 1**). The definitive diagnosis is made by polysomnography, a sleep study that may be performed in a sleep laboratory or at home. These studies quantify the amount of apneic events in which there is complete obstruction of airflow for at least 10 seconds, as well as the number of hypopneic episodes, in which there is partial obstruction of airflow with oxygen desaturation of at least 3% lasting for 10 seconds or more. By measuring these events, an apnea-hypopnea index is calculated by adding all apneas and hypopneas and then dividing by total sleep time. An apnea-hypopnea index of 15 or more events per hour, or 5 or more events per hour in the presence of symptoms or cardiovascular comorbidities, is diagnostic for OSA.[7] An example of an apneic event during polysomnography is illustrated in **Fig. 2**.[9]

IMPACT OF TREATMENT OF OBSTRUCTIVE SLEEP APNEA ON CARDIOVASCULAR DISEASE

Lifestyle modifications may be considered the initial treatment for mild OSA. Obesity results in fatty deposits around the neck, which contribute to pharyngeal collapse.

Weight loss may decrease critical closing pressures of the airway and be curative for some individuals, but is very difficult to achieve and maintain. Behavioral therapy

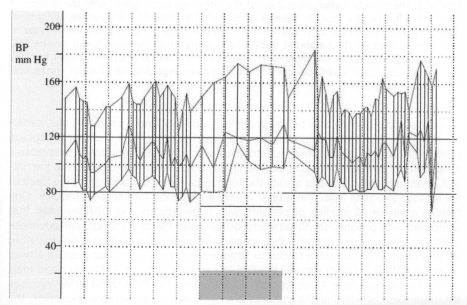

Fig. 1. Plot of BP from 24-hour ambulatory BP monitor with BP in millimeters on the vertical (y-axis) and time on the horizontal (x-axis). The sleep period is represented by a gray rectangle on the x-axis. Each systolic, mean diastolic BP reading is connected by a vertical line. Mean wake period BP is 150/88 ± 12/10 mm Hg. Mean sleep period BP is 166/94 mm Hg ± 9/14 mm Hg. This is a paradoxic BP response or reverse dip.

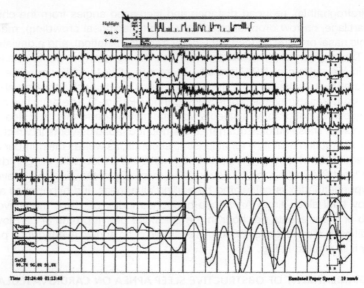

Fig. 2. The upper box (*arrow*) summarizes the total sleep pattern from midnight (0.00 hour) to 9:00 AM (AWK = awake, REM = rapid-eye movement, and sleep stages 1–4). The frequent spikes indicate a disruptive sleep pattern. The vertical line between 0.00 hour and 3:00 AM is detailed in the figure (1:13 AM). It is represented in the first 5 lines by electroencephalogram (EEG) tracings, followed by the nasal/oral airflow tracing, the thorax and abdomen motion tracings, and the oxygen saturation measurements in the lower left corner of the illustration. The nasal/oral airflow tracing shows significant absence of airflow in the boxed region labeled B. There is also paradoxic motion of the abdomen as compared with the motion of the thorax (illustrated in box C). These findings indicate obstructive airflow. Oxygen saturation decreases from 99.7% to 91.8%. Immediately after this period is a sudden increase in airway movement on the nasal/oral tracing with concomitant arousal signals on the EEG tracings (illustrated in the box labeled A). The abdominal and thoracic movement tracings are now synchronized. Over the course of this polysomnography, 68 of these apneic episodes were recorded.

includes avoidance of alcohol before going to sleep, avoidance of sedative use, avoidance of sleep deprivation, and sleeping in a lateral position, thus avoiding the supine position, in which upper airway obstruction occurs most commonly. Mandibular advancement devices hold the mandible slightly down and forward relative to the natural, relaxed position and this results the tongue being farther away from the back of the airway. This may relieve apnea or improve breathing for some individuals. One meta-analysis of 51 studies of patients with hypertension and OSA reported that compared with patients on placebo or not receiving therapy, mandibular advancement devices were associated with a small, but significant reduction in both systolic BP and diastolic BP to levels similar to what is seen with continuous positive airway pressure (CPAP).[10] CPAP remains the first-line treatment for OSA. Randomized trials and meta-analyses have found that effective treatment of OSA using CPAP reduces BP, regardless of whether the patients are hypertensive at baseline. However, the reduction in systemic BP due to positive airway pressure therapy is usually small. In a 2014 meta-analysis that included 30 randomized trials and more than 1900 patients, CPAP therapy was associated with a mean net lowering in systolic BP of 2.6 mm Hg.[11] The 2017 American College of Cardiology/American Heart Association (ACC/AHA)

Guidelines indicate in adults with hypertension and OSA, that the effectiveness of CPAP to reduce BP is not well established.[12] The BP lowering effect of CPAP may be less than that observed with antihypertensive medication. In a randomized cross-over trial of 23 patients with both untreated hypertension and untreated OSA, antihypertensive medication (valsartan 160 mg per day) lowered mean 24-hour BP significantly more than CPAP therapy (−9.0 vs −2.1 mm Hg).[13] In another small randomized clinical trial, spironolactone reduced the severity of OSA and reduced BP in individuals with resistant hypertension and with moderate-to-severe OSA. Thirty patients were enrolled in a prospective, randomized, open trial, with 15 in the treatment group, receiving 20 to 40 mg daily of spironolactone in addition to their usual antihypertensive therapy and 15 receiving usual therapy. After 12 weeks of follow-up, apnea-hypopnea index, hypopnea index, oxygen desaturation index, clinical BP, ambulatory BP, and plasma aldosterone level were reduced significantly in the spironolactone-treated group compared with the control group.[14] This study suggested a potential role for spironolactone not only as a treatment for hypertension, but also as a treatment for OSA. Observational data suggest that treatment of OSA with positive airway pressure may reduce the incidence of cardiovascular events, including events related to coronary artery disease; however, this has not yet been confirmed by randomized clinical trials.[15] In one multicenter randomized trial of 725 patients with moderate-to-severe OSA, but no history of cardiovascular events, randomly assigned to receive CPAP therapy or no active intervention, there was no significant difference in the rate of systemic hypertension or cardiovascular events (nonfatal myocardial infarction, nonfatal stroke, transient ischemic attack, hospitalization for unstable angina/arrhythmia, or cardiovascular death) after a median follow-up of 4 years.[16] Surgical approaches to OSA include uvulo-palato-pharyngoplasty (UPPP) and genio-glossal/mandibular advancement in adults, and tonsillectomy/adenoidectomy in children. UPPP is often ineffective, with up to 50% recurrence rate of OSA in 2 years. This procedure should be used only as a last resort except in patients with severe, specific craniofacial abnormalities.[17] Bariatric surgery in obese patients with OSA may result in improvement in more than 75% of patients and a remission rate of 40% after 2 years.[18]

ELECTROPHYSIOLOGICAL EFFECTS OF OBSTRUCTIVE SLEEP APNEA
Atrial Fibrillation and Obstructive Sleep Apnea

Atrial fibrillation (AF) is the most common cardiac arrhythmia in the general population with a prevalence of 1% to 2%.[19,20] The prevalence increases with age to more than 30% of individuals older than 80 years.[21,22] AF carries significant morbidity, mortality, and health care costs. OSA is exceedingly prevalent in patients with AF.[23] Adults with OSA have almost 2 to 4 times increased risk of developing AF.[24] Similarly, adults with AF have a high prevalence of OSA reported in some trials up to 39%.[25–27] As noted previously with respect to hypertension, OSA may not be the cause of AF in all of these individuals. Their coexistence may in part be due to common risk factors, including advanced age, obesity, diabetes, hypertension, and structural heart disease. The relationship between AF and OSA is multifactorial; however, there may a direct causal relationship that is mutually perpetuating. A significant independent association between the 2 disorders exists.[28] This includes sympathetic and parasympathetic system regulation and cardiac electrical and structural remodeling, particularly of the atria, as shown in **Fig. 3**.[29–31]

During an apneic episode, when there is collapse of the pharyngeal airway leading to interruption of ventilation, vagal efferent output is enhanced, which leads to

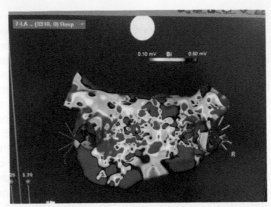

Fig. 3. The posterior wall of the left atrium in a patient with OSA presenting for an AF ablation. There are patchy areas of low voltage as shown by the shades of red and yellow compared with the purple areas of normal voltage.

transient bradycardia as well as a shortened atrial effective refractory period. Episodic hypoxemia during sleep apnea in animal models results in surges of the sympathetic nervous system, thus reducing the induction threshold for AF.[32] However, the pathophysiology is beyond just neurohormonal activation. Sympathetic ganglion blockade provides only incomplete protection against AF associated with apnea.[33-35] There is also electrical and structural remodeling of atrial tissue due to stretch mediated shortening of atrial refractoriness with resultant susceptibility to excitatory stimuli. Furthermore, collagen deposition and changes in gap junction function have been described in individuals with OSA.[36,37] Repetitive apneic episodes resulting in exaggerated changes in intrathoracic pressure lead to left atrial dilatation and fibrosis.[38,39] Electrophysiology studies of these atria in patients with OSA show areas of slow conduction, reduced atrial electrogram amplitude, and complex fractionated atrial electrograms, correlating with the electrical remodeling, as shown in **Fig. 3**. Atrial electrical remodeling, structural remodeling, and neuro-hormonal activation during apneic episodes provide the milieu for the induction of AF.[36,37] Treatment of AF is more difficult in patients with OSA. In the ORBIT-AF trial, patients with OSA had significantly worse symptoms and were more likely to be on rhythm control therapy.[40] Individuals with OSA had more episodes of recurrent AF, even after catheter ablation.[41-44] Treatment of OSA is indispensable for proper management of AF and maintenance of sinus rhythm. The cohort of patients treated with CPAP in the ORBIT-AF trial were less likely to progress to persistent AF compared with those not treated with CPAP.[11] In addition, other trials have shown less AF after catheter ablation in those patients with OSA treated with CPAP compared with a 57% risk of recurrence of AF in those not treated with CPAP.[43]

Current guidelines recommend treating OSA with CPAP for rhythm control of AF, particularly after catheter ablation. It is especially important in diagnosing and treating suspected OSA in any patient who presents with symptomatic AF and is a candidate for ablation.[45] Suspected OSA should be evaluated in those individuals with drug-refractory AF and those with recurrent AF after cardioversion or catheter ablation.

Premature Ventricular Contractions, Nonsustained Ventricular Tachycardia, and Obstructive Sleep Apnea

Most studies focus on the relationship of AF with OSA. However, there is an increasing body of evidence linking OSA with ventricular arrhythmias (VAs), particularly premature ventricular contractions (PVCs) and nonsustained ventricular tachycardia (NSVT). VAs have been reported in up to two-thirds of patients with OSA.[46–48] VAs are more common during apneic episodes.[49–51] The mechanisms are similar to those causing the induction of AF in adults with OSA. As with AF, neurohormonal changes, such as enhanced parasympathetic activation during, and sympathetic surges create the arrhythmogenic substrate necessary for VAs.[48] Exaggerated intrathoracic pressure changes cause myocardial stretch, leading to the structural changes in the ventricles similar to the atria. Increased systemic inflammation and endothelial dysfunction from repetitive apneic episodes may directly trigger VAs. These mechanisms also lead to hypertension, ventricular hypertrophy, myocardial fibrosis, ventricular dysfunction, and coronary artery disease, all of which may further predispose these patients to arrhythmia.[52] The frequency of PVCs correlates with the degree of sympathetic tone during waking hours. PVC frequency decreases during normal rapid-eye movement (REM) sleep. Thus, sympatho-vagal balance plays a role in the frequency of PVCs in adults with OSA.[53] NSVT may also be seen with OSA; however, not to the same degree as with PVCs. Abe and colleagues[54] showed that PVCs are more frequent in the more severe forms of OSA. NSVT, however, is not consistently more common in patients with OSA. One study by Mehra and colleagues[55] did find NSVT to be more common in individuals with sleep-disordered breathing (SDB). However, PVCs and OSA have a stronger link. Furthermore, Koshino and colleagues[56] found that 51% of individuals with idiopathic PVCs without heart failure were found to have OSA. This strengthens the idea that of all the VAs, PVCs were more clearly associated with OSA. Other VAs do occur. A study of intracardiac defibrillator (ICD) therapy, including shocks and antitachycardia pacing, in patients with SDB found that VAs were more common during apnea/hypopnea than with normal breathing.[57,58] The presence of SDB was an independent predictor of ICD therapy and the severity of OSA correlated with an increased risk of VAs.[59]

Sudden Cardiac Death and Obstructive Sleep Apnea

In 2005, a study by Gami and colleagues[60] looked at the association of OSA and sudden cardiac death (SCD). The investigators reviewed the death certificates of 112 people who died during sleep and found that 46% of those who died between midnight and 6 AM had OSA. In 2013, a longitudinal study of 10,000 patients found that VAs were not the sole cause of death in patients with OSA. Acute myocardial infarction and pulmonary embolism were also included.[61]

SINUS NODE DYSFUNCTION, ATRIOVENTRICULAR BLOCK, AND OBSTRUCTIVE SLEEP APNEA

Sinus node dysfunction and atrioventricular (AV) block have been linked to patients with OSA. The mechanism is similar to that attributed to AF and VAs, involving electrical and structural remodeling of the myocardial tissue. Fibrosis and dilation of the atria provoke areas of low voltage and slow conduction, resulting in sinus node dysfunction and AV block. Simantirakis and colleagues[62] reported a 22% prevalence of bradycardia with significant pauses on implantable loop recorders in patients with OSA. An observational study by Garrigue and colleagues,[63] showed a 59% prevalence of undiagnosed OSA in patients with permanent pacemakers. Becker and colleagues, found AV block and sinus arrest in 30% of patients with OSA.[64]

There is currently no conclusive evidence that connects the prevalence or severity of electrophysiological effects, including AF, VAs, heart block, and SCD with the treatment of OSA. However, there have been observational trials suggesting that CPAP is an effective strategy in limiting the arrhythmogenic complications of OSA. Larger prospective trials are needed to firmly establish the true role of CPAP in limiting the electrophysiological sequelae of OSA.

CLINICS CARE POINTS

- OSA may be a cause of resistant hypertension.
- OSA is a contributing factor in patients with atrial fibrillation, PVCs and NSVT.
- OSA may be diagnosed with polysomnography.
- OSA may cause a blunted or paradoxical increase in sleep BP.
- Spironolactone may provide benefit for OSA independent of BP lowering effect.
- Treatment of OSA with CPAP may help lower BP, and help maintain sinus rhythm in patients with atrial fibrillation.

DISCLOSURE

The authors have nothing to disclose

REFERENCES

1. Somers VK, White DP, Amin RA, et al. Sleep apnea and cardiovascular disease: an American Heart Association/American College of Cardiology Foundation scientific statement from the American Heart Association council for high BP research professional education committee, council on clinical cardiology, stroke council, and council on cardiovascular nursing. J Am Coll Cardiol 2008;52: 686–717.
2. Punjabi NM. The epidemiology of adult obstructive sleep apnea. Proc Am Thorac Soc 2008;5(2):136–43.
3. Benjafield AV, Ayas NT, Eastwood P, et al. Estimation of the global prevalence and burden of obstructive sleep apnea: literature-based analysis. Lancet Respir Med 2019;7(8):687–98.
4. Young T, Peppard P, Palta M, et al. Population-based study of sleep-disordered breathing as a risk factor for hypertension. Arch Intern Med 1997;157:1746–52.
5. Nieto FJ, Young TB, Lind BK, et al. Association of sleep-disordered breathing, sleep apnea, and hypertension in a large community-based study. Sleep Heart Health Study. JAMA 2000;283:1829–36.
6. Gonçalves SC, Martinez D, Gus M, et al. Obstructive sleep apnea and resistant hypertension: a case-control study. Chest 2007;132(6):1858.
7. Silke R. Mechanisms of cardiovascular disease in obstructive sleep apnea. J Thorac Dis 2018;10(34):S4201–11.
8. Semelka M, Wilson J, Floyd R. Diagnosis and treatment of obstructive sleep apnea in adults. Am Fam Physician 2016;94(5):355–60.
9. Diamond JA, DePalo L. Resistant hypertension in a young man with asthma. Am J Hypertens 2002;15(2):199–200.
10. Bratton DJ, Gaisl T, Wons AM, et al. CPAP vs mandibular advancement devices and BP in patients with obstructive sleep apnea: a systematic review and meta-analysis. JAMA 2015;314(21):2280–93.
11. Fava C, Dorigoni S, Dalle Vedove F, et al. Effect of CPAP on BP in patients with OSA/hypopnea a systematic review and meta-analysis. Chest 2014;145(4):762.

12. Whelton PK, Carey RM, Aronow WS, et al. 2017 Acc/AHA/AAPA/ABC/ACPM/ AGS/APhA/ASH/ASPC/NMA/CNA guideline for the prevention, detection, evaluation, and management of high BP in adults: a report of the American College of Cardiology/American Heart Association Task Force on Clinical Practice Guidelines. J Am Coll Cardiol 2018;71(19):e127–248.

13. Pépin JL, Tamisier R, Barone-Rochette G, et al. Comparison of continuous positive airway pressure and valsartan in hypertensive patients with sleep apnea. Am J Respir Crit Care Med 2010;182(7):954.

14. Yang L, Zhang H, Cai M, et al. Effect of spironolactone on patients with resistant hypertension and obstructive sleep apnea. Clin Exp Hypertens 2016;38(5): 464–8.

15. Marin JM, Carrizo SJ, Vicente E, et al. Long-term cardiovascular outcomes in men with obstructive sleep apnoea-hypopnoea with or without treatment with continuous positive airway pressure: an observational study. Lancet 2005;365(9464): 1046.

16. Barbé F, Durán-Cantolla J, Sánchez-de-la-Torre M, et al. Effect of continuous positive airway pressure on the incidence of hypertension and cardiovascular events in non-sleepy patients with obstructive sleep apnea: a randomized controlled trial. JAMA 2012;307(20):2161–8.

17. Sundaram S, Bridgman SA, Lim J, et al. Surgery for obstructive sleep apnoea. Cochrane Database Syst Rev 2005;(4):CD001004.

18. Sarkhosh K, Switzer NJ, El-Hadi M, et al. The impact of bariatric surgery on obstructive sleep apnea: a systematic review. Obes Surg 2013;23(3):414–23.

19. Go AS, Hylek EM, Phillips KA, et al. Prevalence of diagnosed atrial fibrillation in adults: national implications for rhythm management and stroke prevention: the Anticoagulation and Risk Factors in Atrial Fibrillation (ATRIA) Study. JAMA 2001;285:2370–5.

20. Tietjens JR, Claman D, Kezirian EJ, et al. Obstructive sleep apnea in cardiovascular disease: a review of the literature and proposed multidisciplinary clinical management strategy. J Am H Assoc 2019;8:e010440.

21. Marulanda-Londono E, Chaturvedi S. The interplay between obstructive sleep apnea and atrial fibrillation. Front Neurol 2017;8:668.

22. January CT, Wann LS, Alpert JS, et al. 2014 AHA/ACC/HRS guideline for the management of patients with atrial fibrillation: executive summary: a report of the American College of Cardiology/American Heart Association Task Force on practice guidelines and the Heart Rhythm Society. Circulation 2014;130(23): 2071–104.

23. Shahar E, Whitney CW, Redline S, et al. Sleep-disordered breathing and cardiovascular disease: cross-sectional results of the Sleep Heart Health Study. Am J Respir Crit Care Med 2001;163:19–25.

24. Somers VK, White DP, Amin R, et al. Sleep apnea and cardiovascular disease: an American Heart Association/American College of Cardiology Foundation scientific statement from the American Heart Association Council for High BP Research Professional Education Committee, Council on Clinical Cardiology, Stroke Council, and Council on Cardiovascular Nursing. In collaboration with the National Heart, Lung, and Blood Institute National Center on Sleep Disorders Research (National Institutes of Health). Circulation 2008;118(10):1080–111.

25. Albuquerque FN, Calvin AD, Sert Kuniyoshi FH, et al. Sleep disordered breathing and excessive daytime sleepiness in patients with atrial fibrillation. Chest 2012; 141:967–73.

26. Bitter T, Langer C, Vogt J, et al. Sleep disordered breathing in patients with atrial fibrillation and normal systolic left ventricular function. Dtsch Arztebl Int 2009;106: 164–70.
27. Gami AS, Pressman G, Caples SM, et al. Association of atrial fibrillation and obstructive sleep apnea. Circulation 2004;110:364–7.
28. Drager LF, Bortolotto LA, Pedrosa RP, et al. Left atrial diameter is independently associated with arterial stiffness in patients with obstructive sleep apnea: potential implications for atrial fibrillation. Int J Cardiol 2010;144:257–259.
29. Leung RS. Sleep-disordered breathing: autonomic mechanisms and arrhythmias. Prog Cardiovasc Dis 2009;51:324–38.
30. Force ESCT, Gorenek B, Pelliccia A, et al. European Heart Rhythm Association (EHRA)/European Association of Cardiovascular Prevention and Rehabilitation (EACPR) position paper on how to prevent atrial fibrillation endorsed by the Heart Rhythm Society (HRS) and Asia Pacific Heart Rhythm Society (APHRS). European Journal of Preventive Cardiology 2016;24(1):4–40.
31. De Jong AM, Maass AH, Oberdorf-Maass SU, et al. Mechanisms of atrial structural changes caused by stretch occurring before and during early atrial fibrillation. Cardiovasc Res 2011;89:754–65.
32. May AM, Van Wagoner DR, Mehra R. OSA and cardiac arrhythmogenesis: mechanistic insights. Chest 2017;151:225–41.
33. Ghias M, Scherlag BJ, Lu Z, et al. The role of ganglionated plexi in apnea-related atrial fibrillation. J Am Coll Cardiol 2009;54:2075–83.
34. Linz D, Mahfoud F, Schotten U, et al. Renal sympathetic denervation suppresses postapneic BP rises and atrial fibrillation in a model for sleep apnea. Hypertension 2012;60:172–8.
35. Linz D, Hohl M, Khoshkish S, et al. Low-level but not high-level baroreceptor stimulation inhibits atrial fibrillation in a pig model of sleep apnea. J Cardiovasc Electrophysiol 2016;27:1086–92.
36. Iwasaki YK, Kato T, Xiong F, et al. Atrial fibrillation promotion with long-term repetitive obstructive sleep apnea in a rat model. J Am Coll Cardiol 2014;64:2013–23.
37. Linz D, Schotten U, Neuberger HR, et al. Negative tracheal pressure during obstructive respiratory events promotes atrial fibrillation by vagal activation. Heart Rhythm 2011;8:1436–43.
38. Drager LF, Bortolotto LA, Pedrosa RP, et al. Left atrial diameter is independently associated with arterial stiffness in patients with obstructive sleep apnea: potential implications for atrial fibrillation. Int J Cardiol 2010;144:257–9.
39. Dimitri H, Ng M, Brooks AG, et al. Atrial remodeling in obstructive sleep apnea: implications for atrial fibrillation. Heart Rhythm 2012;9:321–7.
40. Holmqvist F, Guan N, Zhu Z, et al, ORBIT-AF Investigators. Impact of obstructive sleep apnea and continuous positive airway pressure therapy on outcomes in patients with atrial fibrillation—results from the Outcomes Registry for Better Informed Treatment of Atrial Fibrillation (ORBIT-AF). Am Heart J 2015;169:647–54.
41. Kanagala R, Murali NS, Friedman PA, et al. Obstructive sleep apnea and the recurrence of atrial fibrillation. Circulation 2003;107:2589–94.
42. Naruse Y, Tada H, Satoh M, et al. Concomitant obstructive sleep apnea increases the recurrence of atrial fibrillation following radiofrequency catheter ablation of atrial fibrillation: clinical impact of continuous positive airway pressure therapy. Heart Rhythm 2013;10:331–7.
43. Li L, Wang ZW, Li J, et al. Efficacy of catheter ablation of atrial fibrillation in patients with obstructive sleep apnea with and without continuous positive airway

pressure treatment: a meta-analysis of observational studies. Europace 2014;16: 1309–14.

44. Ng CY, Liu T, Shehata M, et al. Meta-analysis of obstructive sleep apnea as predictor of atrial fibrillation recurrence after catheter ablation. Am J Cardiol 2011; 108:47–51.

45. Calkins H, Hindricks G, Cappato R, et al. 2017 HRS/EHRA/ECAS/APHRS/SOL-AECE expert consensus statement on catheter and surgical ablation of atrial fibrillation: executive summary. J Arrhythm 2017;33:369–409.

46. Guilleminault C, Connolly SJ, Winkle RA. Cardiac arrhythmia and conduction disturbances during sleep in 400 patients with sleep apnea syndrome. Am J Cardiol 1983;52:490–4.

47. Hoffstein V, Mateika S. Cardiac arrhythmias, snoring, and sleep apnea. Chest 1994;106:466–71.

48. Marinheiro R, Parreira L, Amador P, et al. Ventricular arrhythmias in patients with obstructive sleep apnea. Curr Cardiol Rev 2019;15(1):64–74.

49. Shepard JW Jr, Garrison MW, Grither DA, et al. Relationship of ventricular ectopy to oxyhemoglobin desaturation in patients with obstructive sleep apnea. Chest 1985;88(3):335–40.

50. Harbison J, O'Reilly P, McNicholas WT. Cardiac rhythm disturbances in the obstructive sleep apnea syndrome: effects of nasal continuous positive airway pressure therapy. Chest 2000;118(3):591–5.

51. Javaheri S. Effects of continuous positive airway pressure on sleep apnea and ventricular irritability in patients with heart failure. Circulation 2000;101:392–7.

52. May AM, VanWagoner DR, Mehra R. Obstructive sleep apnea and cardiac arrhythmogenesis: mechanistic insights. Chest 2017;151(1):225–41.

53. Muller JE, Tofler GH, Verrier RL. Sympathetic activity as the cause of the morning increase in cardiac events. A likely culprit, but the evidence remains circumstantial. Circulation 1995;91(10):2508–9.

54. Abe H, Takahashi M, Yaegashi H, et al. Efficacy of continuous positive airway pressure on arrhythmias in obstructive sleep apnea patients. Heart Vessels 2010;25:63–9.

55. Mehra R, Benjamin EJ, Shahar E, et al. Association of nocturnal arrhythmias with sleep-disordered breathing: the sleep heart health study. Am J Respir Crit Care Med 2006;173:910–6.

56. Koshino Y, Satoh M, Katayose Y, et al. Sleep apnea and ventricular arrhythmias: clinical outcome, electrophysiologic characteristics, and follow-up after catheter ablation. J Cardiol 2010;55(2):211–6.

57. Fichter J, Bauer D, Arampatzis S, et al. Sleep-related breathing disorders are associated with ventricular arrhythmias in patients with an implantable cardioverter-defibrillator. Chest 2002;122(2):558–61.

58. Anselme F, Maounis T, Mantovani G, et al. Severity of sleep apnea syndrome correlates with burden of ventricular tachyarrhythmias in unselected ICD patients [abstract]. Heart Rhythm 2013;10(5):S190.

59. Zeidan-Shwiri T, Aronson D, Atalla K, et al. Circadian pattern of life-threatening ventricular arrhythmia in patients with sleep disordered breathing and implantable cardioverter-defibrillators. Heart Rhythm 2011;8(5):657–62.

60. Gami AS, Howard DE, Olson EJ, et al. Day-night pattern of sudden death in obstructive sleep apnea. N Engl J Med 2005;352(12):1206–14.

61. Gami AS, Olson EJ, Shen WK, et al. Obstructive sleep apnea and the risk of sudden cardiac death: a longitudinal study of 10,701 adults. J Am Coll Cardiol 2013; 62(7):610–6.

62. Simantirakis EN, Schiza SI, Marketou ME, et al. Severe bradyarrhythmias in patients with sleep apnea: the effect of continuous positive airway pressure treatment: a long-term evaluation using an insertable loop recorder. Eur Heart J 2004;25:1070–6.
63. Garrigue S, Pépin JL, Delaye P, et al. High prevalence of sleep apnea syndrome in patients with long-term pacing: the European Multicenter Polysomnographic Study. Circulation 2007;115:1703–9.
64. Becker H, Brandenburg U, Peter JH, et al. Reversal of sinus arrest and atrioventricular conduction block in patients with sleep apnea during nasal continuous positive airway pressure. Am J Respir Crit Care Med 1995;151:215–8.

Management of Dyslipidemia in Endocrine Diseases

Lisa R. Tannock, MD*

KEYWORDS

- Lipids • Cardiovascular • Endocrine • Dyslipidemia

KEY POINTS

- Treatment of dyslipidemia decreases cardiovascular risk.
- Many endocrine diseases are associated with dyslipidemia.
- Many endocrine diseases can affect cardiovascular risk, but are not considered when assessing risk.

INTRODUCTION/HISTORY/DEFINITIONS/BACKGROUND

Most lipid management guidelines recommend assessment of lipid levels and cardiovascular risk factors within an individual, then based on estimated cardiovascular disease (CVD) risk, suggest lipid-lowering therapy and/or lipid goals.[1] Overall, this approach works well. However, one of the limitations is that the cardiovascular risk factors typically included in risk calculators and guidelines are somewhat limited: smoking, hypertension, diabetes, age, sex, and race are the typical factors. In some guidelines additional factors, such as family history of premature CVD events, chronic inflammatory disorders, chronic kidney disease, and premature menopause (age <40 years), are often also noted as risk-enhancing factors. However, these factors are fairly difficult to turn into a quantitative risk, and thus often not included in risk calculators, and may be overlooked by providers.

Most endocrine disorders are chronic in nature, and thus even a minor effect to increase risk for CVD can lead to a significant impact when duration of exposure is considered. Although robust therapies exist for many endocrine disorders (whether it be suppression of excess hormone amounts, or replacement of hormone deficiencies), the therapies do not perfectly restore normal physiology. Thus, individuals with endocrine disorders are at potential increased CVD risk, and maximizing

This article originally appeared in *Endocrinology and Metabolism Clinics*, Volume 51, Issue 3, September 2022.

Division of Endocrinology, Diabetes, and Metabolism, University of Kentucky, Department of Veterans Affairs, MN145, 780 Rose Street, Lexington, KY 40536, USA

* Corresponding author.

E-mail address: Lisa.Tannock@uky.edu

Clinics Collections 13 (2023) 223–236
https://doi.org/10.1016/j.ccol.2023.02.010
2352-7986/23/Published by Elsevier Inc.

strategies to reduce that risk are needed. The Endocrine Society recently published a guideline explicitly assessing the lipid profile and CVD risk and thus indications for lipid-lowering therapy in individuals with endocrine diseases.[2] This new guideline suggests that some endocrine diseases, including hyperthyroidism, hypothyroidism, Cushing disease, chronic glucocorticoid therapy with doses greater than physiologic needs, obesity, postmenopausal hormone-replacement therapy use, and premature menopause, should be included in the list of risk enhancing factors. This article reviews various endocrine conditions that can impact lipid levels and/or CVD risk.

CASE STUDY

A 47-year-old woman presents to clinic to establish care. She has recently moved to your region. She was diagnosed with autoimmune adrenal insufficiency at age 12, and takes glucocorticoid-replacement therapy. She currently takes 20 mg every morning and 5 to 10 mg in the afternoon. She tells you that her previous endocrinologist kept attempting to reduce her hydrocortisone dose, but every time she decreased the dose she suffered severe fatigue and would go back up to this dose. She states she was trained in sick day management, and doubles the dose for 2 to 4 days each time she has nausea, vomiting, fever, or severe fatigue. She estimates that she doubles her dose at least five times each year.

At age 22 she presented with Graves disease, was treated with radioactive iodine ablation, and subsequently became hypothyroid treated with levothyroxine. Her current dose is 150 μg daily. She was diagnosed with endometriosis in her teens. She had one pregnancy complicated by preeclampsia at age 32, and had hysterectomy and oophorectomy at age 37. She took estrogen for 2 to 3 years afterward, but then discontinued it because she did not see the need. She has struggled with her weight for years, but has recently put on about 10 lb (4.5 kg) with the stress of the move, and her current weight is 216 lb (98.2 kg). She reports her height as 5 ft, 6 inches (1.67 m); and her body mass index is 34.9 kg/m². She has long-standing depression controlled with citalopram 40 mg daily. She has never smoked.

Her current medications are:

Hydrocortisone, 25 to 30 mg daily
Levothyroxine, 150 μg daily
Multivitamin, one daily
Citalopram, 40 mg daily.

Her blood pressure is 132/74 mm Hg. Her pulse is 82 beats per minute. Her examination is notable for generalized obesity with numerous pale striae on her abdomen. Her thyroid is not palpable. The remainder of the examination is normal.

Fasting laboratory studies are as follows:

Metabolic panel normal, with fasting glucose 97 mg/dL and estimated glomerular filtration rate greater than 60 mL/min/m²
Hemogram, normal
Thyroid-stimulating hormone 6.9 mIU/mL (normal range, 0.5–5.0 mIU/mL); free T4 0.6 ng/dL (normal range, 0.8–1.8 ng/dL)
Total cholesterol (TC) 234 mg/dL
Low-density lipoprotein cholesterol (LDL-c) 148 mg/dL
High-density lipoprotein cholesterol (HDL-c) 32 mg/dL
Triglycerides (TG) 268 mg/dL

The ASCVD risk calculator estimates her 10-year risk as 2.8%.

Clinical Questions

Does the ASCVD risk calculator 10-year risk estimate reassure you? Are there any other factors you need to consider?

DISCUSSION

On the surface, this patient seems to have several endocrine issues that need to be addressed, but cardiovascular risk does not seem to be one. She is obese, has premature menopause, inadequately treated hypothyroidism, and overtreated adrenal insufficiency. Managing these chronic conditions is important, and would likely be addressed by most endocrinologists. However, the 10-year CVD risk estimate may seem reassuring, and it would not be surprising if most providers did not consider CVD risk reduction and lipid-lowering therapy as high priorities. The recent guidelines published by the Endocrine Society suggest that her endocrine comorbidities may impact her cardiovascular risk, and should be considered.[2] In the following sections we address these (and others) one by one.

Changes in Lipids with Hyperthyroidism and Hypothyroidism

Altered thyroid hormone levels can have profound effects on lipoprotein metabolism and thus lipid levels. Thyroid hormone decreases intestinal absorption of cholesterol; increases biliary secretion leading to decreased hepatic cholesterol content and compensatory increase in LDL-receptors; increases HMG-CoA reductase activity; and increases enzymes involved in LDL metabolism including lipoprotein lipase, hepatic lipase, cholesteryl ester transfer protein and lecithin cholesterol acyltransferase.[3–7] Thus, hyperthyroidism tends to lead to accelerated metabolism of lipoprotein particles such that TC and LDL-c are often low, whereas TG and HDL-c are not usually affected. Conversely, hypothyroidism tends to lead to elevated TC, LDL-c, HDL-c, and TG. The Endocrine Society meta-analysis[8] found that treatment of hyperthyroidism (with surgery, radioactive iodine, or antithyroid medication) led to significant increases in TC and LDL-c and HDL-c with restoration of euthyroid state; however, this was only true in overt hyperthyroidism and not in subclinical hyperthyroidism. Treatment of overt hypothyroidism correspondingly led to significant decreases of TC, LDL-c, HDL-c, and TG.[8] Indeed, levothyroxine has been studied as a therapy for elevated lipid levels (**Table 1**).[9]

Whether hyperthyroidism or hypothyroidism directly influence CVD (rather than indirectly, via dyslipidemia) is unknown. Epidemiologic studies suggest that coronary disease prevalence is increased in hypothyroidism compared with euthyroid controls.[10,11] Hypothyroidism can affect cardiac contractility and exacerbate angina; however, it is not clear if there are direct pathophysiologic changes related to thyroid hormone abnormalities, or if the association is mediated through dyslipidemia.

Table 1
Change in lipid parameters after treatment of thyroid disease

Mean % Change with Treatment	TC	LDL-c	HDL-c	TG
Overt hypothyroidism	↓22%	↓24%	↓7%	↓18%
Subclinical hypothyroidism	↓5%	↓8%	0%	↓4%
Overt hyperthyroidism	↑28%	↑35%	↑12%	↑7%
Subclinical hyperthyroidism	↑5%	↑6%	0%	↓30%

Data adapted from a meta-analysis of n=3-72 studies per parameter, with total patients from 104-4588 per parameter.[8]

Considerations for clinical management

The Endocrine Society guidelines recommend screening for hypothyroidism as a cause of dyslipidemia and deferring treatment decisions until after restoration of euthyroid status when a patient has either hyperthyroidism or hypothyroidism. These recommendations are prudent and will help avoid unnecessary lipid-lowering therapy in the setting of hypothyroidism (if the repeated lipid panel shows resolution of hyperlipidemia), and avoid a missed therapeutic opportunity in the setting of hyperthyroidism if the lipid panel is falsely reassuring when the patient is hyperthyroid.

Thus, for the case vignette presented, it would be prudent to adjust her levothyroxine dose, and repeat the lipid panel 6 to 8 weeks later when she would be expected to be euthyroid. Although her freeT4 is only marginally low, restoration of euthyroid state could lead to some improvement in her dyslipidemia.

Changes in Lipids with Glucocorticoid Excess or Therapy

Elevated glucocorticoid levels (whether endogenous, such as in Cushing syndrome, or exogenous, as in the case vignette) can lead to elevations in TC, LDL-c, and TG. Glucocorticoids stimulate preadipocyte differentiation and increased adipose tissue, especially visceral adipose, and also promote fatty acid and cholesterol synthesis in the liver, leading to hepatic steatosis.[12] Chronic elevations in glucocorticoids increase metabolic syndrome prevalence, with associated hypertension, insulin resistance, and prothrombotic state, all of which contribute to increased CVD risk. Patients cured of Cushing syndrome typically experience improvements in dyslipidemia, and reduced obesity, hypertension, and insulin resistance.[13] For patients using exogenous steroids the literature is conflicted, but at least one study indicates a glucocorticoid dose-dependent increase in TC, LDL-c, and TG levels.[14,15] Furthermore, several studies suggest increased CVD in patients using exogenous glucocorticoids, particularly for those with iatrogenic hypercortisolism and Cushing syndrome.[16–19]

Considerations for clinical management

The Endocrine Society guidelines address lipid screening and management in settings of excess endogenous or exogenous glucocorticoids. The guidelines recommend screening lipid levels in adults with Cushing syndrome and those on chronic glucocorticoid therapy greater than standard physiologic replacement doses. The guidelines go on to suggest statin therapy in addition to lifestyle modification in adults with persistent Cushing syndrome to reduce CVD risk, regardless of cardiovascular risk score. There is not any evidence to guide recommendation of lipid lowering therapies (statins) in individuals with exogenous glucocorticoids greater than physiologic doses, but certainly, there is accumulating evidence that supraphysiologic doses of glucocorticoids convey health risks. Thus, at a minimum it is prudent to recommend decreasing glucocorticoid doses, which may help decrease lipid levels and CVD risk.

Thus, for the case vignette presented, it would be prudent to taper her hydrocortisone dose down, review sick day rules to minimize excessive dosing, and repeat the lipid panel when stable on a lower dose. Collectively, her use of glucocorticoid therapy should be considered along with other risk factors when making a decision about lipid-lowering therapy.

Changes in Lipids with Obesity

Obesity prevalence is high and rising, and thus a common concern for health care providers. In particular, when obesity is mainly central it often exists as part of the metabolic syndrome (elevated TG, reduced HDL, increased waist circumference, hyperglycemia, increased blood pressure) where dyslipidemia is highly prevalent, and robust evidence indicates an increased risk for CVD. Even without metabolic syndrome, obesity is associated with elevations in TG and decreases in HDL-c, and although LDL-c may not be elevated, the particles are often small and dense, which are thought to be more atherogenic.[20–22] In addition, delayed lipoprotein metabolism leads to prolonged and exacerbated postprandial hyperglycemia.[23–25] Furthermore, elevated body mass index, or increased waist circumference or waist/hip ratio are predictors of CVD mortality.[24,26–28]

Considerations for clinical management

Weight loss, whether induced by caloric restriction, medications, or surgery, leads to improvements in the lipid profile. Five percent body weight reduction can lead to improvements in several comorbidities of obesity.[29] There is a corresponding improvement in lipids with increased weight loss, so that 3-kg weight loss is associated with a TG decrease of 15 mg/dL (0.17 mmol/L), but weight loss of 5 to 8 kg is associated with decreases in LDL-c of −5 mg/dL (−0.13 mmol/L) and increases in HDL-c of 2 to 3 mg/dL (0.5–0.8 mmol/L).[30] A meta-analysis showed that the most consistent and favorable effect of weight loss is a lowering of TG.[31] When patients are actively undergoing weight loss several changes in lipid levels can occur, including paradoxic drops in HDL-c during active weight loss[32,33]; thus, the Endocrine Society recommends reassessment of lipids after weight loss once weight has stabilized.

Lipid-lowering therapy with statins has been clearly shown to decrease CVD events in patients with and without obesity. Although LDL-c is not always high in obesity, statins (which target LDL-c) are highly efficacious in lowering CVD risk.[34,35] Conversely, fibrates (which target TG) have not been consistently shown to decrease CVD risk. Thus, if there are indications for lipid-lowering therapy then most guidelines recommend statins as the first-line therapy. Of note, when TG are elevated to the extent that pancreatitis is a risk there is uniform agreement of using fibrates to lower TG.

Thus, for the case vignette presented, it would be appropriate to screen her for metabolic syndrome (based on information provided she does have metabolic syndrome because she has high TG, low HDL-c, and high systolic blood pressure; even without knowing her fasting glucose or waist circumference), and counsel her on weight loss strategies. The Endocrine Society recommends use of a risk calculator to assess 10-year CVD risk, and initiation of lipid-lowering therapy if indicated by the calculator. In this vignette the 10-year CVD risk was 2.8%, and thus she does not clearly meet recommendations for lipid-lowering therapy. However, as discussed throughout this article, the risk calculator does not adjust for potential CVD impact of her combined metabolic disorders, and may underestimate her risk.

Changes in Lipids with Menopause

Although the changes in lipid levels from premenopause to postmenopause are fairly small, epidemiologic evidence consistently indicates an increase in CVD risk. Studies have yielded variable results, but in general the lipid panel shows decreases in HDL-c, increases in TC, and a shift in LDL particle size toward a small, dense phenotype; collectively these are proatherogenic changes. The mechanisms behind shifts in lipid levels likely relate to the decrease in estrogen. Estrogen affects VLDL synthesis, insulin sensitivity, LDL-receptors, and PCSK9.[36,37] Estrogen-replacement therapy leads to increases in HDL-c and decreases in LDL-c; however, progestins tend to decrease HDL-c.[38,39] In patients with an underlying predisposition to hypertriglyceridemia (because of genetics or other risk factors, such as diabetes, obesity, or insulin resistance) estrogen therapy can cause significant increases in TG levels and increase risk for pancreatitis. However, although this is not uncommonly seen in specific individuals, population-based studies have not found a significant increase of pancreatitis with estrogen therapy.[40]

Considerations for clinical management

Several decades ago the standard of care was to recommend hormone-replacement therapy (estrogen, with or without progestins for uterine protection) with the expectation this would decrease CVD risk in postmenopausal women. However, several large randomized controlled trials of estrogen ($\pm$ progestins) found increased CVD events, thought to be caused by increased thrombosis, especially when introduced late after onset of menopause (>60 years, or >10 years since last menstrual period).[41,42] Thus, most guidelines recommend caution for initiation of estrogen, especially in older women.

When menopause occurs early, regardless of whether it is spontaneous or surgically induced, CVD risk is increased: a younger age at menopause seems to be an independent risk factor for CVD.[43-46] The estimate is that the risk of ASCVD is 1.5-fold higher in women with menopause less than 40 years, and 1.3-fold higher in women with menopause occurring at age 40 to 44 years, compared with women who entered menopause at age 50 to 51 years.[46] Several recent guidelines now recognize early menopause as a cardiovascular risk factor. Statin therapy in postmenopausal women has been shown to lower CVD risk, for women using or not using hormone-replacement therapy.[47,48] As further evidence, a meta-analysis of estrogen therapy in younger women reported a significant reduction in CVD.[49] Thus, the Endocrine Society recommends use of statin therapy in postmenopausal women with dyslipidemia, or those on hormone therapy with other risk factors for CVD, and encourages consideration of CVD risk in patients who enter menopause early.

Thus, for the case vignette presented, there are several factors to consider. Her hypothyroidism is undertreated, her glucocorticoid dose is supraphysiologic, she has obesity, and she has early menopause. Although the 10-year risk calculator estimates her risk as fairly low (2.8%) none of these factors are included in that calculator. Collectively, this patient has several endocrine comorbidities that each confer increased CVD risk, and initiation of statin therapy would be expected to help reduce her risk. However, if the provider does not consider each of these comorbidities, the therapeutic opportunity may be missed.

OTHER LIPID-INFLUENCING ENDOCRINE DIAGNOSES

Beyond the topics raised by the case vignette, the Endocrine Society addressed several other endocrine diagnoses that affect lipid levels and CVD risk. These are summarized next.

Changes in Lipids with Polycystic Ovary Syndrome

Polycystic ovary syndrome (PCOS) is characterized by insulin resistance and often a similar lipid profile to that seen in metabolic syndrome: increased TG, low HDL-c, and normal or increased LDL-c.[50,51] In addition, increased levels of Lp(a) may be seen, particularly in nonobese women with PCOS.[52-54] The dyslipidemia exists throughout the reproductive years, tends to be worse in anovulatory women,[53,55] and may be further exacerbated after the onset of menopause. Thus, although the dyslipidemia may be mild, it may be of long duration. Despite the dyslipidemia, it is not clear if there is increased ASCVD risk in PCOS per se, or if the risk is explained by the obesity and metabolic syndrome components.[56]

Considerations for clinical management

Unlike the impact on dyslipidemia in obesity and metabolic syndrome, weight loss achieved via lifestyle therapy (diet and exercise) in PCOS seems to have minimal effects on the dyslipidemia, although improvements in body composition, insulin resistance, and ovulation are seen.[57,58] Other common therapies used in PCOS include metformin and oral contraceptives. Metformin monotherapy seems to have minimal effects on the dyslipidemia in PCOS, although metformin in combination with other medications, such as statins, thiazolidinediones, oral contraceptives, or inositol, can induce improvements.[59–61] However, treatment with oral contraceptives confers the risk of further elevations in TG in susceptible women, although beneficial effects of estrogen on LDL-c and HDL-c are seen.[62]

There have been several trials determining the effect of lipid-lowering medications (mainly statins) in PCOS; collectively, statins are efficacious at lipid-lowering in women with PCOS,[63–67] but cardiovascular outcomes and reproductive outcomes remain unclear.

The Endocrine Society recommends obtaining a lipid panel in all women with PCOS, but using lipid-lowering therapies only as indicated for lipid lowering, and not for the treatment of hyperandrogenism or infertility.

Changes in Lipids with Male Hypogonadism and Testosterone Therapy

Men with hypogonadism tend to have elevations in LDL-c and TG with lower levels of HDL-c[68]; however, repletion of testosterone tends to have minimal effects on lipid levels.[69,70] Thus, use of testosterone therapy is not recommended as a treatment of dyslipidemia. Furthermore, illicit use of testosterone or other androgens is not uncommon, and elevated (supraphysiologic) androgen levels can dramatically suppress HDL-c, increase ApoB and decrease Lp(a).[71,72]

Considerations for clinical management

Although hypogonadism is associated with increased CVD risk,[73] there are multiple factors involved, including insulin resistance, obesity, increased prevalence of metabolic syndrome, and increased free fatty acids, in addition to the dyslipidemia. However, it remains controversial if testosterone therapy alters CVD risk, with some benefit perhaps seen in appropriate dosing of certain subpopulations, but no global benefit.[74]

The Endocrine Society recommends using testosterone therapy for hypogonadism symptoms, but not as a treatment of dyslipidemia or CVD risk. Moreover, in patients with very low HDL-c but without high TG, androgen abuse should be considered as a cause of the dyslipidemia.

Changes in Lipids with Gender-Affirming Hormone Therapy

The use of gender-affirming hormone therapy is increasing, but there is still a paucity of long-term outcome data to guide CVD recommendations. Numerous small studies and a meta-analysis reported an increase in TG and LDL-c and a drop in HDL-c with use of testosterone therapy for transmen.[75–77] In transwomen treated with estrogen therapy most studies have reported an increase in TG with use of oral estrogens, but not with use of transdermal estrogens.[77] Although an increase in HDL-c may be expected, this has not always been confirmed.

Considerations for clinical management

There are minimal data to guide use of lipid-lowering therapy in the transgender population. The Endocrine Society recommends evaluation of CVD risk using the same guidelines as in cisgender adults.

Changes in Lipids with Growth Hormone Deficiency or Growth Hormone Excess

In the setting of growth hormone deficiency, elevations in TC and LDL-c are commonly seen, whereas TG and HDL-c changes are variable.[78–80] Conversely, in growth hormone excess, such as seen in acromegaly, increased TG is commonly observed with variable effects on cholesterol and LDL-c levels.[81,82] Growth hormone inhibits hepatic lipase and lipoprotein lipase activity[81,83] and can increase hepatic LDL-R expression and decrease PCSK9 expression.[84,85]

Considerations for clinical management

Hypopituitarism, of which growth hormone deficiency is the most common hormone abnormality, is associated with increased premature mortality, including increased risk of CVD.[86–88] Growth hormone deficiency itself may affect the myocardial and endothelial tissue, cardiac performance, and coronary calcification, although the direct mechanisms linking growth hormone deficiency and CVD are not fully understood. Although long-term growth hormone therapy improves the dyslipidemia in growth hormone deficiency[89–91] it is not clear that growth hormone therapy can decrease mortality.[92]

SUMMARY

Numerous endocrine disorders affect lipid levels, and thus may confer risk for CVD. Because the current CVD risk calculators that are widely used to guide lipid-lowering therapy decisions do not consider endocrine comorbidities, CVD risk may be underestimated, and thus lipid-lowering therapy may be underused in these populations. Consideration of the additional impact of endocrine diseases when assessing individuals for dyslipidemia, CVD risk, and lipid lowering therapy is urged.

CLINICS CARE POINTS

- Many endocrine diseases affect lipid levels and thus may confer CVD risk.
- CVD risk calculators do not currently assess the impact of endocrine comorbidities.
- Clinicians should consider impact of endocrine comorbidities on CVD risk when making treatment decisions regarding lipid-lowering medications.

ACKNOWLEDGMENTS

This work was supported in part by funding from the National Institutes of Health R01 HL147381 and the Department of Veterans Affairs BX004275.

DISCLOSURE

Dr L.R. Tannock has no conflicts to disclose.

REFERENCES

1. Grundy SM, Stone NJ, Bailey AL, et al. 2018 AHA/ACC/AACVPR/AAPA/ABC/ACPM/ADA/AGS/APhA/ASPC/NLA/PCNA Guideline on the management of blood cholesterol: a report of the American College of Cardiology/American Heart Association task force on clinical practice guidelines. Circulation 2019;139(25): e1082–143.

2. Newman CB, Blaha MJ, Boord JB, et al. Lipid management in patients with endocrine disorders: an endocrine society clinical practice guideline. J Clin Endocrinol Metab 2020;105(12):dgaa674.

3. Choi JW, Choi HS. The regulatory effects of thyroid hormone on the activity of 3-hydroxy-3-methylglutaryl coenzyme A reductase. Endocr Res 2000;26(1):1–21.

4. Duntas LH, Brenta G. The effect of thyroid disorders on lipid levels and metabolism. Med Clin North Am 2012;96(2):269–81.

5. Kuusi T, Taskinen MR, Nikkila EA. Lipoproteins, lipolytic enzymes, and hormonal status in hypothyroid women at different levels of substitution. J Clin Endocrinol Metab 1988;66(1):51–6.

6. Lithell H, Boberg J, Hellsing K, et al. Serum lipoprotein and apolipoprotein concentrations and tissue lipoprotein-lipase activity in overt and subclinical hypothyroidism: the effect of substitution therapy. Eur J Clin Invest 1981;11(1):3–10.

7. Lopez D, Abisambra Socarras JF, Bedi M, et al. Activation of the hepatic LDL receptor promoter by thyroid hormone. Biochim Biophys Acta 2007;1771(9): 1216–25.

8. Kotwal A, Cortes T, Genere N, et al. Treatment of thyroid dysfunction and serum lipids: a systematic review and meta-analysis. J Clin Endocrinol Metab 2020; 105(12):dgaa672.

9. Tanis BC, Westendorp GJ, Smelt HM. Effect of thyroid substitution on hypercholesterolaemia in patients with subclinical hypothyroidism: a reanalysis of intervention studies. Clin Endocrinol (Oxf) 1996;44(6):643–9.

10. Mya MM, Aronow WS. Subclinical hypothyroidism is associated with coronary artery disease in older persons. J Gerontol A Biol Sci Med Sci 2002;57(10):M658–9.

11. Razvi S, Jabbar A, Pingitore A, et al. Thyroid hormones and cardiovascular function and diseases. J Am Coll Cardiol 2018;71(16):1781–96.

12. Ferrau F, Korbonits M. Metabolic comorbidities in Cushing's syndrome. Eur J Endocrinol 2015;173(4):M133–57.

13. Giordano R, Picu A, Marinazzo E, et al. Metabolic and cardiovascular outcomes in patients with Cushing's syndrome of different aetiologies during active disease and 1 year after remission. Clin Endocrinol (Oxf) 2011;75(3):354–60.

14. Choi HK, Seeger JD. Glucocorticoid use and serum lipid levels in US adults: the Third National Health and Nutrition Examination Survey. Arthritis Rheum 2005; 53(4):528–35.

15. Filipsson H, Monson JP, Koltowska-Haggstrom M, et al. The impact of glucocorticoid replacement regimens on metabolic outcome and comorbidity in hypopituitary patients. J Clin Endocrinol Metab 2006;91(10):3954–61.

16. Fardet L, Petersen I, Nazareth I. Risk of cardiovascular events in people prescribed glucocorticoids with iatrogenic Cushing's syndrome: cohort study. BMJ 2012;345:e4928.

17. Souverein PC, Berard A, Van Staa TP, et al. Use of oral glucocorticoids and risk of cardiovascular and cerebrovascular disease in a population based case-control study. Heart 2004;90(8):859–65.

18. Varas-Lorenzo C, Rodriguez LA, Maguire A, et al. Use of oral corticosteroids and the risk of acute myocardial infarction. Atherosclerosis 2007;192(2):376–83.

19. Wei L, MacDonald TM, Walker BR. Taking glucocorticoids by prescription is associated with subsequent cardiovascular disease. Ann Intern Med 2004;141(10): 764–70.

20. Franssen R, Monajemi H, Stroes ES, et al. Obesity and dyslipidemia. Med Clin North Am 2011;95(5):893–902.

21. Klop B, Elte JW, Cabezas MC. Dyslipidemia in obesity: mechanisms and potential targets. Nutrients 2013;5(4):1218–40.
22. Paredes S, Fonseca L, Ribeiro L, et al. Novel and traditional lipid profiles in metabolic syndrome reveal a high atherogenicity. Sci Rep 2019;9(1):11792.
23. Couillard C, Bergeron N, Prud'homme D, et al. Postprandial triglyceride response in visceral obesity in men. Diabetes 1998;47(6):953–60.
24. Nieves DJ, Cnop M, Retzlaff B, et al. The atherogenic lipoprotein profile associated with obesity and insulin resistance is largely attributable to intra-abdominal fat. Diabetes 2003;52(1):172–9.
25. Taskinen MR, Adiels M, Westerbacka J, et al. Dual metabolic defects are required to produce hypertriglyceridemia in obese subjects. Arterioscler Thromb Vasc Biol 2011;31(9):2144–50.
26. Ohlson LO, Larsson B, Svardsudd K, et al. The influence of body fat distribution on the incidence of diabetes mellitus. 13.5 years of follow-up of the participants in the study of men born in 1913. Diabetes 1985;34(10):1055–8.
27. Ortega FB, Lavie CJ, Blair SN. Obesity and cardiovascular disease. Circ Res 2016;118(11):1752–70.
28. Yusuf S, Hawken S, Ounpuu S, et al. Obesity and the risk of myocardial infarction in 27,000 participants from 52 countries: a case-control study. Lancet 2005; 366(9497):1640–9.
29. Jensen MD, Ryan DH, Apovian CM, et al. 2013 AHA/ACC/TOS guideline for the management of overweight and obesity in adults: a report of the American College of Cardiology/American Heart Association Task Force on Practice Guidelines and The Obesity Society. Circulation 2014;129(25 Suppl 2):S102–38.
30. Zomer E, Gurusamy K, Leach R, et al. Interventions that cause weight loss and the impact on cardiovascular risk factors: a systematic review and meta-analysis. Obes Rev 2016;17(10):1001–11.
31. Hasan B, Nayfeh T, Alzuabi M, et al. Weight loss and serum lipids in overweight and obese adults: a systematic review and meta-analysis. J Clin Endocrinol Metab 2020;105(12):dgaa673.
32. Dattilo AM, Kris-Etherton PM. Effects of weight reduction on blood lipids and lipoproteins: a meta-analysis. Am J Clin Nutr 1992;56(2):320–8.
33. Wadden TA, Anderson DA, Foster GD. Two-year changes in lipids and lipoproteins associated with the maintenance of a 5% to 10% reduction in initial weight: some findings and some questions. Obes Res 1999;7(2):170–8.
34. Won KB, Hur SH, Nam CW, et al. Evaluation of the impact of statin therapy on the obesity paradox in patients with acute myocardial infarction: a propensity score matching analysis from the Korea acute myocardial infarction registry. Medicine (Baltimore) 2017;96(35):e7180.
35. Nicholls SJ, Tuzcu EM, Sipahi I, et al. Effects of obesity on lipid-lowering, anti-inflammatory, and antiatherosclerotic benefits of atorvastatin or pravastatin in patients with coronary artery disease (from the REVERSAL Study). Am J Cardiol 2006;97(11):1553–7.
36. Palmisano BT, Zhu L, Stafford JM. Role of estrogens in the regulation of liver lipid metabolism. Adv Exp Med Biol 2017;1043:227–56.
37. Ghosh M, Galman C, Rudling M, et al. Influence of physiological changes in endogenous estrogen on circulating PCSK9 and LDL cholesterol. J Lipid Res 2015;56(2):463–9.
38. Effects of estrogen or estrogen/progestin regimens on heart disease risk factors in postmenopausal women. The Postmenopausal Estrogen/Progestin

Interventions (PEPI) Trial. The Writing Group for the PEPI Trial. JAMA 1995;273(3): 199–208.

39. Godsland IF. Effects of postmenopausal hormone replacement therapy on lipid, lipoprotein, and apolipoprotein (a) concentrations: analysis of studies published from 1974-2000. Fertil Steril 2001;75(5):898–915.

40. Tetsche MS, Jacobsen J, Norgaard M, et al. Postmenopausal hormone replacement therapy and risk of acute pancreatitis: a population-based case-control study. Am J Gastroenterol 2007;102(2):275–8.

41. Hulley S, Grady D, Bush T, et al. Randomized trial of estrogen plus progestin for secondary prevention of coronary heart disease in postmenopausal women. Heart and Estrogen/progestin Replacement Study (HERS) Research Group. JAMA 1998;280(7):605–13.

42. Manson JE, Hsia J, Johnson KC, et al. Estrogen plus progestin and the risk of coronary heart disease. N Engl J Med 2003;349(6):523–34.

43. Lubiszewska B, Kruk M, Broda G, et al. The impact of early menopause on risk of coronary artery disease (PREmature Coronary Artery Disease In Women–PRECADIW case-control study). Eur J Prev Cardiol 2012;19(1):95–101.

44. Muka T, Oliver-Williams C, Kunutsor S, et al. Association of age at onset of menopause and time since onset of menopause with cardiovascular outcomes, intermediate vascular traits, and all-cause mortality: a systematic review and meta-analysis. JAMA Cardiol 2016;1(7):767–76.

45. Wellons M, Ouyang P, Schreiner PJ, et al. Early menopause predicts future coronary heart disease and stroke: the Multi-Ethnic Study of Atherosclerosis. Menopause 2012;19(10):1081–7.

46. Zhu D, Chung HF, Dobson AJ, et al. Age at natural menopause and risk of incident cardiovascular disease: a pooled analysis of individual patient data. Lancet Public Health 2019;4(11):e553–64.

47. Herrington DM, Vittinghoff E, Lin F, et al. Statin therapy, cardiovascular events, and total mortality in the Heart and Estrogen/Progestin Replacement Study (HERS). Circulation 2002;105(25):2962–7.

48. Berglind IA, Andersen M, Citarella A, et al. Hormone therapy and risk of cardiovascular outcomes and mortality in women treated with statins. Menopause 2015; 22(4):369–76.

49. Salpeter SR, Walsh JM, Greyber E, et al. Brief report: coronary heart disease events associated with hormone therapy in younger and older women. A meta-analysis. J Gen Intern Med 2006;21(4):363–6.

50. Legro RS, Kunselman AR, Dunaif A. Prevalence and predictors of dyslipidemia in women with polycystic ovary syndrome. Am J Med 2001;111(8):607–13.

51. Berneis K, Rizzo M, Lazzarini V, et al. Atherogenic lipoprotein phenotype and low-density lipoproteins size and subclasses in women with polycystic ovary syndrome. J Clin Endocrinol Metab 2007;92(1):186–9.

52. Berneis K, Rizzo M, Hersberger M, et al. Atherogenic forms of dyslipidaemia in women with polycystic ovary syndrome. Int J Clin Pract 2009;63(1):56–62.

53. Rizzo M, Berneis K, Hersberger M, et al. Milder forms of atherogenic dyslipidemia in ovulatory versus anovulatory polycystic ovary syndrome phenotype. Hum Reprod 2009;24(9):2286–92.

54. Enkhmaa B, Anuurad E, Zhang W, et al. Lipoprotein(a) and apolipoprotein(a) in polycystic ovary syndrome. Clin Endocrinol (Oxf) 2016;84(2):229–35.

55. Kim JJ, Chae SJ, Choi YM, et al. Atherogenic changes in low-density lipoprotein particle profiles were not observed in non-obese women with polycystic ovary syndrome. Hum Reprod 2013;28(5):1354–60.

56. Fauser BC, Tarlatzis BC, Rebar RW, et al. Consensus on women's health aspects of polycystic ovary syndrome (PCOS): the Amsterdam ESHRE/ASRM-Sponsored 3rd PCOS Consensus Workshop Group. Fertil Steril 2012;97(1):28–38.e25.

57. Moran LJ, Hutchison SK, Norman RJ, et al. Lifestyle changes in women with polycystic ovary syndrome. Cochrane Database Syst Rev 2011;(7):CD007506.

58. Haqq L, McFarlane J, Dieberg G, et al. The effect of lifestyle intervention on body composition, glycemic control, and cardiorespiratory fitness in polycystic ovarian syndrome: a systematic review and meta-analysis. Int J Sport Nutr Exerc Metab 2015;25(6):533–40.

59. Wang A, Mo T, Li Q, et al. The effectiveness of metformin, oral contraceptives, and lifestyle modification in improving the metabolism of overweight women with polycystic ovary syndrome: a network meta-analysis. Endocrine 2019; 64(2):220–32.

60. Zhao H, Xing C, Zhang J, et al. Comparative efficacy of oral insulin sensitizers metformin, thiazolidinediones, inositol, and berberine in improving endocrine and metabolic profiles in women with PCOS: a network meta-analysis. Reprod Health 2021;18(1):171.

61. Liu Y, Shao Y, Xie J, et al. The efficacy and safety of metformin combined with simvastatin in the treatment of polycystic ovary syndrome: a meta-analysis and systematic review. Medicine (Baltimore) 2021;100(31):e26622.

62. Herink M, Ito MK. Medication induced changes in lipid and lipoproteins. In: Feingold KR, Anawalt B, Boyce A, et al, editors. Endotext. 2000.

63. Banaszewska B, Pawelczyk L, Spaczynski RZ, et al. Effects of simvastatin and oral contraceptive agent on polycystic ovary syndrome: prospective, randomized, crossover trial. J Clin Endocrinol Metab 2007;92(2):456–61.

64. Puurunen J, Piltonen T, Puukka K, et al. Statin therapy worsens insulin sensitivity in women with polycystic ovary syndrome (PCOS): a prospective, randomized, double-blind, placebo-controlled study. J Clin Endocrinol Metab 2013;98(12): 4798–807.

65. Raja-Khan N, Kunselman AR, Hogeman CS, et al. Effects of atorvastatin on vascular function, inflammation, and androgens in women with polycystic ovary syndrome: a double-blind, randomized, placebo-controlled trial. Fertil Steril 2011;95(5):1849–52.

66. Raval AD, Hunter T, Stuckey B, et al. Statins for women with polycystic ovary syndrome not actively trying to conceive. Cochrane Database Syst Rev 2011;(10):CD008565.

67. Sathyapalan T, Kilpatrick ES, Coady AM, et al. The effect of atorvastatin in patients with polycystic ovary syndrome: a randomized double-blind placebo-controlled study. J Clin Endocrinol Metab 2009;94(1):103–8.

68. Feingold KR, Brinton EA, Grunfeld C. The effect of endocrine disorders on lipids and lipoproteins. In: Feingold KR, Anawalt B, Boyce A, et al, editors. Endotext. 2000.

69. Huo S, Scialli AR, McGarvey S, et al. Treatment of men for "low testosterone": a systematic review. PLoS One 2016;11(9):e0162480.

70. Pizzocaro A, Vena W, Condorelli R, et al. Testosterone treatment in male patients with Klinefelter syndrome: a systematic review and meta-analysis. J Endocrinol Invest 2020;43(12):1675–87.

71. Kuipers H, Wijnen JA, Hartgens F, et al. Influence of anabolic steroids on body composition, blood pressure, lipid profile and liver functions in body builders. Int J Sports Med 1991;12(4):413–8.

72. Hartgens F, Rietjens G, Keizer HA, et al. Effects of androgenic-anabolic steroids on apolipoproteins and lipoprotein (a). Br J Sports Med 2004;38(3):253–9.

73. Corona G, Rastrelli G, Di Pasquale G, et al. Endogenous testosterone levels and cardiovascular risk: meta-analysis of observational studies. J Sex Med 2018; 15(9):1260–71.

74. Corona G, Rastrelli G, Di Pasquale G, et al. Testosterone and cardiovascular risk: meta-analysis of interventional studies. J Sex Med 2018;15(6):820–38.

75. Velho I, Fighera TM, Ziegelmann PK, et al. Effects of testosterone therapy on BMI, blood pressure, and laboratory profile of transgender men: a systematic review. Andrology 2017;5(5):881–8.

76. Irwig MS. Testosterone therapy for transgender men. Lancet Diabetes Endocrinol 2017;5(4):301–11.

77. Maraka S, Singh Ospina N, Rodriguez-Gutierrez R, et al. Sex steroids and cardio-vascular outcomes in transgender individuals: a systematic review and meta-analysis. J Clin Endocrinol Metab 2017;102(11):3914–23.

78. Abdu TA, Neary R, Elhadd TA, et al. Coronary risk in growth hormone deficient hypopituitary adults: increased predicted risk is due largely to lipid profile abnor-malities. Clin Endocrinol (Oxf) 2001;55(2):209–16.

79. Beshyah SA, Johnston DG. Cardiovascular disease and risk factors in adults with hypopituitarism. Clin Endocrinol (Oxf) 1999;50(1):1–15.

80. de Boer H, Blok GJ, Van der Veen EA. Clinical aspects of growth hormone defi-ciency in adults. Endocr Rev 1995;16(1):63–86.

81. Takeda R, Tatami R, Ueda K, et al. The incidence and pathogenesis of hyperlipi-daemia in 16 consecutive acromegalic patients. Acta Endocrinol (Copenh) 1982; 100(3):358–62.

82. Beentjes JA, van Tol A, Sluiter WJ, et al. Low plasma lecithin:cholesterol acyl-transferase and lipid transfer protein activities in growth hormone deficient and acromegalic men: role in altered high density lipoproteins. Atherosclerosis 2000;153(2):491–8.

83. Tan KC, Shiu SW, Janus ED, et al. LDL subfractions in acromegaly: relation to growth hormone and insulin-like growth factor-I. Atherosclerosis 1997;129(1): 59–65.

84. Rudling M, Parini P, Angelin B. Effects of growth hormone on hepatic cholesterol metabolism. Lessons from studies in rats and humans. Growth Horm IGF Res 1999;9(Suppl A):1–7.

85. Persson L, Cao G, Stahle L, et al. Circulating proprotein convertase subtilisin kexin type 9 has a diurnal rhythm synchronous with cholesterol synthesis and is reduced by fasting in humans. Arterioscler Thromb Vasc Biol 2010;30(12): 2666–72.

86. Nielsen EH, Lindholm J, Laurberg P. Excess mortality in women with pituitary dis-ease: a meta-analysis. Clin Endocrinol (Oxf) 2007;67(5):693–7.

87. Pappachan JM, Raskauskiene D, Kutty VR, et al. Excess mortality associated with hypopituitarism in adults: a meta-analysis of observational studies. J Clin En-docrinol Metab 2015;100(4):1405–11.

88. Rosen T, Bengtsson BA. Premature mortality due to cardiovascular disease in hy-popituitarism. Lancet 1990;336(8710):285–8.

89. Deepak D, Daousi C, Javadpour M, et al. The influence of growth hormone replacement on peripheral inflammatory and cardiovascular risk markers in adults with severe growth hormone deficiency. Growth Horm IGF Res 2010; 20(3):220–5.

90. Maison P, Griffin S, Nicoue-Beglah M, et al. Impact of growth hormone (GH) treatment on cardiovascular risk factors in GH-deficient adults: a metaanalysis of blinded, randomized, placebo-controlled trials. J Clin Endocrinol Metab 2004; 89(5):2192–9.
91. Newman CB, Carmichael JD, Kleinberg DL. Effects of low dose versus high dose human growth hormone on body composition and lipids in adults with GH deficiency: a meta-analysis of placebo-controlled randomized trials. Pituitary 2015; 18(3):297–305.
92. van Bunderen CC, van Nieuwpoort IC, Arwert LI, et al. Does growth hormone replacement therapy reduce mortality in adults with growth hormone deficiency? Data from the Dutch National Registry of Growth Hormone Treatment in adults. J Clin Endocrinol Metab 2011;96(10):3151–9.

Role of Lipid Management in Women's Health Preventive Care

Pardis Hosseinzadeh, MD, Robert Wild, MD, MPH, PhD*

KEYWORDS

• Women's health • Lipids • Dyslipidemia • Hypertriglyceridemia

KEY POINTS

- Understanding opportunities to diagnose and manage dyslipidemia across a woman's life span has major implications for cardiovascular disease risk prevention for the entire population.
- Obstetricians/gynecologists are uniquely positioned to raise awareness on the early diagnose and management of dyslipidemias and thus impact the overall health of the women they care for throughout different stages in life.
- Contraceptives can impact one's lipid profile and care should be taken when counseling for different options regarding baseline comorbidities, including the dyslipidemias.

INTRODUCTION

Dyslipidemia and its sequelae such as atherosclerosis can affect a woman throughout her life and lead to long-term comorbidities for both the mother and the child.[1] Many women rely only on their obstetrician/gynecologists (OB/GYN) for primary care during their reproductive ages. Acknowledging the principle that lipid awareness is critical throughout the life of the individual is therefore paramount for OB/GYNs. This article aims to discuss some unique women's health issues that are important in lipid management because of the epidemic of the metabolic syndrome and obesity in our society. Practitioners caring for women of reproductive age are ideally placed to help decrease atherosclerosis development for the entire population by screening for and managing abnormal lipid levels during gestation.[1]

Atherosclerotic cardiovascular disease (ASCVD), which increases with age, is caused by multiple interrelating factors such as hypertension, diabetes mellitus, dyslipidemia, and obesity. Some of these factors relate to one's lifestyle and are

This article originally appeared in *Obstetrics and Gynecology Clinics*, Volume 48 Issue 1, March 2021.

Section of Reproductive Endocrinology and Infertility, Department of Obstetrics and Gynecology, University of Oklahoma Health and Sciences Center, 800 Stanton L. Young Boulevard, Suite 2000, Oklahoma City, OK 73104, USA
* Corresponding author.
E-mail address: robert-wild@ouhsc.edu

considered modifiable; others are nonmodifiable. We now know that 90% of women have at least 1 risk factor for developing heart disease, although ASCVD is recognized an average of 10 years later than for their same age male counterparts. This factor has led to an inadvertent decreased emphasis on atherosclerosis prevention for women. Given that dyslipidemia imparts the highest population-adjusted cardiovascular risk for women at 47%, a working knowledge of issues important for managing dyslipidemia is essential for OB/GYNs who serve as the primary care provider for majority of women of childbearing age.[2] Recognition of high-risk areas and how lipids are affected by major reproductive events affecting women's health should be areas of high priority.

Understanding the opportunities to decrease dyslipidemia before, during, and after pregnancy has major implication for ASCVD risk prevention for the entire population. Understanding how contraceptive and hormone choices affect clinical lipid management for women is essential.

PREGNANCY
Alterations of Lipid Values in Pregnancy

As pregnancy progresses, lipids levels steadily increase during the pregnancy with a noticeable increase in the third trimester.[3] This lipid metabolism throughout pregnancy allows for proper nutrients for the fetus. The natural increase reflects the increasing insulin resistance for the mother as pregnancy progresses through term. Total cholesterol (TC), low-density lipoprotein cholesterol (LDL-C), high-density lipoprotein cholesterol (HDL-C), and triglycerides (TG) average values have been measured in normal women followed before, during, and after pregnancy in a large cohort of women proceeding through normal pregnancy and delivery (**Fig. 1**).[4] Most of the women are of young reproductive age and as such their values before pregnancy are in the normal range for nonpregnant women.

Understanding lipids alteration pattern throughout pregnancy and postpartum is essential. As depicted in **Fig. 1**, there may be a decrease in levels in the first 8 weeks of gestation and then a noticeable increase discerned by the end of the first trimester. There begins a steady increase throughout pregnancy in the major lipoprotein lipids. By the third trimester, levels peak to maximize near term.[4] It is important to note that

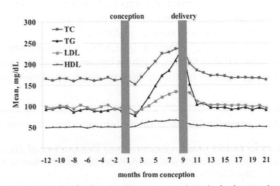

Fig. 1. TC, triglycerides (TG), high-density lipoprotein (HDL) cholesterol, and low-density lipoprotein (LDL) cholesterol 1 year before, during, and after pregnancy. (*From* Wiznitzer A, Mayer A, Novack V, et al. Association of lipid levels during gestation with preeclampsia and gestational diabetes mellitus: a population-based study. Am J Obstet Gynecol 2009;201(5):482.e1–8; with permission.)

the values in this population do not exceed 250 mg/dL at any time during pregnancy. TC seems to return to prepregnancy levels within 1 year,[5] and in some populations these peak values are lower (Chinese). Levels of HDL-C decrease postpartum and remains lower than prepregnancy for multiple years. With less consistent evidence TG can remain elevated.[5] TG levels decrease rapidly in the postpartum period, whereas LDL levels remain elevated for at least 6 to 7 weeks.[6] Postpartum factors can also influence this return. Lactation is associated with an earlier or more complete return.[7]

The sequential average fasting lipid and lipoproteins measured in the different population is shown in **Fig. 2**. **Fig. 2** illustrates mean lipid levels also; however, these measurements also include persons with pregnancy complications. Likewise, TG and TC increase to term; however, values exceed 300 mg/dL[6]. There is also a significant increase in TG content in all circulating lipoprotein fractions during pregnancy.[3]

Fig. 3 shows the first trimester maternal TG in relationship to pregnancy complications. TG levels exceeding 250 mg/dL are associated with pregnancy-induced hypertension, preeclampsia, gestational diabetes, and large for gestational age babies.[8]

Screening for Dyslipidemia in Pregnancy

The prevalence of dyslipidemia during pregnancy varies significantly depending on which criteria are used; however, it is higher with comorbidities.[9] Many women have out of normal range undiscovered dyslipidemia before pregnancy. The early identification of any woman at risk for severe gestational hypertriglyceridemia is essential. Ideally, this process happens at the preconception counseling visit or soon after pregnancy diagnosis.

Women with a history of pancreatitis or abdominal pain associated with prior estrogen use and those with a family history of hypertriglyceridemia are at risk during pregnancy. Individuals with known hypertriglyceridemia should have their TG levels monitored during pregnancy. Signs suggestive of hypertriglyceridemia include eruptive xanthomata skin lesions, lipemia retinalis, and hepatosplenomegaly. Not all patients with severe hypertriglyceridemia have these signs, however. The dyslipidemia is often associated with other health conditions, making that woman at risk for obstetric and fetal complications. These include uncontrolled diabetes mellitus, polycystic ovarian syndrome (PCOS), and genetic lipid disorders. These put the mother at risk for problems, they put her offspring at risk, and possibly put future generations at

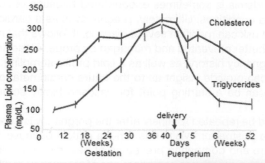

Fig. 2. Pregnancy, lipids, and lipoproteins. Fasting lipids were measured serially throughout pregnancy, at delivery, and in the puerperium and at 12 months. Results are standard error of the mean and include normal and complicated pregnancies. (*Adapted from* Potter JM, Nestel PJ. The hyperlipidemia of pregnancy in normal and complicated pregnancies. Am J Obstet Gynecol 1979;133(2):165–70; with permission.)

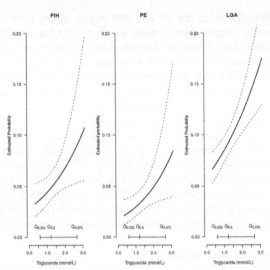

Fig. 3. First trimester maternal TG relationships. The estimated probability of PIH, preeclampsia, and LGA. TG levels in the first trimester of pregnancy are a significant, but modest, contributor in the expression of PIH, PE, induced preterm birth, and children to be born large for gestational age. With this observation, inclusion of a lipid profile may be considered in early pregnancy and in the preconception screening. 1 mmol/L of TG = 135 mg/dL; 2 mmol/L of TG = 176 mg/dL. Q0.025, Q0.5, and Q0.875 represent the 2.5th, 50th, and 97.5th percentiles of the studied population. PIH, pregnancy induced hypertension; PE, preeclampsia; LGA, large for gestational age. (*Adapted from* Vrijkotte TG, Krukziener N, Hutten BA, et al. Maternal lipid profile during early pregnancy and pregnancy complications and outcomes: the ABCD study. J Clin Endocrinol Metab 2012;97(11):3917–25; with permission.)

risk. High levels of maternal TC and/or TG are associated with preterm birth,[10] pregnancy-induced hypertension,[11] and large for gestational age.[12] Conversely, decreased levels of TC during pregnancy are associated with preterm birth,[13] with a greater risk for a small for gestational age fetus.[10] Familial hyperlipidemia (FH) is more common than any of the genetic diseases routinely screened for in pregnancy,[14] yet there are currently no obstetrician recommendations in place to screen for FH. Severe hypertriglyceridemia is sometimes encountered because of screening for other genetic or acquired conditions. Ultimately, pregnancy is as a cardiometabolic stress test where those at risk can manifest severe disease. It follows that maternal and fetal complications are better prevented and managed by proper screening with a detailed metabolic and pregnancy history, as well as a lipid profile sampling. A careful cardiometabolic history can provide insight as to the future cardiometabolic risk of mother and child. It also can be a starting point for cascade family screening initiated by the OB/GYN.

Screening should be repeated routinely after the pregnancy is concluded, usually at the 6-week routine postpartum visit. This time is critical because of transitioning in provider health care and competing pressures of new mothers, who can be lost to follow-up. Women who experience complications of pregnancy or who gain excessive weight before or during pregnancy likely have abnormal cardiometabolic profiles.[15] In patients whose primary provider changes, continuity plans with attention to a long-term assessment of hyperlipidemia during the extended puerperal period and beyond is prudent. Attention to and avoiding this gap can go a long way in preventing disease.

Hypertriglyceridemia in Pregnancy

The differential diagnosis of hypertriglyceridemia in pregnancy is the same as in a nonpregnant woman, with the exception that OB/GYNs need to be aware of obstetric complications associated with hypertriglyceridemia. The evaluation of hypertriglyceridemia is as in nonpregnant women, with the realization that there is an expected 2- to 3-fold TG level increase by the third trimester. Women diagnosed with gestational diabetes and/or preeclampsia often have abnormal TG levels greater and additive to their persistent hypertriglyceridemia before the pregnancy. In the United States, the average values in persons with these disorders can exceed 300 mg/dL and levels escalate as pregnancy progresses. Hypertriglyceridemia at the end of gestation is associated with the development of dyslipidemia in the postpartum period, and there is a greater risk of the child being large for gestational age[16] and at risk of greater atherosclerosis burden going in to in adult life.[17] The most common etiology for hypertriglyceridemia is poorly controlled or undiscovered diabetes mellitus. Other etiologies include medications that aggravate TG metabolism, psychiatric and/or human immunodeficiency virus medications, illicit drugs, and/or alcohol. Undiagnosed hypothyroidism and/or genetic dyslipidemias lead to hyperlipidemia in pregnancy.

In summary, women with hypertriglyceridemia need a careful analysis of family history for hypertriglyceridemia, pancreatitis, diabetes, hypertension, smoking status, cardiometabolic disease, illicit drugs, or dietary carbohydrate and alcohol intake, as well as the use of prescription medicines and/or supplements. Glycemic, thyroid, hepatic, and renal evaluations are also indicated.

Management of Dyslipidemia Associated with Pregnancy

For women with a diagnosis of dyslipidemia before pregnancy, any lipid level-lowering medications aside from bile acid sequestrates or omega-3 fatty acids should be stopped. Recommendations for the best time to stop statins range from 3 months to 1 month before conception. When an unplanned pregnancy occurs, statins should be stopped immediately when the pregnancy is discovered. These recommendations are based on expert opinion alone, without definitive evidence. Statins have been used in animal models of preeclampsia to revert the angiogenic imbalance, a hallmark of preeclampsia, and restore endothelial dysfunction. This biological plausibility and data from preclinical animal studies support a role for statins in preeclampsia prevention.[18] A recent randomized controlled trial, provides preliminary safety and pharmacokinetic data regarding the use of pravastatin for preventing preeclampsia in high-risk pregnant women. They reported no identifiable safety risks associated with pravastatin use in this cohort.[19]

Despite this finding, and because of animal data that found that very high doses of lipophilic statins caused birth defects, the US Food and Drug Administration (FDA) historically categorized stains as pregnancy category X. **Table 1** provides the pregnancy classification of widely used lipid level-lowering agents. This classification is no longer advised by the FDA, conceding that the potential risk of harm and possible benefits should always be considered. Most cardiologists advise against their use because of unknowns and potential liability.

Unfortunately, despite the known benefits of many antihyperlipidemic therapies on atherogenic lipid profiles and clinical outcomes, there is a paucity of studies that have been performed in pregnancy. In fact, pregnant women are routinely excluded from clinical trials. As a result, recommendations on the treatment of significant dyslipidemia in pregnant women are limited.

Table 1	
Historical FDA classification of lipid level-lowering agents and pregnancy classification	
Lipid Level-Lowering Agent	Pregnancy Class
Statins	X
Fibrates	C
Ezetimibe	C
Niacin	C
Cholestyramine	C
Colesevelam	B

Dyslipidemia discovered during pregnancy should be treated with a diet and exercise intervention, as well as glycemic control when associated with diabetes types 1 and 2. Common agents used are glyburide and metformin as well as insulin to control blood glucose. Omega-3 fatty acids are frequently used and are thought to be safe in pregnancy as monotherapy to decrease maternal TG levels. Hypercholesterolemia can be treated with bile acid sequestrates; notably, colesevelam is in pregnancy category B.

Severe hypertriglyceridemia (including at levels associated with pancreatitis) can be treated with omega-3 fatty acids, parenteral nutrition, plasmapheresis, or historically with gemfibrozil in the mid to late trimesters (pregnancy class C medication).[20] It is recommended that lipids be monitored every trimester or within 6 weeks of an intervention to evaluate for compliance, response, and dose adjustment if needed. Close postpartum follow-up of mothers and children with FH or dysmetabolic issues of pregnancy is required. States of severe hypertriglyceridemia, hypertension of pregnancy, preeclampsia, gestational diabetes, and/or albuminuria need to be evaluated for residual cardiometabolic risk.

Familial Hyperlipidemia and Pregnancy

Cholesterol levels increase in pregnancy, with a similar percentage increase in normal women and those with heterozygous FH. Women with FH do not seem to have a higher risk of preterm delivery or to have low birth weight infants or infants with congenital malformation (undetected bias cannot be ruled out).[21] An experienced lipid specialist should be consulted for women with homozygous FH whose care is beyond the OB/GYN scope of practice. Because TG levels increase progressively with each trimester, women with TG levels of 500 mg/dL or greater at the onset of pregnancy may develop severe hypertriglyceridemia during the third trimester, leading to pancreatitis.[22]

A complete lipid profile assessment during each trimester of pregnancy is recommended. For women with FH, following brain natriuretic peptide, or B-type natriuretic peptide, as a useful monitor for potential coronary ischemia has been suggested.[23] FH can be treated with lifestyle interventions, bile acid sequestrants, and monitoring of potential TG level increases in response. If adequate control is not obtained with these regimens, Colesevelam (pregnancy class B medication), and/or LDL apheresis may be necessary.[24] Given the complex nature of treatment in such cases, patients with FH are best followed in tertiary care centers in a multidisciplinary approach setting with experienced OB/GYNs, endocrinologists, and a cardiologists involved.

Dyslipidemia and Breastfeeding

Lactation may attenuate unfavorable metabolic risk factor changes that occur with pregnancy, with effects of masking apparent after weaning. As a modifiable behavior, lactation may affect women's future risk of cardiovascular and metabolic diseases.[25] For disorders with high TG levels, it is advisable to avoid estrogenic oral contraception, even with late breastfeeding. However, breastfeeding does not guarantee lactational anovulation and thereby contraception. Approximately 1 in 3 women ovulate during prolonged breast feeding, highlighting the need to advise patients regarding the best contraceptives despite breastfeeding. Diet, nutritional consultation, and regular exercise should be considered for patients affected with dyslipidemia during and after the pregnancy.

Long-Term Implications of Complications in Pregnancy

Several conditions specific to women (eg, hypertensive disorders during pregnancy, preeclampsia, gestational diabetes mellitus, delivering a preterm or low birth weight infant)[26,27] have been shown to increase ASCVD risk. Contributions of dyslipidemia, obesity, the presence of the metabolic syndrome, or insulin resistance states before pregnancy[28,29] also host important future ASCVD risk scenarios. The accumulated weight gain during successive pregnancies and the inability to effect adequate weight loss during middle age are well-known risk factors for ASCVD.[30] The increase in lipid components during pregnancy, notably TG and their metabolically dangerous atherogenic particle metabolites, may not be corrected postpartum. Thus, after pregnancy and throughout the life course of every woman, a thorough pregnancy history should be obtained, and risk factors and risk-enhancing factors should be identified. Interventions should include aggressive lifestyle counseling to decrease ASCVD risk and, when appropriate, statin therapy, if ASCVD risk estimation indicates that the potential for benefit from statin therapy outweighs the potential for adverse effects.

POLYCYSTIC OVARIAN SYNDROME

PCOS is the most common endocrine disorder among women of reproductive age. Depending on the population and diagnostic criteria used, PCOS affects between 4% and 19% of reproductive-aged women.[31] Women with PCOS are at an increased risk for the metabolic syndrome, diabetes mellitus, complications of pregnancy, and endometrial cancer.[29] Most individuals with PCOS show insulin resistance, which is intensified by obesity and often the pregnant state, potentially leading to attendant complications. In addition, women with PCOS are at greater risk for obstetric complications irrespective of whether they have developed overt metabolic syndrome. Lipid abnormalities are found in women affected by PCOS. A recent study showed that mild hypercholesterolemia is frequently encountered in women with PCOS.[32] Different lipid patterns have been shown to be present in PCOS, including low levels of HDL; high TG, TC, and LDL-C; and significantly higher lipoprotein concentrations.[33] Concomitantly, the HDL-C level is often decreased, TG production increases, and circulating atherogenic small LDL particles increase, all of which are further aggravated if women with PCOS are obese.

Women with PCOS frequently develop dyslipidemia and/or the metabolic syndrome at any age, including at the onset of menses and continuing throughout the adolescent years. The standard medication used to control menses, to decrease endometrial and ovarian cancer risk, and to decrease hirsutism is the combined oral contraceptive (COC).

Depending on which COC is chosen for which clinical manifestation of PCOS, TG levels may increase, HDL-C levels may increase, and LDL-C levels may decrease when COCs are given to women with PCOS who have associated dyslipidemia.

Rarely, a genetic lipid disorder is uncovered when screening for dyslipidemia in women with PCOS. Very high TG levels (ie, >500 mg/dL) are rarely caused by PCOS alone. Using an oral contraceptive can further aggravate hypertriglyceridemia of this magnitude and can precipitate pancreatitis.

Screening for Associated Dyslipidemia in Polycystic Ovarian Syndrome

We recommend that all patients with PCOS, regardless of age, undergo lipid and diabetes screening given the increased prevalence of dyslipidemia and insulin resistance in this population.[18,34] We also recommend an increased frequency of monitoring for such clinical changes compared with the general population, even if the initial values are normal, because the risk of developing these conditions increases with age. Some experts have suggested 2-year screening intervals. Given that normalizing dyslipidemia and glucose intolerance can decrease atherogenesis, OB/GYNs need to be familiar with the principles of management for such conditions throughout the reproductive period. We recommend similar, if not tighter, lipid level goals in dyslipidemia as those used in the metabolic syndrome. The Androgen Excess Society consensus document recommends the target values. These values have been updated according to the American Association of Clinical Endocrinologists and the American College of Endocrinology **Table 2**. Lipid management of women with PCOS (ref#59).

Treatment of Dyslipidemia in Polycystic Ovarian Syndrome

Diet and exercise are the foundations of intervention. The available evidence suggests that lifestyle interventions (diet, exercise, and behavioral interventions) are more effective than minimal treatment for weight loss and for improving insulin resistance and

Table 2
PCOS risk categories and lipid target values

	Risk	LDL Target Values, mg/dL (mmol/L)[a]	Non-HDL Target Values, mg/dL (mmol/L)[a]
PCOS	At optimal	≤100 (2.59)	≤130 (3.37)
PCOS (obesity, hypertension, dyslipidemia, cigarette smoking, IGT, subvascular disease)	At risk	≤100 (2.59)	≤100 (2.59)
PCOS with MetS	High risk	≤100 (2.59)	≤130 (3.37)
PCOS[b] with MetS and T2DM, overt renal disease, or other vascular disease	—	≤70 (1.81)	≤100 (2.59)

Values are based on a 12-hour fast. For secondary prevention post events LDL targets are less than 55 mg/dL.

Abbreviations: IGT, impaired glucose tolerance; MetS, metabolic syndrome; T2DM, type 2 diabetes mellitus.

[a] To convert mg/dL to mmol/L, divide by 39.

[b] Odds for CVD increase with number of MetS components and with other risk factors, smoking, poor diet, inactivity, obesity, family history of premature CVD (men <55 years old or women <65 years old), and subclinical vascular disease.

Adapted from Wild RA, Carmina E, Diamanti-Kandarakis E, et al. Assessment of cardiovascular risk and prevention of cardiovascular disease in women with the polycystic ovary syndrome: a consensus statement by the Androgen Excess and Polycystic Ovary Syndrome (AE-PCOS) Society. J Clin Endocrinol Metab 2010;95(5);2038–49; with permission.

dyslipidemia.[35] The use of medication to control lipids has special considerations for women with PCOS. Therapy should be focused on reversing all components of the metabolic syndrome through diet, exercise, and medication only if needed.[36]

In general, metformin is widely used because of its low cost, long-term safety data, and low side effect profile. However, treatment of type 2 diabetes mellitus is the only approved indication for metformin. Nevertheless, it has been used off-label to treat or prevent several clinical problems associated with PCOS, including oligomenorrhea, hirsutism, anovulatory infertility, prevention of pregnancy complications, and obesity.[37] However, available data do not support the use of metformin for the treatment of hirsutism or as a first-line treatment for ovulation induction, oligomenorrhea, and many other features of PCOS, except insulin resistance. Data regarding the effect of metformin on dyslipidemia are controversial and it has been suggested to improve the lipid profile through an increase in LDL-C and decreased weight, waist circumference, and blood pressure in patients with PCOS.[38] Metformin is not considered as a first-line therapy for dyslipidemia in women with PCOS. Numerous medications have been used for PCOS, including weight loss medications (as of this writing, 8 have been FDA approved). Glucagon-like peptide 1 receptor agonists, sodium glucose cotransporter inhibitors, which have a glucosuria effect that results in a decreased hemoglobin A1C, weight, and systolic blood pressure have been used in women with PCOS with significant comorbidities. Dipeptidyl peptidase 4 inhibitors exert anti hyperglycemic effects by inhibiting dipeptidyl peptidase 4 to enhance glucagon-like peptide 1 and other incretin hormones. They are weight neutral, have modest hemoglobin A1C–lowering effects, and are available in combinations with metformin, a sodium glucose cotransporter inhibitor, and thiazolidinediones. Pioglitazone has been used in PCOS; however, weight gain, bone fracture risk in postmenopausal women, and an increased risk of chronic edema and heart failure have limited the use of all thiazolidinediones. Of the numerous diet interventions available, Heart Healthy, Mediterranean, and the Dietary Approaches to Stop Hypertension diets have shown short-term improved lipid and other biomarker effects for women with PCOS.[39] High carbohydrate diets tend to aggravate insulin resistance and severely restricting low carbohydrate diets acutely offer weight loss; however, this is not sustainable with long-term lipid reduction and normalization. Weight loss should be targeted in all overweight women with PCOS by decreasing caloric intake in the setting of adequate nutritional intake and healthy food choices, irrespective of diet composition.[40] There is no perfect diet for all patients and national nutritional guidelines should be followed to encourage diets that work for a given individual.

Statins are an ideal choice to treat elevated LDL-C and are the most important primary and secondary prevention medications for cardiovascular diseases (CVD). Statins are used in women with PCOS to treat their metabolic syndrome as well as to decrease testosterone and androstenedione levels. Statins decrease LDL-C and non–HDL-C levels. In 1 clinical trial, atorvastatin therapy improved chronic inflammation and the lipid profile and also decreased the testosterone level in women with PCOS.[41] However, statins impair insulin sensitivity.[42] Because women with PCOS are at an increased risk of developing type 2 diabetes mellitus, statin therapy should be initiated from the generally accepted American Health association or American college of Cardiology or National Lipid Association guidelines, criteria after individual risk assessment of ASCVD risk, and not solely in the setting of a diagnosis of PCOS.[43]

Among the statins, atorvastatin, simvastatin, and lovastatin are the most commonly used statins and can inhibit DNA synthesis and growth of follicular mesenchymal cells. Other statins have a lower risk of minor side effects and are commonly substituted. Simvastatin has been shown to improve menstrual cyclicity and to decrease hirsutism, acne, and ovarian volume. The decrease in ovarian volume likely occurs in parallel with a decrease reduction in the number of theca cells, resulting in decreased androgen production.[44] Given the current categorization of statins use in pregnancy owing to concern for teratogenic risk, women who are at risk of becoming pregnant must be counseled extensively[45] as to the need for a reliable form of contraception. Stains can be useful in treating fatty liver, which is common in women with PCOS who have the metabolic syndrome.[46]

Other lipid level-lowering medications used successfully in women with PCOS include. Nicotinic acid, also known as vitamin B_3, is involved in lipid metabolism through the conversion to nicotinamide. Nicotinic acid inhibits hydrolysis, reduces the release of nonesterified fatty acids into the liver, and subsequently decrease the hepatic synthesis and release of very low-density lipoprotein TGs by binding to nicotinic receptors in adipose tissue. Moreover, nicotinic acid can improve the lipid profile by lowering LDL particles and increasing HDL in the serum of PCOS patients as TG are lowered.[47]

CONTRACEPTION

Family planning optimizes pregnancy and maternal outcomes. OB/GYNs must have insight into the effects of contraceptive type on lipid metabolism and the effects of lipid management because of contraceptive choice, keeping in mind the risks associated with being pregnant if contraception is not used.

Most surveys show that approximately 50% of pregnancies are unexpected in the United States.[48] No contraceptive method fits everyone. The risk of complications associated with pregnancy, contraceptive efficacy in preventing pregnancy (which most often carries greater risk to the mother if the contraceptive is not used or fails), as well as the cardiometabolic impact of the method chosen are important considerations.

Screening for lipid levels should be kept up to date, commensurate with childhood, adolescent, and adult guidelines for population screening (see the National Lipid Association guidelines). Special thought must be used to identify persons with FH, hypertriglyceridemia, or rare genetic forms of hyperlipidemia on routine screening and/or family history. A detailed metabolic and pregnancy history provides insight as to the cardiometabolic future risk of the mother and her children.

Lipid Changes with Different Forms of Contraception

Combined oral contraceptives

COCs have multiple tissue effects, including estrogenic, progestational, androgenic, antiestrogenic, and antiandrogenic effects. All forms decrease the risk for endometrial and ovarian cancers. The major risk associated with all COCs is thromboembolic disease. Women with various medical comorbidities including obesity, older age, and tobacco use are at an increased risk for these cardiovascular events. There are 2 types of estrogen (ethinyl-estradiol and mestranol) used in the United States. Various doses of estrogen within COCs are available. Higher estrogen doses carry a greater risk of thromboembolic events. Few 50-mg estrogen-containing pills are available on the market today for this reason. At present, most COCs contain 35 mg of ethinyl-estradiol or less and there are multiple types of progestins used in the COCs currently marketed.

In healthy women, COC use decreases insulin sensitivity, but in general, this decrease is not clinically significant.[49] Evidence for the effects of COCs on insulin sensitivity in women with PCOS is conflicting. Studies have reported improvement,[50] worsening,[51] or no change[52] in insulin sensitivity. Nevertheless, there is no evidence that COC use influences the risk of developing diabetes or affects glycemic control.[53]

COCs can negatively impact lipid and carbohydrate metabolism, but usually not with a clinically meaningful effect size. For certain subgroups, such as those with PCOS, these changes can be significant.[54] The estrogenic effect of COCs increases levels of TGs and HDL-C and decreases levels of LDL-C. Androgenic progestins (such as norgestrel and levonorgestrel) can increase LDL-C levels and decrease HDL-C levels. The progestational effect is lipid neutral. For example, desogestrel, a third-generation COC that uses low-dose norethindrone, decrease LDL-C levels and increases HDL-C levels. In addition, the more overall estrogenic a COC is, the more it seems to increase TG and HDL levels. This effect carries a greater risk of precipitating pancreatitis in scenarios in which baseline TG levels are increased and increase further with estrogenic COC use. Transdermal or vaginal combination contraceptives (estrogenic plus progestin) do not decrease the risk of a thrombotic event compared with COCs. Transdermal estrogenic do not aggravate TG levels.

Intrauterine devices

Persons with known severe hyperlipidemia can be given a progestin-impregnated intrauterine device (level 2 recommendation). Less overall bleeding is noted with this method, but irregular and unpredictable bleeding is common. A nonhormonal option is the copper intrauterine device, which can be used for up to 10 years per device and is a lipid-neutral option. In regards to progestin-only intrauterine devices, randomized comparative studies have shown that this method is safe regarding effects on lipid metabolism, blood pressure, and liver function tests.[55,56]

Progestin only

Oral, implantable, or injectable progestins are widely used, especially for persons at risk of noncompliance. In general, progestin-only methods are lipid neutral. There is some evidence that injectable depo-medroxyprogesterone is associated with weight gain. Weight gain is associated with creating or aggravating a current metabolic syndrome with the associated risks of diabetes and mixed dyslipidemia. Despite this finding, implantable and injectable progestin forms of contraception are extremely efficacious for preventing pregnancy. Newer and older progestin-only oral contraceptives are available and are often used when estrogenic preparations are contraindicated or when the risk/benefit ratio is a concern with a COC. However, progestin-only formulations are associated with increased breakthrough bleeding and decreased contraceptive efficacy.

Permanent Sterilization

Male and female permanent sterilization procedures are widely used and highly effective forms of contraception. Although nonhormonal and thus lipid neutral, permanent sterilization can unfortunately lead to loss of general-care follow-up as patients are no longer seeking medical care for pregnancy. As primary care providers offering such contraceptive options, it is prudent to recognize the importance of continuing screening for ASCVD risk factors.

MENOPAUSE TRANSITION
Lipid Changes During Menopause

With the onset of waning of ovarian function, lipid changes are noticeable on both a population and an individual basis. The changes tend to occur primarily during the later phases of menopause transition. The magnitude of change toward dyslipidemia is like and additive to the changes that occur with aging. The relative odds of having an LDL-C level of 130 mg/dL before to after menopause has been reported to be 2.1 (95% confidence interval, 1.5–2.9).[57]

An increase in serum cholesterol in postmenopausal women is generally considered as result of a decrease in serum estradiol and a decrease in the number of LDL-C receptors. Changes in body fat distribution are also observed during this transitional time.[58]

Fig. 4 shows the natural changes of the major lipid and apolipoprotein lipid levels using cross-sectional panel design analysis as these women transitioned through the menopause years, studied in the multiethnic Study of Women's Health Across the Nation (SWAN) dataset. Note that the levels are assessed and measured as annual mean data comparing years before and after the final menstrual period. Menopause is defined in retrospect as 1 year with no menses during this transition. Day 0 in the graphs is labeled and standardized as the final menstrual period. Importantly, apolipoprotein B levels increase noticeably.

The absolute risk for CVD increases substantially in midlife for women. Rates associated with an adverse effect on lipid metabolism increase at the time of menopause. Those persons with significant risk factors before menopause are additionally affected. A high LDL-C level is a strong predictor of CVD risk in women younger than 65 years and a low HDL-C level is a stronger predictor of CHD mortality in women than in men and particularly so in women 65 years of age and older.[59] In the Framingham Heart Study, the 8-year risk of heart disease was 7% for women with a total/HDL-C ratio of less than 5%, 12% for those with ratios of 5% to 7%, and 20% for those with ratios of greater than 7.[60] It is important for OB/GYNs to identify these individuals early to plan for the best control of these same risk factors during the menopause transition.[57,61]

In addition, there is a link to an increased prevalence of the metabolic syndrome.[62] With expert treatment, it has been shown that carotid atherosclerosis is observed more frequently beginning in the menopause transition, and a significant number of women also possess coronary calcium deposition before this time.[63]

Annual rates of change in carotid intima media thickness and adventitial diameter have been reported, as noted in **Fig. 5**. The rate of change at the late perimenopausal stage significantly differs from that at the premenopausal stage. The rate of change at the late perimenopausal stage significantly differs from that at the early perimenopausal

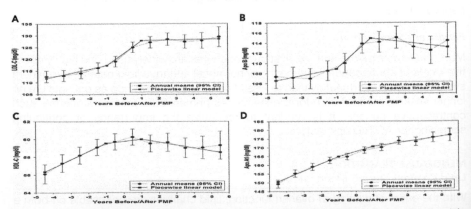

Fig. 4. Lipids annual and estimated means pattern of LDL-C (*A*), apolipoprotein (Apo) B (*B*), HDL-C (*C*), and Apo A-I (*D*) across the SWAN study follow-up period.

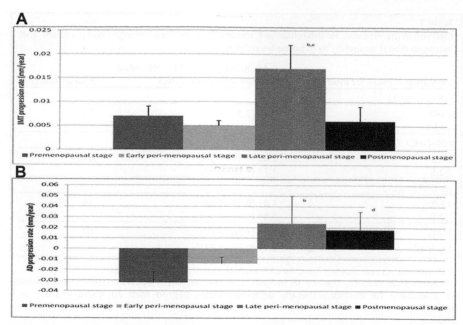

Fig. 5. Annual rates of change in (*A*) carotid intima media thickness (IMT) and (*B*) adventitial diameter (AD). (*From* El Khoudary SR, Wildman RP, Matthews K, et al. Progression rates of carotid intima-media thickness and adventitial diameter during the menopausal transition. Menopause 2013;20(1):8–14; with permission.)

stage. The rate of change at the postmenopausal stage significantly differs from that at the premenopausal stage ($P<.05$).

Considerations for Hormone Replacement Therapy

The hormonal changes of menopause are associated with an increasingly atherogenic lipid profile. This factor provides both an opportunity and a challenge for the aggressive management of dyslipidemia. Menopausal hormone replacement therapy is primarily indicated to control menopause-related quality-of-life issues. Replacement therapy should not be prescribed to reduce cardiovascular events (ie, for prevention or treatment of vascular diseases). Identifying appropriate candidates for menopausal hormone therapy is challenging given the complex profile of risks and benefits associated with treatment.[64,65] Most professional societies agree that hormone therapy should not be used for chronic disease prevention. Note the results from an analysis of the Women's Health Initiative (WHI), in which oral estrogen plus progestin and estrogen alone were used in the randomized clinical trial (**Table 3**). Accordingly, there is a black box warning by the FDA for women with known coronary artery disease, thromboembolic disorders, or who have had a cerebrovascular accident because these preparations carry thrombotic risk and critical events in persons with these disorders involving thrombotic pathophysiology.

The WHI, a 15-year longitudinal study of morbidity and mortality in more than 160,000 healthy, postmenopausal women (average age 63 years at baseline), found a lack of a cardioprotective effect associated with hormone replacement therapy.[66] Although estrogen replacement did decrease LDL-C and increase HDL-C, it also increased TG and small, dense LDL particles, 2 of the 3 components that characterize

Table 3
CHD risk in the Women's Health Initiative hormone therapy trials (estrogen and progestin and estrogen alone) according to baseline levels of biomarkers

Biomarker P Value for Interaction	Odds Ratio (95% CL) for Hormone Therapy Treatment Effect	P for Interaction
LDL-C (mg/dL)		
<130	0.66 (0.34–1.27)	.03
≥130		
LDL-C/HDL-C ratio		
<2.5	0.66 (0.34–1.27)	.002
≥2.5	1.73 (1.18–2.53)	
Hs-CRP (mg/dL)		
<2.0	1.01 (0.63–1.62)	.16
≥2.0	1.58 (1.05–2.39)	
MetS	2.26 (1.26–4.07)	.03
No MetS	0.97 (0.58–1.61)	–

Abbreviations: CL, confidence limit; hs-CRP, high-sensitivity C-reactive protein.
Adapted from Wild RA, Manson JE. Insights from the Women's Health Initiative: individualizing risk assessment for hormone therapy decisions. Semin Reprod Med 2014;32(6):433–37; with permission.

atherogenic dyslipidemia.[67] Based on this, WHI findings are consistent with previous trials in which hormone replacement therapy was not shown to protect against ASCVD or cerebrovascular accident. This analysis suggests that persons at higher risk for CVD events (increased dyslipidemia or the presence of the metabolic syndrome or with a family history of thrombotic disease) are more likely to have this risk aggravated by the administration of oral hormone replacement therapy. Findings from the WHI and other randomized trials suggest that a woman's age, proximity to menopause, underlying cardiovascular risk factor status, and various biological characteristics may modify health outcomes with hormone therapy.

The message is clear: assessing CVD risk before hormone therapy is given for menopausal symptoms is prudent to identify persons who may be at increased adverse event risk with oral hormone therapy.

An emerging body of evidence suggests that it may be possible to assess an individual's risk and, therefore, better predict who is likely to have favorable outcomes versus adverse effects when taking hormone therapy. There are also several biomarkers under study to determine whether they provide incremental risk prediction for CVD in women taking hormone therapy. However, thus far none have been shown to provide added risk prediction and currently they are not recommended for clinical use. Several risk estimators are available to estimate risk, including the Framingham Risk Assessment tool (https://www.framinghamstudy.org/risk-functions/coronary-heart-disease/hard-10-year-risk.php), the Reynold Risk Score, which includes C-reactive protein (https://www.reynold'sriskscore.org), and the Multi-Ethnic Study Atherosclerosis 10-year risk score (https://mesa-nhlbi.org/MESACHDRiks/MesaRiskScore/RiskScore.aspx), which are increasingly validated for women 40 years and older. Many of these estimators are embedded within the electronic medical records systems. Thus, once a woman is identified as a potential candidate for hormone therapy because of moderate to severe menopausal symptoms or other indications, risk stratification may be an important tool for minimizing patient CVD risk factors and for assessing suitability for hormone therapy.[64,65,68]

This individualized approach holds great promise for improving the safety of hormone therapy. A treatment decision to provide symptom relief should be made with a patient's full understanding of the potential risks and benefits, and considering her personal preferences. To better integrate patient values, practical considerations, and emerging clinical experience, recent research from observational studies and randomized clinical trials on hormone therapy should be considered.

Systemic estrogens induce a dose-dependent decrease in TC and LDL-C, as well as an increase in HDL-C concentrations; these effects are more prominent with oral administration. Micronized progesterone or dydrogesterone are the preferred progestogens owing to their neutral effect on the lipid profile. Using the lowest effective dose of hormone therapy is recommended, regardless of the clinical scenario. In general, doses of less than 0.3 mg of oral conjugated estrogen daily do not control hot flashes for most women. However, this dose is protective against bone loss from estrogen deficiency osteopenia.[64] Transdermal rather than oral estrogens should be used in women with hypertriglyceridemia. Delivering the medication transdermally may be associated with fewer adverse events than when given by the oral route.[69] Tissue effects may differ depending on whether there is a first-pass hepatic effect, as is the case with oral estrogen. Ospemifene, an oral selective estrogen receptor modulator, and vaginal dehydroepiandrosterone are both recently FDA approved for the treatment of moderate to severe symptomatic vulvovaginal atrophy in postmenopausal women who are not candidates for vaginal estrogen therapy. Ospemifene exerts a favorable effect on the lipid profile, but data are scant regarding dehydroepiandrosterone.[70]

With vaginal and transdermal preparations, there is less of an effect on clotting factors, lipid metabolism, inflammatory biomarkers, and sex hormone–binding globulin synthesis. Differences in the dose, route, and formulations, in conjunction with genetic metabolic differences, may lead to different outcomes. Observational studies, although limited in number, suggest that transdermal delivery may be associated with a lower risk of venous thromboembolism and stroke than with oral estrogen administration; however, these studies do not prove a cause–effect relationship.[71] Randomized clinical trial evidence is needed to answer this question more definitively.

SUMMARY

Advances in research, technology, and pharmacology increase the options available for women, but this rapidly changing knowledge-based presents a challenge for clinicians. Moreover, the delivery of care for women has been historically fragmented. To overcome this barriers, multidisciplinary curriculums in women's health education have been created. Care for women is optimized by education on a range of medical concerns provided by experts from a wide variety of medical specialties. Given the complexity of care, interdisciplinary approaches are becoming an increasingly important aspect of care by health care providers, with needs that cross many areas of medical expertise.

DISCLOSURE

The authors have nothing to disclose.

REFERENCES

1. de Oliveira Y, Cavalcante RGS, Cavalcanti Neto MP, et al. Oral administration of Lactobacillus fermentum post-weaning improves the lipid profile and autonomic

dysfunction in rat offspring exposed to maternal dyslipidemia. Food Funct 2020; 11(6):5581–94.

2. Eckel RH, Jakicic JM, Ard JD, et al. 2013 AHA/ACC guideline on lifestyle management to reduce cardiovascular risk: a report of the American College of Cardiology/American Heart Association Task Force on Practice Guidelines. Circulation 2014;129(25 Suppl 2):S76–99.

3. Piechota W, Staszewski A. Reference ranges of lipids and apolipoproteins in pregnancy. Eur J Obstet Gynecol Reprod Biol 1992;45(1):27–35.

4. Wiznitzer A, Mayer A, Novack V, et al. Association of lipid levels during gestation with preeclampsia and gestational diabetes mellitus: a population-based study. Am J Obstet Gynecol 2009;201(5):482.e1-8.

5. Mankuta D, Elami-Suzin M, Elhayani A, et al. Lipid profile in consecutive pregnancies. Lipids Health Dis 2010;9:58.

6. Potter JM, Nestel PJ. The hyperlipidemia of pregnancy in normal and complicated pregnancies. Am J Obstet Gynecol 1979;133(2):165–70.

7. Stuebe AM, Rich-Edwards JW. The reset hypothesis: lactation and maternal metabolism. Am J Perinatol 2009;26(1):81–8.

8. Vrijkotte TG, Krukziener N, Hutten BA, et al. Maternal lipid profile during early pregnancy and pregnancy complications and outcomes: the ABCD study. J Clin Endocrinol Metab 2012;97(11):3917–25.

9. Feitosa ACR, Barreto LT, Silva IMD, et al. Impact of the use of different diagnostic criteria in the prevalence of dyslipidemia in pregnant women. Arq Bras Cardiol 2017;109(1):30–8.

10. Catov JM, Ness RB, Wellons MF, et al. Prepregnancy lipids related to preterm birth risk: the coronary artery risk development in young adults study. J Clin Endocrinol Metab 2010;95(8):3711–8.

11. Jan MR, Nazli R, Shah J, et al. A study of lipoproteins in normal and pregnancy induced hypertensive women in tertiary care hospitals of the north west frontier province-Pakistan. Hypertens Pregnancy 2012;31(2):292–9.

12. Kushtagi P, Arvapally S. Maternal mid-pregnancy serum triglyceride levels and neonatal birth weight. Int J Gynaecol Obstet 2009;106(3):258–9.

13. Edison RJ, Berg K, Remaley A, et al. Adverse birth outcome among mothers with low serum cholesterol. Pediatrics 2007;120(4):723–33.

14. Nordestgaard BG, Chapman MJ, Humphries SE, et al. Familial hypercholesterolaemia is underdiagnosed and undertreated in the general population: guidance for clinicians to prevent coronary heart disease: consensus statement of the European Atherosclerosis Society. Eur Heart J 2013;34(45):3478–3490a.

15. Smith GN, Walker MC, Liu A, et al. A history of preeclampsia identifies women who have underlying cardiovascular risk factors. Am J Obstet Gynecol 2009; 200(1):58.e1-8.

16. Son GH, Kwon JY, Kim YH, et al. Maternal serum triglycerides as predictive factors for large-for-gestational age newborns in women with gestational diabetes mellitus. Acta Obstet Gynecol Scand 2010;89(5):700–4.

17. Brown HL, Warner JJ, Gianos E, et al. Promoting risk identification and reduction of cardiovascular disease in women through collaboration with obstetricians and gynecologists: a presidential advisory from the American Heart Association and the American College of Obstetricians and Gynecologists. Circulation 2018; 137(24):e843–52.

18. Costantine MM, Cleary K, Eunice Kennedy Shriver National Institute of Child Health and Human Development Obstetric–Fetal Pharmacology Research Units

Network. Pravastatin for the prevention of preeclampsia in high-risk pregnant women. Obstet Gynecol 2013;121(2 Pt 1):349–53.

19. Costantine MM, Cleary K, Hebert MF, et al. Safety and pharmacokinetics of pravastatin used for the prevention of preeclampsia in high-risk pregnant women: a pilot randomized controlled trial. Am J Obstet Gynecol 2016; 214(6):720.e1-7.

20. Goldberg AS, Hegele RA. Severe hypertriglyceridemia in pregnancy. J Clin Endocrinol Metab 2012;97(8):2589–96.

21. Toleikyte I, Retterstol K, Leren TP, et al. Pregnancy outcomes in familial hypercholesterolemia: a registry-based study. Circulation 2011;124(15):1606–14.

22. Jeon HR, Kim SY, Cho YJ, et al. Hypertriglyceridemia-induced acute pancreatitis in pregnancy causing maternal death. Obstet Gynecol Sci 2016;59(2):148–51.

23. Tanous D, Siu SC, Mason J, et al. B-type natriuretic peptide in pregnant women with heart disease. J Am Coll Cardiol 2010;56(15):1247–53.

24. Kusters DM, Homsma SJ, Hutten BA, et al. Dilemmas in treatment of women with familial hypercholesterolaemia during pregnancy. Neth J Med 2010;68(1): 299–303.

25. Zarrati M, Shidfar F, Moradof M, et al. Relationship between breast feeding and obesity in children with low birth weight. Iran Red Crescent Med J 2013;15(8): 676–82.

26. Grandi SM, Vallee-Pouliot K, Reynier P, et al. Hypertensive disorders in pregnancy and the risk of subsequent cardiovascular disease. Paediatr Perinat Epidemiol 2017;31(5):412–21.

27. Shostrom DCV, Sun Y, Oleson JJ, et al. History of gestational diabetes mellitus in relation to cardiovascular disease and cardiovascular risk factors in US women. Front Endocrinol 2017;8:144.

28. Charlton F, Tooher J, Rye KA, et al. Cardiovascular risk, lipids and pregnancy: preeclampsia and the risk of later life cardiovascular disease. Heart Lung Circ 2014;23(3):203–12.

29. Kjerulff LE, Sanchez-Ramos L, Duffy D. Pregnancy outcomes in women with polycystic ovary syndrome: a metaanalysis. Am J Obstet Gynecol 2011;204(6): 558.e1-6.

30. Gunderson EP. Childbearing and obesity in women: weight before, during, and after pregnancy. Obstet Gynecol Clin North Am 2009;36(2):317–32, ix.

31. Yildiz BO, Bozdag G, Yapici Z, et al. Prevalence, phenotype and cardiometabolic risk of polycystic ovary syndrome under different diagnostic criteria. Hum Reprod 2012;27(10):3067–73.

32. Pergialiotis V, Trakakis E, Chrelias C, et al. The impact of mild hypercholesterolemia on glycemic and hormonal profiles, menstrual characteristics and the ovarian morphology of women with polycystic ovarian syndrome. Horm Mol Biol Clin Invest 2018;34(3):20180002.

33. Ghaffarzad A, Amani R, Mehrzad Sadaghiani M, et al. Correlation of serum lipoprotein ratios with insulin resistance in infertile women with polycystic ovarian syndrome: a case control study. Int J Fertil Steril 2016;10(1):29–35.

34. Moran LJ, Misso ML, Wild RA, et al. Impaired glucose tolerance, type 2 diabetes and metabolic syndrome in polycystic ovary syndrome: a systematic review and meta-analysis. Hum Reprod Update 2010;16(4):347–63.

35. Moran LJ, Hutchison SK, Norman RJ, et al. Lifestyle changes in women with polycystic ovary syndrome. Cochrane Database Syst Rev 2011;(2):CD007506.

36. Diabetes Prevention Program Research G, Knowler WC, Fowler SE, et al. 10-year follow-up of diabetes incidence and weight loss in the diabetes prevention program outcomes study. Lancet 2009;374(9702):1677–86.

37. Nestler JE. Metformin for the treatment of the polycystic ovary syndrome. N Engl J Med 2008;358(1):47–54.

38. Kumar DRN, Seshadri KG, Pandurangi M. Effect of metformin-sustained release therapy on low-density lipoprotein size and adiponectin in the south Indian women with polycystic ovary syndrome. Indian J Endocrinol Metab 2017;21(5): 679–83.

39. Asemi Z, Esmaillzadeh A. DASH diet, insulin resistance, and serum hs-CRP in polycystic ovary syndrome: a randomized controlled clinical trial. Horm Metab Res 2015;47(3):232–8.

40. Moran LJ, Ko H, Misso M, et al. Dietary composition in the treatment of polycystic ovary syndrome: a systematic review to inform evidence-based guidelines. J Acad Nutr Diet 2013;113(4):520–45.

41. Duleba AJ, Banaszewska B, Spaczynski RZ, et al. Simvastatin improves biochemical parameters in women with polycystic ovary syndrome: results of a prospective, randomized trial. Fertil Steril 2006;85(4):996–1001.

42. Hyun MH, Jang JW, Choi BG, et al. Risk of insulin resistance with statin therapy in individuals without dyslipidemia: a propensity-matched analysis in a registry population. Clin Exp Pharmacol Physiol 2020;47(6):947–54.

43. Puurunen J, Piltonen T, Puukka K, et al. Statin therapy worsens insulin sensitivity in women with polycystic ovary syndrome (PCOS): a prospective, randomized, double-blind, placebo-controlled study. J Clin Endocrinol Metab 2013;98(12): 4798–807.

44. Banaszewska B, Pawelczyk L, Spaczynski RZ, et al. Effects of simvastatin and metformin on polycystic ovary syndrome after six months of treatment. J Clin Endocrinol Metab 2011;96(11):3493–501.

45. Zarek J, Koren G. The fetal safety of statins: a systematic review and meta-analysis. J Obstet Gynaecol Can 2014;36(6):506–9.

46. Setji TL, Brown AJ. Polycystic ovary syndrome: update on diagnosis and treatment. Am J Med 2014;127(10):912–9.

47. Aye MM, Kilpatrick ES, Afolabi P, et al. Postprandial effects of long-term niacin/laropiprant use on glucose and lipid metabolism and on cardiovascular risk in patients with polycystic ovary syndrome. Diabetes Obes Metab 2014;16(6):545–52.

48. Sanga K, Mola G, Wattimena J, et al. Unintended pregnancy amongst women attending antenatal clinics at the Port Moresby General Hospital. Aust N Z J Obstet Gynaecol 2014;54(4):360–5.

49. Wang A, Mo T, Li Q, et al. The effectiveness of metformin, oral contraceptives, and lifestyle modification in improving the metabolism of overweight women with polycystic ovary syndrome: a network meta-analysis. Endocrine 2019; 64(2):220–32.

50. Pasquali R, Gambineri A, Anconetani B, et al. The natural history of the metabolic syndrome in young women with the polycystic ovary syndrome and the effect of long-term oestrogen-progestagen treatment. Clin Endocrinol 1999;50(4):517–27.

51. Korytkowski MT, Mokan M, Horwitz MJ, et al. Metabolic effects of oral contraceptives in women with polycystic ovary syndrome. J Clin Endocrinol Metab 1995; 80(11):3327–34.

52. Cibula D, Sindelka G, Hill M, et al. Insulin sensitivity in non-obese women with polycystic ovary syndrome during treatment with oral contraceptives containing low-androgenic progestin. Hum Reprod 2002;17(1):76–82.

53. Gourdy P. Diabetes and oral contraception. Best Pract Res Clin Endocrinol Metab 2013;27(1):67–76.

54. Bargiota A, Diamanti-Kandarakis E. The effects of old, new and emerging medicines on metabolic aberrations in PCOS. Ther Adv Endocrinol Metab 2012; 3(1):27–47.

55. Ng YW, Liang S, Singh K. Effects of Mirena (levonorgestrel-releasing intrauterine system) and Ortho Gynae T380 intrauterine copper device on lipid metabolism–a randomized comparative study. Contraception 2009;79(1):24–8.

56. Kayikcioglu F, Gunes M, Ozdegirmenci O, et al. Effects of levonorgestrel-releasing intrauterine system on glucose and lipid metabolism: a 1-year follow-up study. Contraception 2006;73(5):528–31.

57. Derby CA, Crawford SL, Pasternak RC, et al. Lipid changes during the menopause transition in relation to age and weight: the Study of Women's Health Across the Nation. Am J Epidemiol 2009;169(11):1352–61.

58. Park JK, Lim YH, Kim KS, et al. Changes in body fat distribution through menopause increase blood pressure independently of total body fat in middle-aged women: the Korean National Health and Nutrition Examination Survey 2007-2010. Hypertens Res 2013;36(5):444–9.

59. Garber AJ, Abrahamson MJ, Barzilay JI, et al. Consensus Statement by the American Association of Clinical Endocrinologists and American College of Endocrinology on the comprehensive type 2 diabetes management algorithm - 2018 executive summary. Endocr Pract 2018;24(1):91–120.

60. Trinder M, Uddin MM, Finneran P, et al. Clinical utility of lipoprotein(a) and LPA genetic risk score in risk prediction of incident atherosclerotic cardiovascular disease. JAMA Cardiol 2020;e205398 [Epub ahead of print].

61. Matthews KA, Gibson CJ, El Khoudary SR, et al. Changes in cardiovascular risk factors by hysterectomy status with and without oophorectomy: Study of Women's Health Across the Nation. J Am Coll Cardiol 2013;62(3):191–200.

62. Mendes KG, Theodoro H, Rodrigues AD, et al. Prevalence of metabolic syndrome and its components in the menopausal transition: a systematic review. Cad Saude Publica 2012;28(8):1423–37 [in Portuguese].

63. El Khoudary SR, Wildman RP, Matthews K, et al. Progression rates of carotid intima-media thickness and adventitial diameter during the menopausal transition. Menopause 2013;20(1):8–14.

64. Mizunuma H, Shiraki M, Shintani M, et al. Randomized trial comparing low-dose hormone replacement therapy and HRT plus 1alpha-OH-vitamin D3 (alfacalcidol) for treatment of postmenopausal bone loss. J Bone Miner Metab 2006; 24(1):11–5.

65. Wild RA, Manson JE. Insights from the Women's Health Initiative: individualizing risk assessment for hormone therapy decisions. Semin Reprod Med 2014; 32(6):433–7.

66. Rossouw JE, Anderson GL, Prentice RL, et al. Risks and benefits of estrogen plus progestin in healthy postmenopausal women: principal results From the Women's Health Initiative randomized controlled trial. JAMA 2002;288(3):321–33.

67. Blum CB, Adult Treatment Panel IIIoTNCEP. Perspectives: some thoughts on the adult treatment panel III report. Prev Cardiol 2002;5(2):87–9, 93.

68. Mosca L, Appel LJ, Benjamin EJ, et al. Evidence-based guidelines for cardiovascular disease prevention in women. Circulation 2004;109(5):672–93.

69. North American Menopause S. The 2012 hormone therapy position statement of: the North American Menopause Society. Menopause 2012;19(3):257–71.

70. Anagnostis P, Bitzer J, Cano A, et al. Menopause symptom management in women with dyslipidemias: an EMAS clinical guide. Maturitas 2020;135:82–8.
71. Canonico M, Oger E, Plu-Bureau G, et al. Hormone therapy and venous thromboembolism among postmenopausal women: impact of the route of estrogen administration and progestogens: the ESTHER study. Circulation 2007;115(7): 840–5.

New and Emerging Therapies for Dyslipidemia

Alberto Zambon, MD, PhD[a],*, Maurizio Averna, MD[b],
Laura D'Erasmo, MD, PhD[c], Marcello Arca, MD[c],
Alberico Catapano, MD, PhD[d,e]

KEYWORDS

- Atherosclerotic cardiovascular disease (ASCVD) • Inclisiran • SiRNA
- Selective PPAR alpha modulators • SPPARM • Volanesorsen
- Angiopoietin-like protein 3 • ANGPTL3

KEY POINTS

- Genetic studies have informed on biological pathways modulating lipid and lipoprotein metabolism, which have been exploited to design new drugs
- Inhibition of PCSK9 expression by long-acting siRNA is effective in lowering LDL-C
- Bi-annual administration of long-acting siRNA will improve adherence and represents a novel therapeutic strategy in high and very high CV risk patients
- Selective PPARa modulator (SPPARM) pemafibrate might represent a new option for combination LLT to decrease the risk of macro and microvascular complications in diabetes.
- Targeting ANGPTL3 is showing highly effective in reducing LDL-C and total triglycerides
- Targeting ApoCIII reduces TGRL by an LPL-independent mechanism

INTRODUCTION

Atherosclerotic cardiovascular disease (ASCVD) continues to represent a growing global health challenge. Despite guideline-recommended treatment of ASCVD risk, including antihypertensive, high-intensity statin therapy, and antiaggregant agents, high-risk patients, especially those with established ASCVD and patients with type 2 diabetes, continue to experience cardiovascular events.[1]

This article originally appeared in *Endocrinology and Metabolism Clinics*, Volume 51, Issue 3, September 2022.

[a] University of Padova, Clinica Medica 1, Department of Medicine - DIMED, Via Giustiniani 2, Padova 35128, Italy; [b] Policlinico, Paolo Giaccone, Via del Vespro 149, Palermo 90127, Italy; [c] Department of Translational and Precision Medicine, University of Rome, Viale dell' Università 37, Sapienza 00161, Italy; [d] Department of Pharmacological and Biomolecular Sciences, Università degli Studi di Milano, Via G. Balzaretti 9, Milan 20133, Italy; [e] IRCCS MultiMedica, Via Milanese 300, Sesto San Giovanni (MI) 200099, Italy
* Corresponding author.
E-mail address: alberto.zambon@unipd.it

Clinics Collections 13 (2023) 257–275
https://doi.org/10.1016/j.ccol.2023.02.007
2352-7986/23/© 2023 Elsevier Inc. All rights reserved.

Robust and growing evidence from epidemiologic and genetic studies, as well as randomized clinical trials, suggest that triglyceride (TG)-rich VLDL (very-low-density lipoprotein) and their remnants, lipoprotein (a) [Lp(a)], and inflammation are causally related to risk of ASCVD in individuals already treated with statin therapy (**Fig. 1**).

Recent years have brought significant developments in lipid and atherosclerosis research. Several lipid drugs owe their existence, in part, to human genetic evidence.[2] Although statins remain the mainstay of guideline-recommended lipid-lowering strategies, new and effective lipid-lowering therapies (LLT) are, or will be soon, available to lower risk of ASCVD events by further reducing atherogenic apoB-containing particles, such as LDL but also Lp(a), TG-rich VLDL, and their remnants (see **Fig. 1**).

These emerging therapeutic strategies will likely translate into a significant clinical benefit for individuals with severe dyslipidemias that are resistant to existing treatments, those who experience intolerable or harmful adverse effects from existing therapies, and most importantly for patients at significant residual ASCVD risk, despite apparently acceptable response to the current standard of care. Here, the authors briefly review the mechanisms, the effect on lipid parameters, and safety profiles of some of the most promising new lipid-lowering approaches that will be soon available in our daily clinical practice.

Inclisiran

The primary and secondary prevention of ASCVD is based on the achievement of the goals for the major risk factors recommended by the Guidelines.[3] LDL-cholesterol (LDL-C) is considered a causal factor of ASCVD, and the evidence collected suggests that the strategies aimed to reduce LDL-C are the most effective in reducing cardiovascular morbidity and mortality. Statins alone, and in combination with ezetimibe, have represented the conventional drug strategies to reduce ASCVD events, and recently the discovery of the role of PCSK9 as one of the main regulators of the LDL receptor degradation pathway[4,5] has prompted the development of novel approaches targeting this protein, which increase the number of LDL receptors and reduce plasma levels of LDL-C. The inhibition of PCSK9 by monoclonal antibodies is today a well-established strategy sustained by a large body of evidence based on efficacy, safety, and CVD outcomes trials (review). Evolocumab and alirocumab

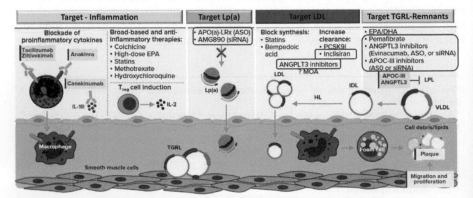

Fig. 1. Current and emerging therapeutic strategies to reduce cardiovascular risk. (*Adapted from* Hussain A, Ballantyne CM. New Approaches for the Prevention and Treatment of Cardiovascular Disease: Focus on Lipoproteins and Inflammation. Annu Rev Med. 2021 Jan 27;72:431-446.)

have received approval from regulatory authorities and are currently used in real-world clinical settings. The anti-PCSK9 monoclonal antibodies inhibit the circulating PSK9 protein without interfering with the molecular mechanisms of PCSK9 gene expression, transcription, and translation.[6]

The pharmacologic development of inclisiran represents a new and promising approach to target PCSK9 at the RNA level in the liver. Inclisiran is a small interfering RNA (siRNA) molecule obtained by chemical synthesis and shares the mechanism of action with the siRNA family by interfering with the expression of the PCSK9 gene, as its complementary nucleotide sequences produce the degradation of PCSK9 messenger RNA (mRNA) once transcripted, preventing its translation.

The appealing features of inclisiran are the durability—it is a long-acting siRNA— and the liver specificity conferred by the conjugation to triantennary N-acetyl galactosamine carbohydrates that bind to asialoglycoprotein receptors highly abundant in hepatocytes.[7–9]

In 2020 and 2021, inclisiran was approved in Europe and the United States for reducing LDL-C in adults with primary hypercholesterolemia (heterozygous familial and nonfamilial) or mixed dyslipidemia, as an adjunct to diet, and in combination with a statin or a statin plus other LLT, who are unable to reach LDL-C goals. Inclisiran is also approved for adults on other LLT who cannot tolerate a statin or for whom a statin is contraindicated. The dose is 284 mg sc to be repeated at 3 months, 6 months, and subsequently every 6 months. Inclisiran, 284 mg, is equivalent to inclisiran sodium salt, 300 mg.

Phase I Trials

In 2014[9] a phase I trial demonstrated the safety and efficacy of ALN-PCS (inclisiran). Thirty-two healthy volunteers with plasma LDL-C levels of 3 mmol/L or higher were allocated in 6 single-dose cohorts with a ratio 3:1 to receive inclisiran intravenously or placebo. The incidence of adverse events (AEs) was not different in treatment and placebo groups, and the pharmacodynamic studies showed that the plasma increase of ALN-PCS was dose dependent. The plasma levels of PCSK9 and LDL-C were significantly reduced with the highest dose of ALN-PCS (0·4 mg/kg) by 70% and 40%, respectively. In 2017 the results of a phase I trial, aimed to assess safety and efficacy of single- and multiple-dose regimens of inclisiran administered subcutaneously, were published.[10] No serious AEs were registered and the more frequent AEs (≥5% of the inclisiran treated subjects) were cough, musculoskeletal pain, and nasopharyngitis. The highest reduction of PCSK9 plasma levels (74.5%), which was maintained at day 180, was seen in the group treated with a single 300 mg dose. In the multiple dose arm of the trial, plasma LDL-C and PCSK9 levels were reduced by about 60% and 80%, respectively. LDL-C levels remained reduced at day 180 with doses of 300 mg or higher.

The Orion/Victorion Program

The clinical development of inclisiran has been conducted by the Orion/Victorion program.[11] The Orion-1 and -2 (phase II trials) and Orion-8, -9, -10, and -11 (phase III trials)[12] have been completed. In these studies, the efficacy and safety of inclisiran have been tested in several categories of patients such as the following: (1) patients with ASCVD or ASCVD risk equivalents and elevated LDL-C (Orion-1 and Orion-11); (2) patients with familial homozygous hypercholesterolemia (HoFH) (ORION-2); (3) patients with familial heterozygous hypercholesterolemia (HeFH) (Orion-9); (4) patients with ASCVD and elevated LDL-C (Orion-10).

Inclisiran sodium has been used at single or multiple subcutaneous injections (Orion-1) or at a dose of 300 mg subcutaneously at day 1, day 90, and then every 6 months (Orion- 9, -10, and 11).

PATIENTS WITH ATHEROSCLEROTIC CARDIOVASCULAR DISEASE OR ATHEROSCLEROTIC CARDIOVASCULAR DISEASE RISK EQUIVALENT AND ELEVATED LEVEL OF LDL-C (ORION-1, -10, AND -11)

Inclisiran at a dose of 284 mg subcutaneously every 6 months for 18 months reduced LDL-C by about 50% at day 540 in about 1500 patients, with placebo-corrected reduction in PCSK9 plasma levels of about 80%.[13] The safety and tolerability were good.

PATIENTS WITH HOMOZYGOUS HYPERCHOLESTEROLEMIA (ORION-2) AND HETEROZYGOUS HYPERCHOLESTEROLEMIA (ORION-9)

Inclisiran has been studied in 2 "difficult-to-treat settings" HoFH and HeFH; in the Orion-2 pilot study, 4 patients with a genetic or clinical diagnosis of HoFH (untreated LDL-C >500 mg/d–13 mmol/L) completed the study. The background treatment was combination therapy for high-intensity statin plus ezetimibe. Inclisiran sodium was administered at a dose of 300 mg subcutaneously on day 1 and eventually repeated based on the reduction of PCSK9 levels. All 4 patients showed a durable reduction of PCSK9 plasma levels (up to 80%) and 3 out of 4 a durable reduction of LDL-C (up to 37%). The results of the Orion-9 trial that enrolled 481 HeFH subjects have shown that inclisiran significantly reduced LDL-C levels by about 48% and that the effect was sustained up to day 540 with an LDL-C reduction of about 44%. A dose of 300 mg, or a placebo, was administered subcutaneously on days 1, 90, 270, and 450. No differences of AEs or serious AEs in comparison with the placebo group were found.

The other Orion/Victorion trials are still in the recruiting phase.

Outcome Trials

The ORION-4 trial[14] is the large ongoing outcome trial that will evaluate the effect of inclisiran on MACE; at the end of the enrolment period, 15,000 subjects older than 55 years with ASCVD will be randomized to inclisiran sodium, 300 mg, subcutaneously every 180 days or placebo. The primary endpoint is the 5-year occurrence of coronary heart disease death, myocardial infarction, fatal or nonfatal ischemic stroke, and urgent coronary revascularization procedures. The other outcome trial—VICTORION-2 PREVENT—in 16,000 patients with established ACVD[15] has a composite primary endpoint of cardiovascular death, nonfatal myocardial infarction, and nonfatal ischemic stroke. In this trial, inclisiran sodium will be administered subcutaneously at the dose of 300 mg subcutaneously injected on day 1, day 90, and every 6 months until the end of the study.

Conclusions

Taken together, all these studies show that inclisiran, a long-acting siRNA belonging to the family of "sirans," is effective in lowering LDL-C in several populations of patients at high and very high risk of cardiovascular disease: patients with HoFH, HeFH, ASCVD, and ASCVD risk equivalent, including patients with diabetes. The appealing feature is the frequency of administration (twice/year) that will likely be associated with a much greater adherence than currently available lipid-lowering approaches (ie, statins and ezetimibe) allowing for a better time-averaged LDL-C reduction in the medium long term. In about 60% of patients a durable LDL-C reduction greater than 50% was obtained. A pooled analysis has shown that inclisiran is safe and well tolerated even in patients with chronic kidney disease and a creatinine clearance level of 15 to 29 mL/min, and the rate of AEs was not different from the placebo arm with the exception for minor and transient injection site reactions. In addition, no AEs have been reported for platelet counts or immunogenicity.[12] The ongoing trials will answer several relevant questions regarding the impact of inclisiran on therapeutic adherence and ASCVD clinical events, the safety and efficacy in special populations such as children and older people, the clinical use in postacute coronary syndromes, and, not less relevant, economic sustainability.

SELECTIVE PEROXISOME PROLIFERATOR–ACTIVATED RECEPTOR ALPHA MODULATORS

Growing evidence has established that triglyceride-rich lipoproteins (TRLs) and their remnants are also causal factors in ASCVD, and their contribution to atherothrombotic processes seems statistically independent of, and additional to, that of LDL.[16,17] A key investigational drug to address the residual vascular risk related to TRL remnants is a member of the nuclear peroxisome proliferator–activated receptors (PPARs) family, PPAR alpha (PPARα). PPARα, is mainly expressed in metabolically active tissues, such as the liver, kidney, heart, muscle, and macrophages, and has a key role in modulating the expression of genes involved in fatty acid oxidation, lipoprotein metabolism, and inflammation.[18,19] Guidelines recommend fibrates (PPARα agonists) and omega-3 fatty acids for the management of hypertriglyceridemia, usually as an add-on to primary statin treatment.[3] Clinicians are, however, well aware that current PPARα agonists, that is, fenofibrate, have proved disappointing in cardiovascular outcome studies either as monotherapy (FIELD)[20] or against a background of best evidence-based treatment including statin therapy,[21] with the possible exception of subgroups of patients with elevated baseline triglyceride levels (TG > 200 mg/dL–2.3 mmol/L). Pemafibrate is a selective PPARα modulator (SPPARM) that has been shown to reduce TG levels and elevate HDL-C levels. It is approved in Japan for use in dyslipidemia and is still undergoing phase III trials in the United States and Europe.

Preclinical Studies

Preclinical studies have revealed that enhanced potency, selectivity, and cofactor binding profile differentiate this novel SPPARMα agent, pemafibrate, from traditional nonselective PPARα agonists (**Fig. 2**). Compared with fenofibrate, pemafibrate resulted in greater TG lowering and elevation in HDL-C in animals with hypertriglyceridemia and more effective attenuation of postprandial hypertriglyceridemia, by suppressing the postprandial increase in chylomicrons and accumulation of chylomicron remnants.[22] Clinically relevant genes regulated by this SPPARMα agonist include those involved in regulation of lipoprotein metabolism, such as VLDLR and ABCA1. In addition, pemafibrate has been associated with an increased expression of genes involved in the regulation of the innate immune system (mannose-binding lectin 2), inflammation, and fibroblast growth factor (FGF),[23] a metabolic regulator with favorable effects on glucose- and lipid-mediated energy metabolism (FGF21), implying the potential for effects beyond lipid metabolism. Finally, this SPPARMα agonist may produce beneficial microvascular benefits, with evidence of reduction of diabetic nephropathy in diabetic db/db mice, attributed, at least partly, to inhibition of renal lipid content and oxidative stress.[24] Interestingly, the positive effect on microvascular complications supports data from FIELD[20] and ACCORD[21] where the use of

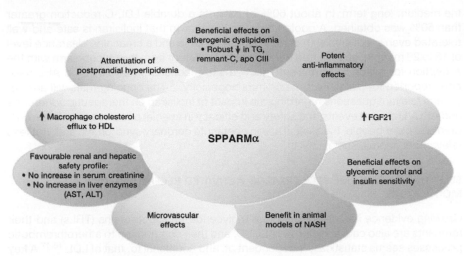

Fig. 2. Unique pharmacologic profile of pemafibrate (SPPARMα). (*From* Fruchart JC, Santos RD, Aguilar-Salinas C, Aikawa M, Al Rasadi K, Amarenco P, Barter PJ, Ceska R, Corsini A, Després JP, Duriez P, Eckel RH, Ezhov MV, Farnier M, Ginsberg HN, Hermans MP, Ishibashi S, Karpe F, Kodama T, Koenig W, Krempf M, Lim S, Lorenzatti AJ, McPherson R, Nuñez-Cortes JM, Nordestgaard BG, Ogawa H, Packard CJ, Plutzky J, Ponte-Negretti CI, Pradhan A, Ray KK, Reiner Ž, Ridker PM, Ruscica M, Sadikot S, Shimano H, Sritara P, Stock JK, Su TC, Susekov AV, Tartar A, Taskinen MR, Tenenbaum A, Tokgözoğlu LS, Tomlinson B, Tybjærg-Hansen A, Valensi P, Vrablík M, Wahli W, Watts GF, Yamashita S, Yokote K, Zambon A, Libby P. The selective peroxisome proliferator-activated receptor alpha modulator (SPPARMα) paradigm: conceptual framework and therapeutic potential : A consensus statement from the International Atherosclerosis Society (IAS) and the Residual Risk Reduction Initiative (R3i) Foundation. Cardiovasc Diabetol. 2019 Jun 4;18(1):71.)

fenofibrate in patients with type 2 diabetes was associated with a significant reduction in the progression of microvascular complications such as diabetic retinopathy and worsening of the albumin/creatinine ratio.

Clinical Trial Evidence and Safety

A phase II dose-ranging trial in Japanese patients with elevated TG ($\geq$2.3 mmol/L) and low HDL-C (<1.3 mmol/L) showed that, after 12 weeks, this agent produced reductions from baseline in TG (up to 42.7%), VLDL-cholesterol (up to 48.4%), remnant-cholesterol (up to 50.1%), apoB-48 (up to 55.9%), and apolipoprotein C-III (apoC-III) (up to 34.6%), compared with both placebo and micronized fenofibrate 100 mg/d, with maximal effects at a dose of 0.2 to 0.4 mg daily.[25] Phase II/III trials in Japanese and European patients with elevated TG with or without type 2 diabetes mellitus (T2DM) confirmed the lipid-modifying activity of this SPPARMα agonist, in particular robust and sustained lowering of remnant cholesterol (by up to 80%) and TG and apoC-III (by ~50%). Treatment with pemafibrate, 0.2 to 0.4 mg/d, significantly reduced the postprandial area under the curve for TG, apoB-48, and remnant cholesterol for patients with and without T2DM.

Across published trials, this SPPARMα agonist was generally well tolerated both as monotherapy and in combination with statins, particularly with respect to renal and hepatic safety signals[26] with no difference as compared with the placebo groups. Importantly, and in contrast to studies with fenofibrate, which showed reversible increases in serum creatinine,[20,21] pemafibrate at any studied dose showed no increase in serum creatinine in studies up to 52 weeks in patients with or without preexisting renal dysfunction.[26]

Therefore, pemafibrate may offer a novel approach to target residual cardiovascular risk in high-risk patients with atherogenic dyslipidemia, especially those with T2DM, on a background of best evidence-based treatment including statin therapy.

The PROMINENT study (Pemafibrate to Reduce cardiovascular OutcoMes by reducing triglycerides IN diabetic patiENTs) will address this critical question.[27] PROMINENT has been designed with the goal of evaluating cardiovascular outcomes in more than 10,000 patients with elevated TG (baseline 200–500 mg/dL) and reduced HDL-C (≤55 mg/dL). Thus, unlike the previous fibrate trials, PROMINENT will specifically target a hypertriglyceridemic population. Patients will be randomized to pemafibrate, 0.2 mg, BID versus placebo in addition to optimized statin therapy and followed-up for 4 years.[27] The primary endpoint is a composite of nonfatal myocardial infarction, nonfatal ischemic stroke, hospitalization for unstable angina requiring urgent coronary revascularization, and cardiovascular death. The trial should take 4 to 5 years to be completed. Within PROMINENT, a prospective nested substudy will investigate whether pemafibrate will significantly slow the progression of diabetic retinopathy in patients with nonproliferative diabetic retinopathy.[28] PROMINENT will determine whether therapeutic application of the SPPARMα concept translates to reduction in cardiovascular events in high-risk patients with T2DM already receiving evidence-based treatment. The results will provide additional information on the combination of LLT for elevated apoB-containing lipoproteins. A prior study, Reduction of Cardiovascular Events with Icosapent Ethyl-Intervention (REDUCE-IT), showed significant cardiovascular event reduction in patients with elevated TG taking statins when treated with 2 g twice daily of highly purified eicosapentaenoic acid ethyl ester.[29]

APOLIPOPROTEIN C-III TARGETING APPROACHES

Apolipoprotein C-III (apoC-III) has a key role in triglyceride-rich lipoprotein metabolism. ApoC-III is a 79 amino acid protein expressed mainly in the liver and intestine and found primarily on chylomicrons and VLDL. ApoC-III inhibits lipoprotein lipase (LPL) activity.

Robust data show that high levels of apoC-III lead to hypertriglyceridemia and, thereby, may influence the risk of cardiovascular disease. In humans, loss-of-function (LOF) mutations in apoC-III have been associated with low TG levels and reduced risk of atherosclerotic disease (**Fig. 3**).[30] Moreover, recent findings indicate that apoC-III might also modulate glucose homeostasis, monocyte adhesion, activation of inflammatory pathways, and modulation of the coagulation cascade.[31] These observations highlight the possibility of therapeutically targeting apoC-III in hypertriglyceridemia. Based on these findings, significant efforts have been undertaken to find a therapy specifically targeting apoC-III.[32]

Volanesorsen

Volanesorsen, a second-generation chimeric antisense inhibitor of Apo-CIII production, binds to apoC-III mRNA, triggering degradation by RNase H1.[31] ApoC-III inhibits LPL and hepatic uptake of TG-rich particles, which can lead to hypertriglyceridemia. Inhibition of apoC-III production thus allows for increased uptake of TG particles and reduces TG levels. It is administered as a subcutaneous once weekly injection with a follow-up dose after 3 months. It is eliminated by the kidneys after being metabolized by tissue endonucleases and exonucleases. The efficacy of volanesorsen was first

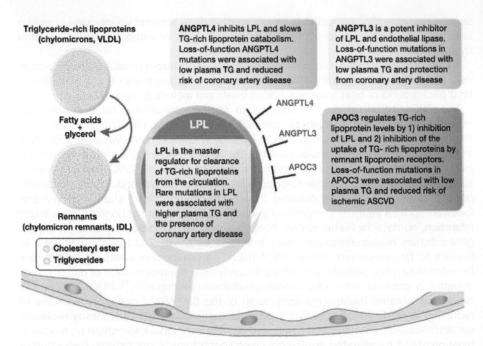

Fig. 3. Novel approaches for the management of hypertriglyceridemia and key targets in the regulation of triglyceride-rich lipoprotein metabolism: apolipoprotein C-III (encoded by *APOC3*), angiopoietin-like proteins (ANGPTL) 3 and 4. (*From* Fruchart JC, Santos RD, Aguilar-Salinas C, Aikawa M, Al Rasadi K, Amarenco P, Barter PJ, Ceska R, Corsini A, Després JP, Duriez P, Eckel RH, Ezhov MV, Farnier M, Ginsberg HN, Hermans MP, Ishibashi S, Karpe F, Kodama T, Koenig W, Krempf M, Lim S, Lorenzatti AJ, McPherson R, Nuñez-Cortes JM, Nordestgaard BG, Ogawa H, Packard CJ, Plutzky J, Ponte-Negretti CI, Pradhan A, Ray KK, Reiner Ž, Ridker PM, Ruscica M, Sadikot S, Shimano H, Sritara P, Stock JK, Su TC, Susekov AV, Tartar A, Taskinen MR, Tenenbaum A, Tokgözoğlu LS, Tomlinson B, Tybjærg-Hansen A, Valensi P, Vrablík M, Wahli W, Watts GF, Yamashita S, Yokote K, Zambon A, Libby P. The selective peroxisome proliferator-activated receptor alpha modulator (SPPARMα) paradigm: conceptual framework and therapeutic potential : A consensus statement from the International Atherosclerosis Society (IAS) and the Residual Risk Reduction Initiative (R3i) Foundation. Cardiovasc Diabetol. 2019 Jun 4;18(1):71.)

published from a study of 3 patients with a rare syndrome of familial chylomicronemia syndrome (FCS). FCS is a rare autosomal recessive disease generally caused by mutations in the gene encoding LPL or genes encoding proteins involved in LPL function (see Alan Chait's article, "Hypertriglyceridemia," in this issue); FCS is characterized by elevated levels of plasma chylomicrons, resulting in severe hypertriglyceridemia and increased risk of recurrent acute pancreatitis and other complications.[33] In this study, TG were found to decrease by 56% to 86% through LPL-independent pathways.[34] All patients achieved TG levels less than 500 mg/dL (<5.7 mmol/L) with treatment. TG levels in chylomicrons, apoB-48 levels, and non-HDL-C were also reduced.

Phase II Clinical Trials

Subsequent phase II studies showed similar TG reductions (40%–80%) compared with placebo when used as monotherapy or in combination with statins/fibrates.[35] In a phase II clinical trial of patients with hypertriglyceridemia (www.clinicaltrials.gov:

NCT01529424), volanesorsen, 300 mg, given weekly reduced plasma apoC-III and TG levels by 79.6% and 70.9%, respectively.[36] In 80 patients from phase II studies treated for 85 days or less, volanesorsen, 300 mg, was associated with greater than 80% reductions in apoC-III in various lipoprotein classes. In 15 adults with T2DM and hypertriglyceridemia treated for 15 weeks, volanesorsen reduced TG by 69%, with significant improvements in glycemia, glucose disposal, and insulin sensitivity.[37] In a study of 17 patients with hypertriglyceridemia, volanesorsen significantly reduced TG, apoC-II, and apoC-III and increased apoA-I and apoA-II.

Phase III Clinical Trials

Two phase III randomized, double-blind, placebo-controlled trials have been completed. APPROACH (www.clinicaltrials.gov:NCT02211209) evaluated 66 patients with FCS who had fasting TG greater than or equal to 8.4 mmol/L ($\geq$750 mg/dL).[38] Participants were randomized to 52 weeks of weekly subcutaneous volanesorsen, 300 mg, or matching placebo. At 3 months, TG decreased by 77% in 33 volanesorsen-treated patients but increased by 18% in 33 placebo-treated patients ($P < .0001$); the effect was sustained during 52 weeks. There were 3 placebo-treated patients with 4 acute pancreatitis events, whereas 1 volanesorsen-treated patient had 1 event 9 days after the end of therapy. The most common AE was injection-site reactions, most of which were mild to moderate (mean of 11.8% of all volanesorsen injections). However, declines in platelet counts led to 5 early terminations; 2 patients had platelet count less than 25 000/μL, which recovered after cessation of volanesorsen. The COMPASS study (clinicaltrials.gov: NCT02300233) randomized 113 patients with fasting TG greater than or equal to 500 mg/dL ($\geq$5.7 mmol/L; mean TG, 1261 $\pm$ 955 mg/dL or 14.3 $\pm$ 10.8 mmol/L) in a 2:1 ratio to receive either volanesorsen, 300 mg, or placebo subcutaneously once weekly for 26 weeks.[39] Patients treated with volanesorsen achieved a 71.8% reduction in TG from baseline after 3 months, compared with a 0.8% reduction in placebo-treated patients ($P < .0001$). Treatment effects were sustained after 26 weeks. Pancreatitis episodes were reduced on treatment, with 5 events in 3 patients occurring with placebo arm versus none with volanesorsen ($P = .036$). In contrast to APPROACH, there were no serious platelet events in the COMPASS study. However, injection-site reactions, nasopharyngitis, fatigue, arthralgias, myalgias, and thrombocytopenia are important AEs observed in trials.

Although the mechanism of the thrombocytopenia is unclear, development of a next-generation N-acetylgalactosamine (GalNac)-conjugated antisense oligonucleotide (ASO) targeting apoC-III may mitigate this risk. In a double-blind, placebo-controlled, dose-escalation phase I/IIa study in healthy volunteers with TG levels greater than or equal to 200 mg/dL, multiple doses of AKCEA-APO-CIII-LRx resulted in mean reductions of apoC-III of 83% and TGs of 65%, as well as significant reductions in total cholesterol, ApoB, non–HDL-C, and VLDL-C and increases in HDL-C. AKCEA-APO-CIIIL therapy was well tolerated with no flulike reactions, no platelet count reductions, and no liver or renal safety signals.[40] An ongoing multicenter, randomized, placebo-controlled, double-blind, phase II/III trial, BROADEN study (NCT02639286), has been planned to determine the benefit of volanesorsen in patients with familial partial lipodystrophy.[41] The primary objective of this study is to evaluate the efficacy and safety of volanesorsen therapy compared with placebo in reducing TG levels after 3 months of drug therapy. The study will last 52 weeks and involve 60 patients.

Because of the potential severity of side effects, caution is needed when evaluating the benefit/risk of medications under development for hypertriglyceridemia.

Nevertheless, data strongly support the importance of apoC-III as a modulator of the lipolytic cascade and its inhibition as a major strategy for the development of new therapies for hypertriglyceridemia. It remains to be established if this approach may be useful also in controlling the residual cardiovascular risk associated with elevated TG and metabolic disorders.

On 28 February 2019, the Committee for Medicinal Products for Human Use of the European Medicines Agency recommended the conditional marketing authorization of volanesorsen for patients with genetically confirmed FCS and at high risk of pancreatitis, in whom the response to diet and TG reduction therapy is inadequate.[42] Volanesorsen has not been approved by the FDA because of safety concerns—low platelet counts and bleeding.

A phase I single and multiple dose-escalating study to evaluate the safety, tolerability, pharmacokinetics, and pharmacodynamic effects of ARO-APO CIII, a GalNAc–siRNA conjugate targeting Apo CIII, in adult healthy volunteers as well as in severely hypertriglyceridemic patients and patients with familial chylomicronemia syndrome is currently ongoing [ClinicalTrials.gov Identifier: NCT03783377].[43]

ANGIOPOIETIN-LIKE PROTEIN 3 TARGETING APPROACHES
The Role of Angiopoietin-like Protein 3 in Lipoprotein Metabolism

ANGPTL3 is a glycoprotein of 45 kDa protein that is only synthesized and secreted by the liver.[44,45] It belongs to a family of secretory proteins with structural homologies with angiopoietins, the key factors that regulate angiogenesis.[44] It is composed by an N-terminal coiled-coil domain, which is the functional portion of the protein, and a fibrinogen-like C-terminal domain.[44,45] Original studies conducted in mice have clearly established that ANGPTL3 is an important regulator of plasma TG levels due to its role as circulating inhibitor of LPL (see **Fig. 3**), the enzyme catalyzing the hydrolysis of TG contained in circulating VLDL and chylomicrons.[44,45] Furthermore, ANGPTL3 raises plasma HDL-C levels by inhibiting endothelial lipase.[44,45] Genome-wide association studies in humans have linked single nucleotide polymorphisms near to and within the *ANGPTL3* gene to TG variation in the population.[46] Later, homozygous LOF mutations in the ANGPTL3 gene were found to cause a lipid phenotype in humans, defined as familial combined hypolipidemia (FHBL2, OMIM #605019).[47,48] Noteworthy, this human model of ANGPTL3 deficiency has provided the unique opportunity to study ANGPTL3 function and the favorable consequences associated with its absence.[44] FHBL2 is characterized by a marked reduction of ApoA1- and ApoB-containing lipoprotein VLDL and LDL, an increase in LPL activity, and a markedly accelerated removal of TG-rich lipoproteins with an almost abolished postprandial lipemia.[48–52] The mechanism determining LDL-C reduction in ANGPLT3 deficiency is still unknown, even though it seems to be independent from the LDLR pathway. Indeed, Mendelian randomization studies have shown that subjects carrying LOF variants in *ANGPTL3* exhibit a reduced risk of atherosclerotic cardiovascular disease.[44] Altogether, these data have clearly established the rationale for developing pharmacologic strategies to inactivate ANGPTL3 and, thereby, to reduce plasma levels of atherogenic lipoproteins and cardiovascular risk.

Strategies to Pharmacologically Inactivate Angiopoietin-like Protein 3

To date, 2 different approaches have been used to inactivate ANGPTL3[53–55]: the administration of a human mAb against ANGPTL3 (REGN1500—evinacumab) or an ASO targeting Angptl3 (vupanorsen). The main difference between these treatments is that vupanorsen acts inside the nucleus of the hepatocyte, whereas evinacumab inhibits circulating ANGPTL3. Nevertheless, in animal models both therapies have been found to decrease TG, LDL-C, and HDL-C. Therefore, several clinical trials have been developed to evaluate the effectiveness and safety of these investigational drugs in humans.[53–55]

Evinacumab

Evinacumab is a fully humanized antibody that binds with high-affinity ANGPTL3. Phase I clinical trials have showed that the administration of evinacumab (75–250 mg subcutaneously or 5–20 mg/kg intravenously) to 83 healthy human volunteers with mild-to-moderate hypertriglyceridemia (150–450 mg/dL) or LDL-C greater than or equal to 100 mg/dL was associated with a dose-dependent, placebo-adjusted reduction of TG and LDL-C up to 76% and 23%, respectively.[53–55] Later, evinacumab was tested in a phase II, open-label, proof-of-concept study involving 9 patients with HoFH. HoFH is a rare autosomal dominant genetic disorder causing severe elevation of LDL-C and, consequently, accelerated atherosclerosis.[54,55] Results showed that the addition of evinacumab to background LLT determined in these patients a reduction in LDL-C, TG, and HDL-C levels by about 50%, 47%, and 36%, respectively.[53–55] Given these promising results, the Evinacumab Lipid Study in Patients with Homozygous Familial Hypercholesterolemia (ELIPSE HoFH trial), a phase III, double-blind, placebo-controlled trial, was conducted to assess the efficacy and safety of evinacumab in 65 patients with HoFH selected irrespectively of the molecular diagnosis and background LLT.[53–55] This trial found that monthly administration of evinacumab, in addition to background LLT, reduced LDL-C by 49%. More importantly, the reduction of LDL-C was independent from the residual LDLR activity with patients with HoFH carrying null/null *LDLR* variants exhibiting LDL-C reductions of about 70% compared with placebo.[53–55] The combined safety analysis of placebo-controlled studies showed that the most common adverse reactions (>3% of patients) after 24 weeks of therapy in patients in the evinacumab group versus placebo were nasopharyngitis (16% vs 13%), influenza-like illness (7% vs 6%), dizziness (6% vs 0%), rhinorrhea (5% vs 0%), nausea (5% vs 2%), extremity pain (4% vs 0% placebo), and asthenia (4% vs 0%).[53–55]

Therefore, evinacumab may offer a safe and effective option to significantly ameliorate atherogenic lipoprotein levels, thus possibly reducing cardiovascular events in patients with HoFH. Indeed, the Food and Drug Administration has approved evinacumab (Evkeeza) injection as an add-on treatment of patients with HoFH aged 12 years and older.[56]

Vupanorsen

Vupanorsen (IONIS-ANGPTL3-LRx or AKCEA-ANGPTL3-LRx) is a second-generation Gal-NAc-conjugated ASO targeting ANGPTL3 mRNA.[53,54] The Gal-NAc conjugation specifically directs the ASO to the liver (where ANGPTL3 is exclusively produced), allowing the use of a lower drug dosage, thus possibly preventing the most common adverse effect observed with ASO, namely thrombocytopenia.[57] Vupanorsen was first tested in a randomized, double-blind, placebo-controlled, phase I clinical trial designed to evaluate the safety, side-effect profile, pharmacokinetics, and pharmacodynamics of single ascending doses (N = 12) and multiple ascending doses (N = 32) of ANGPTL3-LRx in healthy adults aged 18 to 65 years.[53,54] Results of this trial indicated that inhibition of hepatic ANGPTL3 led to lowering of TG, LDL VLDL cholesterol, and apoC-III levels.[53,54] Later, a double-blind, placebo-controlled, dose-ranging, phase II study tested this drug in a broader spectrum of subjects (N = 105): (1) with elevated fasting plasma TG levels (>150 mg/dL), (2) type 2 diabetes with HbA1c greater than 6.5% and less than or equal to 10%, (3) hepatic steatosis.[53,54] Patients were treated for 6 months with placebo or vupanorsen at doses of 40 or 80 mg every 4 weeks (Q4W) or 20 mg every week (QW) given subcutaneously. Results of these trials showed that the maximal TG reduction of 53% from baseline was obtained with the 80 mg Q4W regimen and was associated with an LDL-C reduction of about 7%.[53,54] It must be noted that treatment with vupanorsen was not associated with any significant change in platelet count, and the injection site reactions were generally mild.[53,54]

Currently an ongoing phase II single-center, open-label trial is evaluating the efficacy of vupanorsen for triglyceride reduction in participants with familial chylomicronaemia syndrome (NCT03360747), and a phase II, double-blind, placebo-controlled, parallel group study is studying the efficacy, safety, tolerability, and pharmacokinetics of various doses and regimens of vupanorsen in participants with mixed dyslipidemia (NCT04516291).

It seems that there are differences in the LDL-lowering potency between evinacumab and vupanorsen. Further studies are needed to clarify if the strategy used to inhibit ANGPTL3 (mAb vs ASO) or the treatment protocol used (intravenous vs subcutaneous) might be the basis of the differences in lipid-lowering efficacy of these 2 approaches.

Future Perspectives

In the era of precision medicine, innovative therapeutic approaches targeting non-LDLR pathways as ANGPLT3 are currently in development; this includes RNA-based and gene-editing technologies.

siRNA Against ANGPTL3

ANGPTL3-targeted siRNA (ARO-ANG3) is an N-acetylgalactosamine-conjugated RNA silencing (siRNA) investigational therapy targeting ANGPTL3 mRNA.[58] ARO-ANG3 is administered subcutaneously and specifically directed at the liver, where it induces degradation of ANGPLT3 mRNA. Preliminary results of the phase I study in healthy volunteers have been presented at the European Atherosclerosis Society 2020 meeting.[59] The administration of ARO-ANG3 induced dose-dependent silencing of the ANGPTL3 gene, apparently avoiding off-target effects. This treatment was associated with a marked reduction of all lipoprotein fractions comparable to that observed in FHBL2. Indeed, maximal mean reductions in fasting lipid, lipoprotein, and apolipoprotein concentrations were −71% in TG, −50% in LDL-C, −42% in ApoB, −34% in non-HDL-C, and −47% in HDL-C.

In addition, initial results following repeated doses of ARO-ANG3 in 17 patients with HeFH and presenting LDL-C of 130 mg/dL despite intensive LLT, showed a reduction in LDL-C and TG of about 23% to 37% and 25% to 43%, respectively, at all doses.[60]

An ongoing phase II trial is currently recruiting patients with mixed dyslipidemia to assess the efficacy and safety of ARO-ANG3 in this population (NCT04832971).

CRISPR-Cas9 System for Gene Editing

A great interest is growing around CRISPR-based gene editing, which in recent years has emerged as a promising new strategy for treating patients with genetic disorders, including those with atherogenic dyslipidemia.[61,62] DNA strands at the target site are cleaved by an RNA-guided nuclease. When the standard DNA repair system of the cell attempts to repair the DNA, the engineered donor DNA provided by the CRISPR-Cas9 system is inserted into the target site.[55] As compared with ASO or antibody technologies that transiently reduce levels of the targeted protein, the CRISPR-Cas9 gene editing permanently repairs a mutated gene or inserts a missing gene in the edited cells, possibly inducing long-term therapeutic effects.[55,61,62]

Only preliminary studies on mouse models are available to date. Results have shown that both in-vivo adenoviral-mediated[63] and the nonviral lipid nanoparticle–mediated[64] editing of ANGPTL3 are associated with significantly reduced plasma levels of ANGPTL3, TG, and LDL-C.

Although these data are promising, further studies in humans are needed to establish the efficacy, safety, and durability of this method of inhibition of ANGPTL3.[62]

LIPOPROTEIN (A)-LOWERING APPROACHES: ANTISENSE OLIGONUCLEOTIDE AND SMALL INTERFERING RNA AGAINST APOLIPOPROTEIN (A)

Apolipoprotein B100 (apoB) containing lipoproteins are key players in atherogenesis and contribute causally to cardiovascular disease.[65] The apoB concentration in plasma is an excellent marker of cardiovascular risk.[66] Lp(a) is an apoB-containing lipoprotein bound to a hydrophilic, highly glycosylated protein called apolipoprotein (a) [apo(a)][67,68] (see Wann Jia Loh and Gerald F. Watts' article, "The Inherited Hypercholesterolemias," in this issue).

Epidemiologic, genome-wide association, and Mendelian randomization data[69–73] clearly demonstrate a causal role for Lp(a) in the development of ASCVD. To date, however, the definitive proof that specific interventions lowering Lp(a) reduce the risk of cardiovascular outcomes is missing. Still, some clinicians have a secondary goal of lowering Lp(a) in addition to lowering LDL-C and apoB in high-risk patients, in particular when recurrent ASCVD events occur despite aggressive LDL-C lowering.

Results from studies of dietary intervention show very modest effects on Lp(a) levels.[74] The most effective clinically available intervention for Lp(a) lowering is lipoprotein apheresis where the Lp(a) concentration is acutely lowered by approximately 50% to 85%, in association with comparable reductions in oxidized phospholipids. In addition to lowering Lp(a), lipoprotein apheresis with some systems also lowers LDL concentrations by 60% to 85%.[75,76] Limited clinical trial data suggest that Lp(a) lowering with lipoprotein apheresis may reduce the risk of ASCVD events,[77] but definitive studies are needed.

Currently available LDL-C lowering treatments have minor effects on Lp(a), with statins slightly increasing Lp(a) levels.[1,78] Data from trials of monoclonal antibodies directed against PCSK9 demonstrate dramatic LDL-C lowering by an average of 50% to 60% but a modest Lp(a)-lowering of 25% to 30%. The results of a recent analysis suggest that alirocumab-mediated Lp(a)-lowering independently contributed to major adverse cardiovascular event reduction.[79] Moreover, in patients with recent acute coronary syndrome on optimal statin therapy and LDL-C less than 70 mg/dL, alirocumab only lowered major adverse cardiovascular events in patients with mildly elevated (>13.7 mg/dL) Lp(a); there was no such interaction between Lp(a) levels and alirocumab benefit when LDL-C was greater than or equal to 70 mg/dL.[80] How to interpret these data remains difficult, given the multiple tests and the difficulties in knowing the contribution of Lp(a) cholesterol to the measurement of LDL cholesterol in subjects with high Lp(a) and low LDL. Niacin may dose-dependently lower Lp(a) up to 25% to 40%, but the cardiovascular benefit of this intervention is unknown, and the adverse side-effect profile of niacin in the setting of statins is a concern.[81,82]

Several experimental therapies targeting the apo(a) moiety of Lp(a) are under development.

Two mendelian randomization analyses aimed at estimating the extent of Lp(a) reduction required to observe a clinical benefit showed that large absolute reductions in Lp(a) levels (70–100 mg/dL) may be required to show a CHD risk reduction comparable to that observed with a 1 mmol/L ($\approx$ 39 mg/dL) LDL-C reduction.[83,84] Such large reduction cannot be achieved with conventional LLT but requires RNA therapeutics targeting selectively the hepatic synthesis of apo(a), which are currently under development. An ASO targeting apo(a) mRNA was shown to reduce Lp(a) by up to 80% at the highest dose (corresponding to ≈190 nmol/L, or 75 mg/dL) in patients with elevated Lp(a) levels,[85] with 98% of subjects treated with the ASO reaching on-treatment Lp(a) levels less than 125 nmol/L (<50 mg/dL). The ongoing phase 3 Lp(a) HORIZON outcomes trial will evaluate the effect of the ASO against apo(a) mRNA or placebo in patients after myocardial infarction with high levels of Lp(a).[86] The primary outcome is the time to the first occurrence of major ASCVD events in patients with Lp(a) greater than or equal to 70 mg/dL or greater than or equal to 90 mg/dL; the estimated completion date is June 2022.

Olpasiran is an siRNA designed to reduce the production of Lp(a) by targeting messenger RNA transcription. In a Phase I study (https://clinicaltrials.gov/ct2/show/record/NCT03626662), the safety, tolerability, pharmacokinetics (PK), and pharmacodynamics of olpasiran was evaluated. Adults with plasma concentrations at screening of Lp(a) greater than or equal to 70 to less than or equal to 199 nmol/L (cohorts 1 5) or greater than or equal to 200 nmol/L (cohorts 6 7) were randomized 3:1 to receive a single subcutaneous dose of olpasiran or placebo. The primary endpoints were treatment emergent AEs, safety laboratory analytes, vital signs, and electrocardiograms. Secondary endpoints included PK parameters and percent change from baseline in Lp(a). In olpasiran-allocated subjects, no safety concerns nor clinically relevant changes in liver or renal tests, platelets, or coagulation parameters were identified. In adults with elevated Lp(a) (median Lp(a) = 122 nmol/L [cohorts 1–5] and 253 nmol/L [cohorts 6 and 7]), a single dose of olpasiran significantly reduced Lp(a) with observed approximate median percent reductions of greater than 90% at doses of greater than or equal to 9 mg in a dose-dependent manner. The response persisted for 3 to 6 months at doses of greater than or equal to 9 mg. A phase II study is currently evaluating the efficacy, safety, and tolerability of an N-acetylgalactosamine–conjugated siRNA in 240 subjects with Lp(a) greater than 60 mg/dL (>150 nmol/L) (https://clinicaltrials.gov/ct2/show/record/NCT04270760).[87]

SUMMARY

In conclusion, despite national and international guideline recommendations to use statins as the first-line lipid therapy for ASCVD prevention, clinically relevant residual ASCVD risk, as observed in our daily clinical practice, emphasizes the need for additional therapies. Emerging agents offer options for further LDL-C reduction as well as alternative targets including TG and TG-rich lipoproteins, Lp(a), and inflammation. The clinical benefits in terms of ASCVD are being studied in ongoing clinical trials, including large outcomes studies. Combining many of these strategies will likely improve ASCVD outcomes, highlighting the role of health care professionals in selecting the correct patient population for each treatment modality to maximize benefits with the fewest medications and low sustainable costs.

CLINICS CARE POINTS

- In ASCVD and ASCVD risk equivalent patients Inclisiran is effective and safe in reducing LDL-C up to 50%
- In HeFH patients Inclisiran 300 mg s.c results in a durable reduction of LDL-C

- The efficacy of Inclisiran in reducing the cardiovascular outcomes will be highlighted by the results of the ORION-4 and VICTORION-2 Trials

- Pemafibrate, a selective PPARa modulator (SPPARM) is a "next generation" fibrate characterized by an enhanced potency as TG-lowering agent and greater safety profile compared to traditional non-selective PPARa agonists

- The presence of severe, resistant hypertriglyceridemia is suggestive of familial chylomicronemia syndrome

- The concomitant presence of low cholesterol and reduced HDL-C is suggestive of familial combined hypolipidemia (FHBL2)

- Evinacumab, a fully humanized mAb against ANGPTL3, may offer a safe and effective option to significantly decrease LDL-C and thus possibly reducing cardiovascular events in patients with HoFH independently of the residual LDL receptor activity

- Lp(a) is causal for CVD: the absolute weight of elevated plasma levels and the extent of Lp(a) reduction required to achieve a significant benefit are unknown

- Antisense oligonucleotide targeting apo(a) mRNA and small interfering RNA designed to reduce the production of Lp(a), represent the first specific and highly effective pharmacological approaches reducing plasma Lp(a) up to 80-85%.

REFERENCES

1. Hoogeveen RC, Ballantyne CM. Residual Cardiovascular Risk at Low LDL: Remnants, Lipoprotein(a), and Inflammation. Clin Chem 2021;67(1):143–53.
2. Kathiresan S. Developing medicines that mimic the natural successes of the human genome: lessons from NPC1L1, HMGCR, PCSK9, APOC3, and CETP. J Am Coll Cardiol 2015;65:1562–6.
3. Mach F, Baigent C, et al. 2019 ESC/EAS Guidelines for the management of dyslipidaemias: lipid modification to reduce cardiovascular risk. Eur Heart J 2020; 41(1):111–88.
4. Seidah NG, et al. The secretory proprotein convertase neural apoptosis-regulated convertase 1 (NARC-1): Liver regeneration and neuronal differentiation. Proc Natl Acad Sci USA 2003;100:928–33.
5. Cohen JC, et al. Sequence variations in PCSK9, low LDL, and protection against coronary heart disease. N Engl J Med 2006;354:1264–72.
6. Preis D, et al. Lipid-Modifying Agents,From Statins to PCSK9 Inhibitors. Am Coll Cardiol 2020;75:1945–55.
7. Nair JK, et al. Multivalent N-acetylgalactosamine-conjugated siRNA localizes in hepatocytes and elicits robust RNAi-mediated gene silencing. J Am Chem Soc 2014;136:16958–61.
8. Frank-Kamenetsky M, et al. Therapeutic RNAi targeting PCSK9 acutely lowers plasma cholesterol in rodents and LDL cholesterol in nonhuman primates. Proc Natl Acad Sci U.S.A 2008;105:11915–20.
9. Fitzgerald K, et al. Effect of an RNA interference drug on the synthesis of proprotein convertase subtilisin/kexin type9 (PCSK9) and the concentration of serum LDL cholesterol in healthy volunteers: A randomized, single-blind, placebo-controlled, phase 1 trial. Lancet 2014;383:60–8.
10. Fitzgerald K, et al. A Highly Durable RNAi Therapeutic Inhibitor of PCSK9. N Engl J Med 2017;376:41–51.
11. Henney NC, et al. RNA Silencing in the Management of Dyslipidemias. Curr Atheroscler Rep 2021;23:69.

12. Scott Wright R, et al. Pooled Patient-Level Analysis of Inclisiran Trials in Patients With Familial Hypercholesterolemia or Atherosclerosis. Am Coll Cardiol 2021;77: 1182–93.
13. Ray KK, Wright RS, Kallend D, et al. Two Phase 3 Trials of Inclisiran in Patients with Elevated LDL Cholesterol. NEJM 2020;382:1507–19.
14. NCT03705234 Available at: https://www.clinicaltrials.gov/ct2/show/NCT03705234. Accessed October 20, 2021.
15. NCT04929249 Available at: https://www.clinicaltrials.gov/ct2/show/NCT05030428. Accessed October 20, 2021.
16. Laufs U, Parhofer KG, Ginsberg HN, et al. Clinical review on triglycerides. Eur Heart J 2020;41:99–109.
17. Quispe R, Martin SS, Michos ED, et al. Remnant cholesterol predicts cardiovascular disease beyond LDL and ApoB: a primary prevention study. Eur Heart J 2021;42:4324–32.
18. Fruchart JC, Duriez P, Staels B. Peroxisome proliferator-activated receptor alpha activators regulate genes governing lipoprotein metabolism, vascular inflammation and atherosclerosis. Curr Opin Lipidol 1999;10:245–57.
19. Gervois P, Fruchart JC, Staels B. Drug Insight: mechanisms of action and therapeutic applications for agonists of peroxisome proliferator-activated receptors. Nat Clin Pract Endocrinol Metabol 2007;3:14556.
20. Keech A, Simes RJ, Barter P, et al. Effects of long-term fenofibrate therapy on cardiovascular events in 9795 people with type 2 diabetes mellitus (the FIELD study): randomized controlled trial. Lancet 2005;366(9500):1849–61.
21. ACCORD Study Group, Ginsberg HN, Elam MB, Lovato LC, et al. Effects of combination lipid therapy in type 2 diabetes mellitus. N Engl J Med 2010;362: 1563e74.
22. Sairyo M, Kobayashi T, Masuda D, et al. A novel selective PPAR Modulator (SPPARM), K-877 (pemafibrate), attenuates postprandial hypertriglyceridemia in mice. J Atheroscler Thromb 2018;25:142–52.
23. Raza-Iqbal S, Tanaka T, Anai M, et al. Transcriptome analysis of K-877 (a novel Selective PPARα Modulator (SPPARMα))-regulated genes in primary human hepatocytes and the mouse liver. J Atheroscler Thromb 2015;22:754–72.
24. Maki T, Maeda Y, Sonoda N, et al. Renoprotective effect of a novel selective PPARα modulator K-877 in db/db mice: a role of diacylglycerol-protein kinase C-NAD(P)H oxidase pathway. Metabolism 2017;71:33–45.
25. Ishibashi S, Yamashita S, Arai H, et al. Effects of K-877, a novel selective PPARα modulator (SPPARMα), in dyslipidaemic patients: a randomized, double blind, active- and placebo controlled,phase 2 trial. Atherosclerosis 2016;249:36–43.
26. Yokote K, Yamashita S, Arai H, et al. A pooled analysis of pemafibrate Phase II/III clinical trials indicated significant improvement in glycemic and liver function-related parameters. Atheroscler Suppl 2018;32:155.
27. Pradhan AD, Paynter NP, Everett BM, et al. Rationale and design of the pemafibrate to Reduce Cardiovascular Outcomes by Reducing Triglycerides in Patients with Diabetes (PROMINENT) study. Am Heart J 2018;206:80–93.
28. PROMINENT-Eye Ancillary Study (Protocol AD). ClinicalTrials.gov IdentifierNCT03345901. https://clinicaltrials.gov/ct2/show/NCT03345901. Accessed 7 Aug 2018.
29. Bhatt DL, Steg PG, Miller M, et al. Cardiovascular risk reduction with icosapent ethyl for hypertriglyceridemia. N Engl J Med 2019;380(1):11–22.
30. Crosby J, Peloso GM, Auer PL, et al. TG and HDL Working Group of the Exome Sequencing Project, National Heart, Lung, and Blood Institute. Loss-of-function

mutations in APOC3, triglycerides, and coronary disease. N Engl J Med 2014; 371(1):22–31.

31. Norata GD, Tsimikas S, Pirillo A, et al. Apolipoprotein C-III: from pathophysiology to pharmacology. Trends Pharmacol Sci 2015;36:675–87.

32. D'Erasmo L, Gallo A, Di Costanzo A, et al. Evaluation of efficacy and safety of antisense inhibition of apolipoprotein C-III with volanesorsen in patients with severe hypertriglyceridemia. Expert Opin Pharmacother 2020;21(14):1675–84.

33. Chait A, Brunzell JD. Chylomicronemia syndrome. Adv Intern Med 1992;37: 249–73.

34. Gaudet D, Brisson D, Tremblay K, et al. Targeting APOC3 in the familial chylomicronemia syndrome. N Engl J Med 2014;371(23):2200–6.

35. Yang X, Lee SR, Choi YS, et al. Reduction in lipoprotein-associated apoC-III levels following volanesorsen therapy: phase 2 randomized trial results. J Lipid Res 2016;57(4):706–13.

36. Gaudet D, Alexander VJ, Baker BF, et al. Antisense inhibition of apolipoprotein C-III in patients with hypertriglyceridemia. N Engl J Med 2015;373:438–47.

37. Digenio A, Dunbar RL, Alexander VJ, et al. Antisense-mediated lowering of plasma apolipoprotein C-III by volanesorsen improves dyslipidemia and insulin sensitivity in type 2 diabetes. Diabetes Care 2016;39(8):1408–15.

38. Gaudet D, Digenio A, Alexander VJ, et al. The APPROACH study: a randomized double-blind placebo-controlled, phase 3 study of volanesorsen administered subcutaneously to patients with FCS. Athero Suppl 2017;263:e10.

39. Gouni-Berthold I, Alexander V, Digenio A, et al. Apolipoprotein C-III Inhibition with volanesorsen in patients with hypertriglyceridemia (COMPASS): a randomized, double-blind, placebo-controlled trial. Athero Suppl 2017;28:e1–2.

40. Alexander VJ, Digenio A, Xia S, et al. Inhibition of apolipoprotein C-III with GalNac conjugated antisense drug potently lowes fasting serum apolipoprotein C-III and triglyceride levels in healthy volunteers with elevated triglycerides. J Am Coll Cardiol 2018;71:A1724.

41. The BROADEN study: a study of volanesorsen (Formerly ISIS-APOCIIIRx) in patients with familial partial lipodystrophy. Available at: https://clinicaltrials.gov/ct2/show/NCT02527343.

42. European Medicines Agency. 2018. Available at: https://www.ema.europa.eu/en/medicines/human/EPAR/waylivra. Accessed November 19, 2021.

43. Butler AA, Price GA, Graham JL, et al. Fructose-induced hypertriglyceridemia in rhesus macaques is attenuated with fish oil or ApoC3 RNA interference. J Lipid Res 2019;60:805–18.

44. Arca M, D'Erasmo L, Minicocci I. Familial combined hypolipidemia: angiopoietin-like protein-3 deficiency. Curr Opin Lipidol 2020;31(2):41–8.

45. Bini S, D'Erasmo L, Di Costanzo A, et al. The Interplay between Angiopoietin-Like Proteins and Adipose Tissue: Another Piece of the Relationship between Adiposopathy and Cardiometabolic Diseases? Int J Mol Sci 2021;22(2):742.

46. Kathiresan S, Melander O, Guiducci C, et al. Six new loci associated with blood low-density lipoprotein cholesterol, high-density lipoprotein cholesterol or triglycerides in humans. Nat Genet 2008;40(2):189–97. Erratum in: Nat Genet. 2008 Nov;40(11):1384.

47. Musunuru K, Pirruccello JP, Do R, et al. Exome sequencing, ANGPTL3 mutations, and familial combined hypolipidemia. N Engl J Med 2010;363(23):2220–7.

48. Minicocci I, Montali A, Robciuc MR, et al. Mutations in the ANGPTL3 gene and familial combined hypolipidemia: a clinical and biochemical characterization. J Clin Endocrinol Metab 2012;97(7):E1266–75.

49. Minicocci I, Santini S, Cantisani V, et al. Clinical characteristics, and plasma lipids in subjects with familial combined hypolipidemia: a pooled analysis. J Lipid Res 2013;54(12):3481–90.

50. Minicocci I, Tikka A, Poggiogalle E, et al. Effects of angiopoietin-like protein 3 deficiency on postprandial lipid and lipoprotein metabolism. J Lipid Res 2016; 57(6):1097–107.

51. Tikkanen E, Minicocci I, Hällfors J, et al. Metabolomic Signature of Angiopoietin-Like Protein 3 Deficiency in Fasting and Postprandial State. Arterioscler Thromb Vasc Biol 2019;39(4):665–74.

52. Ruhanen H, Haridas PAN, Minicocci I, et al. ANGPTL3 deficiency alters the lipid profile and metabolism of cultured hepatocytes and human lipoproteins. Biochim Biophys Acta Mol Cell Biol Lipids 2020;1865(7):158679.

53. Kersten S. ANGPTL3 as therapeutic target. Curr Opin Lipidol 2021;32(6):335–41.

54. D'Erasmo L, Bini S, Arca M. Rare Treatments for Rare Dyslipidemias: New Perspectives in the Treatment of Homozygous Familial Hypercholesterolemia (HoFH) and Familial Chylomicronemia Syndrome (FCS). Curr Atheroscler Rep 2021;23(11):65.

55. Cesaro A, Fimiani F, Gragnano F, et al. New Frontiers in the Treatment of Homozygous Familial Hypercholesterolemia. Heart Failure Clin 2022;18(1):177–88.

56. Available at: https://www.fda.gov/drugs/news-events-human-drugs/fda-approves-add-therapy-patients-genetic-form-severely-high-cholesterol-0. Accessed 17 November 2021.

57. Debacker AJ, Voutila J, Catley M, et al. Delivery of Oligonucleotides to the Liver with GalNAc: From Research to Registered Therapeutic Drug. Mol Ther 2020; 28(8):1759–71.

58. Ruotsalainen AK, Mäkinen P, Ylä-Herttuala S. Novel RNAi-Based Therapies for Atherosclerosis. Curr Atheroscler Rep 2021;23(8):45.

59. Available at: https://doi.org/10.1093/ehjci/ehaa946.3331. Accessed November 19, 2021.

60. Available at: https://doi.org/10.1161/circ.142.suppl_3.15751. Accessed November 19, 2021.

61. Sander JD, Joung JK. CRISPR-Cas systems for editing, regulating and targeting genomes. Nat Biotechnol 2014;32(4):347–55.

62. Behr M, Zhou J, Xu B, et al. In vivo delivery of CRISPR-Cas9 therapeutics: Progress and challenges. Acta Pharm Sin B 2021;11(8):2150–71.

63. Chadwick AC, Evitt NH, Lv W, et al. Reduced Blood Lipid Levels With In Vivo CRISPR-Cas9 Base Editing of ANGPTL3. Circulation 2018;137(9):975–7.

64. Qiu M, Glass Z, Chen J, et al. Lipid nanoparticle-mediated codelivery of Cas9 mRNA and single-guide RNA achieves liver-specific in vivo genome editing of Angptl3. Proc Natl Acad Sci U S A 2021;118(10). https://doi.org/10.1073/pnas. 2020401118. e2020401118.

65. Sniderman AD, Thanassoulis G, Glavinovic T, et al. Apolipoprotein B Particles and Cardiovascular Disease: A Narrative Review. JAMA Cardiol 2019;4:1287–95.

66. Grundy SM, Stone NJ. Elevated apolipoprotein B as a risk-enhancing factor in 2018 cholesterol guidelines. J Clin Lipidol 2019;13:356–9.

67. Berg K. A New Serum Type System in Man–the Lp System. Acta Pathol Microbiol Scand 1963;59:369–82.

68. Kostner KM, Kostner GM. Lipoprotein (a): a historical appraisal. J Lipid Res 2017; 58:1–14.

69. Erqou S, Kaptoge S, Perry PL, et al. Lipoprotein(a) concentration and the risk of coronary heart disease, stroke, and nonvascular mortality. Jama 2009;302:412–23.

70. Bennet A, Di Angelantonio E, Erqou S, et al. Lipoprotein(a) levels and risk of future coronary heart disease: large-scale prospective data. Arch Intern Med 2008;168:598–608.

71. Afshar M, Kamstrup PR, Williams K, et al. Estimating the Population Impact of Lp(a) Lowering on the Incidence of Myocardial Infarction and Aortic Stenosis-Brief Report. Arterioscler Thromb Vasc Biol 2016;36:2421–3.

72. Saleheen D, Haycock PC, Zhao W, et al. Apolipoprotein(a) isoform size, lipoprotein(a) concentration, and coronary artery disease: a mendelian randomisation analysis. Lancet Diabetes Endocrinol 2017;5:524–33.

73. Clarke R, Peden JF, Hopewell JC, et al. Genetic variants associated with Lp(a) lipoprotein level and coronary disease. N Engl J Med 2009;361:2518–28.

74. Enkhmaa B, Petersen KS, Kris-Etherton PM, et al. Diet and Lp(a): Does Dietary Change Modify Residual Cardiovascular Risk Conferred by Lp(a)? Nutrients 2020;12.

75. Waldmann E, Parhofer KG. Lipoprotein apheresis to treat elevated lipoprotein (a). J Lipid Res 2016;57:1751–7.

76. Pokrovsky SN, Afanasieva OI, Ezhov MV. Therapeutic Apheresis for Management of Lp(a) Hyperlipoproteinemia. Curr Atheroscler Rep 2020;22:68.

77. Roeseler E, Julius U, Heigl F, et al. Lipoprotein Apheresis for Lipoprotein(a)-Associated Cardiovascular Disease: Prospective 5 Years of Follow-Up and Apolipoprotein(a) Characterization. Arterioscler Thromb Vasc Biol 2016;36:2019–27.

78. Fras Z. Increased cardiovascular risk associated with hyperlipoproteinemia (a) and the challenges of current and future therapeutic possibilities. Anatol J Cardiol 2020;23:60–9.

79. Bittner VA, Szarek M, Aylward PE, et al. Effect of Alirocumab on Lipoprotein(a) and Cardiovascular Risk After Acute Coronary Syndrome. J Am Coll Cardiol 2020;75:133–44.

80. Schwartz GG, Szarek M, Bittner VA, et al. Lipoprotein(a) and Benefit of PCSK9 Inhibition in Patients With Nominally Controlled LDL Cholesterol. J Am Coll Cardiol 2021;78:421–33.

81. Landray MJ, Haynes R, Hopewell JC, et al. Effects of extended-release niacin with laropiprant in high-risk patients. N Engl J Med 2014;371:203–12.

82. Albers JJ, Slee A, O'Brien KD, et al. Relationship of apolipoproteins A-1 and B, and lipoprotein(a) to cardiovascular outcomes: the AIM-HIGH trial (Atherothrombosis Intervention in Metabolic Syndrome with Low HDL/High Triglyceride and Impact on Global Health Outcomes). J Am Coll Cardiol 2013;62:1575–9.

83. Burgess S, Ference BA, Staley JR, et al. Association of LPA variants with risk of coronary disease and the implications for lipoprotein(a)-lowering therapies: a Mendelian randomization analysis. JAMA Cardiol 2018;3:619–27.

84. Lamina C, Kronenberg F, Lp GC. Estimation of the Required Lipoprotein(a)-Lowering Therapeutic Effect Size for Reduction in Coronary Heart Disease Outcomes: A Mendelian Randomization Analysis. JAMA Cardiol 2019;4:575–9.

85. Tsimikas S, Karwatowska-Prokopczuk E, Gouni-Berthold I, et al. Lipoprotein(a) Reduction in Persons with Cardiovascular Disease. N Engl J Med 2020;382:244–55.

86. Tsimikas S, Moriarty PM, Stroes ES. Emerging RNA Therapeutics to Lower Blood Levels of Lp(a) 2021. J Am Coll Cardiol 2021;77:1576–89.

87. Available at: https://clinicaltrials.gov/ct2/show/record/NCT04270760. Accessed on November 21, 2021.

LDL Cholesterol—How Low Can We Go?

Jonathan A. Tobert, MD, PhD

KEYWORDS

- LDL cholesterol • Hypocholesterolemia • Guidelines • Safety
- Cardiovascular risk reduction

KEY POINTS

- Most if not all mammalian nucleated cells can produce cholesterol, so LDL particles are needed only to recycle it.
- Normal human newborns have very low LDL cholesterol, showing that it is physiologic.
- Randomized controlled trials have shown that lowering LDL cholesterol below 70 mg/dL reduces the risk of atherosclerotic vascular events with minimal adverse effects.
- There is no known threshold below which lowering LDL cholesterol is harmful.
- Reducing LDL cholesterol below 40 mg/dL is often feasible with combination therapy and can be considered in patients who have had 2 or more major vascular events, but below 25 mg/dL further reduction may provide little if any further benefit.

INTRODUCTION

Forty years ago, 300 mg/dL was generally considered the upper limit of normal for total plasma cholesterol in Western countries. In that era, the risks associated with high concentrations of plasma and low-density lipoprotein cholesterol (LDL-C) were only beginning to be appreciated and were vigorously debated, so the normal range was based on population statistics, not biology. In 1984, an NIH Consensus Conference concluded that lowering elevated LDL-C with diet and drugs would reduce the risk of coronary heart disease (CHD). Efforts to educate physicians and the public about the importance of treating hypercholesterolemia followed. However, the effectiveness of diet and the available drugs was limited. The 1987 introduction of lovastatin, the first statin, was a radical advance. Lovastatin is generally well tolerated and could produce a 40% mean reduction in LDL-C at its maximal dose, and subsequently atorvastatin and rosuvastatin expanded that to about 55%. The cholesterol absorption inhibitor

This article originally appeared in *Endocrinology and Metabolism Clinics*, Volume 51, Issue 3, September 2022.
Nuffield Department of Population Health, University of Oxford, Richard Doll Building, Old Road Campus, Oxford OX3 7LF, UK
E-mail address: jonathan.tobert@cantab.net

Abbreviation	
LDL	low-density lipoprotein

ezetimibe, introduced in 2001, lowers LDL-C by a further 20% when added to a statin. From 2015 onwards, adding a PCSK9 inhibitor to high-intensity statin treatment (atorvastatin or rosuvastatin at maximal or near-maximal doses) with or without ezetimibe made possible the reduction of LDL-C to well below 1 mmol/L (38.7 mg/dL) in many patients.

Doubts about the value of lowering LDL-C, and the safety of doing so, were largely quenched in 1994 with the publication of the Scandinavian Simvastatin Survival Study (4S), in which a 30% reduction in total mortality ($P = .0003$) was demonstrated.[1] The 25 years that followed saw a steady stream of large-scale randomized controlled trials (RCTs) of statins and other lipid-modifying agents,[2] including those mentioned earlier, which collectively showed that the reduction in the risk of myocardial infarction and ischemic stroke, and other atherosclerotic events, was proportional to the absolute reduction in LDL-C, with a reduction of 1 mmol/L ($\sim$ 40 mg/dL) producing an average reduction in risk of 22%.[2] The PCSK9 monoclonal antibodies alirocumab and evolocumab, introduced in 2015, lower LDL-C by about 50% when added to a statin. This has created a new question: is there any level of LDL-C below which reducing it does not produce any worthwhile cardiovascular risk reduction and/or creates an unacceptable increase in adverse effects[3,4]?

In cardiovascular outcome trials with both alirocumab[5] and evolocumab[6] compared to placebo on a background of statin therapy, the mean on-treatment value of LDL-C was around 40 mg/dL ($\sim$ 1 mmol/L). Neither study raised any safety concerns. Indeed, current European guidelines[7] suggest 1 mmol/L ($\sim$ 40 mg/dL) as the target of treatment in patients who have suffered 2 or more major atherosclerotic events.

CHOLESTEROL TRANSPORT

Very low-density lipoprotein (VLDL) is synthesized in the liver and released into the circulation to transport triglycerides and fat-soluble vitamins to tissues. VLDL particles also contain liver-derived esterified cholesterol, which stabilizes them. Lipoprotein lipase liberates fatty acids from triglycerides in VLDL and chylomicrons, thus converting VLDL into remnant lipoproteins and subsequently LDL. Cholesterol is required for the formation of cell membranes and bile acids, and for steroidogenesis, but nucleated mammalian cells can synthesize cholesterol from acetate.[8] Intricate control mechanisms enable cells to synthesize cholesterol when it is depleted.[8,9] But circulating LDL can penetrate the vascular endothelium, which may lead to atherosclerotic lesions and eventually serious outcomes, including myocardial infarction and ischemic stroke. A high concentration of LDL particles is the primary cause of atherosclerosis.

LDL is what remains after most of the triglyceride in VLDL particles has been lipolyzed. Thus, LDL is essentially a byproduct. Removal of LDL from the circulation is accomplished predominantly by the LDL receptors on the surface of hepatocytes, which bind the apolipoprotein B component of LDL. LDL is then taken up mostly into the liver but also peripheral tissues, and the apolipoprotein B it contains is catabolized, while the cholesterol is either recycled into VLDL, used for steroidogenesis and to produce bile acids, or incorporated into cell membranes. Some cholesterol is excreted in the bile, and enterohepatic recirculation returns most intestinal cholesterol to the liver via chylomicrons. Dietary cholesterol is superfluous, as indicated by the health of vegans. A simplified diagram of these pathways is shown in **Fig. 1**,

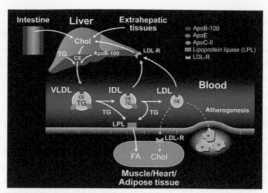

Fig. 1. A simplified diagram of cholesterol transport. (*From* Feingold KR. Introduction to Lipids and Lipoproteins. [Updated 2021 Jan 19]. In: Feingold KR, Anawalt B, Boyce A, et al., editors. Endotext [Internet]. South Dartmouth (MA): MDText.com, Inc.; 2000-. https://www.ncbi.nlm.nih.gov/books/NBK305896/. 2021).

reproduced from Feingold,[10] and Kenneth R Feingold's article, "Lipid and Lipoprotein Metabolism," in this issue provides in-depth information beyond the scope of this article, as do Goldstein and Brown,[8] who led much of the effort to work out these pathways. In this article, very low LDL-C is somewhat arbitrarily defined as a concentration less than 40 mg/dL (1 mmol/L). The conversion factor is 38.7, approximated to 40 in the case of 1 mmol/L. When this article cites the work of authors who use the SI system, SI values are provided with traditional units in parentheses.

Cholesterol is an essential component of mammalian cell membranes, and nucleated cells have the capacity to synthesize it.[8] Because LDL has no essential function other than recycling cholesterol back to the liver,[8,9] very low LDL-C—defined here as less than 40 mg/dL (approximately 1 mmol/L)—should be compatible with health, as long as the other components of the lipidome are within normal limits. This should be true regardless of whether very low LDL-C is the result of normal physiology, or mutations that are associated with these very low levels, or is reduced to very low levels by drug treatment. We shall examine in turn each of these 3 components of the hypothesis that very low LDL-C is not harmful.

LOW CHOLESTEROL STATES
Neonatal Human Physiology

It has long been known that LDL-C concentrations are much lower in neonates than in young children or adults. For example, Khoury and colleagues[11] reported mean LDL-C in 122 cord blood samples of 23 mg/dL with a standard deviation of 10 mg/dL, indicating that about one-third of the newborns had LDL-C at or below 13 mg/dL (0.34 mmol/L). Plasma triglycerides and apolipoprotein B were also much lower than in children or adults. This very low level of LDL-C is compatible with the rapid growth of the near-term fetus because, as previously mentioned, mammalian nucleated cells are capable of cholesterol biosynthesis; in particular, the large quantities of cholesterol required for fetal cerebral development are produced within the brain. VLDL production appears to be minimal in the intrauterine environment, in which nutrients are supplied via the placenta and not the gastrointestinal system, so that few LDL particles are formed. Concentrations of LDL-C, triglycerides, and apolipoprotein B rise rapidly in the days following birth,[11] when the infant must process breast milk and later solid food.

Mutations

Mutations of the LDL receptor have been a key resource in the elucidation of the mechanisms that control circulating levels of LDL. Homozygosity for loss of function LDL receptor mutations prevents receptor-mediated uptake of LDL into hepatocytes and other cells, leading to LDL-C concentrations of 500 mg/dL or higher. This condition, homozygous familial hypercholesterolemia (FH), is found in approximately one in a million individuals, whereas heterozygous FH occurs in about one in 300 and typically leads to untreated LDL-C levels of 250 mg/dL or higher. If untreated, patients with homozygous FH frequently succumb as children or adolescents due to myocardial infarctions and other atherosclerotic events, whereas in untreated heterozygous FH, these events typically occur in midlife. The lethality of homozygous FH in children, who have no other risk factors for atherosclerosis, was strong evidence for the pathogenicity of LDL-C and the physiologic requirement for pathways to control it. Elucidation of the LDL receptor control mechanisms[12] led to the award of the 1985 Nobel Prize in Physiology or Medicine to Michael Brown and Joseph Goldstein.

Mutations that are associated with low LDL-C concentrations have been useful but have not led to such clear-cut results. Familial hypobetalipoproteinemia[13] generally results from mutant alleles coding for apolipoprotein B that disrupt the production of VLDL, the precursor of LDL-C. Plasma concentrations of LDL-C fall to around 30 mg/dL. Although most patients with heterozygous mutant alleles are generally healthy, they are at risk of fatty liver, chronic diarrhea, steatorrhea, and deficiency of fat-soluble vitamins.[14] However, all apolipoprotein B containing lipoproteins are depleted, not just LDL, so the relevance of familial hypobetalipoproteinemia to the question at hand is limited.

Heterozygous genetic variants that cause loss of function of PCSK9 have a frequency of 2% to 3% in the United States and are associated with moderate reductions of LDL-C, not large enough to bring LDL-C down to very low levels.[15] Nevertheless, these variants have a disproportionately large beneficial effect on the risk of CHD, presumably because the LDL-C reduction is lifelong, in contrast to a few years in cardiovascular outcome trials. Reports of individuals homozygous for PCSK9 loss of function mutations are minimal. Details of one subject with undetectable circulating PCSK9 were published in 2006.[16] Genetic analysis indicated that she was a compound heterozygote with 2 loss-of-function PCSK9 mutant alleles. At that time, she was an apparently healthy, fertile, college-educated African-American woman who worked as an aerobics instructor. Liver and renal function tests were normal. Her LDL-C was 14 mg/dL, whereas HDL-cholesterol and triglycerides were well within the normal range. Another subject with very low LDL-C, 0.4 mmol/L (15 mg/dL), and homozygosity for the C679X loss-of-function variant was found in a study of 653 women attending antenatal clinics in Zimbabwe[17]; further details have not been published. Identifying and where possible studying more subjects who are homozygotes or compound heterozygotes for loss-of-function variants would be of great interest; but if such individuals are not only very rare but also typically healthy, and have a very low rate of CHD and other atherosclerotic events later in life,[15] they are unlikely to come to the attention of geneticists or lipid specialists.

Studies of PCSK9 human genetics, therefore, suggest that this enzyme is not essential for health. The apparent normality of PCSK9-knockout mice is consistent with this conclusion.[18] The implication is that the very low levels of LDL-C that follow from the absence of PCSK9 are compatible with health, at least in a well-nourished population under contemporary conditions. Possibly under earlier evolutionary conditions there might have been a greater need for PCSK9, which serves as an additional regulator of cholesterol homeostasis.

Drug Treatment

As with all drugs, the adverse effects of lipid-lowering drugs are dose-related, but there is no evidence that these are augmented at low achieved LDL-C concentrations. For example, cerivastatin was removed from the market in 2001 because of a much higher frequency of rhabdomyolysis compared with other statins,[19] particularly when taken with concomitant gemfibrozil. But cerivastatin was a moderate efficacy statin, reducing LDL-C by only about 40% on average at the maximal 0.8 mg dose, and target LDL-C levels were less aggressive than today. In contrast, the most commonly used statin, atorvastatin, reduces LDL-C by about 55% at its maximal dose and it rarely causes rhabdomyolysis.

Statins are the bedrock of lipid-lowering therapy. The most effective statins, atorvastatin and rosuvastatin, produce a mean reduction in LDL-C of about 55%, which is not usually sufficient to lower LDL-C much below 70 mg/dL when used as monotherapy. However, the addition of monoclonal antibodies against PCSK9, alirocumab or evolocumab, or the small interfering RNA inclisiran,[20] that blocks PCSK9 transcription, will often reduce LDL-C below 40 mg/dL. The adverse effects of statins and the safety of the LDL-C reductions produced have been a subject of intense interest for many years. However, the currently marketed statins have a history going back to 1987 and an excellent safety profile,[21] as discussed in Connie B. Newman's article, "Safety of Statins and Non-Statins for Treatment of Dyslipidemia," in this issue. The well-established adverse effects of statins are serious muscle injury, including rhabdomyolysis, with an incidence less than 0.1%, and a 0.2% risk of newly diagnosed diabetes.[22] Both of these adverse effects appear to be caused by statins directly, as opposed to indirectly via the lipid-lowering they produce; the main evidence for this is that PCSK9 inhibitors lower LDL-C at least as much as statins and, to date at least, do not appear to cause rhabdomyolysis or newly diagnosed diabetes.[23,24]

Unexplained muscle symptoms without significant elevation of creatine kinase are commonly reported by statin-treated patients and are a barrier to therapy, but in RCTs, the incidence of these symptoms is consistently very similar in the statin and placebo groups (see Connie B. Newman's article, "Safety of Statins and Non-Statins for Treatment of Dyslipidemia," in this issue). Furthermore, several studies have shown that statin intolerance due to muscle symptoms is not reproducible under double-blind conditions.[21,22,25,26] Consequently these symptoms are mostly attributed to the nocebo effect.

The safety of lipid-lowering agents is discussed in detail in Connie B. Newman's article, "Safety of Statins and Non-Statins for Treatment of Dyslipidemia," in this issue. Here we consider only adverse effects arising from treatment that produces very low concentrations of LDL-C. The ODYSSEY-Outcomes protocol specified blinded replacement of active alirocumab with placebo if LDL-C fell below 15 mg/dL on 2 occasions.[5] This occurred in 730 patients, who had a median duration on active treatment of 6.8 months. There was no excess of neurocognitive disorders or new-onset diabetes in patients who achieved LDL-C levels less than 15 mg/dL, and there were no cases of hemorrhagic stroke. In FOURIER,[24] comparing evolocumab versus placebo, 1335 (5%) patients allocated to evolocumab had an on-treatment LDL-C concentration of less than $0 \cdot 4$ mmol/L (15 mg/dL) and 504 (2%) less than $0 \cdot 26$ mmol/L (10 mg/dL). No safety signal was detected in either of these groups.

Inclisiran is a recently approved double-stranded small interfering RNA (siRNA) that suppresses hepatic PCSK9 translation. It reduces the concentration of circulating

PCSK9 by 80% to 90%, which leads to LDL reductions of about 50%, similar to that achieved by the PCSK9 monoclonal antibodies.[20] This siRNA is given subcutaneously at 6-month intervals, with an extra dose at month 3. It too has an excellent safety profile,[27] although ORION-4, a cardiovascular outcome study, is still in progress, so treatment duration in RCTs is still relatively short, less than 2 years. In a pooled analysis of phase 3 studies with inclisiran that included 3660 participants,[27] 52% of patients randomized achieved LDL-C values below 50 mg/dL and 14% below 25 mg/dL. No safety signal emerged, except for injection site reactions and a slightly higher incidence of bronchitis in the inclisiran group (4.3% vs 2.7%).

Overall, experience to date indicates that bringing LDL-C down to below 40 mg/dL involves little if any additional risk compared with less aggressive targets. Longer follow-up of patients with these low and ultralow concentrations of LDL-C may be informative, but as of 2021, there is no good evidence of a threshold below which new adverse effects emerge.

This is encouraging, but possibly not the last word. Two decades passed before statins were found to increase the risk of new-onset diabetes, for example, and the mechanism of the hallmark adverse effect of statins, myopathy/rhabdomyolysis, is still unclear. The biology of PCSK9 is complex and an active field of research.[9] Experience with PCSK9 inhibitors has not raised any major concerns, but these agents have been available for prescription for less than 5 years, compared with nearly 35 years for statins. There is even less experience with inclisiran.

UTILITY OF REDUCING LDL-C BELOW 40 MG/dL

Having arrived at the conclusion that there is no detectable hazard arising from very low LDL-C concentrations, the next question to consider is whether reducing LDL-C to below 40 mg/dL confers additional cardiovascular benefit, with the caveat that measurement of low (<100 mg/dL) concentrations of LDL-C by the traditional Friedewald equation is subject to clinically important inaccuracies (see Lucero and colleagues' article, "Lipoprotein Assessment in the 21st Century," in this issue). In particular, when plasma triglyceride concentration exceeds 150 mg/dL, the relative contribution of VLDL-C to the estimate of low LDL-C is appreciable and underestimation of LDL-C results.[28] Various methods, particularly the Martin/Hopkins equation[29] and the Sampson-NIH equation,[30] can be used to increase the accuracy of LDL-C estimation by adjustments to the relationship of VLDL-C to triglycerides. Alternatively, LDL-C can be measured directly by various chemical methods, but the methods are proprietary and may not be well validated. A further source of error is the inclusion of cholesterol in lipoprotein(a) when measuring LDL-C. In a patient with low LDL-C and high lipoprotein(a), this can lead to substantial overestimation of LDL-C. Lucero and colleagues' article, "Lipoprotein Assessment in the 21st Century," in this issue provides a full discussion of these analytical issues.

More than 30 large-scale cardiovascular outcome trials have provided data on cardiovascular risk reduction and LDL-C reduction, with statins in most cases but also PCSK9 inhibitors, the cholesterol absorption inhibitor ezetimibe, and CETP inhibitors. The 2010 meta-analysis by the Cholesterol Treatment Trialists Collaboration (CTTC)[2] was confined to statins and included a subgroup with baseline LDL-C less than 2 mmol/L (77 mg/dL). The overall number of patients with major vascular events was 24,323 and the overall reduction in major vascular events was 22% per 1 mmol/L LDL-C lowering, with very similar reductions in all the subgroups determined by baseline LDL-C, all the way down to the subgroup with the lowest LDL-C, less than 2 mmol/L (77 mg/dL). In this subgroup, the risk reduction was also 22% per 1 mmol/L

LDL-C lowering, but with a much wider confidence interval, because the subgroup included only 1922 participants with endpoint events, 8% of the total.

Subgroup analyses[23,24,31] addressing the utility and safety of on-treatment very low LDL-C concentrations are available from various cardiovascular outcome trials. Whenever an RCT population is divided into subgroups defined by postrandomization characteristics (as opposed to baseline values), the rigor of randomization is lost and bias may well be introduced, requiring careful application of statistical techniques to minimize it. Therefore, interpretation should be cautious. One such study is a prespecified analysis of ODYSSEY Outcomes,[23] the cardiovascular outcome trial for alirocumab in patients with acute coronary syndrome. The authors considered and listed numerous possible sources of bias and used propensity scoring to match the placebo control groups to the groups allocated to active treatment. Sensitivity analyses were used for confirmation.

The subgroups were 3 prespecified strata of LDL-C in patients allocated to active treatment, measured at 4 months after randomization: less than 25 (n = 3357), 25 to 50 (n = 3692), or greater than 50 mg/dL (n = 2197). LDL-C was calculated using the Friedewald equation unless the calculated value was less than 15 mg/dL or the concurrent triglyceride level was greater than 400 mg/dL, in which case LDL-C was measured directly by preparative ultracentrifugation and β-quantitation. The primary endpoint, major vascular events, was a composite of nonfatal myocardial infarction, ischemic stroke, or hospitalization for unstable angina.

The treatment benefit of alirocumab was similar in patients in the lowest and middle strata, and less in the upper stratum, in which adherence to study medication was relatively poor. The respective primary endpoint hazard ratios were 0.74, 0.74, and 0.87. This suggests that lowering LDL-C to 25 to 50 mg/dL is optimal in patients with atherosclerotic vascular disease and that further reduction of LDL-C in a patient with a level of about 25 mg/dL may be unproductive, no matter how high their cardiovascular risk. This is consistent with current guidelines. However, a large prespecified 2017 subgroup analysis of FOURIER,[24] also based on on-treatment values of LDL-C, reported no detectable utility threshold with evolocumab all the way down to 0.2 mmol/L (8 mg/dL). Both FOURIER and ODYSSEY Outcomes compared PCSK9 monoclonal antibodies, evolocumab or alirocumab, respectively, versus placebo in patients on statin therapy. The statistical methodology of the FOURIER subgroup analysis,[24] including adjustment for covariates, was different from that used in the subgroup analysis of ODYSSEY Outcomes. This might account for its different conclusions; indeed, the authors of a 2021 reanalysis[32] of the FOURIER subgroup results acknowledged the possibility of confounding in the original subgroup analysis.[24] Using statistical methodology that preserved randomization, they found that lowering LDL-C to ≤40 mg/dL proportionally reduced cardiovascular risk, but they did not claim evidence for benefit of reducing LDL-C to any particular value below 40 mg/dL. Thus, the results of FOURIER and ODYSSEY Outcomes are no longer inconsistent.

DISCUSSION

ODYSSEY Outcomes demonstrate a possible threshold of 25 mg/dL below which further lowering of LDL-C does not further reduce the risk of major atherosclerotic vascular events. This is consistent with FOURIER and is plausible, as we cannot assume that the CTTC meta-analysis[2] 22% reduction in cardiovascular risk per 1 mmol/L reduction of LDL-C holds down to very low levels. Even if it does hold, lowering LDL-C by 50% from 25 mg/dL would provide an absolute reduction of only 12.5 mg/dL (0.32 mmol/L) and an expected risk reduction of only 7%. A patient whose

LDL-C is 25 mg/dL is probably already taking a high-intensity statin and a PCSK9 inhibitor. To obtain a yet further 50% reduction might require the addition of inclisiran or some other equally effective but not yet developed agent. Interventions targeting risk factors other than LDL-C, such as lipoprotein(a), seem a more promising avenue for reducing residual risk. A small interfering RNA that produces a 90% reduction in lipoprotein(a) concentration is currently being tested in a large-scale cardiovascular outcome trial (NCT04023552).[33] Trial completion is scheduled for 2024.

There is no evidence for a threshold below which lowering LDL-C leads to adverse effects, nor does the biology of LDL lead to any expectation of a threshold. Nevertheless, evidence for rare but serious adverse effects could emerge in long-term studies when large numbers of patients are treated down to around 25 mg/dL or below. If that happens, experience with statins indicates that interpretation should be cautious. At various times concerns arose that statins might increase the risk of cataracts, breast cancer, or neurocognitive adverse effects. None of these concerns survived critical scrutiny and the acquisition of more data.[21,22]

To put the question that titles this article into perspective, residual uncertainty about reducing LDL-C below 25 mg/dL is far less of a barrier to treatment than the reluctance of many patients, even those at high risk with LDL-C far above 25 mg/dL, to take a statin, as discussed in Connie B. Newman's article, "Safety of Statins and Non-Statins for Treatment of Dyslipidemia," in this issue.

SUMMARY

The cardiovascular benefit and safety of reducing LDL-C to about 40 mg/dL (1 mmol/L) has been demonstrated in large-scale RCTs. The current therapeutic armamentarium makes further reduction of LDL-C achievable in some high-risk patients, but clinicians should be aware that the benefit of further reduction of LDL-C to below 25 mg/dL has not been established. If there is a hazard related to reducing LDL-C to very low levels, as of 2021 it has not been detected.

CLINICAL PEARLS

- In patients who have had 2 or more atherosclerotic events or are otherwise at very high risk, consider treatment to lower LDL cholesterol below 40 mg/dL.
- There is no evidence for any threshold below which further lowering of LDL cholesterol is harmful, but below 25 mg/dL, the reduction of cardiovascular risk is likely to be small if not nonexistent.

DISCLOSURE

The author has nothing to disclose.

REFERENCES

1. Scandinavian Simvastatin Survival Study Group. Randomised trial of cholesterol lowering in 4444 patients with coronary heart disease: the Scandinavian Simvastatin Survival Study (4S). Lancet 1994;344:1383–9.
2. Cholesterol Treatment Trialists' (CTT) Collaboration. Efficacy and safety of more intensive lowering of LDL cholesterol: a meta-analysis of data from 170,000 participants in 26 randomised trials. Lancet 2010;376:1670–81.
3. Olsson AG, Angelin B, Assmann G, et al. Can LDL cholesterol be too low? Possible risks of extremely low levels. J Intern Med 2017;281(6):534–53.

4. Gotto AM Jr. Low-density lipoprotein cholesterol and cardiovascular risk reduction: how low is low enough without causing harm? JAMA Cardiol 2018;3(9): 802–3.
5. Schwartz GG, Steg PG, Szarek M, et al. Alirocumab and cardiovascular outcomes after acute coronary syndrome. N Engl J Med 2018;379(22):2097–107.
6. Sabatine MS, Giugliano RP, Keech AC, et al. Evolocumab and clinical outcomes in patients with cardiovascular disease. N Engl J Med 2017;376(18):1713–22.
7. Mach F, Baigent C, Catapano AL, et al. 2019 ESC/EAS Guidelines for the management of dyslipidaemias: lipid modification to reduce cardiovascular risk: The Task Force for the management of dyslipidaemias of the European Society of Cardiology (ESC) and European Atherosclerosis Society (EAS). Eur Heart J 2019;41(1):111–88.
8. Goldstein JL, Brown MS. A century of cholesterol and coronaries: from plaques to genes to statins. Cell 2015;161(1):161–72.
9. Shapiro MD, Tavori H, Fazio S. PCSK9. Circ Res 2018;122(10):1420–38.
10. Feingold KR. Introduction to Lipids and Lipoproteins. [Updated 2021 Jan 19]. In: Feingold KR, Anawalt B, Boyce A, et al, editors. Endotext [Internet]. South Dartmouth (MA): MDText.com, Inc.; 2000. Available from: https://www.ncbi.nlm.nih.gov/books/NBK305896/.
11. Khoury J, Henriksen T, Christophersen B, et al. Effect of a cholesterol-lowering diet on maternal, cord, and neonatal lipids, and pregnancy outcome: a randomized clinical trial. Am J Obstet Gynecol 2005;193(4):1292–301.
12. Brown MS, Goldstein JL. A receptor-mediated pathway for cholesterol homeostasis. Science 1986;232(4746):34–47.
13. Jakubowski B, Shao Y, McNeal C, et al. Monogenic and polygenic causes of low and extremely low LDL-C levels in patients referred to specialty lipid clinics: Genetics of low LDL-C. J Clin Lipidol 2021;15(5):658–64.
14. Rimbert A, Vanhoye X, Coulibaly D, et al. Phenotypic differences between polygenic and monogenic hypobetalipoproteinemia. Arterioscler Thromb Vasc Biol 2021;41(1):e63–71.
15. Cohen JC, Boerwinkle E, Mosley TH Jr, et al. Sequence variations in PCSK9, low LDL, and protection against coronary heart disease. N Engl J Med 2006;354(12): 1264–72.
16. Zhao Z, Tuakli-Wosornu Y, Lagace TA, et al. Molecular characterization of loss-of-function mutations in PCSK9 and identification of a compound heterozygote. Am J Hum Genet 2006;79(3):514–23.
17. Hooper AJ, Marais AD, Tanyanyiwa DM, et al. The C679X mutation in PCSK9 is present and lowers blood cholesterol in a Southern African population. Atherosclerosis 2007;193(2):445–8.
18. Rashid S, Curtis DE, Garuti R, et al. Decreased plasma cholesterol and hypersensitivity to statins in mice lacking PCSK9. Proc Natl Acad Sci U S A 2005;102(15): 5374–9.
19. Tobert JA. Lovastatin and beyond: the history of the HMG-CoA reductase inhibitors. Nat Rev Drug Discov 2003;2(7):517–26.
20. Ray KK, Landmesser U, Leiter LA, et al. Inclisiran in patients at high cardiovascular risk with elevated LDL cholesterol. N Engl J Med 2017;376(15):1430–40.
21. Collins R, Reith C, Emberson J, et al. Interpretation of the evidence for the efficacy and safety of statin therapy. Lancet 2016;388(10059):2532–61.
22. Newman CB, Preiss D, Tobert JA, et al. Statin safety and associated adverse events: a scientific statement from the american heart association. Arterioscler Thromb Vasc Biol 2019;39(2):e38–81.

23. Schwartz GG, Gabriel Steg P, Bhatt DL, et al. Clinical efficacy and safety of alirocumab after acute coronary syndrome according to achieved level of low-density lipoprotein cholesterol: a propensity score-matched analysis of the ODYSSEY OUTCOMES trial. Circulation 2021;143(11):1109–22.

24. Giugliano RP, Pedersen TR, Park JG, et al. Clinical efficacy and safety of achieving very low LDL-cholesterol concentrations with the PCSK9 inhibitor evolocumab: a prespecified secondary analysis of the FOURIER trial. Lancet 2017; 390(10106):1962–71.

25. Herrett E, Williamson E, Brack K, et al. Statin treatment and muscle symptoms: series of randomised, placebo controlled n-of-1 trials. BMJ 2021;372:n135.

26. Wood FA, Howard JP, Finegold JA, et al. N-of-1 trial of a statin, placebo, or no treatment to assess side effects. N Engl J Med 2020;383(22):2182–4.

27. Wright RS, Ray KK, Raal FJ, et al. Pooled patient-level analysis of inclisiran trials in patients with familial hypercholesterolemia or atherosclerosis. J Am Coll Cardiol 2021;77(9):1182–93.

28. Martin SS, Blaha MJ, Elshazly MB, et al. Friedewald-estimated versus directly measured low-density lipoprotein cholesterol and treatment implications. J Am Coll Cardiol 2013;62(8):732–9.

29. Martin SS, Blaha MJ, Elshazly MB, et al. Comparison of a novel method vs the Friedewald equation for estimating low-density lipoprotein cholesterol levels from the standard lipid profile. JAMA 2013;310(19):2061–8.

30. Sampson M, Ling C, Sun Q, et al. A New equation for calculation of low-density lipoprotein cholesterol in patients with normolipidemia and/or hypertriglyceridemia. JAMA Cardiol 2020;5(5):540–8.

31. Everett BM, Mora S, Glynn RJ, et al. Safety profile of subjects treated to very low low-density lipoprotein cholesterol levels (<30 mg/dl) with rosuvastatin 20 mg daily (from JUPITER). Am J Cardiol 2014;114(11):1682–9.

32. Marston NA, Giugliano RP, Park JG, et al. Cardiovascular benefit of lowering low-density lipoprotein cholesterol below 40 mg/dL. Circulation 2021;144(21):1732–4.

33. Plakogiannis R, Sorbera M, Fischetti B, et al. The role of antisense therapies targeting lipoprotein(a). J Cardiovasc Pharmacol 2021;78(1):e5–11.

High-Density Lipoprotein and Cardiovascular Disease—Where do We Stand?

Iulia Iatan, PhD, MD, Hong Y Choi, PhD, Jacques Genest, MD*

KEYWORDS

- High-density lipoproteins • ATP-binding cassette transporters • Cholesterol
- Atherosclerosis • Genetics

KEY POINTS

- The epidemiologic association between high-density lipoprotein cholesterol (HDL-C) and cardiovascular disease is strong and coherent.
- Strong biological plausibility for HDL as a therapeutic target.
- Mendelian randomization does not support HDL-C as a causal risk factor.
- Severe HDL deficiency can be associated with atherosclerosis.
- The clinical trial data on HDL-C raising drugs is neutral.

INTRODUCTION. BRIEF HISTORY OF HIGH-DENSITY LIPOPROTEIN DISCOVERY, NOMENCLATURE, AND COMPLEXITY

High-density lipoproteins (HDL) were described over 50 years ago following the identification of lipoproteins by thin layer chromatography and density ultracentrifugation. An inverse link between coronary artery disease (CAD)—myocardial infarctions (MI)—and the cholesterol content of HDL was soon established, and the strength of this association was confirmed in multiple, independent studies. The Emerging Risk Factor Collaborative Studies firmly established HDL cholesterol (HDL-C) as a strong, coherent, and independent cardiovascular risk factor.[1] Basic research into the putative protective effects of HDL revealed pleiotropic effects in cellular and plasma membrane cholesterol homeostasis, modulation of inflammation and oxidative stress, arterial endothelial function, endothelial progenitor cell proliferation, and apoptosis.

This article originally appeared in *Endocrinology and Metabolism Clinics,* Volume 51, Issue 3, September 2022.
Research Institute of the McGill University Health Center, 1001 Decarie Boulevard, Bloc E, EM12212, Montreal, Quebec H4A 3J1, Canada
* Corresponding author. Research Institute of the McGill University Health Center, 1001 Decarie Boulevard, Bloc E, EM12212, Montreal, Quebec H4A 3J1, Canada.
E-mail address: jacques.genest@mcgill.ca

Clinics Collections 13 (2023) 287–302
https://doi.org/10.1016/j.ccol.2023.02.005
2352-7986/23/

Abbreviations	
ATP	Adenosine triphosphate
ABCA1	ATP binding cassette transporter A1
HDL	Hidh density lipoproteins
ASCVD	Atheroscelrosit cardiovascular disease
DSC1	Desmocollin 1
RCT	Reverse cholesterol transport
LCAT	Lecithin:cholesterol acyltransferase
CETP	Cholesteryl ester transfer protein
SR-B1	Scavenger receptor B1
S1P	Sphingosine-1-phosphate
GWAS	Genome-wide association studies

These data markedly strengthened the role of HDL in preventing atherosclerosis. Drugs were soon developed to increase HDL-C.

Yet, these findings have not translated into clinical benefit. Here, the authors review the epidemiology of HDL and cardiovascular disease (CVD), discuss the effects of HDL on the pathogenesis of atherosclerosis, review the genetic disorders of HDL and their relation to CVD, and the clinical trials conducted thus far. They finally discuss future directions for translational research into the biology of HDL and potential clinical applications.

Refinements in analytical techniques signifies that HDL particles have become increasingly complex. It is important to understand the extraordinary diversity of HDL particles, their content, and dynamic interactions in plasma, lymph, and vascular wall environments. As such, defining HDL requires a deeper look at measurement and analytical techniques. Clinicians and epidemiologists have focused on the cholesterol content (free cholesterol and cholesteryl esters) within HDL. Measurement techniques for HDL particles have evolved considerably since the days of ultracentrifugation and the measurement of cholesterol and triglycerides.[2] Briefly, preparative and analytical techniques examine HDL by size and density in a salt solution, by chromatography or magnetic resonance, and by charge and size in 2-dimensional electrophoresis (**Fig. 1**). Although the time-honored definition includes a specific density range with respect to plasma (1.063<d < 1.210 g/mL), size (5–20 nm), and the presence of apolipoprotein A-I (apoA-I), HDL particles carry a very complex proteome with at least 90 separate proteins that are generally recognized by most research laboratories and perhaps as many as greater than 800 different proteins thus far identified.[3] The HDL proteome may shift toward an inflammatory phenotype, depending on the milieu created by such circumstances such as acute coronary syndromes and inflammatory diseases.[4–6] The HDL lipidome is also very complex. Although cholesterol and cholesteryl esters are a major source of lipids, comprising ~50% of lipids, sphingolipids, especially sphingomyelin and several species of phospholipids (phosphatidyl serine and phosphatidyl choline), lysophospholipids, and sulfatides are found.[7] Serna and colleagues identified 172 lipid species within HDL particles.[8] Lastly, the identification of circulating small and circular RNAs that are carried within HDL particles and influence their metabolic fate expands their potential physiologic roles[9,10] (**Table 1**). Cellular export of microRNAs (miRNAs) to HDL is regulated, at least in part, by sphingomyelinase. Interestingly, the miRNA profile varies distinctly according to specific physiologic states such as atherosclerosis, inflammation and hyperlipidemia.

It must be noted that "Reconstituted" HDL particles used in clinical trials are composed of a fixed molar (or mass) ratio of apoA-I, phosphatidyl choline, and free

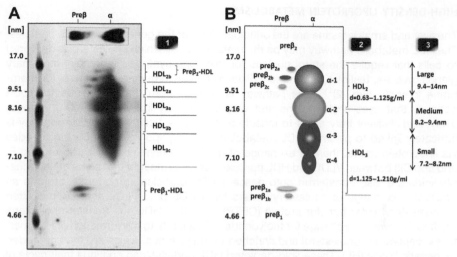

Fig. 1. Analytical techniques for HDL lipids. (*A-1*) Representative 2-dimensional gradient gel electrophoresis where HDL particles are separated by charge (horizontal dimension) and by size (vertical dimension). HDL particle size varies between 7 and 17 nm; lipid-poor (nascent) HDL particles comprising mostly apoA-I and some phospholipids are termed pre-β HDL. (*B*) Stylized diagram showing discrete HDL particles separated in HDL2 and HDL3 (*B-2*) or by large, medium, and small HDL particles when analyzed by nuclear magnetic resonance (NMR) (*B-3*). (*Modified from* Hafiane A, Genest J. High density lipoproteins: Measurement techniques and potential biomarkers of cardiovascular risk. BBA Clin. 2015 Jan 31;3:175–88.)

cholesterol. These particles may exhibit some of the characteristics of HDL particles in terms of density and electrophoretic mobility, but likely do not exist in nature, nor are they likely to present the 3-dimensional configuration of its protein, apoA-I, essential for various cellular interactions.

Table 1
Characteristics and components of high-density lipoprotein

Origin	Density (g/mL)	Size (nm)
Major: liver, intestine Minor: macrophage foam cells	1.063–1.210	5–20
PROTEIN	LIPIDS	RNA
40%–55% weight	[Chol] 0.9–1.6 mmol/L (35–62 mg/dL) [Trig] 0.1–0.2 (mmol/L) (9–18 mg/dL)	miRNA, circular RNA
Major: ApoA-I, A-II	<ul><li>Cholesteryl esters</li><li>Triglycerides</li><li>Free cholesterolphosphatidyletanolamine</li><li>Phosphatidylinositol</li><li>Sulfatides</li><li>Phosphatidylcholine</li><li>Lysophosphatidylcholine sphingomyelin</li></ul>	From multiple cell types
At least 90 proteins reliably identified in HDL particles[3]	At least 171 lipid species identified in HDL[8]	>100[10]

HIGH-DENSITY LIPOPROTEIN METABOLISM

The liver and small intestine are the principal sites for the generation of HDL particles. The HDL metabolic pathway may be the major route by which cholesterol is delivered to cells that require the sterol nucleus for hormone synthesis (adrenals, mammary glands, ovaries, testicles) and rapidly dividing tissues requiring cholesterol for membrane integrity (**Fig. 2**)[11]. This pathway is distinct from the triglyceride transport pathway that uses chylomicrons and very-low-density lipoprotein (VLDL), respectively, and delivers fatty acids to muscle and adipose tissues. The HDL pathway is intricately linked to plasma VLDL metabolism. During lipolysis of VLDL triglycerides via lipoprotein lipase, there is exchange of apolipoproteins (especially apo-I, apo E, and apo CII) between VLDL and HDL particles, and it is thought that some of the phospholipids are also transferred onto nascent HDL particles. Importantly, there is an equimolar exchange of cholesteryl esters from HDL onto VLDL and IDL mediated by cholesteryl ester transfer protein (CETP) such that HDL can transfer cholesterol back to the liver, in exchange for triglycerides. This leads to the formation of HDL particles, depleted in cholesterol and enriched in triglycerides, which are then degraded by hepatic lipase (HL). These lipid-depleted HDL particles can continue their cycle of cellular cholesterol uptake.

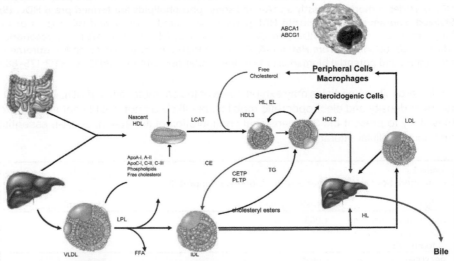

Fig. 2. HDL metabolism in plasma. The intestine and the liver are the main source of HDL particles (*blue arrows*). Nascent HDL particles (lipid-poor apoA-I phospholipid complexes) come in contact with cells expressing the ABCA1 transporter, which acts predominantly as a phospholipid transfer protein from the plasma membrane onto nascent HDL. Cholesterol efflux requires ABCA1 but seems to occur in distinct lipid rafts within the membrane. Further lipidation is mediated via ABCG1. In plasma, several lipases, including LCAT, mediate the conversion of cholesterol into cholesteryl esters, increasing the size of HDL. HDL cholesterol can be transferred via CETP onto triglyceride-rich lipoproteins in exchange for triglyceride. HDL can also bind to hepatocytes via the SR-B1 receptor. Hepatic cholesterol can then be converted to bile acids. The reverse cholesterol transport pathway (*red arrows*) proposes that HDL particles can also remove cholesterol from cells such as macrophages or smooth muscle cells within arterial wall and return it to the liver for disposal. (*Modified from* Genest J, Libby P. Chapter 48: Lipoprotein Disorders and Cardiovascular Disease. In: Zipes DP, Libby P, Bonow RO, Mann DL, Tomaselli GF, and Braunwald E. eds. Braunwald's Heart Diseas: A Textbook if Cardiovascular Medicine. 11th[th] ed. Elsevier; 2019:960-982.)

A second pathway, that of "reverse cholesterol transport (RCT)" is a mechanism by which excess cellular cholesterol from peripheral cells (including lipid laden macrophages and smooth muscle cells in the arterial wall) is transferred onto lipid-poor nascent HDL particles containing apoA-I and delivered to the liver for secretion as bile acids.

HDL biogenesis, or the formation of HDL particles, occurs when lipid-free or lipid-poor apoA-I comes in contact with the ATP-binding cassette transporter A-1 (ABCA1). The transfer of plasma membrane phospholipids onto apoA-I alters its 3-dimensional structure; cholesterol lipidation seems to occur by lateral transfer on the plasma membrane.[12] These particles become substrate for the ABCG1 transporter present on many cell types including hepatic, macrophages, and vascular endothelial cells. Circulating HDL particles undergo multiple changes, especially the enzymatic conversion of free cholesterol into cholesteryl esters by lecithin:cholesterol acyltransferase (LCAT), the transfer of these cholesteryl esters onto VLDL particles in exchange for triglycerides by CETP. Multiple enzymes, such as sphingomyelinase and other phospholipases, alter the phospholipid moiety of HDL, thus altering some functional aspect. The scavenger receptor B1 (SR-B1) mediates the bidirectional movement of cholesterol between HDL and cells. Here, the authors review the pleiotropic effects of HDL particles on pathologic processes such as atherosclerosis, inflammation, and infections, thus providing biological plausibility for targeting this pathway. Casting doubt on the protective role of HDL, Frikke-Schmidt and colleagues published the first of many reports using Mendelian randomization, showing that the relationship between genetic variants of the ABCA1 gene associated with decreased HDL-C levels and atherosclerosis ASCVD is not robust.[13] Clinical trials aimed at raising HDL-C and further described later also failed to change relevant clinical outcomes such as major adverse cardiovascular events. A more granular picture thus emerges that HDL-C might be a biomarker of cardiovascular health that does not reflect the many biological functions of HDL particles. The future in HDL research and translational medicine will therefore consist in identifying reproducible and upscalable biomarkers of HDL function, novel pharmacologic agents that promote the beneficial effects of HDL function and alter clinical outcomes.

MECHANISMS BY WHICH HIGH-DENSITY LIPOPROTEIN MIGHT BE ATHEROPROTECTIVE

HDL plays key roles in pathways related to the development of atherosclerotic disease including RCT, antioxidation and antiinflammation, endothelial function, as well as in other physiologic systems including immune system modulation, cellular apoptosis, and endothelial progenitor cell homeostasis (Fig. 3). It must be kept in mind that many physiologic effects described here have been studied in in-vitro systems and the physiologic relevance is, for the most part, not fully understood.

The RCT pathway is thought to be the major pathway by which HDL prevents atherosclerosis; this might be because it is the most extensively studied. It must be noted that HDL-mediated cellular cholesterol efflux is only weakly correlated with the cholesterol mass of HDL and depends more on the HDL proteome and lipidome. To exert antiatherosclerosis effects, plasma circulating HDL must cross the endothelium, to mediate cholesterol efflux from macrophages and smooth muscle cells and exert antioxidant and antiinflammatory functions. Transendothelial HDL transport is a highly regulated process involving several receptor and enzymes, including SR-B1, ABCA1, and ABCG1 transporters, as well as endothelial lipase. Furthermore,

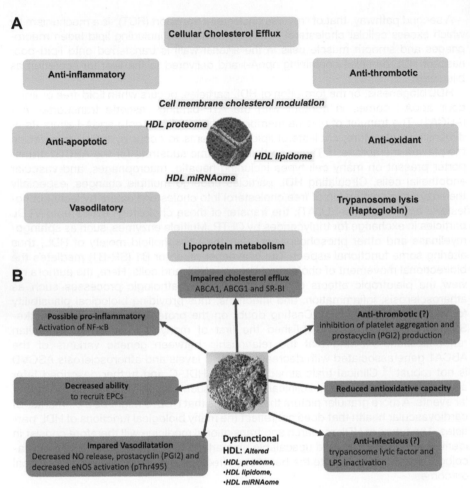

Fig. 3. Pleiotropic effects of HDL. (*A*) HDL particles contribute to a wide variety of physiologic processes. Individual components of HDL (proteins, lipids and RNA), as well as the ability to modulate plasma membrane cholesterol content mediate these effects. (*B*) Dysfunctional HDL are encountered in acute and chronic inflammatory states, diabetes, and metabolic syndrome and may contribute to the pathogenesis of atherosclerosis. (*Modified from* Schwertani A, Choi HY, Genest J. HDLs and the pathogenesis of atherosclerosis. Curr Opin Cardiol. 2018 May;33(3):311-316.)

HDL helps maintain endothelial barrier integrity by stimulating the proliferation and migration of endothelial progenitor and endothelial cells, by promoting intercellular junction closure to prevent transmigration of inflammatory cells, and by enhancing nitric oxide and prostacyclin production.[14–17]

From large population studies, the potential role of HDL as an important modulator of inflammation is emerging. Madsen and colleagues examined the incidence of autoimmune disease in 117,341 subjects from the general population of the Copenhagen Heart study and concluded that a low HDL-C level is associated with a high risk of autoimmune disease.[18] Although causality cannot be inferred, this finding suggests that HDL may modulate the emergence of inflammatory diseases. Studies of patients with systemic inflammation, including acute coronary syndromes, have revealed a shift of HDL proteins toward an inflammatory phenotype. It follows that these "altered HDL" may become dysfunctional and thus contribute to atherosclerosis disease progression, rather than its prevention (see **Fig. 3**B).[4–6,18,19]

Plasma from patients with acute inflammatory conditions (eg, acute coronary syndromes) or chronic inflammatory conditions reveal a striking shift in the proteome and lipidome of HDL particles, especially oxidized phospholipids, and these lead to dysfunctional HDL particles that cause—rather than prevent—atherosclerosis. ApoA-I and nascent HDL modulate plasma membrane function and may alter the composition of membrane microdomains, such as lipid rafts. Most cells contain these domains, including immune cells that express key receptors involved in their activation. However, dysfunctional HDL particles may lead to the disruption of B- and T-cell receptors and Toll-like receptors and subsequent activation of monocytes and macrophages and cytokine production.[20,21]

HDL-associated sphingosine-1-phosphate (S1P) has also multiple roles in regulating the immune response. S1P seems to have an immunoregulatory role during infection by reducing proinflammatory cytokine secretion by dendritic cells and favoring the production of regulatory cytokines such as interleukin-10. S1P was further shown to inhibit macrophage activation in response to TLR2 ligation and nitric oxide–induced damage and to influence dendritic cell trafficking, lymphocyte trafficking, and antigen presentation.[20] Deficient or dysfunctional HDL might lose its immunomodulatory properties or participate in inflammatory reactions, thus tipping the balance toward autoimmunity in susceptible individuals.

EPIDEMIOLOGY AND GENETICS OF HIGH-DENSITY LIPOPROTEIN IN RELATION TO CARDIOVASCULAR DISEASE

To date, HDL-C has been evaluated as a risk marker in multiple studies, including 68 long-term population-based studies involving more than 302,430 individuals from Europe and North America.[1] In multivariate models adjusted for both nonlipid and lipid risk factors, HDL-C was shown to be inversely correlated with CAD events. For every 0.39 mmol/L increase in HDL-C concentration, the risk of a CAD event was reduced by 22% (95% confidence interval [CI], 18%–26%).[15] Despite this, after decades of belief that HDL protected from atherosclerosis, the "HDL hypothesis" has been put into question, as there still lacks unequivocal evidence of a beneficial effect of HDL-raising treatments on cardiovascular end points.[22,23] This was demonstrated in several studies, including a meta-analysis of 95 clinical trials involving greater than 300,000 individuals, suggested that on-trial HDL-C concentrations were not significantly related to CAD events.[24] Investigations using statins also showed that by aggressively lowering LDL-C (<2.0 mmol/L), HDL-C levels no longer predicted residual cardiovascular risk.[25] These findings, combined with Mendelian randomization data on genetic HDL deficiency states, stirs controversy on the validity of HDL-C as a therapeutic target.[13] Mendelian randomization principles assume that the existence of a causal relationship between HDL-C and CAD would imply that association between a gene variant and HDL-C levels will translate into the CAD risk expected from the effect on HDL-C. Using this approach, however, several genetic studies[26–28] have casted doubt on a direct protective effect of HDL-C on atherosclerotic risk, as gene variants affecting HDL-C levels do not necessarily correlate with a corresponding effect on heart disease. For example, subjects with genetic forms of HDL deficiency, such as apoA-I Milano, or some mutations at ABCA1 and LCAT, are not necessarily associated with premature CAD, whereas mutations in the HL or the CETP genes—leading to high HDL-C—may not be protective.[29] In some cases, elevated HDL-C levels are paradoxically associated with increased cardiovascular and overall mortality, suggesting a U-shaped relationship between mortality and HDL-C concentrations.[30] As such, these observations indicate that the relationship between CAD and HDL-C remains more complex than originally thought.

INHERITED DISORDERS OF HIGH-DENSITY LIPOPROTEIN METABOLISM AND THEIR RELATIONSHIP TO ATHEROSCLEROSIS

It must be emphasized that plasma levels of HDL-C are highly related to lifestyle. Yet, HDL-C concentrations are also under strong genetic control, with heritability estimates ranging between 40% and 80% across multiple populations. Genetic determinants include both rare large-effect variants and common small-effect variants.[28,31] As such, several monogenic disorders have been described, with very low (<5th percentile age-sex matched) or high (>90th percentile age-sex matched) HDL-C levels. Genes implicated in monogenic disorders associated with these low HDL-C concentrations include *APOA1*, *LCAT*, and *ABCA1*, whereas those associated with elevated HDL-C levels include *CETP*, *SCARB1*, and *LIPC*.[28,32,33,55]

Low High-Density Lipoprotein Cholesterol States

Apolipoprotein A-I deficiency

ApoA-I is the main apolipoprotein of HDL, accounting for 70% of the protein mass. Primary defects affecting the production of HDL particles can be caused by variants in the apoAI-apoCIII-apoAIV-apoAV gene complex. Complete apoA-I deficiency resulting from homozygous or compound heterozygous mutations is a rare condition leading to undetectable plasma apoA-I levels accompanied by tuberoeruptive xanthomas, marked decrease in HDL-C, and an increased risk of premature ASCVD. Heterozygous mutations within apoA-I have also been described, with at least 47 variants affecting apoA-I structure, some leading to a marked reduction in apoA-I and HDL-C levels, and concomitant coronary artery disease, whereas others with low HDL but no incidence of heart disease. In line with these observations, some rare variants of apoA-I, such as apoA-I Milano and apoA-I Paris, are paradoxically associated with low HDL-C concentrations and reduced risk of ASCVD and longevity.[34]

ATP-binding cassette transporter A-1 deficiency

The identification of ABCA1 as the rate-limiting step in HDL biogenesis and the first step of the RCT pathway has triggered a great deal of investigation into its role as a genetic factor in atherosclerosis. Tangier disease (TD) is a rare form of severe HDL deficiency due to homozygous or compound heterozygous mutations at the *ABCA1* gene. The major biochemical abnormality is a near-absence of HDL-C due to impaired cholesterol efflux to lipid-free Apo-I, mild to moderate increased triglyceride levels, and a marked decrease in LDL-C. The association of TD and premature CAD is however tenuous and has been subject to considerable debate over the years, as ABCA1 deficiency is not clearly associated with an increased risk of CVD, possibly due to low LDL-C levels. In individuals with heterozygous ABCA1 mutations, however, the association with CAD seems less ambiguous.[35] Although the risk of heart disease in individuals with heterozygous ABCA1 mutations was increased 3-fold compared with unaffected controls, a more recent study also showed that carriers of 1 or 2 loss-of-function *ABCA1* mutations with significantly low HDL-C but similar LDL-C levels displayed a larger atherosclerotic burden compared with their unaffected relatives.[36] In contrast, additional insights into the effects of ABCA1 genetic variation on CAD have been described by Frikke-Schmidt in Mendelian randomization analyses of the Copenhagen City Heart Study; this revealed that lower plasma HDL-C levels owing to heterozygous, rare *ABCA1* loss-of-function mutations were not associated with increased risk of CVD end points.[13]

Lecithin:cholesterol acyltransferase deficiency

Naturally occurring mutations in LCAT are another rare cause of low HDL-C levels. Classic homozygous or familial LCAT deficiency results from a complete loss of LCAT activity, whereas Fish-eye disease (partial LCAT deficiency) is associated with a change in the substrate specificity of LCAT that retains its activity to esterify free cholesterol of apoB-containing lipoproteins but becomes inactive toward HDL. This property leads to higher LDL-C levels in Fish-eye disease and thus acceleration of atherosclerosis, relative to complete LCAT deficiency, where a decreased risk of CAD has been observed.[29] As such, the absence of an association between homozygous LCAT deficiency and increased risk of CVD has been attributed to concomitant low levels of serum LDL-C, as well as an increase in endothelial nitric oxide production. Of note however, in Mendelian randomization studies, Haase and colleagues investigated the effect of S208 T, a homozygous loss-of-function variant of LCAT, in 2 Danish cohorts. The investigators identified that a 13% decrease in plasma HDL-C levels predicts an 18% increased risk of MI but genetically decreased HDL-C concentrations, associated with the S208 T variant, did not.[26]

High High-Density Lipoprotein States

Cholesteryl ester transfer protein *deficiency*

Complete loss of CETP activity associated with homozygous *CETP* gene variants leads to increased HDL-C and a reduction in LDL-C, due to impaired transfer of cholesteryl esters from HDL to LDL. Based on epidemiologic observations, this mechanism of action was expected to reduce atherosclerosis by generating antiatherogenic lipoprotein profiles. Yet, this promise has not been realized in clinical outcome trials of CETP inhibitors. In fact, a recent meta-analysis of 11 randomized controlled trials examined the effects of CETP inhibitors on major cardiovascular events and all-cause mortality, showing a nonsignificant reduction in the risk of nonfatal myocardial infarction (−7%) and death from cardiovascular causes (−8%).[37] As such, despite the limited cardiovascular benefits of CETP inhibitors and their off-target toxic effects, data from multiple large human genetic studies and animal investigations suggest that CETP deficiency is protective against atherosclerosis.[38,39] Moreover, several loss-of-function SNPs in the *CETP* gene that are associated with increased HDL-C and concomitant decreases in TG and LDL-C are also associated with corresponding risk reductions in CAD and MI.

Hepatic lipase and endothelial lipase deficiency

Complete HL deficiency due to rare loss-of-function variants in *LIPC* alleles is associated with 2- to 3-fold increase in HDL-C and ApoA-I concentrations.[29] Concurrently however, it is also associated with elevations in apoB-containing lipoproteins, as well as atherogenic remnant particles, explaining the increase in premature CHD in some families with HL deficiency. Similarly, endothelial lipase (EL) deficiency also induces hyperalphalipoproteinemia and increases HDL-C, but without decreasing MI risk. Voight and colleagues performed 2 Mendelian randomization analyses, using both an SNP in *EL* (LIPG Asn396Ser) and a genetic score consisting of 14 common SNPs known to exclusively associate with increased HDL-C. Both approaches failed to show any association with a reduced risk of MI.[27] These data challenge the concept that raising plasma HDL-C will uniformly translate into CVD risk reduction.

Scavenger receptor B1 deficiency

SR-B1 mediates the selective uptake of CE from HDL into hepatocytes and steroidogenic tissues. The atheroprotective effects of SR-BI are therefore primarily attributable to its role in cholesterol efflux from lipid-laden macrophages to HDL and in the delivery of HDL CE to the liver. Interestingly though, SR-B1 knockout mice exhibit increased atherosclerosis despite having higher levels of HDL-C, a process that was attributed to a critical block in the RCT to the liver (see **Fig. 2**). In humans, several studies have described genetic *SCARB1* variants associated with HDL-C levels. In a kindred with the P297S missense variant in *SCARB1*, carriers showed an increase in HDL-C levels, although no differences in carotid intima-media thickness were observed. Similarly, a recent study showed that elevated HDL-C due to pathogenic variants in *SCARB1* carriers were not predictive of CAD.[40]

Genome-wide association studies and complex genetic determinants of high-density lipoprotein cholesterol

Genome-wide association studies (GWAS) have previously confirmed multiple loci that modulate HDL-C in man, as well as identified novel genomic regions for HDL-C.[29,41] The Global Lipid Genetics Consortium Collaboration GWAS initially identified 47 loci primarily associated with HDL-C levels in more than 100,000 individuals, with a subsequent additional 30 loci associated with HDL-C found in 196,000 individuals.[42] The strongest associations included common variants in *ABCA1*, *CETP*, *LCAT*, *LIPG*, and *LPL* genes and in the *apoAI–apoCIII–apoAIV– apoAV* gene cluster. These common variants can be present in up to 50% of the general population, in contrast with rare variants in the same genes underlying monogenic dyslipidemias, occurring in less than 1% of the population. Furthermore, despite statistical significant associations between these common genetic variants and HDL-C plasma concentrations, cumulatively, they only account for a small proportion (10%–15%) of the total variance in serum HDL-C levels.

Why have current clinical trials of high-density lipoprotein cholesterol raising failed?

The "HDL hypothesis" postulates that the association between low HDL-C and ASCVD should provide a therapeutic goal, namely, that raising HDL-C would be beneficial. However, the effects of a therapeutic modality that exclusively raises HDL-C (without affecting other lipoproteins of pathways) has proved elusive. To date, therefore, clinicians had to rely on inference from clinical trials to assess whether raising HDL-C decreases ASCVD outcomes.

FIBRATES

The fibric acid derivatives, or fibrates, activate peroxisome proliferator-activated receptor alpha (PPARα) and enhance lipoprotein lipase activity, in part, by decreasing the expression of its inhibitor, apoCIII. This, in turn, decreases plasma triglyceride levels and raises HDL-C. Early trials using bezafibrate or gemfibrozil yielded positive results on some components of major cardiac adverse events (MACE). However, in the statin era, the FIELD (Fenofibrate Intervention and Event Lowering in Diabetes) and ACCORD (Action to Control Cardiovascular Risk in Diabetes—also with fenofibrate) trials failed to reduce cardiovascular outcomes in diabetic patients, despite a significant increase in HDL-C.[38,39] Newer PPARα and γ, such as aleglitazar, also failed to change outcomes in diabetic patients. Pemafibrate is a selective PPARα modulator with quantitatively better triglyceride lowering and HDL-C raising than fenofibrate.[43] It remains to be determined however if, in combination with statin therapy, this will decrease MACE.

NIACIN

Niacin has been used for over 60 years to treat lipoprotein disorders and was used in early clinical trials. The AIM-HIGH (Atherothrombosis Intervention in Metabolic Syndrome with Low HDL Cholesterol/High Triglyceride and Impact on Global Health Outcomes) was a relatively modest trial of 3300 patients with ASCVD and residual dyslipidemia that did not meet its primary outcome of reducing ASCVD risk. The large HPS2-THRIVE (Heart Protection Study-2 Treatment of HDL to Reduce the Incidence of Vascular Events) randomized 25,673 high-risk patients taking simvastatin to placebo or the combination of niacin and laropiprant (an inhibitor of prostaglandin D2), thought to mediate the cutaneous flushing reaction seen with niacin. Although no beneficial effects on ASCVD risk were observed, an increase in complications led to the withdrawal of the combination drug and a decrease in the use of niacin clinically.

CHOLESTERYL ESTER TRANSFER PROTEIN INHIBITORS

Inhibitors of CETP were developed to increase HDL-C, by interfering with the exchange of cholesteryl esters from HDL particles to triglyceride-rich lipoproteins in exchange for triglycerides in an equimolar ratio. Trials with torcetrapib, dalcetrapib, and evacetrapib ended because of toxicity or futility.[68] The REVEAL trial (Heart Protection-3 Randomized Evaluation of the Effects of Anacetrapib Through Lipid-modification) randomized 30,449 patients with ASCVD on atorvastatin with atherosclerotic vascular disease who were receiving intensive atorvastatin therapy to placebo or anacetrapib,100 mg/d. After a median follow-up of 4 years, the primary outcome was reduced by an absolute rate of 1.0% (rate ratio, 0.91; 95% CI 0.85–0.97; P = .004). HDL-C increased by 104% and non-HDL-C decreased by 18% (0,44 mmol/L or 17 mg/dL). Although there were no differences in the risk of death, cancer, or serious adverse events, this very modest benefit was likely explained by the slight reduction in non-HDL-C.[37,44,45] Obicetrapib is currently investigated as a lipid-modifying drug, mostly for patients intolerant to statins.

APOLIPOPROTEIN A-I INFUSIONS

Based on animal models, it was proposed that the intravenous injection of proteoliposomes containing apoA-I combined with a fixed molar ratio of phospholipids—usually phosphatidylcholine (lecithin) and free cholesterol ("reconstituted" HDL particle)—would either stabilize atherosclerotic plaques in acute coronary syndromes or promote the regression of established plaques. Unfortunately, this approach has not met clinical success. It is likely that the apoA-I provided in this fashion transiently enters the plasma apoA-I pool but this effect seems physiologically insufficient.[46–48]

APOLIPOPROTEIN A-I MIMETICS

Novel agents that increase apoA-I protein or function include apoA-I mimetics, HDL mimetics, and RVX 208 (Apabetalone), a bromodomain and extraterminal (BET) antagonist that raises the transcriptional regulation of apoA-I, showed promise in animal models and early phase clinical trials. However, in the BETonMACE trial, Apabetalone failed to meet its primary end point.[49]

Overall, this brief overview of clinical trials shows the futility of raising HDL-C as a therapeutic target. It is now time to put to rest the "HDL hypothesis" and consider plasma levels of HDL-C as a biomarker of cardiovascular health, rather than a goal of therapy.

WHERE DO WE GO FROM HERE?

There is agreement that modulation of HDL functions for therapeutic purposes shows considerable promise. The future lies in the identification of novel biomarkers of HDL function that predict outcomes and in that of new targets that act in the arterial *subendothelium*. It is well known that ApoA-I accumulates in the arterial subendothelial layer[50] and subsequently becomes trapped. Therefore, developing biomarkers of HDL biogenesis (the ability of apoA-I or lipid-poor HDL to remove cellular cholesterol) that can be scaled up to a clinical test will be essential.[51,52] There are however challenges to developing these biomarkers of HDL function, such as cell-based cholesterol efflux and inflammatory indices mediated by HDL, as compared with the current static biochemical measurements. The standardization, validation, and large-throughput commercialization can be considered important barriers to their implementation into clinical practice. As of now, the validity of these measurements and their commercial availability remain obstacles to a realistic transition to clinical medicine.[17]

The failure of translating the HDL hypothesis into clinical benefit has demonstrated that HDL-C does not necessarily reflect HDL function. This has led us to rethink of *the primary* HDL function contributing to cardiovascular health. ASCVD is a chronic inflammatory process initiated by cholesterol deposition in the subendothelial space of arteries; therefore, removal of cholesterol accumulated in the atherosclerotic plaque is believed to be the most beneficial effect of HDL. The formation and maturation of HDL particles are coupled with cellular cholesterol removal occurring through cholesterol efflux pathways, and thus the HDL biogenic process has been reviewed as the most clinically relevant therapeutic target for the development of HDL-directed therapies. There are 4 major cholesterol efflux pathways, and the one mediated by ABCA1 is responsible for the formation of nascent HDL particles (**Fig. 4**). Although ABCA1-and ABCG1-dependent cholesterol efflux are unidirectional in the removal of excess cellular cholesterol, SR-BI and aqueous diffusion are involved in both cholesterol influx as well as efflux (see **Fig. 4**). Although the ABCA1- and ABCG1-dependent unidirectional pathways have long been attractive targets to develop drugs promoting cholesterol efflux, it has been challenging to identify druggable molecular targets in the pathways. Recent efforts to characterize plasma membrane microdomains involved in ABCA1-dependent cholesterol efflux allowed us to identify desmocollin-1 (DSC1) as a negative regulator of the ABCA1 pathway.[53] The DSC1 action mechanism was to bind apoA-I so as to prevent apoA-I lipidation by ABCA1. The apoA-I binding site in DSC1 was highly druggable and was successfully targeted with small molecules.[54] The potency and efficacy of a small molecule, docetaxel, in promoting ABCA1-dependent cholesterol efflux have suggested that the ABCA1 pathway may be therapeutically modulated.[54] In addition to small molecules, peptides and antibodies may also be developed to inhibit apoA-I–DSC1 interactions, proposing DSC1 as a viable therapeutic target. As seen in **Fig. 4**, nascent HDL particles can acquire additional cholesterol via the other cholesterol efflux pathways, suggesting that identification of druggable molecular targets in the ABCA1 pathway may provide us with new opportunities to develop HDL-directed therapies.

Another issue of consideration with therapeutic strategies aimed at enhancing atheroprotective HDL function is the absence of methods to assess HDL function in clinical practice. Although cell-based cholesterol efflux assays are useful research tools, they are not only far from clinical practice but also different from measuring cholesterol efflux in the atherosclerotic plaque. It will be ideal to identify circulating biomarkers that directly reflect cholesterol efflux activity in the plaque, but such studies have

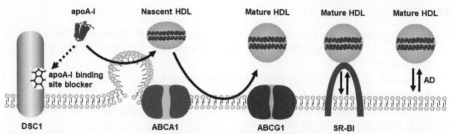

Fig. 4. The HDL biogenic process and four major cholesterol efflux pathways. ABCA1 creates a plasma membrane microdomain to facilitate efflux of cellular phospholipids and cholesterol to lipid-free or lipid-poor apolipoproteins such as apoA-I. The lipidated apoA-I is called a nascent HDL particle. An apoA-I binding protein DSC1 sequesters apoA-I to prevent the formation of nascent HDL; therefore, blocking of the apoA-I binding site in DSC1 promotes ABCA1-dependent HDL formation. Nascent HDL particles are matured by acquiring additional cholesterol via ABCG1-dependent cholesterol efflux. ABCG1 facilitates cholesterol efflux by increasing the pool of cholesterol available for efflux in the outer leaflet of the plasma membrane. Matured HDL particles are able to acquire more cholesterol via SR-BI–dependent cholesterol efflux and aqueous diffusion. These 2 pathways are however involved in both efflux and influx of cholesterol, and thus it is difficult to therapeutically modulate them.

not been reported due to lack of drugs with which such studies can be performed. DSC1 is abundantly expressed in the atherosclerotic plaque,[53] and docetaxel is an efficient DSC1-targeting agent, thus it will be interesting to investigate if administration of docetaxel reduces atherosclerosis and releases lipid and/or inflammatory biomarkers into the circulation.

In conclusion, the future lies in the identification of new druggable targets in cholesterol efflux pathways in the atherosclerotic plaque along with discovery of biomarkers that can accurately predict atheroprotective HDL function. Development of DSC1-targeting strategies may be a good starting point.

CLINICS CARE POINTS

- A low HDL-C should trigger the search for a suboptimal lifestyle (obesity, lack of exercise, poorly controlled diabetes).
- Patients should be counseled that their low HDL-C in itself is not a reason for treatment with medications.
- Rare forms of HDL deficiency should be evaluated in a specialized lipid clinic.
- Targeting HDL function remains a sound therapeutic avenue but will require rigorous clinical outcomes.

DISCLOSURE

J. Genest and H. Choi: funded by a project grant from the Canadian Institutes of Health Research on Desmocollin 1 (DSC1) and atherosclerosis (PJT-165924). J. Genest and H. Choi have filed Patent Cooperation Treaty (PCT) and United States patent applications entitled "Desmocollin 1 Inhibitors for the Prevention or Treatment of atherosclerosis" (PCT/CA2018/050,669 and US application no. 16/619,789). I. Iatan: no disclosures.

REFERENCES

1. Emerging Risk Factors Collaboration, Di Angelantonio E, Sarwar N, Perry P, et al. Major lipids, apolipoproteins, and risk of vascular disease. JAMA 2009;302: 1993–2000.
2. Hafiane A, Genest J. High Density Lipoproteins: Measurement Techniques and Potential Biomarkers of Cardiovascular Risk. BBA Clin 2015;3:175–88.
3. Davidson S. Available at: https://homepages.uc.edu/~davidswm/HDLproteome.html. Accessed October 2021.
4. Vaisar T, Pennathur S, Green PS, et al. Shotgun proteomics implicates protease inhibition and complement activation in the antiinflammatory properties of HDL. J Clin Invest 2007;117:746–56.
5. de la Llera Moya M, McGillicuddy FC, Hinkle CC, et al. Inflammation modulates human HDL composition and function in vivo. Atherosclerosis 2012;222:390–4.
6. Alwaili K, Bailey D, Awan Z, et al. The HDL proteome in acute coronary syndromes shifts to an inflammatory profile. Biochim Biophys Acta 2012;1821: 405–15.
7. Kontush A, Lhomme M, Chapman MJ. Unraveling the complexities of the HDL lipidome. J Lipid Res 2013;54:2950–63.
8. Serna J, García-Seisdedos D, Alcázar A, et al. Quantitative lipidomic analysis of plasma and plasma lipoproteins using MALDI-TOF mass spectrometry. Chem Phys Lipids 2015;189:7–18.
9. Rayner KJ, Esau CC, Hussain FN, et al. Inhibition of miR-33a/b in non-human primates raises plasma HDL and lowers VLDL triglycerides. Nature 2011;478(7369): 404–7.
10. Vickers KC, Michell DL. HDL-small RNA Export, Transport, and Functional Delivery in Atherosclerosis. Curr Atheroscler Rep 2021;23(7):38.
11. Genest J, Libby P. Chapter 48: Lipoprotein Disorders and CAD and Guidelines: Management of Lipid. In: Braunwald E, Libby P, Zipes D, et al, editors. Braunwald's heart disease 11th Edition. New York: Saunders; 2019.
12. Iatan I, Bailey D, Ruel I, et al. Membrane microdomains modulate oligomeric ABCA1 function: impact on apoAI-mediated lipid removal and phosphatidylcholine biosynthesis. J Lipid Res 2011;52(11):2043–55, 21846716.
13. Frikke-Schmidt R. Genetic variation in the ABCA1 gene, HDL cholesterol, and risk of ischemic heart disease in the general population. Atherosclerosis 2010;208(2): 305–16.
14. Jang E, Robert J, Rohrer L, et al. Transendothelial transport of lipoproteins. Atherosclerosis 2020;315:111–25.
15. Rosenson RS, Brewer HB, Ansell BJ, et al. Dysfunctional HDL and atherosclerotic cardiovascular disease. Sci Rep 2020;10(1):19223.
16. Robert J, Osto Elena, Arnold von Eckardstein. The Endothelium Is Both a Target and a Barrier of HDL's Protective Functions. Cells 2021;10(5):1041. PMID: 33924941.
17. Allard-Ratick MP, Kindya BR, Khambhati J, et al. HDL: Fact, fiction, or function? HDL cholesterol and cardiovascular risk. Eur J Prev Cardiol 2021;28(2):166–73.
18. Annema W, von Eckardstein A. Dysfunctional high-density lipoproteins in coronary heart disease: implications for diagnostics and therapy. Transl Res 2016; 173:30–57.
19. Madsen CM, Varbo A, Nordestgaard B. Low HDL cholesterol and high risk of autoimmune disease: two population-based cohort studies including 117341 individuals. Clin Chem 2019;65:644–52.

20. Schwertani A, Choi H, Genest J. High-density Lipoproteins and the Pathogenesis of Atherosclerosis. Curr Opin Cardiol 2018;33(3):311–6.
21. Gupta N, DeFranco AL. Lipid Rafts and B cell signaling. Semin Cell Dev Biol 2007;18:616–26.
22. Catapano AL, Pirillo A, Bonacina F, et al. HDL in innate and adaptive immunity. Cardiovasc Res 2014;103:372–83. 15.
23. Libby P. The changing landscape of atherosclerosis. Nature 2021;592(7855): 524–33.
24. Riaz H, Khan SU, Rahman H, et al. Effects of high-density lipoprotein targeting treatments on cardiovascular outcomes: A systematic review and meta-analysis. Eur J Prev Cardiol 2019;26(5):533–43.
25. Briel M, Ferreira-Gonzalez I, You JJ, et al. Association between change in high density lipoprotein cholesterol and cardiovascular disease morbidity and mortality: systematic review and meta-regression analysis. BMJ 2009;338:b92.
26. Mora S, Glynn RJ, Boekholdt SM, et al. On-treatment non-high-density lipoprotein cholesterol, apolipoprotein B, triglycerides, and lipid ratios in relation to residual vascular risk after treatment with potent statin therapy: JUPITER (justification for the use of statins in prevention: an intervention trial evaluating rosuvastatin). J Am Coll Cardiol 2012;59(17):1521–8.
27. Haase CL, Tybjærg-Hansen A, Qayyum AA, et al. LCAT, HDL cholesterol and ischemic cardiovascular disease: a Mendelian randomization study of HDL cholesterol in 54,500 individuals. J Clin Endocrinol Metab 2012;97(2):E248–56.
28. Voight BF, Peloso GM, Orho-Melander M, et al. Plasma HDL cholesterol and risk of myocardial infarction: a mendelian randomisation study. Lancet 2012;380: 572–80.
29. Brewer HB Jr, Barter PJ, Björkegren JLM, et al. HDL and atherosclerotic cardiovascular disease: genetic insights into complex biology. Nat Rev Cardiol 2018; 15(1):9–19.
30. Weissglas-Volkov D, Pajukanta P. Genetic causes of high and low serum HDL-cholesterol. J Lipid Res 2010;51(8):2032–57.
31. Ko DT, Alter DA, Guo H, et al. High-Density Lipoprotein Cholesterol and Cause-Specific Mortality in Individuals Without Previous Cardiovascular Conditions: The CANHEART Study. J Am Coll Cardiol 2016;68(19):2073–83.
32. Schaefer EJ, Anthanont P, Diffenderfer MR, et al. Diagnosis and treatment of high density lipoprotein deficiency. Prog Cardiovasc Dis 2016;59:97–106.
33. Geller AS, Polisecki EY, Diffenderfer MR, et al. Genetic and secondary causes of severe HDL deficiency and cardiovascular disease. J Lipid Res 2018;59: 2421–35.
34. Casula M, Colpani O, Xie S, et al. HDL in Atherosclerotic Cardiovascular Disease: In Search of a Role. Cells 2021;10(8):1869.
35. Chiesa G, Sirtori CR. Apolipoprotein A-I(Milano): current perspectives. Curr Opin Lipidol 2003;14(2):159–63.
36. Hooper AJ, Hegele RA, Burnett JR. Tangier disease: update for 2020. Curr Opin Lipidol 2020;31(2):80–4.
37. Westerterp M, Bochem AE, Yvan-Charvet L, et al. ATP-binding cassette transporters, atherosclerosis, and inflammation. Circ Res 2014;114(1):157–70.
38. Taheri H, Filion KB, Windle SB, et al. Cholesteryl Ester Transfer Protein Inhibitors and Cardiovascular Outcomes: A Systematic Review and Meta-Analysis of Randomized Controlled Trials. Cardiology 2020;145(4):236–50.
39. Rader DJ, Tall AR. The not-so-simple HDL story: Is it time to revise the HDL cholesterol hypothesis? Nat Med 2012;18(9):1344–6.

40. Tall AR, Dader DJ. Trials and Tribulations of CETP Inhibitors. Circ Res 2017;65: 607–8.
41. Helgadottir A, Gretarsdottir S, Thorleifsson G, et al. Variants with large effects on blood lipids and the role of cholesterol and triglycerides in coronary disease. Nat Genet 2016;48(6):634–9.
42. Helgadottir A, Sulem P, Thorgeirsson G, et al. Rare SCARB1 mutations associate with high-density lipoprotein cholesterol but not with coronary artery disease. Eur Heart J 2018;39(23):2172–8.
43. Willer CJ, Schmidt EM, Sengupta S, et al. Global Lipids Genetics Consortium. Discovery and refinement of loci associated with lipid levels. Nat Genet 2013; 45(11):1274–83.
44. Yamashita S, Masuda D, Matsuzawa Y. Pemafibrate, a New Selective PPARalpha Modulator: Drug Concept and Its Clinical Applications for Dyslipidemia and Metabolic Diseases. Curr Atheroscler Rep 2020;22(1):5.
45. Genest J, Choi HY. Novel Approaches for HDL-directed therapies. Curr Atheroscler Rep 2017;19(12):55.
46. Barter P, Genest J. HDL Cholesterol and ASCVD Risk Stratification – A Debate. Atheroscler 2019. https://doi.org/10.1016/j.atherosclerosis.2019.01.001.
47. Nicholls SJ, Andrews J, Kastelein JJP, et al. Effect of Serial Infusions of CER-001, a Pre-beta High-Density Lipoprotein Mimetic, on Coronary Atherosclerosis in Patients Following Acute Coronary Syndromes in the CER-001 Atherosclerosis Regression Acute Coronary Syndrome Trial: A Randomized Clinical Trial. JAMA Cardiol 2018;3(9):815–22.
48. Nicholls SJ, Puri R, Ballantyne CM, et al. Effect of Infusion of High-Density Lipoprotein Mimetic Containing Recombinant Apolipoprotein A-I Milano on Coronary Disease in Patients With an Acute Coronary Syndrome in the MILANO-PILOT Trial: A Randomized Clinical Trial. JAMA Cardiol 2018;3(9):806–14.
49. Gibson CM, Kastelein JJP, Phillips AT, et al. Rationale and design of ApoA-I Event Reducing in Ischemic Syndromes II (AEGIS-II): A phase 3, multicenter, double-blind, randomized, placebo-controlled, parallel-group study to investigate the efficacy and safety of CSL112 in subjects after acute myocardial infarction. Am Heart J 2021;231:121–7.
50. Neele AE, Willemsen L, Chen HJ, et al. Targeting epigenetics as atherosclerosis treatment: an updated view. Curr Opin Lipidol 2020;31(6):324–30.
51. DiDonato JA, Huang Y, Aulak KS, et al. Function and distribution of apolipoprotein A1 in the artery wall are markedly distinct from those in plasma. Circulation 2013; 128(15):1644–55.
52. Khera AV, Demler OV, Adelman SJ, et al. Cholesterol Efflux Capacity, HDL Particle Number, and Incident Cardiovascular Events. An Analysis from the JUPITER Trial. Circulation 2017;135(25):2494–504.
53. Wang N, Westerterp M. ABC Transporters, Cholesterol Efflux, and Implications for Cardiovascular Diseases. Adv Exp Med Biol 2020;1276:67–83.
54. Choi H, Ruel I, Malina A, et al. Desmocollin 1 is abundantly expressed in atherosclerosis and impairs HDL biogenesis. Eur Heart J 2018;39(14):1194–202.
55. Choi HY, Ruel I, Genest J. Chemical compounds targeting desmocollin 1: a new paradigm for HDL-directed therapies. Front Pharmacol 2021;12:679456, eCollection 2021.

Current Status of Pharmacologic and Nonpharmacologic Therapy in Heart Failure with Preserved Ejection Fraction

Mi-Na Kim, MD, PhD, Seong-Mi Park, MD, PhD*

KEYWORDS

• Heart failure • Preserved ejection fraction • Therapy

KEY POINTS

- Heart failure with preserved ejection fraction (HFpEF) is heterogenous systemic disorder that has various phenotype and multiple comorbidities.
- Several therapies for various phenotypes and pathophysiology of HFpEF have been introduced and studied, although the guideline directed medical therapy of HF with reduced EF had shown a limited clinical benefit.
- Several therapies for various phenotypes and pathophysiology of HFpEF have been introduced and studied, although the guideline directed medical therapy of HF with reduced EF had shown a limited clinical benefit.
- The pressure monitoring was demonetrated to reduced HF hospitalization, and several non-pharmacological therapies that are targeting various phenotype and pathophysiology of HEpEF, such as interatrial septal shunt, pacing therapies, left ventricular expander and pericardiectomy, have been introduced and currently studied.

INTRODUCTION

Heart failure with preserved ejection fraction (HFpEF) is now the most common form of heart failure (HF) and accounts for about half the HF cases.[1] It is a growing burden to the health care system because of the increasing prevalence, substantial comorbidities, and unfavorable prognosis.[2] HFpEF is now one of the greatest unmet needs in cardiology[3] because it lacks proven therapy to reduce mortality and morbidity compared with remarkable developments and revolutionized changes in the treatment of HF with reduced ejection fraction (HFrEF). HFpEF is considered to be a systemic

This article originally appeared in *Heart Failure Clinics*, Volume 17, Issue 3, July 2021.
Division of Cardiology, Department of Internal Medicine, Korea University Medicine, Korea University Anam Hospital, Goryeodae-ro 73, Seongbuk-gu, Seoul 02841, Republic of Korea
* Corresponding author.
E-mail address: smparkmd@korea.ac.kr

syndrome with diverse phenotypes, various pathophysiologies, and multiple comorbidities. The diagnosis of HFpEF has become more refined and sophisticated. Numerous pharmacologic and nonpharmacologic therapies for each phenotype or pathophysiology have been suggested and investigated in the HFpEF population.[4] This article summarizes pharmacologic and nonpharmacologic therapies and reviews recent clinical trials in patients with HFpEF and also provides therapeutic options for unmanageable HFpEF.

DIVERSE PATHOPHYSIOLOGY OF HEART FAILURE WITH PRESERVED EJECTION FRACTION AND ITS PHENOTYPE

HFpEF has been considered a diastolic HF for the past 20 years. Left ventricle (LV) diastolic dysfunction caused by impaired relaxation and increased chamber stiffness leads to an increase in LV filling pressure. Increased LV filling pressure at rest or during exercise promotes the development of dyspnea and exercise intolerance. Numerous efforts to elucidate the pathophysiology and define the phenotype of HFpEF have led to a paradigm shift to a systemic syndrome that results from an interplay of coexisting significant abnormalities, including left atrium (LA) dysfunction, subtle LV systolic dysfunction, pulmonary hypertension with right ventricle (RV) dysfunction, extrinsic restraint by epicardial fat, microvascular dysfunction, chronotropic incompetence, skeletal muscle dysfunction, altered ventriculoarterial coupling, and abnormal cardiorenal relationship, besides LV diastolic dysfunction.[5] These abnormalities might be generated and affected by systemic inflammation, endothelial dysfunction, and oxidative stress induced by multiple risk factors and comorbidities of HFpEF, such as coronary artery disease (CAD), hypertension, obesity, diabetes, atrial fibrillation (AF), anemia, renal dysfunction, sleep apnea, and chronic lung disease.[6–8] The oxidative stress induced by systemic inflammation reduces the bioavailability of nitric oxide (NO) and produces highly reactive superoxide in the endothelium. The endothelium is changed to be favorable for vasoconstriction and prothrombotic status.[7] Impaired NO bioavailability influences the NO–cyclic guanosine monophosphate (cGMP)–protein kinase G (PKG) pathway in the myocardium. Because of decreased PKG activity by downregulation of the NO-cGMP-PKG pathway, cardiomyocytes are stiffened.[6,9] Furthermore, interstitial fibrosis occurs because of increased collagen secretion by myofibroblasts activated by an increased level of transforming growth factor-β (TGF-β) released from macrophage.[10] Moreover, upregulated galetin-3 in HFpEF is another important mediator of myocardial fibrosis.[11] Also, systemic inflammation leads to impaired myocardial energetics via altered structure and impaired function of mitochondria, change in energy metabolism, and intracellular calcium overload. These cardiometabolic abnormalities are regarded as another pathophysiology in HFpEF even though these concepts are derived from studies in HFrEF.[12]

A schematic diagram of comorbidities, pathophysiology, and representative phenotypes of HFpEF is presented in **Fig. 1**.

EFFORTS TO INCREASE THE ACCURACY OF HEART FAILURE WITH PRESERVED EJECTION FRACTION DIAGNOSIS

HF is a clinical syndrome caused by structural or functional impairment of contraction or filling of the heart. According to current guidelines, the diagnosis of HF is based on a combination of the presence of symptoms and signs of HF and increased natriuretic peptide levels. Subsequently, HFpEF is classified according to LV ejection fraction (LVEF).[13–15] However, the diagnostic algorithm of current guidelines is limited when diagnosing HFpEF, a clinical syndrome that has numerous causes and various

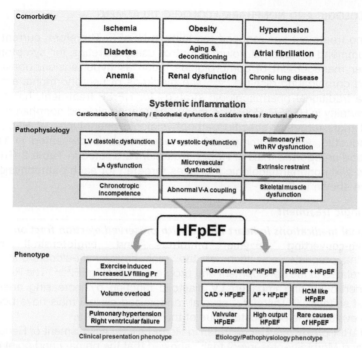

Fig. 1. Comorbidities, pathophysiology, and phenotypes of HFpEF. HCM, hypertrophic cardiomyopathy; HT, hypertension; PH, pulmonary hypertension; Pr, pressure; RHF, right heart failure, V-A, ventriculoarterial.

and distinct phenotypes.[16] Recently, new diagnostic algorithms for providing the probability of HFpEF were proposed.[17,18] The H_2FPEF score is obtained by the sum of scores applicable to 6 variables including 2 echocardiographic (representative of increased LV filling pressure and pulmonary hypertension) and 4 clinical variables that are major comorbidities or causes of HFpEF (age, obesity, hypertension, and AF).[17] The HFA-PEFF diagnostic algorithm suggested by the Heart Failure Association of the European Society of Cardiology approaches the patients in a stepwise process. This 4-step algorithm is composed of pretest assessment, risk stratification by HFA-PEFF score, functional test in patients with intermediate probability, and evaluation of specific cause. The HFA-PEFF score is composed of echocardiographic parameters and the level of natriuretic peptides, which have different cutoff values by rhythm status or age. These new diagnostic algorithms have been reported to be superior to current guidelines.[19,20] The preevaluation before both score calculations was similar to the diagnostic criteria of the 2016 European Society of Cardiology guidelines. The probability of diagnosing HFpEF and recommendation of additional tests, such as exercise stress echocardiography or invasive hemodynamic measurement with and without exercise, in patients with uncertainty are common findings in both diagnostic algorithms. The H_2FPEF score considers comorbidities of HFpEF, and the HFA-PEFF diagnostic algorithm recommends the comprehensive diagnostic process for HFpEF. However, the diagnosis of HFpEF remains challenging in clinical practice. Additional validation, comparison of diagnostic accuracy, and elucidation of reclassified patients who have a different likelihood by new diagnostic systems should be investigated in the future.[21]

PHARMACOLOGIC AND NONPHARMACOLOGIC TREATMENT

To date, no treatment has reduced mortality in HFpEF. Therefore, current guidelines recommend an optimal volume control using diuretics for symptom relief and proper management of comorbidities, such as hypertension, obesity, diabetes, and chronic lung disease.[13,22] The blockade of neurohormonal activation, which is a traditional pharmacologic strategy for HFrEF treatment, has failed to reduce mortality in HFpEF. However, many pharmacologic and nonpharmacologic treatment trials targeting specific pathophysiologic phenotypes of HFpEF have been conducted, and a summary of the recent trials is presented in **Table 1**. Ongoing and unreported trials of HFpEF treatment are listed in **Table 2**. The pharmacologic and nonpharmacologic therapies targeted for each pathophysiology of HFpEF are shown in **Fig. 2**.

Pharmacologic Treatment

Conventional medications in heart failure with preserved ejection fraction
Angiotensin-converting enzyme inhibitors and angiotensin-II receptor blockers. Inappropriate activation of the renin-angiotensin-aldosterone system (RAAS) is related to the development and progression of HFpEF.[23,24] The RAAS leads to LV hypertrophy and impaired LV diastolic function by increasing arterial and myocardial stiffness.[23] Therefore, several randomized clinical trials have been conducted to evaluate the prognostic value of the RAAS blockade.

The CHARM-preserved (Candesartan in Heart Failure: Assessment of Reduction in Mortality and Morbidity-preserved) trial[25] showed that the primary end point of composite cardiovascular (CV) death or HF hospitalization was not statistically different in candesartan versus placebo (hazard ratio, 0.89; 95% confidence interval [CI], 0.77–1.03; $P = .118$); however, HF hospitalization was significantly reduced by candesartan (hazard ratio, 0.84; 95% CI, 0.07–1.00; $P = .047$). In the PEP-CHF (Perindopril in Elderly People with Chronic Heart Failure) study,[26] perindopril improved HF symptoms and reduced HF rehospitalization at 1-year follow-up, but the benefit of perindopril in HFpEF remains uncertain. Because of the lower event rate than anticipated and the large proportion of withdrawal, the statistical power of the study to show a difference in the primary end point was reduced. The I-PRSERVED (Irbesartan in Heart Failure with Preserved Ejection Fraction) study,[27] irbesartan did not reduce all-cause mortality and CV hospitalization and it did not improve the quality of life (QOL) of HFpEF in long-term follow-up.[28] In conclusion, angiotensin-converting enzyme inhibitors (ACEis) and angiotensin-II receptor blockers (ARBs) did not improve mortality and HF hospitalization in patients with HFpEF except for a weak positive result for HF hospitalization by candesartan.

Mineralocorticoid receptor antagonists. Mineralocorticoid receptor antagonists, including spironolactone and eplerenone, are important cornerstones in HFrEF treatment. Aldosterone leads to myocardial fibrosis and results in increased myocardial stiffness and increased ventricular filling pressure. Therefore, aldosterone could be considered a therapeutic target of HFpEF. In the Aldosterone Receptor Blockade in Diastolic Heart Failure (Aldo-DHF) trial, aldosterone showed a positive decrease in LV mass, N-terminal fragment of pro–brain natriuretic peptide (NT-proBNP) level, and improved diastolic function but failed to improve HF symptoms, exercise capacity, and QOL in the HFpEF population.[29] The Treatment of Preserved Cardiac Function Heart Failure With an Aldosterone Antagonist Trial[30] enrolled 3445 patients with HFpEF (LVEF $\geq$ 45%) randomly assigned to either spironolactone or placebo. At a mean follow-up of 3.3 years, the primary end points (death from CV causes, aborted

Table 1
Results of recently reported randomized control trials of pharmacologic and nonpharmacologic therapies of heart failure with preserved ejection fraction

Trials (Number of Patients)	Interventions	Inclusion Criteria	Mean Follow-up (mo)	Primary End Point	Trial Result
Pharmacologic Treatment					
PARAGON-HF[39] 2019, (n = 4822)	Sacubitril-valsartan	NYHA II–IV LVEF ≥ 45% Increased NPs	35	CV death HF hospitalization	No benefit for the primary end point Reduced primary end point in subgroup (patients with LVEF less than median [≤ 57%] and women)
EDIFY[56] 2017, (n = 179)	Ivabradine	NYHA II–III SR with HR ≥ 70 LVEF ≥ 45% Increased NPs	8	E/e', 6MWD NT-proBNP	No difference in E/e', 6MWD, and NT-proBNP
NEAT-HFpEF[60] 2015, (n = 110)	Isosorbide mononitrate	LVEF ≥ 50% HF with objective evidence (≥1) • HF hospitalization with congestion, increased LVEDP or PCWP, increased NP, LVDD on ECHO	3	Daily activity level	Decreased activity and worsened QOL
INDIE-HFpEF[66] 2018, (n = 105)	Nebulized inorganic nitrate	Age ≥ 40 y LVEF ≥ 50% HF with objective evidence (≥1) • HF hospitalization with congestion, increased LVEDP or PCWP, increased NP, LVDD on ECHO	3	Peak O_2 consumption	No improvement in exercise capacity

(continued on next page)

Table 1
(continued)

Trials (Number of Patients)	Interventions	Inclusion Criteria	Mean Follow-up (mo)	Primary End Point	Trial Result
RELAX[69] 2016, (n = 216)	Sildenafil	HFpEF with RVD and RV-RA coupling NYHA II–IV LVEF ≥ 50%	6	Peak O$_2$uptake	No improvement of RV function, exercise capacity, and ventilatory efficiency
DILATE-1[72] 2014, (n = 21)	Riociguat	HFpEF with PH LVEF ≥ 50%, mPAP ≥ 25 mm Hg PAWP >15 mm Hg at rest	6	Peak decrease in mPAP	No significant effect on mPAP
SOCRATES-PRESERVED[73] 2017, (n = 477)	Vericiguat	NYHA II–IV LVEF ≥ 45% Increased NPs history of HFH or intravenous diuretics within 4 wk	3	Change of NT-proBNP and LAV	No significant change in NT-proBNP and LAV
CAPACITY HFpEF[74] 2020, (n = 196)	Praliciguat	LVEF ≥ 40% Impaired peak Vo$_2$ ≥2 condition associated with NO deficiency	3	Peak VO$_2$	No improvement in Peak VO$_2$ consumption
VITALITY-HFpEF[75] 2020, (n = 789)	Vericiguat	NYHA II–III LVEF ≥ 45% Recent decompensation within 6 mo	6	KCCQ change	No improvement in KCCQ
EMPERIAL-preserved[98] unpublished, (n = 315)	Empagliflozin	NYHA II–IV LVEF ≥ 40%	3	6MWD	No improvement in 6MWD
Nonpharmacologic Treatment					
CHAMPION[101] 2011, (n = 119)	Wireless implantable hemodynamic monitoring	HF with NYHA III LVEF ≥ 40%	6	HF hospitalization	Reduction of HF hospitalization

Study	Intervention	Criteria		Outcome	Result
REDUCELAP-HF I[104] 2018, (n = 94)	Interatrial shunt device	NYHA III, IV LVEF ≥ 40% Exercise PCWP ≥ 25 mm Hg, PCWP-RAP gradient ≥ 5 mm Hg	1	Exercise PCWP	Reduction of PCWP during exercise
Ex-DHF[115] 2011, (n = 64)	Endurance/resistance training	Age ≥ 45 y NYHA II–III LVEF ≥ 50% CV risk factor	3	Peak Vo_2	Improvement in exercise capacity and QOL
SECRET-1[118] 2016, (n = 200)	Caloric restriction Aerobic exercise training	HF with obesity Age ≥ 60 y BMI ≥ 30 LVEF ≥ 50%	1	Peak Vo_2 Disease-specific QOL	Increased peak O_2uptake both caloric restriction and aerobic exercise training with addictive value

Abbreviations: 6MWD, 6-minute walking distance; BMI, body mass index; CV, cardiovascular; ECHO, echocardiography; HFH, heart failure hospitalization; HR, heart rate; KCCQ, Kansas City Cardiomyopathy Questionnaire; LAV, left atrial volume; LVDD, LV diastolic dysfunction; LVEDP, LV end-diastolic pressure; mPAP, mean peak arterial pressure; NO, nitric oxide; NP, natriuretic peptide; NT-proBNP, N-terminal pro–brain natriuretic peptide; NYHA, New York Heart Association; PAP, pulmonary artery pressure; PAWP, pulmonary artery wedge pressure; PCWP, pulmonary capillary wedge pressure; QOL, quality of life; RA, right atrium; RAP, right atrial pressure; RVD, RV dysfunction; SR, sinus rhythm; VO_2, peak oxygen consumption.

Table 2
Ongoing or unreported trials of pharmacologic and nonpharmacologic treatment of heart failure with preserved ejection fraction

Name ClinicalTrials.gov Identifier	Intervention	Study Size	Primary End Point	Study Completion
Pharmacologic Treatment				
SPIRRIT-HFPEF NCT02901184	Spironolactone	3500	CV mortality or HF hospitalization	June 2022
PARAGLIDE-HF NCT03988634	Sacubitril/valsartan	800	Proportional change in NT-proBNP	September 2021
PRISTINE-HF NCT04128891	Sacubitril/valsartan	60	Microvascular function and ischemia	February 2024
NCT03928158	Sacubitril/valsartan	60	6MWD	November 2020
KNO3CK OUT HFPEF NCT02840799	KNO₃ KCl	76	Peak Vo₂	December 2020
PIROUETTE NCT02932566	Pirfenidone	200	Myocardial ECV, measuring using CMR	Complete
Regress-HFpEF NCT02941705	Cardiosphere-derived cells	40	Safety	June 2021
CELLpEF NCT02923609	CD34+ cell	30	Change of E/e'	March 2022
NCT02814097	Elamipretide	46	Change of E/e' during exercise	Complete
NCT02914665	Elamipretide	308	NT-proBNP	Complete
HELP NCT03541603	Levosimendan	38	Exercise PCWP	Complete
ILO-HOPE NCT03620526	Iloprost	34	Exercise pulmonary wedge pressure	NA
DELIVER NCT03619213	Dapagliflozin	6100	CV mortality, HF hospitalization, urgent HF visit	November 2021
EMPEROR-Preserved NCT03057951	Empagliflozin	5988	CV mortality or HF hospitalization	April 2021
PRESERVED-HF NCT03030235	Dapagliflozin	320	KCCQ change	February 2021
EMPERIAL-preserved NCT03448406	Empagliflozin	315	6MWD	Complete
FAIR-HFpEF NCT03074591	Ferric carboxymaltose	200	6MWD	July 2021
Nonpharmacologic Treatment				
GUIDE-HF NCT03387813	CardioMEMS HF system	3600	HF hospitalization, intravenous diuretics visit, all-cause mortality	April 2023
REDUCE LAP-HF II NCT03088033	Interatrial septal shunt	608	CV mortality, stroke, HF	August 2027

(*continued on next page*)

Name ClinicalTrials.gov Identifier	Intervention	Study Size	Primary End Point	Study Completion
Table 2 *(continued)*				
			hospitalization, or worsening QOL	
RAPID-HF NCT02145351	Rate-adaptive pacing CRT	30	Exercise capacity	May 2021
PREFECTUS NCT03338374	Rate response pacing CRT	10	Diastolic reserve index	June 2020
CCM-HFpEF NCT03240237	CCM	60	KCCQ change	December 2023
LEAD NCT01618981	Left atrial pacing	NA	NA	Complete
NCT02499601	CORolla	10	All-cause mortality Serious adverse events	September 2024
NCT03923673	Pericardiotomy	4	Major adverse CV event	May 2022

Abbreviations: 6MWD, 6-minute walking distance; CD, cluster of differentiation; CCM, cardiac contractility modulation; CMR, cardiac magnetic resonance; CRT, cardiac resynchronization therapy; CV, cardiovascular; ECV, extracellular volume; HF, heart failure; KCCQ, Kansas City Cardiomyopathy Questionnaire; NA, not available; NT-proBNP, N-terminal pro-brain natriuretic peptide; Peak VO_2, peak oxygen consumption; PCWP, pulmonary capillary wedge pressure; QOL, quality of life.

cardiac arrest, or HF hospitalization) were not different between the groups (hazard ratio, 0.89; 95% CI, 0.77–1.04; P = .14). However, HF hospitalization was moderately decreased in the spironolactone-treated group (hazard ratio, 0.83; 95% CI, 0.69–0.99; P = .04). In subgroup and post hoc analysis, the primary outcome was related to increased natriuretic peptide level at baseline[30] and significant regional variation of primary outcome existed between the Americas (United States, Canada, Brazil, and Argentina) and Russia and Georgia.[31] In the Americas, spironolactone reduced primary end points (hazard ratio, 0.82; 95% CI, 0.69–0.98; P = .026) but not in Russia or Georgia. The presumed reasons for regional variation were the difference in severity at baseline, determinant of patient enrollment (eg, an increased natriuretic peptide in the Americas vs clinical judgment in Russia and Georgia), and lower medication compliance in Russia and Georgia shown by measuring canrenone, an active metabolite of spironolactone.[32] For this reason, reevaluation of the clinical efficacy of spironolactone is required. The ongoing SPIRRIT (Spironolactone Initiation Registry Randomized Interventional Trial in Heart Failure with Preserved Ejection Fraction; NCT02901184) might clarify the therapeutic efficacy of spironolactone.

Angiotensin receptor neprilysin inhibitors. The angiotensin receptor neprilysin inhibitor (ARNI) sacubitril-valsartan is a combination of RAAS blockers and upregulators of the endogenous natriuretic peptide pathway. Sacubitril-valsartan is an upcoming and revolutionizing disease-modifying agent in HFrEF. Inhibition of neprilysin not only augments endogenous natriuretic peptides but also other vasoactive peptides, including

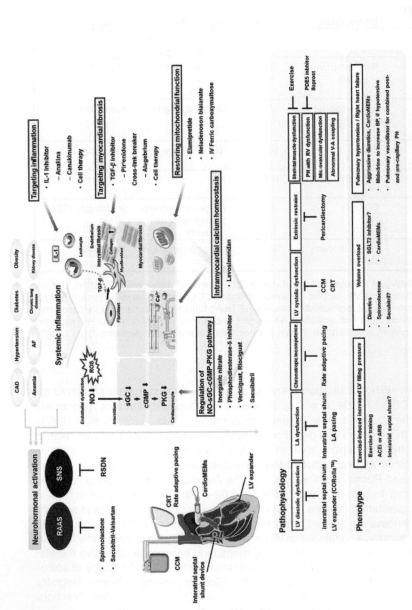

Fig. 2. Pharmacologic and nonpharmacologic therapies according to the pathophysiology of HFpEF. Descriptions of each medication and device therapy are presented in the text. Most of these therapies, except for CardioMEMS, are targeted or associated with the pathophysiology of HFpEF. CardioMEMS is implanted in the pulmonary artery and monitors changes in pulmonary arterial pressure. It would be effective to the phenotype of volume overload and pulmonary hypertension with RV dysfunction in HFpEF. CCM, cardiac contractility modulation; CRT, cardiac resynchronization therapy; IL, interleukin; RAAS, renin-angiotensin-aldosterone system; ROS, reactive oxygen species; RSDN, renal sympathetic denervation; PDE, phosphodiesterase; sGC, soluble guanylyl cyclase; SNS, sympathetic nervous system.

cGMP, that are decreased and related to myocardial stiffness in HFpEF.[33] In patients with HFpEF, sacubitril-valsartan was associated with a larger reduction of natriuretic peptide levels, LA reverse remodeling, and greater symptom improvement than valsartan in a phase II study (PARAMOUNT).[34] This finding might be beneficial to patients with HFpEF. Therefore, the PARAGON-HF[35] (Prospective Comparison of ARNI with ARB Global Outcomes in HF with Preserved Ejection Fraction) trial was conducted to determine the efficacy of sacubitril-valsartan in HFpEF. A total of 4822 patients with New York Heart Association (NYHA) II to IV HF and LVEF greater than or equal to 45% were randomly assigned to sacubitril-valsartan or valsartan. Despite the numerically lower event rate of the primary end points (CV mortality and HF hospitalization), the efficacy of sacubitril-valsartan did not achieve statistical significance (hazard ratio, 0.87; 95% CI, 0.75–1.01; $P = .06$). In subgroup analysis, sacubitril-valsartan showed the benefit of reducing the primary outcome in female patients with LVEF to less than the median (≤57%). In a prespecified analysis of outcomes by sex in the PARAGON-HF trial, the beneficial effect from sacubitril-valsartan to reduce primary composite outcome was greater in women than in men (relative risk [RR], 0.73; 95% CI, 0.59–0.90 in women vs RR, 1.03; 95% CI, 0.84–1.25; P interaction = 0.017).[36] Because of advanced myocardial remodeling even in the same LV systolic function, more progressive age-related arterial stiffening in women, and differences in natriuretic peptide signaling, sacubitril-valsartan might be effective in women, but not in men.[36,37] Recently, the pooled analysis of combined data from PARADIGM-HF (Prospective Comparison of ARNI With ACEI to Determine Impact on Global Mortality and Morbidity in Heart Failure)[38] and PARAGON-HF[35] trials showed that treatment benefit existed for LVEF less than 42.5% and it was maximized in patients with lower LVEF.[39] Sacubitril-valsartan was effective in women with LVEF less than or equal to 60%; however, the threshold of LVEF to lose efficacy of sacubitril-valsartan was 45% to 50% in men. In post hoc analysis,[8] the effect of sacubitril-valsartan for reduction of the primary end point was maximal in patients recently admitted (within 30 days of prior hospitalization) who had a high risk of rehospitalization and CV death, and it gradually decreased with increasing time from the previous admission. Early administration of sacubitril-valsartan after stabilization within 30 days after hospitalization might have amplified the benefit of sacubitril-valsartan.

The role of RAAS inhibitors in HFpEF is controversial. However, some evidence suggests that RAAS inhibitors might be efficient in HFpEF.[30,35] In a meta-analysis to investigate the efficacy of RAAS inhibitors in HFpEF, only spironolactone reduced HF hospitalization, but it did not decrease mortality.[40] In a recent meta-analysis evaluating the effect of RAAS inhibitors on the outcome of HFpEF that included the five trials mentioned above (CHARM-preserved, PEP-CHF, I-PRESERVED, TOPCAT, PARAGON-HF),[41] sacubitril-valsartan was superior to placebo and ARB in reduce HF hospitalization, althouth the RAAS inhibitors did not decrease all-cause mortality and CV mortality. In this context, the ongoing PARAGIDE-HF (Changes in NT-proBNP and Outcomes, Safety, and Tolerability in HFpEF Patients With Acute Decompensated Heart Failure Who Have Been Stabilized During Hospitalization and Initiated In-hospital or Within 30 Days Postdischarge; NCT03988634) study might determine the clinical efficacy of sacubitril-valsartan for HF rehospitalization.

However, the application of RAAS blockade in patients with HFpEF should be made carefully and applied appropriately to each patient. The LVEF cutoff of trials mentioned earlier was greater than or equal to 40% in 2 trials[25,26] and greater than or equal to 45% in 3 trials.[27,30,35] Therefore, a considerable portion of registered patients to trials might belong to HF with mid-ranged EF (HFmrEF) and the proportion of HFmrEF and HFpEF in trials could be different from each other. The RAAS activation is less prominent in HFpEF rather than in HFmrEF and HFrEF and a considerable proportion of patients in trials had already been taking RAAS inhibitors at enrollment due to their comorbidities, hence the effectiveness of RAAS inhibitors might appear to be limited in HFpEF.

β-Blockers. β-Blockers (BBs) are another cornerstone of HFrEF treatment[13] because of improved mortality and HF hospitalization. The increased heart rate (HR) by sympathetic overactivation causes shortening of LV diastolic filling time and leads to increased ventricular filling pressure and exercise intolerance. Thus, HR reduction and reversal of sympathetic overactivation might be beneficial in HFpEF. The increased HR in sinus rhythm, not in AF, is closely associated with poor outcome in HFpEF.[42,43] Thus, several investigations were conducted to evaluate the clinical efficacy of HFpEF. In observational data, BBs showed a modest benefit for survival.[43,44] However, nebivolol did not reduce mortality in patients with HFpEF (LVEF>35%) in prospecified subanalysis of the SENIORS (Study of Effects of Nebivolol Intervention on Outcomes and Rehospitalization in Seniors With Heart Failure).[45] Nebivolol did not improve HF symptoms, exercise capacity, or QOL in the ELANDD (Effects of the Long-term Administration of Nebivolol on the Clinical Symptoms, Exercise Capacity, and Left Ventricular Function of Patients with Diastolic Dysfunction) study.[42] In the Japanese Diastolic Heart Failure (J-DHF) study,[46] carvedilol was not effective in reducing CV death and HF hospitalization in patients with HFpEF (LVEF>40%). In several meta-analyses, the effect of BBs on CV outcome in HFpEF was controversial.[40,47,48] The positive result to reduce mortality in HFpEF was predominantly derived from observational data.[47] In a meta-analysis of 11 randomized controlled trials (RCTs), BBs did not improve prognosis in HFpEF.[48] The prespecified TOPCAT trial to evaluate the effect of BB use on CV outcomes found that BB was associated with increased HF hospitalization and was not associated with CV mortality in HFpEF.[49] A recent meta-analysis revealed that BB had no clear benefit on the severity of HFpEF but it was associated with favorable outcomes in HFpEF with CAD or AF.[50] The conflicting results regarding the efficacy of BB remain to be resolved. These findings might be caused by the differences in the definition of HFpEF, especially LVEF cutoff value, differences in HR at baseline and their changes, and preexisting comorbidities, such as AF and CAD, that could benefit from BB.[51] The use of BB in patients with HFpEF needs to be determined by careful evaluation of the patient conditions and comorbidities.

Ivabradine. Ivabradine is a selective blocker of the funny (I_f) channel in the sinoatrial node, thereby decreasing HR. As mentioned earlier, HR reduction might theoretically be beneficial in patients with HFpEF. However, an EDIFY (Preserved Left Ventricular Ejection Fraction Chronic Heart Failure with Ivabradine Study) study[52] found no beneficial effects on LV diastolic function, exercise capacity, and natriuretic peptide level despite HR reduction. In a recently reported meta-analysis, ivabradine also did not show the benefit of improving exercise capacity.[53] The suppression of HR increase during exercise by ivabradine might contribute to the ineffectiveness of ivabradine in HFpEF.[10]

Digoxin. Digoxin administration might be considered in patients with HFrEF with sinus rhythm symptoms to decrease the risk of hospitalization and in patients with AF to slow a rapid ventricular rate.[13] However, its utility has been decreasing. In the DIG-PEP (The Effects of Digoxin on Morbidity and Mortality in Diastolic Heart Failure) trial, digoxin did not affect mortality and hospitalization in patients with HFpEF (LVEF>45%) sinus rhythm symptoms.[54]

New disease-modifying treatment
Treatment targeting the nitric oxide–soluble guanylyl cyclase—cyclic guanosine monophosphate–protein kinase G pathway. PKGs are intrinsic suppressors of interstitial fibrosis and prevent ventricular hypertrophy via regulation of phosphorylation, structural changes, and oxidation of titin cytoskeletal protein.[4,55] cGMP, a stimulator of PKG, is generated from guanosine triphosphate by guanylyl cyclase (GCs). GCs exist in 2 forms: the soluble form (sGC) stimulated by NO, and the particulate GC (pGC) stimulated by natriuretic peptides.[55]

The downregulation of the NO-sGC-cGMP-PKG pathway is a key mechanism in endothelium-cardiomyocyte signaling altered by systemic inflammation and critical pathophysiology of HFpEF development and progression. Treatments targeting the NO-sGC-cGMP-PKG pathway offer promising therapeutic strategies for HFpEF. Drugs enhancing NO bioavailability, phosphodiesterase-5a (PDE-5) inhibitors, sGC stimulators, and beta 3 adrenergic receptor–selective agonists have been investigated.

Directing nitric oxide donor: organic and inorganic nitrate In the NEAT-HFpEF (Nitrate's Effect on Activity Tolerance in Heart Failure with Preserved Ejection Fraction) trial,[56] organic isosorbide mononitrate did not improve QOL or reduce NT-proBNP level but decreased daily activity and worsened HF symptoms. Excessive hypotension caused by vasodilatation and a decrease in cardiac output by preload reduction[57] were possible causes of the negative outcome of this study. Rapid onset of tolerance and endothelial dysfunction caused by organic nitrates are other possible causes.[58] Inorganic nitrate (NO_3) has a different metabolism of NO via the nitrate-nitrite pathway and might be an important treatment target in HFpEF to improve arterial vasodilatory reserve, increase muscle O_2 delivery, and enhance mitochondrial function in skeletal muscle.[59] In small trials, NO_3 delivered via NO_3-enriched beetroot juice showed an improvement in exercise capacity in the HFpEF population.[60,61] The administration of sodium nitrite via infusion or inhalation improved hemodynamic parameters such as pulmonary artery (PA) pressure during exercise in HFpEF.[59] In contrast with these data, the INDIE-HFpEF (Inorganic Nitrite Delivery to Improve Exercise Capacity in HFpEF) trial[62] showed that inhaled inorganic nitrite failed to improve HF symptoms, exercise capacity, and QOL in patients with HFpEF. Because other administration methods of inorganic nitrite that provide much longer and higher levels of NO achieved positive results, the short-acting nature of inhalation delivery may be the possible cause of the negative result of the INDIE-HFpEF trial. Trials of NO_3 via oral administration in HFpEF, such as KNO3CKOT-HFpEF (Effect of KNO_3 Compared to KCl on Oxygen Uptake in Heart Failure With Preserved Ejection Fraction; NCT02840799) are ongoing.

Phosphodiesterase-5 inhibitors PDE-5 is a metabolizer of NO and cGMP. PDE-5 inhibition is beneficial in HFpEF because of increased cGMP level and cardiac reverse remodeling, and hemodynamic improvement by PDE-5 inhibition has been indicated by experimental and small clinical studies.[63,64] However, in the RELAX (Phosphodiesterase-5 Inhibition to Improve Clinical Status and Exercise Capacity in Heart Failure with Preserved Ejection Fraction) trial,[65] sildenafil did not improve exercise capacity in patients with HFpEF with or without pulmonary hypertension (PH). In patients with HFpEF and postcapillary PH, sildenafil failed to decrease PA pressure and to improve invasive hemodynamics.[66] However, PDE-5 inhibitor is effective in treating precapillary PH and might offer some benefits in combined precapillary and postcapillary PH. Further studies to investigate this possibility are needed.

Soluble guanylyl cyclase stimulators The sGC stimulators (riociguat and vericiguat) enhance cCMP production by acting on NO receptors and are primarily used in the treatment of PH. Recently, a promising result of vericiguat in HFrEF was reported.[67] In HFpEF, sGC stimulators showed limited efficacy in reducing NT-proBNP and LA size in 2 phase 2 trials, DILATE-1 (Acute Hemodynamic Effects of Riociguat in Patients with Pulmonary Hypertension Associated with Diastolic HF)[68] and SOCRATES-PRESERVED (Soluble Guanylate Cyclase Stimulator in Heart Failure Patients with Preserved EF).[69] Furthermore, according to recently reported data (CAPACITY HFpEF [A Study of the Effect of IW-1973 on the Exercise Capacity of Patients With Heart Failure With Preserved Ejection Fraction] trial and VITALITY-HFpEF [Evaluate the Efficacy and Safety of the Oral sGC Stimulator Vericiguat to Improve Physical Functioning in Daily Living Activities of Patients With Heart Failure and Preserved Ejection Fraction] trial), sGC stimulators failed to improve exercise capacity and QOL in the HFpEF population.[70,71]

Other cyclic guanosine monophosphate–protein kinase G–stimulating drugs: sacubitril As mentioned earlier, sacubitril could enhance the production of cGMP and PKG via pGC present in the cell membrane. pGC is stimulated by natriuretic peptides and generates cGMP.[55] The currently reported clinical efficacy of sacubitril-valsartan in HFpEF was described earlier. Although some limited data on sacubitril-valsartan suggest that it may improve hard clinical end points such as mortality, it could also affect so-called soft end points, including reverse cardiac remodeling, improvement of clinical symptoms, exercise capacity, and QOL. Several studies are underway to address these topics (NCT03988634, NCT04128891, and NCT03928158).

Treatment targeting inflammation and myocardial fibrosis

Targeting inflammation: an interleukin-1 inhibitor The interleukin-1 (IL-1) family is one of the major cytokines in chronic systemic inflammation and is an important molecule in the development of HFpEF.[72] In particular, increased IL-1β level affects calcium homeostasis in cardiomyocytes, increases reactive oxygen species (ROS) production, decreases energy production, and impairs myocardial contractility.[72] In a pilot study, D-HART (Diastolic Heart Failure Anakinra Response Trial), anakinra, a recombinant IL-1 antagonist, administered for 2 weeks improved peak oxygen consumption in a small number of patients with HFpEF.[73] However, this favorable outcome was not proved in expanded D-HART2 (Diastolic Heart Failure Anakinra Response Trial 2). Anakinra failed to improve aerobic exercise capacity or ventilatory efficiency even though it reduced C-reactive protein (CRP) levels for 12 weeks.[74] In the Cardiovascular Risk Reduction Study [education in recurrent major CV disease events], which was a large RCT to investigate the efficacy of canakinumab in patients with myocardial infarction and inflammation (CRP level ≥2 mg/L),[75] canakinumab, an IL-1β monoclonal antibody, reduced HF-related hospitalization and mortality in a dose-dependent manner.[76] Further studies are required to elucidate the clinical impact of IL-1 blockade in HFpEF.

Targeting myocardial fibrosis Because interstitial fibrosis and myocyte hypertrophy caused by abandoned deposition of collagen is the major axis of HFpEF pathophysiology, it was hypothesized that antifibrotic therapy used to treat idiopathic pulmonary fibrosis might affect HFpEF.[77] Pirfenidone is an inhibitor of the TGF-β signaling pathway that has shown a favorable effect in IPF[78] by preventing ventricular fibrosis and dysfunction in preclinical tests.[79] The PIROUETTE (Pirfenidone in Patients With Heart Failure and Preserved Left Ventricular Ejection Fraction; NCT02932566) trial evaluating the clinical efficacy of pirfenidone in the HFpEF population has been completed but the results have not been published yet.

Other agents affecting myocardial fibrosis target advanced glycation end products (AGEs). AGEs are molecules formed by nonenzymatic reactions between proteins and carbohydrates.[80] Excessive AGE accumulation in myocardial tissue induces cross-linking with other matrix proteins, such as collagen, and leads to interstitial stiffness and progression of myocardial stiffness. Therefore, AGEs are considered a therapeutic target in HFpEF.[80] Alagebrium is an AGE cross-link breaker that improved LV hypertrophy and LV diastolic dysfunction in patients with diastolic HF.[80]

Cell therapy Cell therapy may be used to decrease inflammation and prevent myocardial fibrosis in HFpEF. In a murine experiment and a pilot study, cell therapy using cardiosphere-derived cells or cluster of differentiation (CD) 34+ cells improved LV diastolic dysfunction. At present, cell therapy in patients with HFpEF is under investigation in 2 clinical studies (NCT02941705, NCT02923609). However, these studies do not aim to evaluate the clinical efficacy of cell therapy; therefore, further studies in this area of development are needed.

Treatment targeting cardiometabolic properties

Targeting mitochondria to preserve and restore mitochondrial function SS-31 (elamipretide) is a variant of Szeto-Schiller (SS) peptides, which act as cardioprotective antioxidants, reduce ROS production in mitochondria, and prevent maladaptive remodeling.[81] Results of 2 long-term phase II trials to evaluate the efficacy of elamipretide in HFpEF are pending (NCT02814097, NCT02914665). Preclinical studies indicated that partial adenosine A1 receptor (A1R) agonists prevented mitochondrial dysfunction of cardiomyocytes under hypoxic conditions by mitochondrial permeability transition.[82] However, the partial A1R agonist neladenoson bialanate failed to improve exercise capacity, QOL, and NT-proBNP level.[82]

Targeting intramyocardial calcium homeostasis Levosimendan is a well-known inodilator in HFrEF that has a positive inotropic action on myocytes by calcium sensitization of troponin C and induces peripheral vasodilation by opening ATP-sensitive potassium channels on vascular smooth muscle cells.[83] It affects ATP-sensitive potassium channels on mitochondria and has cardioprotective[83] and phosphodiesterase-3 inhibition effects. In HFrEF, levosimendan has shown encouraging results in improving hemodynamics, cardiac reverse remodeling, and renal protection.[83–85] The NCT03541603 clinical study is underway to examine the effect of levosimendan on hemodynamics in patients with group 2 PH HFpEF; results will be reported in the future.

Prostacyclin analogue, iloprost

Iloprost, an inhaled synthetic prostacyclin analogue used for pulmonary arterial hypertension, mediates vasodilation of the systemic and pulmonary arteries leading to decreased pulmonary vascular resistance. It also prohibits the proliferation of vascular smooth muscle. The ILO-HOPE (Inhaled Iloprost and Exercise Hemodynamics and Ventricular Performance in Heart Failure with Preserved Ejection Fraction; NCT03620526) phase 2 trial has recruited patients with HFpEF and group 2 PH to investigate the therapeutic effect of iloprost. In the subgroup analysis of the ILO-HOPE trial, inhalation of iloprost before exercise improved subtle LV systolic function, such as global longitudinal strain, and LV diastolic parameters, including E/strain rate and estimated PA pressure.[86]

Sodium-glucose cotransporter-2 inhibitors

The sodium-glucose cotransporter-2 inhibitor empagliflozin (SGLT2 inhibitors: dapagliflozin, empagliflozin, and canagliflozin) has been reported to produce a significant reduction in HF hospitalization and mortality benefit in patients with type 2 diabetes and high CV risk.[87-89] In the DAPA-HF (Study to Evaluate the Effect of Dapagliflozin on the Incidence of Worsening Heart Failure or Cardiovascular Death in Patients With Chronic Heart Failure) trial, dapagliflozin significantly reduced worsening of HF or CV death in patients with HFrEF irrespective of the presence of diabetes.[90] The beneficial effect of SGLT2 inhibitors might be derived from the decrease in intravascular volume via osmotic diuresis and natriuresis without RAAS activation and inhibition of the sodium-hydrogen exchanger in the heart and kidney.[91,92] This treatment might help relieve diuretic resistance in HF and prevent myocardial fibrosis, hypertrophy, and dysfunction.[92] Moreover, SGLT2 inhibitors improve myocardial energetics by enhancing metabolic efficiency and myocardial energy supply.[91] It was shown that SGLT2 inhibitors Induce the decroase of oxidative stress, an increase of endothelial function, and vascular compliance.[93] These properties of SGLT2 inhibitors could be favorable for the treatment of HFpEF; however, their effectiveness in HFpEF is uncertain. Two ongoing large RCTs aim to elucidate the efficacy of SGLT2 inhibitors in reducing CV mortality and HF hospitalization in patients with HFpEF irrespective of diabetes (DELIVER [Dapagliflozin Evaluation to Improve the Lives of Patients with Preserved Ejection Fraction Heart Failure; NCT03619213] and EMPEROR-Preserved [Empagliflozin Outcome Trial in Patients with Chronic Heart Failure with Preserved Ejection Fraction; NCT03057951]). In contrast, EMPERIAL-preserved (Exercise Ability and Heart Failure Symptoms, in Patients with Chronic Heart Failure with Preserved Ejection Fraction; NCT03448406)[94] failed to show an effect of empagliflozin to improve exercise capacity in HFpEF and HFrEF. The PRESERVED-HF (Dapagliflozin in Preserved Ejection Fraction Heart Failure; NCT03030235) trial is ongoing and is expected to determine the effect of dapagliflozin treatment on exercise capacity.

Nonpharmacologic Treatment

Pressure monitoring

Increased LV filling pressure is a well-known pathophysiology of HFpEF symptoms and signs and is related to HF hospitalization and poor prognosis of HFpEF. A therapeutic strategy of hemodynamic monitoring with early therapeutic intervention could improve clinical outcomes in HFpEF as well as in HFrEF. The CardioMEMS heart sensor (Abbott, Sylmar, CA) is a wireless pressure sensor implanted in the PA that monitors PA pressure and heart rate. The CardioMEMS Heart Sensor Allows Monitoring of Pressure to Improve Outcomes in NYHA Class III Heart Failure Patients trial showed that PA pressure–guided pharmacologic therapy significantly reduced HF hospitalization regardless of LVEF.[95] The results of CardioMEMS postapproval study confirmed the beneficial effect of long-term hemodynamically guided therapy, showing that HF, as well as all-cause hospitalizations, was significantly reduced in patients treated with hemodynamically guided therapy.[96] These clinical benefits were reproduced in another RCT (MEMS-HF; CardioMEMS European Monitoring Study for Heart Failure).[97] A planned large RCT, GUIDE-HF (Hemodynamic-Guided Management of Heart Failure; NCT03387813) aims to confirm the reduced HF hospitalization, all-cause mortality, and intravenous diuretic visits over a 1-year duration.

Interatrial septal shunt

The interatrial septal shunt is targeted to reduce the high LV filling pressure and LA pressure. In the REDUCE LAP-HF I (Reduce Elevated Left Atrial Pressure in Patients with Heart Failure), 44 patients with HFpEF (LVEF ≥ 40%) were enrolled and randomized to an interatrial shunt device (DC Devices, Inc, Tewksbury, MA) or sham control.[98] An interatrial septal shunt was effective in decreasing pulmonary capillary wedge pressure (PCWP) during exercise for 1 month, and the efficacy lasted for long-term follow-up without significant complication.[98,99] The interatrial shunt is a potential therapeutic option for HFpEF with increased LA filling pressure caused by LA dysfunction, even though further studies to evaluate the long-term clinical efficacy are required. In this respect, the REDUCE LAP-HF II (NCT03088033) trial is currently underway to identify the effects of interatrial septal shunt on clinical outcomes including CV mortality, stroke, HF worsening and hospitalization, and QOL over 1 year.

Rate-adaptive pacing
Chronotropic incompetence plays a key role in impaired cardiac output reserve. Restoring the normal response of HR by pacemaker could provide a benefit to patients with HFpEF. Two clinical trials are currently testing the clinical and structural efficacy of rate-adaptive pacing (RAPID-HF [Efficacy Study of Pacemakers to Treat Slow Heart Rate in Patients with Heart Failure], NCT02145351, and PREFECTUS [Cardiac Resynchronization Therapy vs Rate-responsive Pacing in Heart Failure With Preserved Ejection Fraction], NCT03338374).

Cardiac contractility modulation
Cardiac contractility modulation (CCM) is a device therapy for HF that delivers an electrical signal to the RV septal wall in the absolute myocardial refractory period.[100] CCM signals induce mild augmentation of LV contractile strength via alteration of myocardial calcium handling and have some favorable biochemical and molecular effects irrespective of stimulation site.[101] In HFrEF, CCM has been shown to increase functional capacity and improve QOL.[101] The mechanism of action of CCM influences certain processes that are also involved in the pathophysiology of HFpEF. At present, CCM-HFpEF (CCM in HF with Preserved Ejection Fraction) is investigating the effect of CCM on QOL in HFpEF (NCT03240237).

Cardiac resynchronization therapy
In HFpEF, LV dyssynchrony is associated with subtle LV systolic and diastolic functions and increased LV filling pressure.[102] Although limited consensus exists on LV dyssynchrony as one of the pathophysiologies of HFpEF,[103] the clinical role of cardiac resynchronization therapy in HFpEF is being evaluated in 2 ongoing clinical trials (NCT03338374 and NCT02145351).

Left atrial pacing
LA dysfunction is not just a bystander or by-product of increased LV filling pressure but is another key mechanism of HFpEF.[94] Patients with HFpEF have impaired LA systolic and diastolic functions and increased intra-atrial dyssynchrony.[104] Therefore, biatrial resynchronization could be a new treatment target of HFpEF.[105] In a pilot study of patients with symptomatic HFpEF and atrial dyssynchrony, LA pacing showed an improvement in symptoms and echocardiographic parameters.[106,107] The LEAD trial (Left Atrial Pacing in Diastolic Heart Failure; NCT01618981) for the evaluation of clinical efficacy of LA pacing has now been completed; results should be available soon.

Left ventricular expander
The CORolla device (Corassist Cardiovascular Ltd, Herzliya, Israel) is designed to increase LV diastolic volume and improve LV diastolic relaxation. The device, consisting of a wire with an elastic spring, is implanted in the LV, and it absorbs energy during systole and releases it during diastole to increase LV filling. The study to evaluate

the safety and feasibility of the CORolla device in patients with NYHA III/IV HFpEF is currently ongoing (NCT 02499601).

Pericardiectomy

If cardiac volume increases and is greater than the reserve volume of pericardial space, the contact pressure by pericardial structure on the surface of the heart also increases. This constraint of the pericardial structure increases further and is transmitted to cardiac chambers, ultimately increasing intracavitary filling pressure.[108] In the experimental data, pericardiectomy was shown to improve diastolic compliance of LV[109] and to blunt the increment of LV filling pressure by volume loading.[110] Pericardiectomy had an impact in attenuating the increase in LV filling pressure in response to volume loading in a human pilot study.[111] The safety and long-term clinical efficacy of minimally invasive pericardiotomy are currently being investigated (NCT03923673).

Renal sympathetic denervation

Renal sympathetic denervation (RSDN) is radiofrequency catheter ablation of the renal sympathetic nerve and is used to treat malignant hypertension. Because RSDN leads to decreased LV mass and improved LV diastolic dysfunction,[112] a clinical trial to test the efficacy of RSDN in HFpEF was conducted.[113] This study was terminated early because of difficulty in recruitment and was underpowered to show the therapeutic value of RSDN. Further studies would be required to delineate the clinical impact of RSDN in HFpEF.

Lifestyle modification

In recent studies, physical inactivity, low fitness, and obesity have been identified as major risk factors for developing HFpEF, and these are potentially modifiable targets for the prevention and management of HFpEF.[114] Exercise including endurance and resistance training improved exercise capacity and QOL in patients with HFpEF.[115,116] Most patients with HFpEF are obese or overweight; the increased body adiposity triggers systemic inflammation and functional impairment of cardiac, vascular, and skeletal muscle.[4] In HFpEF, supervised exercise training was effective in improving exercise capacity and QOL but was ineffective for LV functional improvement.[117] The caloric reduction in older and obese patients with HFpEF significantly improved peak O_2 consumption, symptoms, and QOL, with an additive benefit from a combination of caloric restriction and exercise.[118] However, further investigations to validate the beneficial effect of lifestyle modification and explain their mechanism in HFpEF are required.

SUMMARY

HFpEF is the most common form of HF in an aging society with an unchanged worsening prognosis. Until now, there has been no promising therapy to improve clinical outcomes such as mortality. The results of clinical trials for numerous therapies have been neutral or less effective in meeting their primary outcomes. The limited effectiveness of therapy might be caused by an incomplete understanding of the heterogeneity of HFpEF, lack of universal diagnostic criteria for HFpEF, unconnected pathophysiologic mechanisms, and suboptimal trial designs for statistical power. Further research is required to understand and control the obvious but intricate HFpEF syndrome. Several clinical trials are ongoing to evaluate different therapeutic approaches. Prevention and management of comorbidities and risk factors of HFpEF are of great importance in the absence of proven therapies.

CLINICS CARE POINTS

- HFpEF is systemic disorder in which are intertwined various pathophysiology and multiple comorbidity. To date, neither pharmacologic nor nonpharmacologic treatment has been reported obviously to improve clinical outcomes.

- Although previous studies have not shown consistent results for the clinical efficacy of blockade of the RAAS, candesartan reduced HF hospitalization in the CHARM-preserved trial.

- In the TOPCAT trial, an aldosterone antagonist was effective to reduce heart failure hospitalization (HFH) in patients with increased natriuretic peptide levels at baseline. However, the cutoff value of LVEF was low (LVEF $\geq 40\%$).

- ARNI was effective to reduce mortality and HFH in female patients with HFpEF in the PARAGON-HF trial. In a recently reported meta-analysis, ARNI was superior to placebo or ARB to decrease HF hospitalization.

- Sodium-glucose cotransporter-2 inhibitor had been expected to be effective to reduce mortality and improve symptoms in patients with HFpEF because of its favorable effect on the pathophysiologic aspect of HFpEF. However, it was recently reported that empagliflozin failed to show efficacy in improving the clinical symptoms of HFpEF.

- In nonpharmacologic therapy, an interatrial shunt device was shown to improve symptoms of HFpEF and QOL. In addition, exercise (not only endurance but also resistance training) improves exercise capacity and QOL in HFpEF.

DISCLOSURE

None.

REFERENCES

1. Kitzman DW, Gardin JM, Gottdiener JS, et al. Importance of heart failure with preserved systolic function in patients > or = 65 years of age. CHS Research Group. Cardiovascular Health Study. Am J Cardiol 2001;87(4):413–9.
2. Heidenreich PA, Albert NM, Allen LA, et al. Forecasting the impact of heart failure in the United States: a policy statement from the American Heart Association. Circ Heart Fail 2013;6(3):606–19.
3. Roh J, Houstis N, Rosenzweig A. Why Don't we have proven treatments for HFpEF? Circ Res 2017;120(8):1243–5.
4. Shah SJ, Kitzman DW, Borlaug BA, et al. Phenotype-Specific treatment of heart failure with preserved ejection fraction: a multiorgan roadmap. Circulation 2016; 134(1):73–90.
5. Kim MN, Park SM. Heart failure with preserved ejection fraction: insights from recent clinical researches. Korean J Intern Med 2020;35(4):1026.
6. Pfeffer MA, Shah AM, Borlaug BA. Heart failure with preserved ejection fraction in perspective. Circ Res 2019;124(11):1598–617.
7. Gevaert AB, Boen JRA, Segers VF, et al. Heart failure with preserved ejection fraction: a review of cardiac and noncardiac pathophysiology. Front Physiol 2019;10:638.
8. Vaduganathan M, Claggett BL, Desai AS, et al. Prior heart failure hospitalization, clinical outcomes, and response to Sacubitril/Valsartan compared with valsartan in HFpEF. J Am Coll Cardiol 2020;75(3):245–54.

9. Franssen C, Chen S, Unger A, et al. Myocardial microvascular inflammatory endothelial activation in heart failure with preserved ejection fraction. JACC Heart Fail 2016;4(4):312–24.

10. Wintrich J, Kindermann I, Ukena C, et al. Therapeutic approaches in heart failure with preserved ejection fraction: past, present, and future. Clin Res Cardiol 2020;109(9):1079–98.

11. Suthahar N, Meijers WC, Silljé HHW, et al. Galectin-3 activation and inhibition in heart failure and cardiovascular disease: an update. Theranostics 2018;8(3):593–609.

12. Lam CSP, Voors AA, de Boer RA, et al. Heart failure with preserved ejection fraction: from mechanisms to therapies. Eur Heart J 2018;39(30):2780–92.

13. Ponikowski P, Voors AA, Anker SD, et al. 2016 ESC Guidelines for the diagnosis and treatment of acute and chronic heart failure: The Task Force for the diagnosis and treatment of acute and chronic heart failure of the European Society of Cardiology (ESC). Developed with the special contribution of the Heart Failure Association (HFA) of the ESC. Eur J Heart Fail 2016;18(8):891–975.

14. Yancy CW, Jessup M, Bozkurt B, et al. 2013 ACCF/AHA guideline for the management of heart failure: a report of the American College of Cardiology Foundation/American Heart Association Task Force on Practice Guidelines. J Am Coll Cardiol 2013;62(16):e147–239.

15. Kim K-J, Cho H-J, Kim M-S, et al. Focused update of 2016 Korean Society of Heart Failure Guidelines for the Management of Chronic Heart Failure. Int J Heart Fail 2019;1(1):4–24.

16. Abergel E, Lafitte S, Mansencal N. Evaluation of left ventricular filling pressure: Updated recommendations lack new evidence and have severe interpretation issues. Arch Cardiovasc Dis 2018;111(12):707–11.

17. Reddy YNV, Carter RE, Obokata M, et al. A simple, evidence-based approach to help guide diagnosis of heart failure with preserved ejection fraction. Circulation 2018;138(9):861–70.

18. Pieske B, Tschope C, de Boer RA, et al. How to diagnose heart failure with preserved ejection fraction: the HFA-PEFF diagnostic algorithm: a consensus recommendation from the Heart Failure Association (HFA) of the European Society of Cardiology (ESC). Eur Heart J 2019;40(40):3297–317.

19. Barandiaran Aizpurua A, Sanders-van Wijk S, Brunner-La Rocca HP, et al. Validation of the HFA-PEFF score for the diagnosis of heart failure with preserved ejection fraction. Eur J Heart Fail 2019. https://doi.org/10.1002/ejhf.1614.

20. Sueta D, Yamamoto E, Nishihara T, et al. H2FPEF score as a prognostic value in HFpEF patients. Am J Hypertens 2019;32(11):1082–90.

21. Kapłon-Cieślicka A, Kupczyńska K, Dobrowolski P, et al. On the search for the right definition of heart failure with preserved ejection fraction. Cardiol J 2020. https://doi.org/10.5603/CJ.a2020.0124.

22. Yancy CW, Januzzi JL Jr, Allen LA, et al. 2017 ACC expert consensus decision pathway for optimization of heart failure treatment: answers to 10 pivotal issues about heart failure with reduced ejection fraction: a report of the American College of Cardiology Task Force on expert consensus decision pathways. J Am Coll Cardiol 2018;71(2):201–30.

23. Jia G, Aroor AR, Hill MA, et al. Role of renin-angiotensin-aldosterone system activation in promoting cardiovascular fibrosis and stiffness. Hypertension 2018;72(3):537–48.

24. Pugliese NR, Masi S, Taddei S. The renin-angiotensin-aldosterone system: a crossroad from arterial hypertension to heart failure. Heart Fail Rev 2020; 25(1):31–42.

25. Yusuf S, Pfeffer MA, Swedberg K, et al. Effects of candesartan in patients with chronic heart failure and preserved left-ventricular ejection fraction: the CHARM-Preserved Trial. Lancet 2003;362(9386):777–81.

26. Cleland JG, Tendera M, Adamus J, et al. The perindopril in elderly people with chronic heart failure (PEP-CHF) study. Eur Heart J 2006;27(19):2338–45.

27. Massie BM, Carson PE, McMurray JJ, et al. Irbesartan in patients with heart failure and preserved ejection fraction. N Engl J Med 2008;359(23):2456–67.

28. Rector TS, Carson PE, Anand IS, et al. Assessment of long-term effects of irbesartan on heart failure with preserved ejection fraction as measured by the minnesota living with heart failure questionnaire in the irbesartan in heart failure with preserved systolic function (I-PRESERVE) trial. Circ Heart Fail 2012;5(2):217–25.

29. Edelmann F, Wachter R, Schmidt AG, et al. Effect of spironolactone on diastolic function and exercise capacity in patients with heart failure with preserved ejection fraction: the Aldo-DHF randomized controlled trial. JAMA 2013;309(8): 781–91.

30. Pitt B, Pfeffer MA, Assmann SF, et al. Spironolactone for heart failure with preserved ejection fraction. N Engl J Med 2014;370(15):1383–92.

31. Pfeffer MA, Claggett B, Assmann SF, et al. Regional variation in patients and outcomes in the Treatment of Preserved Cardiac Function Heart Failure With an Aldosterone Antagonist (TOPCAT) trial. Circulation 2015;131(1):34–42.

32. de Denus S, O'Meara E, Desai AS, et al. Spironolactone metabolites in TOPCAT - new insights into regional variation. N Engl J Med 2017;376(17):1690–2. https:// doi.org/10.1056/NEJMc1612601.

33. Greenberg B. Angiotensin Receptor-Neprilysin Inhibition (ARNI) in heart failure. Int J Heart Fail 2020;2(2):73–90.

34. Solomon SD, Zile M, Pieske B, et al. The angiotensin receptor neprilysin inhibitor LCZ696 in heart failure with preserved ejection fraction: a phase 2 double-blind randomised controlled trial. Lancet 2012;380(9851):1387–95.

35. Solomon SD, McMurray JJV, Anand IS, et al. Angiotensin-Neprilysin inhibition in heart failure with preserved ejection fraction. N Engl J Med 2019;381(17): 1609–20.

36. McMurray JJV, Jackson AM, Lam CSP, et al. Effects of Sacubitril-Valsartan versus valsartan in women compared with men with heart failure and preserved ejection fraction: insights from PARAGON-HF. Circulation 2020;141(5):338–51.

37. Regitz-Zagrosek V. Sex and gender differences in heart failure. Int J Heart Fail 2020;2(3):157–81.

38. McMurray JJ, Packer M, Desai AS, et al. Angiotensin-neprilysin inhibition versus enalapril in heart failure. N Engl J Med 2014;371(11):993–1004.

39. Solomon SD, Vaduganathan M, Brian LC, et al. Sacubitril/Valsartan across the spectrum of ejection fraction in heart failure. Circulation 2020;141(5):352–61.

40. Martin N, Manoharan K, Thomas J, et al. Beta-blockers and inhibitors of the renin-angiotensin aldosterone system for chronic heart failure with preserved ejection fraction. Cochrane database Syst Rev 2018;6:Cd012721.

41. Kuno T, Ueyama H, Fujisaki T, et al. Meta-analysis evaluating the effects of renin-angiotensin-aldosterone system blockade on outcomes of heart failure with preserved ejection fraction. Am J Cardiol 2020. https://doi.org/10.1016/j.amjcard. 2020.01.009.

42. Simpson J, Castagno D, Doughty RN, et al. Is heart rate a risk marker in patients with chronic heart failure and concomitant atrial fibrillation? Results from the MAGGIC meta-analysis. Eur J Heart Fail Nov 2015;17(11):1182–91.

43. Yanagihara K, Kinugasa Y, Sugihara S, et al. Discharge use of carvedilol is associated with higher survival in Japanese elderly patients with heart failure regardless of left ventricular ejection fraction. J Cardiovasc Pharmacol 2013;62(5): 485–90.

44. Gomez-Soto FM, Romero SP, Bernal JA, et al. Mortality and morbidity of newly diagnosed heart failure with preserved systolic function treated with beta-blockers: a propensity-adjusted case-control populational study. Int J Cardiol 2011;146(1):51–5.

45. van Veldhuisen DJ, Cohen-Solal A, Bohm M, et al. Beta-blockade with nebivolol in elderly heart failure patients with impaired and preserved left ventricular ejection fraction: Data From SENIORS (Study of Effects of Nebivolol Intervention on Outcomes and Rehospitalization in Seniors With Heart Failure). J Am Coll Cardiol 2009;53(23):2150–8.

46. Yamamoto K, Origasa H, Hori M. Effects of carvedilol on heart failure with preserved ejection fraction: the Japanese Diastolic Heart Failure Study (J-DHF). Eur J Heart Fail 2013;15(1):110–8.

47. Bavishi C, Chatterjee S, Ather S, et al. Beta-blockers in heart failure with preserved ejection fraction: a meta-analysis. Heart Fail Rev 2015;20(2):193–201.

48. Cleland JGF, Bunting KV, Flather MD, et al. Beta-blockers for heart failure with reduced, mid-range, and preserved ejection fraction: an individual patient-level analysis of double-blind randomized trials. Eur Heart J 2018;39(1):26–35.

49. Silverman DN, Plante TB, Infeld M, et al. Association of beta-blocker use with heart failure hospitalizations and cardiovascular disease mortality among patients with heart failure with a preserved ejection fraction: a secondary analysis of the TOPCAT trial. JAMA Netw Open 2019;2(12):e1916598.

50. Fukuta H, Goto T, Wakami K, et al. Effect of beta-blockers on heart failure severity in patients with heart failure with preserved ejection fraction: a meta-analysis of randomized controlled trials. Heart Fail Rev 2020. https://doi.org/10.1007/s10741-020-10013-5.

51. Cho JY. Beta-blockers in heart failure with preserved ejection fraction: could their use be vindicated as an acceptable option in the future treatment guideline? Korean Circ J 2019;49(3):249–51.

52. Komajda M, Isnard R, Cohen-Solal A, et al. Effect of ivabradine in patients with heart failure with preserved ejection fraction: the EDIFY randomized placebo-controlled trial. Eur J Heart Fail 2017;19(11):1495–503.

53. Conceição LSR, Gois C, Fernandes RES, et al. Effect of ivabradine on exercise capacity in individuals with heart failure with preserved ejection fraction. Heart Fail Rev 2020. https://doi.org/10.1007/s10741-020-10002-8.

54. Ahmed A, Rich MW, Fleg JL, et al. Effects of digoxin on morbidity and mortality in diastolic heart failure: the ancillary digitalis investigation group trial. Circulation 2006;114(5):397–403.

55. Park M, Sandner P, Krieg T. cGMP at the centre of attention: emerging strategies for activating the cardioprotective PKG pathway. Basic Res Cardiol 2018; 113(4):24.

56. Redfield MM, Anstrom KJ, Levine JA, et al. Isosorbide mononitrate in heart failure with preserved ejection fraction. N Engl J Med 2015;373(24):2314–24.

57. Schwartzenberg S, Redfield MM, From AM, et al. Effects of vasodilation in heart failure with preserved or reduced ejection fraction implications of distinct pathophysiologies on response to therapy. J Am Coll Cardiol 2012;59(5):442–51.
58. Upadhya B, Haykowsky MJ, Kitzman DW. Therapy for heart failure with preserved ejection fraction: current status, unique challenges, and future directions. Heart Fail Rev 2018;23(5):609–29.
59. Chirinos JA, Zamani P. The Nitrate-Nitrite-NO pathway and its implications for heart failure and preserved ejection fraction. Curr Heart Fail Rep 2016;13(1): 47–59.
60. Eggebeen J, Kim-Shapiro DB, Haykowsky M, et al. One week of daily dosing with beetroot juice improves submaximal endurance and blood pressure in older patients with heart failure and preserved ejection fraction. JACC Heart Fail 2016;4(6):428–37.
61. Shaltout HA, Eggebeen J, Marsh AP, et al. Effects of supervised exercise and dietary nitrate in older adults with controlled hypertension and/or heart failure with preserved ejection fraction. Nitric Oxide 2017;69:78–90.
62. Borlaug BA, Anstrom KJ, Lewis GD, et al. Effect of inorganic nitrite vs placebo on exercise capacity among patients with heart failure with preserved ejection fraction: the indie-hfpef randomized clinical trial. JAMA 2018;320(17):1764–73.
63. Guazzi M, Vicenzi M, Arena R. Phosphodiesterase 5 inhibition with sildenafil reverses exercise oscillatory breathing in chronic heart failure: a long-term cardiopulmonary exercise testing placebo-controlled study. Eur J Heart Fail 2012; 14(1):82–90.
64. Guazzi M, Vicenzi M, Arena R, et al. Pulmonary hypertension in heart failure with preserved ejection fraction: a target of phosphodiesterase-5 inhibition in a 1-year study. Circulation 2011;124(2):164–74.
65. Redfield MM, Chen HH, Borlaug BA, et al. Effect of Phosphodiesterase-5 inhibition on exercise capacity and clinical status in heart failure with preserved ejection fraction: a randomized clinical trial. JAMA 2013;309(12):1268–77.
66. Hoendermis ES, Liu LC, Hummel YM, et al. Effects of sildenafil on invasive haemodynamics and exercise capacity in heart failure patients with preserved ejection fraction and pulmonary hypertension: a randomized controlled trial. Eur Heart J 2015;36(38):2565–73.
67. Armstrong PW, Pieske B, Anstrom KJ, et al. Vericiguat in patients with heart failure and reduced ejection fraction. N Engl J Med 2020;382(20):1883–93.
68. Bonderman D, Pretsch I, Steringer-Mascherbauer R, et al. Acute hemodynamic effects of riociguat in patients with pulmonary hypertension associated with diastolic heart failure (DILATE-1): a randomized, double-blind, placebo-controlled, single-dose study. Chest 2014;146(5):1274–85.
69. Pieske B, Maggioni AP, Lam CSP, et al. Vericiguat in patients with worsening chronic heart failure and preserved ejection fraction: results of the SOluble guanylate Cyclase stimulatoR in heArT failurE patientS with PRESERVED EF (SOC-RATES-PRESERVED) study. Eur Heart J 2017;38(15):1119–27.
70. Udelson JE, Lewis GD, Shah SJ, et al. Effect of praliciguat on peak rate of oxygen consumption in patients with heart failure with preserved ejection fraction: the CAPACITY HFpEF Randomized Clinical Trial. JAMA 2020;324(15):1522–31.
71. Armstrong PW, Lam CSP, Anstrom KJ, et al. Effect of vericiguat vs placebo on quality of life in patients with heart failure and preserved ejection fraction: the VITALITY-HFpEF Randomized Clinical Trial. JAMA 2020;324(15):1512–21.
72. Szekely Y, Arbel Y. A review of Interleukin-1 in heart disease: where do we stand today? Cardiol Ther 2018;7(1):25–44.

73. Van Tassell BW, Arena R, Biondi-Zoccai G, et al. Effects of interleukin-1 blockade with anakinra on aerobic exercise capacity in patients with heart failure and preserved ejection fraction (from the D-HART pilot study). Am J Cardiol 2014;113(2):321–7.

74. Van Tassell BW, Buckley LF, Carbone S, et al. Interleukin-1 blockade in heart failure with preserved ejection fraction: rationale and design of the Diastolic Heart Failure Anakinra Response Trial 2 (D-HART2). Clin Cardiol 2017;40(9):626–32.

75. Ridker PM, Everett BM, Thuren T, et al. Antiinflammatory therapy with canakinumab for atherosclerotic disease. N Engl J Med 2017;377(12):1119–31.

76. Everett BM, Cornel JH, Lainscak M, et al. Anti-inflammatory therapy with canakinumab for the prevention of hospitalization for heart failure. Circulation 2019; 139(10):1289–99.

77. Graziani F, Varone F, Crea F, et al. Treating heart failure with preserved ejection fraction: learning from pulmonary fibrosis. Eur J Heart Fail 2018;20(10):1385–91.

78. King TE Jr, Bradford WZ, Castro-Bernardini S, et al. A phase 3 trial of pirfenidone in patients with idiopathic pulmonary fibrosis. N Engl J Med 2014; 370(22):2083–92.

79. Mirkovic S, Seymour AM, Fenning A, et al. Attenuation of cardiac fibrosis by pirfenidone and amiloride in DOCA-salt hypertensive rats. Br J Pharmacol 2002; 135(4):961–8.

80. Hartog JW, Voors AA, Bakker SJ, et al. Advanced glycation end-products (AGEs) and heart failure: pathophysiology and clinical implications. Eur J Heart Fail 2007;9(12):1146–55.

81. Kumar AA, Kelly DP, Chirinos JA. Mitochondrial dysfunction in heart failure with preserved ejection fraction. Circulation 2019;139(11):1435–50.

82. Bertero E, Maack C. The Partial AdeNosine A1 receptor agonist in patients with Chronic Heart failure and preserved Ejection fraction (PANACHE) trial. Cardiovasc Res 2019;115(8):e71–3.

83. Cameli M, Incampo E, Navarri R, et al. Effects of levosimendan in heart failure: The role of echocardiography. Echocardiography 2019;36(8):1566–72.

84. Najjar E, Stålhberg M, Hage C, et al. Haemodynamic effects of levosimendan in advanced but stable chronic heart failure. ESC Heart Fail 2018;5(3):302–8.

85. Lannemyr L, Ricksten SE, Rundqvist B, et al. Differential effects of Levosimendan and Dobutamine on glomerular filtration rate in patients with heart failure and renal impairment: a randomized double-blind controlled trial. J Am Heart Assoc 2018;7(16):e008455.

86. Huang CY, Lee JK, Chen ZW, et al. Inhaled prostacyclin on exercise echocardiographic cardiac function in preserved ejection fraction heart failure. Med Sci Sports Exerc 2020;52(2):269–77.

87. Wiviott SD, Raz I, Bonaca MP, et al. Dapagliflozin and cardiovascular outcomes in Type 2 diabetes. N Engl J Med 2019;380(4):347–57.

88. Zinman B, Wanner C, Lachin JM, et al. Empagliflozin, cardiovascular outcomes, and mortality in Type 2 diabetes. N Engl J Med 2015;373(22):2117–28.

89. Neal B, Perkovic V, Mahaffey KW, et al. Canagliflozin and cardiovascular and renal events in Type 2 diabetes. N Engl J Med 2017;377(7):644–57.

90. McMurray JJV, Solomon SD, Inzucchi SE, et al. Dapagliflozin in patients with heart failure and reduced ejection fraction. N Engl J Med 2019;381(21): 1995–2008.

91. Lan NSR, Fegan PG, Yeap BB, et al. The effects of sodium-glucose cotransporter 2 inhibitors on left ventricular function: current evidence and future directions. ESC Heart Fail 2019;6(5):927–35.

92. Packer M, Anker SD, Butler J, et al. Effects of Sodium-Glucose Cotransporter 2 inhibitors for the treatment of patients with heart failure: proposal of a novel mechanism of action. JAMA Cardiol 2017;2(9):1025–9.

93. Kato ET, Kimura T. Sodium-glucose Co-transporters-2 inhibitors and heart failure: state of the art review and future potentials. Int J Heart Fail 2020;2(1):12–22.

94. Obokata M, Borlaug BA. Left atrial dysfunction: the next key target in heart failure with preserved ejection fraction. Eur J Heart Fail 2019;21(4):506–8.

95. Abraham WT, Adamson PB, Bourge RC, et al. Wireless pulmonary artery haemodynamic monitoring in chronic heart failure: a randomised controlled trial. Lancet 2011;377(9766):658–66.

96. Shavelle DM, Desai AS, Abraham WT, et al. Lower rates of heart failure and all-cause hospitalizations during pulmonary artery pressure-guided therapy for ambulatory heart failure: one-year outcomes from the CardioMEMS post-approval study. Circ Heart Fail 2020;13(8):e006863.

97. Angermann CE, Assmus B, Anker SD, et al. Pulmonary artery pressure-guided therapy in ambulatory patients with symptomatic heart failure: the CardioMEMS European Monitoring Study for Heart Failure (MEMS-HF). Eur J Heart Fail 2020. https://doi.org/10.1002/ejhf.1943.

98. Feldman T, Mauri L, Kahwash R, et al. Transcatheter interatrial shunt device for the treatment of heart failure with preserved ejection fraction (REDUCE LAP-HF I [Reduce Elevated Left Atrial Pressure in Patients With Heart Failure]): a Phase 2, Randomized, Sham-Controlled Trial. Circulation 2018;137(4):364–75.

99. Shah SJ, Feldman T, Ricciardi MJ, et al. One-year safety and clinical outcomes of a transcatheter interatrial shunt device for the treatment of heart failure with preserved ejection fraction in the reduce elevated left atrial pressure in patients with heart failure (REDUCE LAP-HF I) trial: a randomized clinical trial. JAMA Cardiol 2018;3(10):968–77.

100. Borggrefe M, Mann DL. Cardiac contractility modulation in 2018. Circulation 2018;138(24):2738–40.

101. Tschöpe C, Kherad B, Klein O, et al. Cardiac contractility modulation: mechanisms of action in heart failure with reduced ejection fraction and beyond. Eur J Heart Fail 2019;21(1):14–22.

102. Santos AB, Kraigher-Krainer E, Bello N, et al. Left ventricular dyssynchrony in patients with heart failure and preserved ejection fraction. Eur Heart J 2014; 35(1):42–7.

103. Biering-Sørensen T, Shah SJ, Anand I, et al. Prognostic importance of left ventricular mechanical dyssynchrony in heart failure with preserved ejection fraction. Eur J Heart Fail 2017;19(8):1043–52.

104. Liu S, Guan Z, Zheng X, et al. Impaired left atrial systolic function and inter-atrial dyssynchrony may contribute to symptoms of heart failure with preserved left ventricular ejection fraction: a comprehensive assessment by echocardiography. Int J Cardiol 2018;257:177–81.

105. Galderisi M, Santoro C, Esposito R. Left atrial function and dyssynchrony: Main characters and not actor appearances in heart failure with preserved ejection fraction. Int J Cardiol 2018;257:222–3.

106. Eicher JC, Laurent G, Mathé A, et al. Atrial dyssynchrony syndrome: an overlooked phenomenon and a potential cause of 'diastolic' heart failure. Eur J Heart Fail 2012;14(3):248–58.

107. Laurent G, Eicher JC, Mathe A, et al. Permanent left atrial pacing therapy may improve symptoms in heart failure patients with preserved ejection fraction and

atrial dyssynchrony: a pilot study prior to a national clinical research programme. Eur J Heart Fail 2013;15(1):85–93.

108. LeWinter MM. Pericardiectomy to treat heart failure with preserved ejection fraction: unrestrained enthusiasm? Circ Heart Fail 2017;10(4):e003971.

109. LeWinter MM, Pavelec R. Influence of the pericardium on left ventricular end-diastolic pressure-segment relations during early and later stages of experimental chronic volume overload in dogs. Circ Res 1982;50(4):501–9.

110. Borlaug BA, Carter RE, Melenovsky V, et al. Percutaneous pericardial resection: a novel potential treatment for heart failure with preserved ejection fraction. Circ Heart Fail 2017;10(4):e003612.

111. Borlaug BA, Schaff HV, Pochettino A, et al. Pericardiotomy enhances left ventricular diastolic reserve with volume loading in humans. Circulation 2018;138(20): 2295–7.

112. Brandt MC, Mahfoud F, Reda S, et al. Renal sympathetic denervation reduces left ventricular hypertrophy and improves cardiac function in patients with resistant hypertension. J Am Coll Cardiol 2012;59(10):901–9.

113. Patel HC, Rosen SD, Hayward C, et al. Renal denervation in heart failure with preserved ejection fraction (RDT-PEF): a randomized controlled trial. Eur J Heart Fail 2016;18(6):703–12.

114. Pandey A, Patel KV, Vaduganathan M, et al. Physical activity, fitness, and obesity in heart failure with preserved ejection fraction. JACC Heart Fail 2018; 6(12):975–82.

115. Edelmann F, Gelbrich G, Dungen HD, et al. Exercise training improves exercise capacity and diastolic function in patients with heart failure with preserved ejection fraction: results of the Ex-DHF (Exercise training in Diastolic Heart Failure) pilot study. J Am Coll Cardiol 2011;58(17):1780–91.

116. Kitzman DW, Brubaker PH, Herrington DM, et al. Effect of endurance exercise training on endothelial function and arterial stiffness in older patients with heart failure and preserved ejection fraction: a randomized, controlled, single-blind trial. J Am Coll Cardiol 2013;62(7):584–92.

117. Fukuta H, Goto T, Wakami K, et al. Effects of exercise training on cardiac function, exercise capacity, and quality of life in heart failure with preserved ejection fraction: a meta-analysis of randomized controlled trials. Heart Fail Rev 2019; 24(4):535–47.

118. Kitzman DW, Brubaker P, Morgan T, et al. Effect of caloric restriction or aerobic exercise training on peak oxygen consumption and quality of life in obese older patients with heart failure with preserved ejection fraction: a randomized clinical trial. JAMA 2016;315(1):36–46.

Telehealth in Heart Failure

Savitri Fedson, MD, MA[a,b,c], Biykem Bozkurt, MD, PhD[a,c,d],*

KEYWORDS

- Telehealth • Heart failure • Telemedicine • Remote monitoring

KEY POINTS

- Telehealth is critically important in heart failure, and represents an opportunity to enhance timely access and follow-up, utilization of technology for diagnostic and management strategies, individualize management, increase opportunities for multidisciplinary care, eliminate social and medical barriers to care, and implement complementary management strategies.
- Telemedical interventional management strategies and telemonitoring have been associated with a reduction in heart failure-related hospitalizations and heart failure-related mortality.
- Despite all the potential benefits of expanded access, telehealth may have limitations especially for vulnerable populations, who are at risk for less access to health care, such as the elderly, those experiencing homelessness or housing instability, migrant workers, may have limitations and barriers in their access to virtual health. Every effort should be conducted for equal access to telehealth, digital technologies, and virtual platform for health equity.

INTRODUCTION

Telehealth is the delivery of health care services and health care information whereby patients and providers are separated by a physical distance. This ranges from the use of technology to send patient data back to providers, to the use of virtual clinic visits with video streaming. The use of some forms of telehealth in cardiology is longstanding. Holter monitors have been in use since 1949, implantable loop recorders since the early 1990s, and the ability to remotely monitor implantable cardioverter-defibrillators is likewise well established. Beyond this, telemedicine has been routinely used by emergency medical services, transmitting electrocardiograms (ECG) to local emergency departments from the field for triage and earlier activation of cardiac catheterization laboratories for acute ST-elevation myocardial infarctions. Despite this, in 2019

This article originally appeared in *Heart Failure Clinics*, Volume 18, Issue 2, April 2022.
[a] Michael E DeBakey VA Medical Center, Houston, TX, USA; [b] Center for Medical Ethics and Health Policy, Baylor College of Medicine, One Baylor Plaza, Houston, TX 77030, USA; [c] Winters Center for Heart Failure Research, One Baylor Plaza, Houston, TX 77030, USA; [d] Cardiovascular Research Institute, Baylor College of Medicine, One Baylor Plaza, Houston, TX 77030, USA
* Corresponding author. MEDVAMC, 2002 Holcombe Boulevard, Houston, TX 77030.
E-mail address: bbozkurt@bcm.edu

Clinics Collections 13 (2023) 329–340
https://doi.org/10.1016/j.ccol.2023.02.002
2352-7986/23/Published by Elsevier Inc.

only 8% of the U.S. population regularly used telehealth for their formal health care services,[1] while at the same time telehealth technologies with mobile health applications and fitness trackers (m-Health) are were used by up to 60% of the population.[2] The COVID-19 pandemic catapulted telemedicine into the mainstream with the necessary transition to a telehealth-based health care delivery model. While this has shown the potential for the delivery of quality care,[3] it has also underscored some of the ongoing challenges to provide health care with mixed modalities.

The need to more widely incorporate telehealth into the management of patients with heart failure (HF) may represent an opportunity to integrate conventional face-to-face provider–patient encounters with complementary management strategies.[4] HF is a chronic progressive disorder that affects nearly 6 million in the United States alone, and 30 million worldwide. With increasing prevalence in the elderly and aging populations, HF management faces challenges that arise from the constellation of symptoms of intravascular volume and congestion, frailty, and cognitive impairment that accompany this disease. Hospital admissions contribute to nearly 80% of the cost burden of HF in the United States and are additionally associated with increased mortality and morbidity. HF has qualities that would be well suited to a telehealth-based approach to health care. It is an episodic disease, with periods of stability punctuated by decompensation and increasing symptoms requiring either medication adjustment, or hospitalization. Each subsequent hospitalization then is accompanied by increased risk for recurrent decompensation and increased mortality, in part because of the transition of care at this pivotal time, and the need for the reinstitution of medication, or medication titration. Relying on face-to-face encounters for this is often impractical, yet there is a need for clinician–patient interaction to achieve this. Furthermore, telehealth can help with access for follow-up for patients who do not have easy access to a health care facility due to distance, transportation limitations, other social or health reasons, unavailability of a specialist and or clinician as long as infrastructure can be supported in an equitable manner.

Despite overwhelming data supporting guideline-directed medical therapy (GDMT) for HF with reduced ejection fraction, the ability to achieve target doses of medication, much less simultaneous use of these classes of medicine has been difficult.[5] Disease management programs have using face-to-face strategies are time and labor-intensive and are often challenging likewise for patients who have limitations with ambulation, transportation, or geographic proximity to their provider. In some studies, slightly over half of those patients readmitted to a hospital within 30 days of hospital discharge had not seen a health care provider since their discharge.[6]

Different strategies to supplement the traditional provider–patient encounter have been studied, with a broad range of outcomes, but with varied benefits in terms of hospitalization or mortality. Some of the challenges of interpreting the studies of telehealth interventions are the varied approaches, which have been used, differences in the study population and the different health care systems they are embedded within. Some interventions have used structured telephone support (STS) which typically uses question prompts for patients about symptoms and health statistics, prompting alerts to providers according to their response. Others use telemonitoring (TM) relying on the transmission of physiologic data to the provider. There has been a trend toward decreasing HF-related hospitalizations and HF-related mortality in many of these trials, with greater benefit demonstrated when there was the incorporation of greater than 3 physiologic data sent via TM.[7–12] The telehealth interventions have demonstrated improvements in HF-related quality of life (QoL) measures, and reduction in depressive symptoms. What comprises these interventions need to be examined more closely.

Forms of Telehealth Commonly used in Heart Failure

Telehealth is critically important in HF, and represents an opportunity to enhance timely access and follow-up, utilization of technology for diagnostic and management strategies, individualize management, increase opportunities for multidisciplinary care, eliminate social and medical barriers to care, and implement complementary management strategies.

Telehealth can be largely divided into 3 areas: clinician-to-clinician communication; the patient interacting with mobile health technologies (m-Health), and lastly clinician–patient interaction (**Fig. 1**; **Table 1**).

Clinician-to-Clinician

The role of telehealth in clinician–clinician communication, or teleconsultation has advanced with technologies, moving beyond standard telephones to e-mail communication, video conferencing, and sharing of video data. These consultations can provide access to HF specialists who can remotely view diagnostic data, whether from standard echocardiogram platforms, or the images from hand-held scanners. They can also form the basis of "hub and spoke" models of care as has been modeled both with HF and with the management of patients with ventricular assist devices (VADs). Integrating teleconsultation forms of telehealth in HF can assist with management during the most vulnerable period of transition from the hospital back to the community-based providers. The varied modalities that comprise telehealth can be incorporated into a model of HF management that then makes use of the concept of the Heart Team, coordinating the efforts of all the clinicians involved in the care of these patients during these transitions of care. E-health, through the sharing of medical records, can incorporate triggered reminders or alerts for the up-titration or initiation of GDMT, to follow-up with laboratory testing or parenteral iron administration. Not only might this work for communication with HF specialists but also for other members of the management team such as pharmacists and palliative care specialists.[13] The efficacy of this type of intervention is currently being studied in the Spanish Heart failure Events reduction with Remote Monitoring and eHealth Support (HER-MeS) trial.

There is a supply mismatch between the number of advanced HF cardiologists and the number of patients with HF of all stages. Telehealth e-consultation can allow those in different communities to have access to providers who can suggest medical optimization, or importantly when it might be appropriate to refer to an advanced HF center.

Patient-Data Capture and Remote Monitoring Through Health Technologies

Remote monitoring (RM) allows for the transfer of patient-generated data from the patient to the health care team in a timely manner, across distances. Currently, the most widespread example of this is through the monitoring of ICD/CRT-D for arrhythmias. The monitoring of thoracic impedance is also available in some devices, but not as integrated into the care team algorithms.

Implantable pulmonary artery sensors (CardioMEMS), in particular, have been shown to decrease HF-related hospitalizations at 6 months, in patients with NYHA III irrespective of ejection fraction in the CHAMPION trial. In addition, there was a benefit in QoL as evidenced by decreased MLWHFQ scores at 6 and 12 months.[14,15] The CHAMPION trial was nonblinded, however, and there was a different level of patient contact between the 2 arms, reinforcing the importance of the human element of processing and responding to the patient-derived data. In the recently published

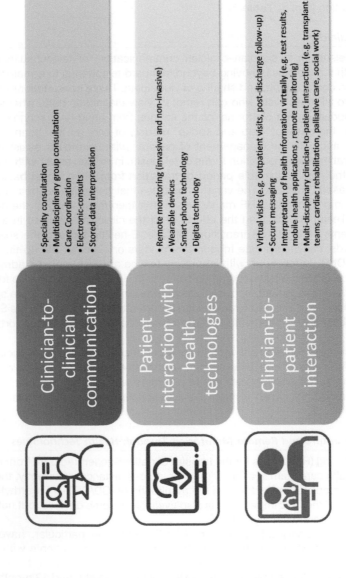

Clinician-to-clinician communication
- Specialty consultation
- Multidisciplinary group consultation
- Care Coordination
- Electronic-consults
- Stored data interpretation

Patient interaction with health technologies
- Remote monitoring (invasive and non-invasive)
- Wearable devices
- Smart-phone technology
- Digital technology

Clinician-to-patient interaction
- Virtual visits (e.g. outpatient visits, post-discharge follow-up)
- Secure messaging
- Interpretation of health information virtually (e.g. test results, mobile health applications, remote monitoring)
- Multi-disciplinary clinician-to-patient interaction (e.g. transplant teams, cardiac rehabilitation, palliative care, social work)

Fig. 1. Forms of telehealth commonly used in heart failure.

Table 1
Forms of telehealth

Types of Telehealth	Explanation
Telehealth	Provision of health care remotely by means of telecommunications technology
Telemedicine	Use of telecommunications to deliver health care at a distance (implies clinical services)
m-Health	Mobile computing, wireless communication, sensors, mobile health apps, social media; electronic stethoscope, hand-held ultrasound
e-Health	Information and communication technology in support of health and health care-related fields, shared electronic medical record
Digital Health	E-learning, remote monitoring, telephonic interventions
Remote Monitoring	Weights, BP, ICD, implantable PA pressure monitoring, thoracic impedance
Teleconsultation	Communication between clinicians across distances, using telehealth

GUIDE-HF trial, implantation of pulmonary artery pressure monitor, in patients with NYHA functional class II–IV HF, with either a recent HF hospitalization or elevated natriuretic peptides did not result in a lower composite endpoint rate of mortality and total HF events compared with the control group in the overall study analysis.[16] However, a pre–COVID-19 impact analysis indicated a possible benefit of hemodynamic-guided management on the primary outcome in the pre–COVID-19 period, primarily driven by a lower HF hospitalization rate compared with the control group.[16]

The assessment of lung congestion using thoracic impedance measures, either with the wearable remote dielectric sensing (ReDS) or the implanted impedance monitors linked to cardiac implantable electric devices, has not been shown to lead to significant decreases in HF hospitalization although more recent studies are more promising, and are ongoing. Part of the limitation of benefit may be linked to the role of patient action to put on the device or to deliberately transmit data.

Wearable devices also permit RM. These are noninvasive sensors that collect data and store them for clinical decision making later. Some are prescribed devices, such as Holter monitors, ambulatory blood pressure monitors, while others are products advertised directly to consumers trying to track or improve their health. m-Health, using smartphone applications also has significant potential uses in HF, with applications tailored to help with medication adherence through automated reminders, monitoring of daily activity.[2,17] However, the integrity of publicly available physiologic tools is not without error, especially at higher heart rates, and in those with darker skin for pulse oximetry.[18] Moreover, there is little regulatory oversight for these m-Health applications. The U.S. Food and Drug Administration does regulate medical devices, but states that the intention of the m-Health app will determine whether it qualifies as a device to be regulated, and the potential risk to patients. Examples of m-Health that might be regulated include electronic stethoscopes or those that monitor heart rate variability from an electrocardiograph.[2,19]

Clinician-to-Patient Communication

Clinician–patient communication using telehealth has historically been based on telephone support, either informally organized or structured (STS) as in the trials. This can involve the incorporation of additional input from RM, or laboratory data, but is both time and personnel intensive. One of the comments regarding the impracticability of the TIM-HF2[9] study was the presence of 24-h coverage of the communication lines to patients. With the social distancing practices during the COVID-19 pandemic, health care delivery relied on telehealth structures between providers and patients with the addition of the virtual video clinic (VVC) visit. The VVC can be based solely on information gathered at the time of the encounter, or can also include additional RM or laboratory data.

The VVC has been the focus of discussion about telehealth, but it is only one piece of health care delivery. There are tips for the preparation of the visit, for the patient as well as for the provider to improve the quality of these visits.[20,21] These also include suggestions on how to create rapport over distance, how to conduct a limited physical examination, and the chance to include advance care planning topics (**Tables 2–4**). The possibility of incorporating the family or caregivers in the clinic appointments can add an important source of information about medical compliance, underreporting of symptoms and functional status, and when nonmedical factors might need to be addressed. Institutions, such as the Veteran's Health Administration (VHA) and Kaiser Permanente were adopters of this virtual platform before the pandemic and provided guidance for structure. The clinical preparation before VVC is no less than for in-person visits as this might require review of m-Health data from other platforms, and often requires the online real-time assessment of vitals by the patient themselves. In a recent randomized controlled trial, outpatient telecare with nurse-led noninvasive assessments reduced the risk of HF hospitalization rates during 12-month follow-up among patients with HF and left ventricular ejection fraction $\leq$49% and history of acute HF within the last 6 months when compared with usual care.[22] According to the study protocol, the nurse-led telehealth intervention included the assessment of presence and intensity of HF symptoms according to NYHA class using predefined questionnaires, measurements of impedance cardiography or thoracic impedance, and treatment recommendations formulated by a cardiologist.[22]

m-Health can also be effective in providing education to patients about symptoms, possible exacerbating factors, and self-management strategies. These can include educational media, text message reminders, or links to other social media sources. Furthermore, m-Health can be used to support decision aids for advanced HF options and for advance care planning, permitting patients and families time to explore their preferences before a provider–patient interaction. These interventions have been studied, again without robust findings but demonstrate the feasibility of integrating these into clinical management.[23]

Table 2
Physical examination

Vital Signs	Weight, Blood Pressure, Temperature, Oxygen Saturation
Skin assessment	New Bruising, rashes
Head, Eyes, Ears, Nose, Throat	Assess symmetry of eye movements, hearing, appearance of scleral icterus
Cardiovascular	
Neck	Jugular Venous distension Bendopnea
	Lower extremity edema, ulcers
Fitness	Sit to stand, gait assessment
Limitations	Touch sensation of skin temperature, perfusion

Table 3 Communication tools for virtual visit	
Communication Concepts	**Example**
Naming	"It sounds like your symptoms are worse."
Understanding	"This helps me understand what you just told me."
Respecting	"I can see that you have really made efforts to improve your diet."
Supporting	"I will work with you to try to get you what you need."
Exploring	"Could you tell me a little more about what you mean when you said that...?"

Telehealth-Cardiac Rehabilitation

Cardio-pulmonary rehabilitation can be provided through telehealth and video visits. Home-based cardiac rehabilitation has been suggested as an alternative for traditional center-based cardiac rehabilitation to help increase access, participation and adherence[24–26] Programs have successfully used components of telehealth to further improve on these home-based programs. Video conferencing can permit the exercise physiologist to provide immediate feedback and demonstration for exercise techniques; assessment of frailty and instability can be assessed watching patients rise from chairs or walk in front of the camera.[27]

Challenges to Telehealth Implementation

For all the potential benefits of expanded access, there remain limitations of telehealth. Those vulnerable populations, who are at risk for less access to health care, such as the elderly, those experiencing homelessness or housing instability, migrant workers, are also vulnerable in their access to virtual health. They may have limited proficiency with technology, or limited broadband access, or few minutes for a telephone-only plan.[28] For patients with dementia or impaired hearing, communication often relies on nonverbal cues such as lip reading, body and facial expressions, which are limited over video interfaces. The delay or lag in the electrical interface,

Table 4 Pros: Cons virtual visit		
	Pros	**Cons**
Access	Improved for those with limited mobility, distance, transportation, child-care needs	Requires technologic literacy, broadband, potential lack of privacy
Environment	Can alert providers to potential safety issues in environment; can "see" the medicine bottles	Lack of privacy; unwillingness to reveal one's home environment
Care Transitions	Continuity of care more easily	
Physical Examination/ Distance	Observation of breathing, orthopnea/bendopnea, visual inspection of neck veins, leg edema, incorporation of physiologic data from remote monitoring	Lack of "therapeutic" touch; Challenging for people relying on nonverbal cues; limited ability to complete examination (skin temperature, pulse characteristics)

interruptions, or ambient noises can also worsen this communication and lead to misunderstandings, frustrations, or an unwillingness to rely on these methods of care delivery. Every effort should be conducted for equal access to telehealth, digital technologies, and virtual platform for health equity. Health care systems should invest in technologies and provide equipment and connectivity to ensure that telehealth does not widen health disparities.

Limitations of Telehealth

For telehealth to be successful, patients and clinicians must be willing and able, and the technology must be available and effective. Some patients and clinicians, especially those with limited infrastructure or access to technology and or virtual connectivity, limited technology comfort may be reluctant to use telehealth. Some patients and clinicians may have physical barriers to use telehealth due to hearing, visual, or other differences. Some may be reluctant to use telehealth due to privacy concerns. Importantly utilization of virtual interactions in lieu of face-to-face visits create concerns regarding lack of ability to perform a full physical examination, have an opportunity for more in-person interaction. Geographic and financial challenges to access Wi-Fi connectivity, computer, smartphone, network, or software platforms remain as major limitations for vulnerable populations creating health inequity. Furthermore, virtual visits do not allow immediate intervention with intravenous therapies, further diagnostic imaging or laboratory studies, or admission to a hospital for higher level of care that may be commonly used in patients with HF. This is a significant concern for patients with worsening symptoms and or hemodynamic instability when an in-person visit may be better than a virtual visit. Due to the limitations of virtual visits, there are also concerns regarding missing important findings that may not be easily visible or discernible by virtual visits, such as subtle changes in physical examination findings, vital signs, or laboratory markers. Actively worsening patients who may require higher levels of care such as additional laboratory and diagnostic tests, intravenous or interventional treatment, and or admission to the hospital may require in-person visits rather than telehealth. Patients with advanced HF symptoms may need to be considered for hybrid models of telehealth including postdischarge telehealth visits, combined with in-person visits when symptoms are worse and or when higher level of care is needed.

Privacy

Additionally, telehealth, and indeed, electronic communication has permeated society, but it is important not to forget the risk to patient privacy, especially on unsecured platforms or networks. The concern for privacy is not only for the patient but also for the provider, because there is no certainty as to whom might be in the virtual clinic room, especially if there is no video feed. There are preferred platforms to use for telehealth encounters, some designed solely for this use, requiring password protection.

The coordinated use of different modalities of telehealth, using the electronic health record to identify at-risk patients, RM for biometric data, and telephone follow-up to maximize medicine titration can be conducted, even before the COVID-19 pandemic.[29] However, as was noted in this single-center study, the patients who participated were younger.

Jurisdiction

One of the additional challenges to telemedicine is the jurisdiction of medical licensure and provider reimbursement. Where does the provider–patient relationship start? In general, for there to be a provider–patient relationship (PPR), a person must "present" themselves for treatment or advice, the provider then provides advice, which the person, now a patient, relies, and acts on. These comprise the relationship but historically, this starts with a traditional face-to-face encounter. It was only with the COVID-19 pandemic that there was an easing of this restriction to allow the initiation of PPR relations to be via telemedicine and temporary waivers in some regulation of telehealth services. Specifically, the need for providers to hold licenses in the states in which they are telepracticing have been waived, whereas before this, to provide telehealth services, a provider had to be licensed in that state, or be in one of the states that grant reciprocity, or practicing though the Veterans Health Administration (VHA) which allows for clinician license portability. Even before COVID-19, there was an increased expansion for the reimbursement of telehealth encounters, specifically for end-stage renal disease, stroke, and substance abuse.[30] As the increased update of VVC visits and other telehealth options, some states have made legislative changes that make permanent some of the pandemic waivers.

RM is not considered to be telehealth; however, to then act or provide advice based on these data is a form of telehealth and would be governed by license restrictions; this has created limitations for provider accessibility in the past. One potential drawback of the patient-derived data using m-Health apps is how to best coordinate provider responses. What is the responsibility of a provider to react to, or act on data that may be inaccurate? Will delays in provider response lead to psychological stress? These are yet unanswered questions and ones that will be challenging given the constraints of both time and personnel that already exist within HF management teams.

Additional barriers to the implantation of telehealth in HF will be provider reimbursement. At present, simple telephone visits, which may be as lengthy as VVC, do not have the same reimbursement, which might push providers aware of those patients who prefer the more simple technology of a telephone.

Because of the clinical challenges of frequent medication titration in the HF population, the social determinants of health can have significant repercussions for models of telehealth, and as telehealth continues to expand there will have to be targeted approaches to help overcome some of the barriers to implementation, which have the potential to worsen some of these disparities. For example, those experiencing homelessness or unstable living conditions might not have access to reliable networks or personal technology to implement the full use of monitoring m-Health applications or e-health education platforms for triggered reminders for medications adherence, or responses to biometric data. Data from experience with telehealth during the COVID-19 pandemic suggest that patients who are older, single, African-American, or of lower socioeconomic status by education and income were less likely to use VVC than telephone visits.[25]

If the HeartTeam relies heavily on these technologies, then a cohort of patients risks falling further behind. As noted earlier, HF is associated with cognitive dysfunction, which can also limit the patient-technology interaction or feeling of ease.[31] The challenge of an appropriate digital prescription is a new element for the HF provider.

Future of telehealth will include the increased use of artificial intelligence in pattern recognition and interpretation of data. Managing the volumes of patient-derived data and either creating alerts for patients directly or to providers is already in practice for implantable PA pressure and thoracic impedance monitors. As more platforms transmit data, integration of these data sets into patient-specific predictions will be a goal. Artificial intelligence may also be used to discover newer tools to help predict compensation in the telehealth area. An example of this might be the analysis of voice characteristics over the telephone to predict decompensation and hospitalization.[32]

Diabetes mellitus is an example of a disease that has been transformed using m-Health with at-home glucose monitoring. HF management has relied on the bathroom scale for years, combined with patient education to also allow for sliding scale diuretic adjustments, but weight changes may seem too late in the spiral of decompensation to prevent hospitalizations effectively. The self-administration of subcutaneous furosemide might be an option for select patients after the integration of their physiologic data. Home-based services, such as phlebotomy for laboratory testing, using home health aides, or nurses as physician extenders, who might be able to assist vulnerable patients with health care visits, being the eyes, ears and literal hands of the HF provider might be a mechanism to combine technology with patient care.

SUMMARY

In HF care, telehealth represents a very important opportunity to enhance timely access and follow-up, expand the utilization of technology platforms for diagnostic and management strategies, individualize management, increase opportunities for multidisciplinary care coordination, and help implement complementary management strategies.

CLINICS CARE POINTS

- Clinicians and health networks should examine strategies to incorporate telehealth in the management of patients with HF. Telehealth represents an opportunity to enhance timely access and follow-up, utilization of technology for diagnostic and management strategies, individualize management, increase opportunities for multidisciplinary care, and implement complementary management strategies.

- Telemedical interventional management strategies and TM have been associated with a reduction in HF-related hospitalizations and HF-related mortality.

- Health care systems should invest in technologies and providing equipment and connectivity to ensure that telehealth does not widen health disparities. Despite all the potential benefits of expanded access, telehealth may have limitations especially for vulnerable populations, who are at risk for less access to health care.

- Patients with advanced HF symptoms may need to be considered for hybrid models of telehealth including postdischarge telehealth visits, combined with in-person visits when symptoms are worse and or when higher level of care is needed.

DISCLOSURE

B. Bozkurt: Consultation for Bayer, Astra Zeneca, Vifor, Relypsa and scPharmaceuticals, Clinical Events Committee for Guide-HF Trial Abbott Pharmaceuticals, Data Safety Monitoring Board for Anthem Trial by LivaNova Pharmaceuticals. S. Fedson: has nothing to disclose.

REFERENCES

1. Vogels EA. About one-in-five Americans use a smart watch or fitness tracker. Pew Research Center. 9-19-2021. Available at: https://www.pewresearch.org/fact-tank/2020/01/09/about-one-in-five-americans-use-a-smart-watch-or-fitness-tracker/. Accessed December 28, 2021.

2. MacKinnon GE, Brittain EL. Mobile Health Technologies in Cardiopulmonary Disease. Chest 2020;157(3):654–64.

3. Analysis of UDS Clinical Quality Measure Performance by Health Center Telehealth Use by Health Information Technology and Evaluation Center. September 22 2020. Available at: https://hiteqcenter.org/Resources/Telehealth-Telemedicine/analysis-of-uds-clinical-quality-measure-performance-by-health-center-telehealth-use. Accessed December 28, 2021.

4. Seferovic PM, Ponikowski P, Anker SD, et al. Clinical practice update on heart failure 2019: pharmacotherapy, procedures, devices and patient management. An expert consensus meeting report of the Heart Failure Association of the European Society of Cardiology. Eur J Heart Fail 2019;21(10):1169–86.

5. Thibodeau JT, Gorodeski EZ. Telehealth for uptitration of guideline-directed medical therapy in heart failure. Circulation 2020;142(16):1507–9.

6. Black JT, Romano PS, Sadeghi B, et al. A remote monitoring and telephone nurse coaching intervention to reduce readmissions among patients with heart failure: study protocol for the better effectiveness after transition - heart failure (BEAT-HF) randomized controlled trial. Trials 2014;15:124.

7. Yun JE, Park JE, Park HY, et al. Comparative effectiveness of telemonitoring versus usual care for heart failure: a systematic review and meta-analysis. J Card Fail 2018;24(1):19–28.

8. Galinier M, Roubille F, Berdague P, et al. Telemonitoring versus standard care in heart failure: a randomised multicentre trial. Eur J Heart Fail 2020;22(6):985–94.

9. Koehler F, Koehler K, Deckwart O, et al. Efficacy of telemedical interventional management in patients with heart failure (TIM-HF2): a randomised, controlled, parallel-group, unmasked trial. Lancet 2018;392(10152):1047–57.

10. Inglis SC, Clark RA, Cleland JG. Telemonitoring in patients with heart failure. N Engl J Med 2011;364(11):1078–9.

11. Ong MK, Romano PS, Edgington S, et al. Effectiveness of remote patient monitoring after discharge of hospitalized patients with heart failure: the better effectiveness after transition – heart failure (BEAT-HF) randomized clinical trial. JAMA Intern Med 2016;176(3):310–8.

12. Inglis SC, Clark RA, Dierckx R, et al. Structured telephone support or non-invasive telemonitoring for patients with heart failure. Cochrane Database Syst Rev 2015;10:CD007228.

13. Huitema AA, Harkness K, Heckman GA, et al. The spoke-hub-and-node model of integrated heart failure care. Can J Cardiol 2018;34(7):863–70.

14. Abraham WT, Stevenson LW, Bourge RC, et al. Sustained efficacy of pulmonary artery pressure to guide adjustment of chronic heart failure therapy: complete follow-up results from the CHAMPION randomised trial. Lancet 2016;387(10017):453–61.

15. Adamson PB, Abraham WT, Stevenson LW, et al. Pulmonary artery pressure-guided heart failure management reduces 30-day readmissions. Circ Heart Fail 2016;9(6).

16. Lindenfeld J, Zile MR, Desai AS, et al. Haemodynamic-guided management of heart failure (GUIDE-HF): a randomised controlled trial. Lancet 2021;398(10304):991–1001.

17. Singhal A, Cowie MR. The role of wearables in heart failure. Curr Heart Fail Rep 2020;17(4):125–32.

18. Nguyen HH, Silva JN. Use of smartphone technology in cardiology. Trends Cardiovasc Med 2016;26(4):376–86.

19. FDA. Policy for device software functions and mobile medical applications. 9-10-2021. Available at: https://www.fda.gov/regulatory-information/search-fda-guidance-documents/policy-device-software-functions-and-mobile-medical-applications. Accessed December 28, 2021.

20. Gorodeski EZ, Goyal P, Cox ZL, et al. Virtual visits for care of patients with heart failure in the Era of COVID-19: A Statement from the Heart Failure Society of America. J Card Fail 2020;26(6):448–56.

21. Orso F, Migliorini M, Herbst A, et al. Protocol for telehealth evaluation and follow-up of patients with chronic heart failure during the COVID-19 Pandemic. J Am Med Dir Assoc 2020;21(12):1803–7.

22. Krzesiński P, Jankowska EA, Siebert J, et al. Effects of an outpatient intervention comprising nurse-led non-invasive assessments, telemedicine support and remote cardiologists' decisions in patients with heart failure (AMULET study): a randomised controlled trial. Eur J Heart Fail 2021. https://doi.org/10.1002/ejhf.2358. Epub ahead of print. PMID: 34617373.

23. Allida S, Du H, Xu X, et al. mHealth education interventions in heart failure. Cochrane Database Syst Rev 2020;7:CD011845.

24. Thomas RJ, Beatty AL, Beckie TM, et al. Home-based cardiac rehabilitation: a scientific statement from the American Association of Cardiovascular and Pulmonary Rehabilitation, the American Heart Association, and the American College of Cardiology. J Am Coll Cardiol 2019;74(1):133–53.

25. Sammour Y, Spertus JA, Shatla I, et al. Comparison of video and telephone visits in outpatients with heart failure. Am J Cardiol 2021;158:153–6.

26. Bozkurt B, Fonarow GC, Goldberg LR, et al. Cardiac rehabilitation for patients with heart failure: JACC Expert Panel. J Am Coll Cardiol 2021;77(11):1454–69.

27. Bryant MS, Fedson SE, Sharafkhaneh A. Using Telehealth Cardiopulmonary Rehabilitation during the COVID-19 Pandemic. J Med Syst 2020;44(7):125.

28. Lam K, Lu AD, Shi Y, et al. Assessing telemedicine unreadiness among older adults in the United States During the COVID-19 Pandemic. JAMA Intern Med 2020;180(10):1389–91.

29. Desai AS, Maclean T, Blood AJ, et al. Remote optimization of guideline-directed medical therapy in patients with heart failure with reduced ejection fraction. JAMA Cardiol 2020;5(12):1430–4.

30. Latifi R, Doarn CR, Merrell RC, eds. Telemedicine, Telehealth and Telepresence: Principles, Strategies, Applications, and New Directions 1st ed. 2021.

31. Rodriguez JA, Betancourt JR, Sequist TD, et al. Differences in the use of telephone and video telemedicine visits during the COVID-19 pandemic. Am J Manag Care 2021;27(1):21–6.

32. Maor E, Tsur N, Barkai G, et al. Noninvasive vocal biomarker is associated with severe acute respiratory syndrome Coronavirus 2 Infection. Mayo Clin Proc Innov Qual Outcomes 2021;5(3):654–62.

Hypertension and Heart Failure
Prevention, Targets, and Treatment

Katherine E. Di Palo, PharmD*, Nicholas J. Barone, BS

KEYWORDS

- Hypertension • Heart failure • Risk reduction • Pharmacotherapy

KEY POINTS

- Given the overt risk of cardiovascular disease development when blood pressure is left uncontrolled, it is imperative to view hypertension as pre–heart failure.
- The complex nature of cardiac remodeling attributed to hypertension can result in diastolic and systolic dysfunction.
- Although all antihypertensive pharmacologic agents inherently decrease blood pressure, there are noted differences between drug classes regarding ability to reduce risk of heart failure onset or progression.

INTRODUCTION

Heart failure continues to represent a major public health burden with prevalence expecting to increase by 46% from 2012 to 2030, resulting in more than 8 million US adults with heart failure.[1] Hypertension is possibly the most powerful, modifiable risk factor for the development of heart failure. In the Framingham Heart Study, hypertension predated disease in 91% of all patients with newly diagnosed heart failure during 20 years of follow-up.[2] Although diastolic dysfunction and heart failure with preserved ejection fraction (HFpEF) are the most common cardiac complications, hypertension also increases risk for myocardial infarction and subsequent heart failure with reduced ejection fraction (HFrEF). Hypertension treatment has been proven to prevent and decrease many clinical presentations related to heart failure, such as increased left ventricular hypertrophy (LVH) and left ventricular mass. This article focuses on mechanistic links, therapeutic goals, and treatment of patients with comorbid hypertension and heart failure.

This article previously appeared in *Cardiology Clinics*, Volume 40, Issue 2, May 2022.
This article originally appeared in *Heart Failure Clinics*, Volume 16, Issue 1, January 2020.
Disclosure: The authors have nothing to disclose.
Office of the Medical Director, Montefiore Medical Center, 111 East 210th Street, Bronx, NY 10467, USA
* Corresponding author.
E-mail address: kdipalo@montefiore.org

Clinics Collections 13 (2023) 341–350
https://doi.org/10.1016/j.ccol.2023.02.004
2352-7986/23/© 2023 Elsevier Inc. All rights reserved.

EPIDEMIOLOGY

Using the new blood pressure threshold of 130 to 139/80 to 89 mm Hg from the 2017 American College of Cardiology (ACC)/American Heart Association (AHA) Hypertension Guidelines it is estimated from 2011 to 2014 National Health and Nutritional Examination Survey (NHANES) data that almost half of US adults 20 years of age or older have hypertension.[1,3] Severe increases in blood pressure directly correlate with higher risks of developing heart failure: the lifetime risk of heart failure doubles in patients with blood pressure greater than or equal to 160/100 mm Hg compared with those with blood pressure less than 140/90 mm Hg.[4] This risk translates to approximately 1 out of every 3 or 4 adults developing heart failure when blood pressure is greater than 160 mm Hg.[5] Similarly, patients with mild hypertension have a 2-fold to 3-fold increased risk of developing LVH compared with normotensive patients, whereas patients with the greatest severity of hypertension have a 10-fold risk.[6] Registry data, epidemiologic studies, and clinical trials signal that hypertension is the most important cause of HFpEF, with a prevalence of 60%-89%.[7]

Differences in hypertension and heart failure incidence based on race, age, and sex are also noted. In the United States, black patients have the highest rate of hypertension, which is more causative of heart failure, in particular HFpEF, than coronary artery disease in this patient population.[8] Black and Hispanic patients also have poorer rates of blood pressure control resulting in longer risk factor exposure.[9] The occurrence of both hypertension and LVH increase significantly with age.[10] LVH is noted in nearly 33% of the male population and 50% of the female population more than 70 years of age.[11] Data from the Framingham Heart Study showed that the hazard for developing heart failure in hypertensive men was about 2-fold compared with 3-fold in hypertensive women, and the population attributable risk for heart failure imparted by hypertension was estimated to be 39% in men and 59% in women.[2] Older women with a long-standing hypertensive history are more likely to present with HFpEF.[12] Although 5-year mortality after initial diagnosis of heart failure is 50%, the combined presence of hypertension and heart failure is associated with even worse outcomes.[1] After the onset of hypertensive heart failure, 5-year mortality is 76% and 69% for men and women respectively.[13]

FROM HYPERTENSION TO HEART FAILURE

The progression from hypertension to heart failure is complex and multifaceted. Briefly, the four degrees of hypertensive heart disease as described by Messerli and colleagues[14] are (1) isolated diastolic dysfunction, (2) diastolic dysfunction with LVH, (3) HFpEF, and (4) HFrEF. Chronic hypertension is the most common cause of asymptomatic diastolic dysfunction, which encompasses abnormalities in diastolic filling, distensibility, or relaxation of the left ventricle (LV).[15] Pressure and volume overload cause different types of LV remodeling and pathophysiologic developments.[14] Cardiac remodeling as a response to principal pressure overload consists of increased cardiac mass at the expense of chamber volume caused by the parallel addition of sarcomeres resulting in concentric LVH. In contrast, cardiac remodeling as a response to principal volume overload consists of increased cardiac mass and chamber volume caused by serial addition of sarcomeres resulting in eccentric LV hypertrophy. These dichotomous remodeling patterns seem to be equally common in patients with hypertension.[16]

The link between hypertension and heart failure is also rooted in changes in the renin-angiotensin-aldosterone system (RAAS), which is overactivated by LV systolic wall stress and further contributes to cardiac hypertrophy. In addition, the sympathetic nervous system plays an idiopathic role in LVH, overt vasoconstriction, and retention of electrolytes such as sodium.[17] Once LVH develops, the risk of developing HFpEF and HFrEF increases dramatically.[18] HFpEF is the more common progression of long-standing hypertension given that diastolic dysfunction is the initial stage of hypertensive heart disease. However, a subset of patients develop systolic dysfunction, which may be the result of a so-called second hit as proposed by Borlaug and Redfield,[19] with an ischemic event often instigating the progression from HFpEF to HFrEF. The presence of hypertension has both a causal and continuous impact on myocardial infarction because risk increases with age and severity.[6] The proposed relationship between hypertension, cardiac remodeling, and heart failure is summarized in **Fig. 1.**

BLOOD PRESSURE TARGETS

Given the overt risk of cardiovascular disease development when blood pressure is left uncontrolled, it is imperative to view hypertension as pre–heart failure. The Staging Classification of Heart Failure (A, B, C, D) introduced by ACC/AHA in 2003 specifically draws attention to the preventive nature of heart failure and the importance of risk factor management.[5,20] For patients with stage A, those at high risk but without structural heart disease or symptoms, chronic pharmacotherapy to reduce both systolic and diastolic hypertension is crucial and has been shown to reduce the risk of incident heart failure by approximately 50%.[21,22] More specifically, a meta-analysis by Verdecchia and colleagues[23] reported that, for each 5-mm Hg reduction in systolic blood pressure (SBP), the risk for heart failure decreases by 24%. Similar results were

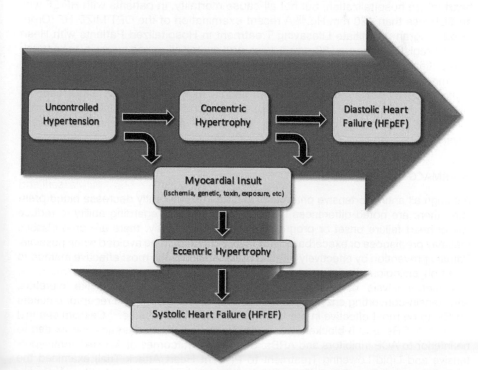

Fig. 1. Proposed mechanism for the progression of hypertensive heart disease to HFpEF or HFrEF. (*Modified from* Borlaug BA, Redfield MM. Diastolic and systolic heart failure are distinct phenotypes within the heart failure spectrum. Circulation 2011;123(18).)

seen in a meta-analysis by Ettehad and colleagues,[24] with every 10-mm Hg reduction SBP significantly reducing the risk of heart failure by 28%.

The results of SPRINT (Systolic Blood Pressure Intervention Trial) revealed a significant reduction in major cardiovascular events, including a 38% lower relative risk of heart failure, by achieving a blood pressure target of less than 120/80 mm Hg among certain patients with high cardiovascular risk.[25] Other findings included greater reduction in LVH as well as resolution of LVH. Stemming from these landmark results, blood pressure goals shifted from conservative (eg, 140/90 mm Hg) toward more aggressive control. The 2017 Focused Update of the 2013 Heart Failure Guidelines included a new section on treating hypertension to reduce the incidence of heart failure as well as treating hypertension in stage C HFrEF and HFpEF. A target of less than 130/80 mm Hg is recommended for all 3 groups and the threshold for therapy initiation is blood pressure greater than or equal to 130/80 mm Hg.[3,26] This target and threshold is also recommended in the 2017 High Blood Pressure Clinical Practice Guideline for patients with other comorbidities such as diabetes mellitus, chronic kidney disease, peripheral artery disease, and stable ischemic heart disease.[3]

Note that randomized clinical trials (RCTs) targeting intensive blood pressure control have not been studied in the heart failure population and SPRINT excluded patients with an ejection fraction less than 35% or a history of symptomatic heart failure within 6 months. The J-shaped relationship between SBP and mortality in hypertensive and high-risk patients, including those with heart failure, has been debated for decades.[27–29] Observational analyses have provided conflicting results. An evaluation of BEST (Beta-Blocker Evaluation of Survival Trial) found an increased risk of heart failure hospitalization, but not all-cause mortality, in patients with HFrEF with an SBP less than 120 mm Hg.[30] A recent examination of the OPTIMIZE-HF (Organized Program to Initiate Lifesaving Treatment in Hospitalized Patients with Heart Failure) registry compared 30-day, 1-year, and overall all-cause mortality in hospitalized patients with HFpEF discharged with an SBP of less than 120 mm Hg versus 120 mm Hg or greater.[31] Lower SBP on discharge was associated with significantly higher risk of all mortality end points in addition to higher risk of heart failure readmission at 30 days. However, the exact cause of this phenomenon is unknown and may be affected by frailty, comorbidities, older age, and more advanced disease severity.[32]

PHARMACOTHERAPY

Although all antihypertensive pharmacologic agents inherently decrease blood pressure, there are noted differences between drug classes regarding ability to reduce risk of heart failure onset or progression. More importantly, there are drug classes that may predispose or exacerbate heart failure and should be avoided when possible. Primary prevention by effectively treating hypertension is the most effective method to divert physiologic remodeling and heart failure.

A meta-analysis of antihypertensive treatment ranked thiazidelike diuretics, angiotensin-converting enzyme (ACE) inhibitors, and angiotensin II receptor blockers (ARBs) to be most effective in preventing new-onset heart failure.[21] Calcium channel blockers (CCBs) and β-blockers were significantly inferior to diuretics and tended to be inferior to ACE inhibitors and ARBs. Secondary outcomes of ALLHAT (Antihypertensive and Lipid-Lowering Treatment to Prevent Heart Attack Trial) examined the role of chlorthalidone, lisinopril, and amlodipine in preventing heart failure.[33] During year 1 of treatment, there was a higher rate of incident heart failure with amlodipine and lisinopril versus chlorthalidone. After 1 year of treatment, risk continued to remain decreased in patients receiving chlorthalidone compared with amlodipine, but longer use of lisinopril was shown to have equivalent risk to chlorthalidone. Results showing the effectiveness of chlorthalidone in reducing LVH was also seen in TOMHS (Treatment of Mild Hypertension Study), which again compared the diuretic with amlodipine and lisinopril as well as doxazosin and acebutolol.[34] Given the prolonged-half life and proven trial data signaling the reduction of heart failure in additional to other cardiovascular diseases, such as stroke, chlorthalidone is the preferential thiazide diuretic, especially because no outcome data are available for hydrochlorothiazide.[3] In patients with stage B heart failure with structural heart disease or LV dysfunction but without heart failure symptoms, β-blockers can reverse remodeling and improve LV function.[35] ACE inhibitors and ARBs can prevent symptomatic heart failure in this setting as well.[36,37] Although sacubitril/valsartan is currently only US Food and Drug Administration approved for the treatment of HFrEF, promising results indicating its effectiveness at blood pressure reduction in patients without heart failure have emerged. Compared with valsartan alone, sacubitril/valsartan showed a greater reduction in systolic and diastolic blood pressure.[38]

RCTs comparing one BP-reducing agent with another for the management of hypertension in patients with comorbid symptomatic heart failure do not exist. Triple therapy to reduce morbidity and mortality in stage C HFrEF includes (1) ACE inhibitors, ARBs or angiotensin II receptor neprilysin inhibitor; (2) select β-blockers; and (3) aldosterone antagonists.[26] Therefore, these agents are guideline recommended as first-line therapy for treatment of comorbid hypertension. For patients who self-identify as black with New York Heart Association (NYHA) class II to III symptoms, hydralazine and isosorbide dinitrate are recommended in addition to the triple-therapy backbone.[39] Therapeutic effect is dose dependent so titration is imperative to maximize blood pressure–reducing ability as well as to achieve positive heart failure outcomes. Target doses for heart failure compared with dose ranges used for hypertension for select agents are listed in **Table 1**. In successful heart failure treatment trials with these agents, it has been observed that SBP usually decreases to a normal range of 110 to 130 mm Hg.[40]

Hypotension, which may or may not be symptomatic, is often a rate-limiting step in guideline-directed medical therapy (GDMT) uptitration and subsequently most patients with advanced HFrEF do not manifest hypertension.[41] However, if additional agents are needed to treat refractory hypertension, careful consideration is warranted to avoid certain agents known to worsen heart failure. Because of its noncardioselective vasodilating properties, carvedilol is more effective in reducing blood pressure compared with the other evidence-based β-blockers metoprolol succinate and bisoprolol.[41] It is therefore reasonable to select or switch to carvedilol as part of GDMT before initiating adjunct therapy with another drug class. If not already indicated, hydralazine can be initiated but other vasodilators, such as minoxidil, should be avoided because there is evidence it affects renin-related salt and fluid retention.[42] Although dihydropyridine CCBs such as amlodipine and felodipine do not improve heart failure, they are efficacious in decreasing blood pressure and seem to be safe to use for patients with HFrEF.[43] However, pedal edema is a common dose-related side effect that is more common in women. Nondihydropyridine CCBs, such as diltiazem and verapamil, should be avoided because of negative inotropic effects. In ALLHAT, patients receiving the alpha-1 antagonist doxazosin had a 2-fold higher risk for heart failure, causing this arm of the trial to stop prematurely. Therefore, this drug class should be avoided in patients with or at risk for heart failure.[44] In addition, moxonidine was associated with increased mortality in patients with heart failure, which may preclude the use of other centrally acting agents such as clonidine.[45]

Table 1
Hypertension dose range and heart failure guideline–directed medical therapy target dose

Drug Class	Hypertension Dose Range	Heart Failure Target Dose
ACE Inhibitors		
Enalapril	5–40 mg daily or twice daily	10–20 mg twice daily
Lisinopril	10–40 mg daily	20–40 mg daily
Ramipril	2.5–20 mg daily or twice daily	10 mg daily
Captopril	12.5–150 mg twice daily or 3 times a day	50 mg 3 times a day
Perindopril	4–16 mg daily	8–16 mg daily
Fosinopril	10–40 mg daily	40 mg daily
ARBs		
Valsartan	80–320 mg daily	160 mg twice daily
Candesartan	8–32 mg daily	32 mg daily
Losartan	50–100 mg daily or twice daily	50–150 mg daily
Aldosterone Antagonists		
Spironolactone	25–100 mg twice daily	25 mg daily or twice daily
Eplerenone	50–100 mg daily or twice daily	50 mg daily
β-Blockers		
Metoprolol succinate	50–200 mg daily	200 mg daily
Bisoprolol	2.5–10 mg daily	10 mg daily
Carvedilol	12.5–50 mg twice daily	50 mg twice daily

Data from Whelton PK, Carey RM, Aronow WS, et al. 2017 ACC/AHA/AAPA/ABC/ACPM/AGS/APhA/ ASH/ASPC/NMA/PCNA guideline for the prevention, detection, evaluation, and management of high blood pressure in adults: executive summary. a report of the American College of Cardiology/American Heart Association Task Force on Clinical Practice Guidelines. Hypertension. 2018;71(6):1269–1324; and Yancy CW, Jessup M, Bozkurt B, et al. 2013 ACCF/AHA guideline for the management of heart failure: a report of the American College of Cardiology Foundation/ American Heart Association Task Force on Practice Guidelines. J Am Coll Cardiol. 2013;62(16):e147–e239.

Despite decades of historical RCTs showing improved outcomes in HFrEF, currently there are no therapeutic options proved to reduce morbidity and mortality in HFpEF. Loop diuretics are a cornerstone for symptom management; however, drugs within this class are usually less effective than thiazidelike diuretics in decreasing blood pressure. ARB and aldosterone antagonist use is suggested to decrease heart failure hospitalizations and can effectively decrease blood pressure through RAAS inhibition.[26] Aldosterone antagonist target doses for hypertension are higher than for heart failure and may increase risk for hyperkalemia, which occurs in a dose-dependent fashion.[46] Refractory hypertension is more common in HFpEF than HFrEF but there is a substantial lack of evidence available to provide recommendations to support or contest therapies such as thiazidelike diuretics, β-blockers, CCBs, or alpha-1 antagonists. Nitrates should be avoided because they may worsen functional status and do not improve quality of life.[39]

Achieving adequate blood pressure control in patients with comorbid HFrEF and HFpEF is vital. However, important considerations of stringent pharmacotherapy to achieve lower blood pressure targets in the setting of maximum-dose GDMT include syncope, orthostatic hypotension, acute kidney injury, and electrolyte disturbances. These adverse drug events may be especially pronounced in older adults, so tapering

---

Box 1
Select fixed-dose combination tablets

ACE inhibitor/calcium channel blocker
  Perindopril/amlodipine

ACE inhibitor/thiazide diuretic
  Lisinopril/hydrochlorothiazide
  Enalapril/hydrochlorothiazide
  Captopril/hydrochlorothiazide
  Fosinopril/hydrochlorothiazide

ARB/calcium channel blocker
  Valsartan/amlodipine

ARB/thiazide diuretic
  Losartan/hydrochlorothiazide
  Valsartan/hydrochlorothiazide
  Candesartan/hydrochlorothiazide

Aldosterone antagonist/thiazide diuretic
  Spironolactone/hydrochlorothiazide

β-Blocker/thiazide diuretic
  Bisoprolol/hydrochlorothiazide
  Metoprolol succinate/hydrochlorothiazide

Calcium channel blocker/thiazide diuretic/ARB
  Amlodipine/hydrochlorothiazide/valsartan

Data from Whelton PK, Carey RM, Aronow WS, et al. 2017 ACC/AHA/AAPA/ABC/ACPM/AGS/ APhA/ASH/ASPC/NMA/PCNA guideline for the prevention, detection, evaluation, and management of high blood pressure in adults: executive summary. a report of the American College of Cardiology/American Heart Association Task Force on Clinical Practice Guidelines. Hypertension. 2018;71(6):1269–1324.

---

should be gradual and additional monitoring may be required. In contrast, low blood pressure levels should not hinder titration of GDMT provided patients are able to tolerate dose increases. When possible, combination therapy should be used to decrease pill burden and polypharmacy,especially in patients with HFpEF. Select fixed-dose combination tablets are detailed in **Box 1**.

LIFESTYLE MODIFICATIONS

Therapeutic lifestyle changes, including sodium cognizance, smoking cessation, and cardiovascular exercise, should be addressed when treating hypertension to prevent heart failure or in patients with established systolic or diastolic dysfunction.[47] Management of other risk factors, such as obesity and sleep apnea, may also help prevent cardiac remodeling. Sodium glucose cotransporter 2 inhibitors represent a paradigm shift in the treatment of diabetes because increasing evidence reveals their ability to reduce cardiovascular risk, including heart failure. This drug class also has important physiologic effects on blood pressure reduction even in patients concomitantly taking antihypertensives.[48]

SUMMARY

The high prevalence of hypertension establishes it as the single greatest risk factor for heart failure from a population health standpoint. Despite this, many patients remain undiagnosed, undertreated, or untreated and fail to achieve control targets. To prevent the seemingly inevitable transition from chronic hypertension to heart failure, blood pressure should be managed in accordance with current clinical practice guidelines and evidence-based therapies should be used when available. Additional RCTs, particularly in patients with HFpEF, are needed to provide strategies for the management of comorbid hypertension and heart failure.

REFERENCES

1. Benjamin EJ, Muntner P, Bittencourt MS. Heart disease and stroke statistics-2019 update: a report from the American Heart Association. Circulation 2019;139(10): e56–528.
2. Levy D, Larson MG, Vasan RS, et al. The progression from hypertension to congestive heart failure. JAMA 1996;275(20):1557–62.
3. Whelton PK, Carey RM, Aronow WS, et al. 2017 ACC/AHA/AAPA/ABC/ACPM/AGS/APhA/ASH/ASPC/NMA/PCNA guideline for the prevention, detection, evaluation, and management of high blood pressure in adults: executive summary. a report of the American College of Cardiology/American Heart Association Task Force on Clinical Practice Guidelines. Hypertension 2018;71(6):1269–324.
4. Lloyd-Jones DM, Larson MG, Leip EP, et al. Lifetime risk for developing congestive heart failure: the Framingham Heart Study. Circulation 2002;106(24):3068–72.
5. Pfeffer MA. Heart failure and hypertension: importance of prevention. Med Clin North Am 2017;101(1):19–28.
6. Vasan RS, Levy D. The role of hypertension in the pathogenesis of heart failure: a clinical mechanistic overview. Arch Intern Med 1996;156(16):1789–96.
7. Bhuiyan T, Maurer MS. Heart failure with preserved ejection fraction: persistent diagnosis, therapeutic enigma. Curr Cardiovasc Risk Rep 2011;5(5):440–9.
8. Carnethon Mercedes R, Pu J, Howard G, et al. Cardiovascular health in African Americans: a scientific statement from the American Heart Association. Circulation 2017;136(21):e393–423.
9. Vivo RP, Krim SR, Cevik C, et al. Heart failure in Hispanics. J Am Coll Cardiol 2009;53(14):1167–75.
10. Lloyd-Jones DM, Evans JC, Levy D. Hypertension in adults across the age spectrum: current outcomes and control in the community. JAMA 2005;294(4):466–72.
11. Levy D, Anderson KM, Savage DD, et al. Echocardiographically detected left ventricular hypertrophy: prevalence and risk factors: the Framingham Heart Study. Ann Intern Med 1988;108(1):7–13.
12. Eisenberg E, Di Palo KE, Piña IL. Sex differences in heart failure. Clin Cardiol 2018;41(2):211–6.
13. Bui AL, Horwich TB, Fonarow GC. Epidemiology and risk profile of heart failure. Nat Rev Cardiol 2010;8:30.
14. Messerli FH, Rimoldi SF, Bangalore S. The transition from hypertension to heart failure: contemporary update. JACC Heart Fail 2017;5(8):543–51.
15. Sorrentino MJ. The evolution from hypertension to heart failure. Heart Fail Clin 2019;15(4):447–53.
16. Ganau A, Devereux RB, Roman MJ, et al. Patterns of left ventricular hypertrophy and geometric remodeling in essential hypertension. J Am Coll Cardiol 1992; 19(7):1550–8.
17. Wright JW, Mizutani S, Harding JW. Pathways involved in the transition from hypertension to hypertrophy to heart failure. Treatment strategies. Heart Fail Rev 2008;13(3):367–75.

18. de Simone G, Gottdiener JS, Chinali M, et al. Left ventricular mass predicts heart failure not related to previous myocardial infarction: the Cardiovascular Health Study. Eur Heart J 2008;29(6):741–7.

19. Borlaug BA, Redfield MM. Diastolic and systolic heart failure are distinct phenotypes within the heart failure spectrum. Circulation 2011;123(18):2006–14.

20. Jessup M, Brozena S. Heart failure. New Engl J Med 2003;348(20):2007–18.

21. Sciarretta S, Palano F, Tocci G, et al. Antihypertensive treatment and development of heart failure in hypertension: a Bayesian network meta-analysis of studies in patients with hypertension and high cardiovascular risk. Arch Intern Med 2011; 171(5):384–94.

22. Staessen JA, Wang J-G, Thijs L. Cardiovascular prevention and blood pressure reduction: a quantitative overview updated until 1 March 2003. J Hypertens 2003;21(6):1055–76.

23. Verdecchia P, Angeli F, Cavallini C, et al. Blood pressure reduction and renin–angiotensin system inhibition for prevention of congestive heart failure: a meta-analysis. Eur Heart J 2009;30(6):679–88.

24. Ettehad D, Emdin CA, Kiran A, et al. Blood pressure lowering for prevention of cardiovascular disease and death: a systematic review and meta-analysis. Lancet 2016;387(10022):957–67.

25. SPRINT Research Group, Wright JT Jr, Williamson JD, Whelton PK, et al. A randomized trial of intensive versus standard blood-pressure control. N Engl J Med 2015;373(22):2103–16.

26. Yancy CW, Jessup M, Bozkurt B, et al. 2017 ACC/AHA/HFSA focused update of the 2013 ACCF/AHA guideline for the management of heart failure: a report of the American College of Cardiology/American Heart Association Task Force on clinical practice guidelines and the Heart Failure Society of America. Circulation 2017;136(6):e137–61.

27. Voko Z, Bots ML, Hofman A, et al. J-shaped relation between blood pressure and stroke in treated hypertensives. Hypertension 1999;34(6):1181–5.

28. Farnett L, Mulrow CD, Linn WD, et al. The J-curve phenomenon and the treatment of hypertension: is there a point beyond which pressure reduction is dangerous? JAMA 1991;265(4):489–95.

29. Banach M, Aronow WS. Blood pressure j-curve: current concepts. Curr Hypertens Rep 2012;14(6):556–66.

30. Desai RV, Banach M, Ahmed MI, et al. Impact of baseline systolic blood pressure on long-term outcomes in patients with advanced chronic systolic heart failure (insights from the BEST trial). Am J Cardiol 2010;106(2):221–7.

31. Tsimploulis A, Lam PH, Arundel C, et al. Systolic blood pressure and outcomes in patients with heart failure with preserved ejection fraction. JAMA Cardiol 2018; 3(4):288–97.

32. Pinho-Gomes AC, Rahimi K. Management of blood pressure in heart failure. Heart 2019;105(8):589–95.

33. Davis BR, Piller LB, Cutler JA, et al. Role of diuretics in the prevention of heart failure: the antihypertensive and lipid-lowering treatment to prevent heart attack trial. Circulation 2006;113(18):2201–10.

34. Liebson PR, Grandits GA, Dianzumba S, et al. Comparison of five antihypertensive monotherapies and placebo for change in left ventricular mass in patients receiving nutritional-hygienic therapy in the Treatment of Mild Hypertension Study (TOMHS). Circulation 1995;91(3):698–706.

35. Colucci WS, Kolias TJ, Adams KF, et al. Metoprolol reverses left ventricular re-modeling in patients with asymptomatic systolic dysfunction: the REversal of VEntricular Remodeling with Toprol-XL (REVERT) trial. Circulation 2007;116(1):49–56.

36. Verdecchia P, Sleight P, Mancia G, et al. Effects of telmisartan, ramipril, and their combination on left ventricular hypertrophy in individuals at high vascular risk in the ongoing telmisartan alone and in combination with ramipril global end point trial and the telmisartan randomized assessment Study in ACE intolerant subjects with cardiovascular disease. Circulation 2009;120(14):1380–9.

37. Investigators* S. Effect of enalapril on mortality and the development of heart failure in asymptomatic patients with reduced left ventricular ejection fractions. N Engl J Med 1992;327(10):685–91.

38. Bavishi C, Messerli FH, Kadosh B, et al. Role of neprilysin inhibitor combinations in hypertension: insights from hypertension and heart failure trials. Eur Heart J 2015;36(30):1967–73.

39. Yancy CW, Jessup M, Bozkurt B, et al. 2013 ACCF/AHA guideline for the management of heart failure: a report of the American College of Cardiology Foundation/American Heart Association Task Force on practice guidelines. J Am Coll Cardiol 2013;62(16):e147–239.

40. Rosendorff C, Black HR, Cannon CP, et al. Treatment of hypertension in the prevention and management of ischemic heart disease: a scientific statement from the American Heart Association Council for High Blood Pressure Research and the Councils on Clinical Cardiology and Epidemiology and Prevention. Circulation 2007;115(21):2761–88.

41. Bozkurt B, Aguilar D, Deswal A, et al. Contributory risk and management of comorbidities of hypertension, obesity, diabetes mellitus, hyperlipidemia, and metabolic syndrome in chronic heart failure: a scientific statement from the American Heart Association. Circulation 2016;134(23):e535–78.

42. Franciosa JA, Jordan RA, Wilen MM, et al. Minoxidil in patients with chronic left heart failure: contrasting hemodynamic and clinical effects in a controlled trial. Circulation 1984;70(1):63–8.

43. Packer M, Carson P, Elkayam U, et al. Effect of amlodipine on the survival of patients with severe chronic heart failure due to a nonischemic cardiomyopathy: results of the PRAISE-2 study (prospective randomized amlodipine survival evaluation 2). JACC Heart Fail 2013;1(4):308–14.

44. ALLHAT Officers and Coordinators for the ALLHAT Collaborative Research Group. The Antihypertensive and Lipid-Lowering Treatment to Prevent Heart Attack Trial. Major outcomes in moderately hypercholesterolemic, hypertensive patients randomized to pravastatin vs usual care: the antihypertensive and lipid-lowering treatment to prevent heart attack trial (ALLHAT-LLT). JAMA 2002; 288:2981–97.

45. Cohn JN, Pfeffer MA, Rouleau J, et al. Adverse mortality effect of central sympathetic inhibition with sustained-release moxonidine in patients with heart failure (MOXCON). Eur J Heart Fail 2003;5(5):659–67.

46. Vardeny O, Claggett B, Anand I, et al. Incidence, predictors, and outcomes related to hypo-and hyperkalemia in patients with severe heart failure treated with a mineralocorticoid receptor antagonist. Circ Heart Fail 2014;7(4):573–9.

47. Georgiopoulou VV, Kalogeropoulos AP, Butler J. Heart failure in hypertension: prevention and treatment. Drugs 2012;72(10):1373–98.

48. Oliva RV, Bakris GL. Blood pressure effects of sodium–glucose co-transport 2 (SGLT2) inhibitors. J Am Soc Hypertens 2014;8(5):330–9.

Atrial Fibrillation and Heart Failure

Epidemiology, Pathophysiology, Prognosis, and Management

Jonathan P. Ariyaratnam, MB BChir[a], Dennis H. Lau, MBBS, PhD[a],
Prashanthan Sanders, MBBS, PhD[a],
Jonathan M. Kalman, MBBS, PhD[b],*

KEYWORDS

- Atrial fibrillation • Heart failure (HF)
- Heart failure with reduced ejection fraction (HFrEF)
- Heart failure with preserved ejection fraction (HFpEF)

KEY POINTS

- Atrial fibrillation (AF) and heart failure (HF) share similar risk factors and frequently coexist.
- The risk of developing AF is higher in patients with HF (both HFrEF and HFpEF). The association between HFpEF and AF appears to be particularly strong.
- Mortality rates are increased when AF coexists with HF. Incident AF confers a particularly increased risk of mortality in patients with HF.
- Management of AF-HFrEF should focus on anticoagulation, rhythm or rate control and risk factor management. There is some evidence that catheter ablation may be effective in AF-HFrEF.
- Strong data to guide management of AF-HFpEF remains lacking. Robust new studies in this area are required.

INTRODUCTION

Atrial fibrillation (AF) and heart failure (HF) are chronic cardiovascular conditions that continue to increase in prevalence worldwide and have been described as global epidemics.[1,2] AF and HF each independently worsen quality of life and increase risk of

This article originally appeared in *Cardiac Electrophysiology Clinics*, Volume 13, Issue 1, March 2021.

[a] Centre for Heart Rhythm Disorders, University of Adelaide and Royal Adelaide Hospital, Adelaide, Australia; [b] Department of Cardiology, Royal Melbourne Hospital, Department of Medicine, University of Melbourne, Melbourne, Australia
* Corresponding author. Department of Cardiology, Royal Melbourne Hospital, Parkville, Victoria 3050, Australia.
E-mail address: jon.kalman@mh.org.au

hospitalization and mortality. In addition, AF and HF commonly coexist (AF-HF), sharing common risk factors and physiologically potentiating the effect of each other. In combination, these conditions appear to have a synergistic effect on outcomes including mortality, emphasizing the need for improved strategies for management of these two conditions in combination.

A significant challenge in HF management is the vast heterogeneity in phenotype. In recent years, HF has been broadly classified into HF with reduced ejection fraction (HFrEF) and HF with preserved ejection fraction (HFpEF), based on left ventricular ejection fraction (LVEF) identified on cardiac imaging. Although HFrEF and HFpEF exhibit the same symptoms and signs, they are increasingly seen as entirely different entities with diverging etiologies, prognostic implications, and management strategies. Furthermore, their interactions with AF (AF-HFrEF and AF-HFpEF) are distinctive. In this review article, we discuss the pathophysiology, epidemiology, prognosis, and evidence-based management of AF-HF, highlighting the significant differences between AF-HFrEF and AF-HFpEF.

HEART FAILURE WITH REDUCED EJECTION FRACTION AND HEART FAILURE WITH PRESERVED EJECTION FRACTION

HFrEF and HFpEF have been shown to contribute equally to the global burden of HF.[3] Simplistically, HFrEF is HF due to impaired left ventricular systolic function, whereas HFpEF is HF due to impaired left ventricular diastolic function. Diagnosis of HFrEF requires symptoms of HF in association with impaired systolic function identified on cardiac imaging. On the other hand, diagnosis of HFpEF is rather more challenging and recently published guidelines highlight the complexities of the diagnosis.[4] Diagnosis of HFpEF is made even more difficult by the presence of AF, as the symptoms of AF and HFpEF commonly overlap (**Fig. 1**). In addition, the echocardiographic and natriuretic peptide measurements used to diagnose diastolic failure are altered by the presence of AF.[5] Many of the studies investigating AF-HFpEF are therefore limited by overly simplistic definitions of HFpEF. Conclusions drawn regarding the prevalence and incidence of AF-HFpEF, the mortality associated with AF-HFpEF, and the optimal management of AF-HFpEF should therefore be tempered by the knowledge that HFpEF may have been overdiagnosed in these studies.

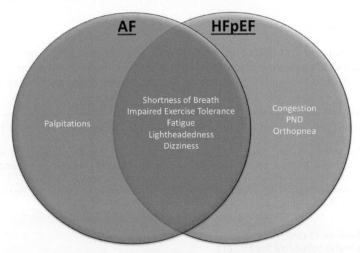

Fig. 1. Overlapping symptoms of AF and HFpEF.

EPIDEMIOLOGY OF ATRIAL FIBRILLATION–HEART FAILURE

The prevalence of HF worldwide is 2% with up to 26 million people affected.[6] Similarly, it is estimated that approximately 33.5 million people have AF.[1] The prevalence of both conditions is increased in men and older age; the prevalence of HF in those older than 75 is 8.4%,[7] whereas the prevalence of AF in those older than 80 is 9%.[8] With aging populations around the world, the burden of both diseases is expected to continue to climb.

The prevalence of each condition is increased in the presence of the other. Patients with AF have a high prevalence of underlying HF, whereas, conversely, patients with HF have a marked association with prevalent AF.[9,10] **Fig. 2** shows the prevalence of AF in major HF registries, highlighting the consistently higher prevalence of AF in HFpEF compared with HFrEF.

The Framingham Heart Study (FHS), in which healthy adults were biennially monitored over their lifetimes for the development of cardiovascular disease, has been particularly useful in monitoring the temporal relationships between AF and HF. In total, 382 participants developed both AF and HF between 1948 and 1995.[11] Of these participants, 38% developed AF first, 41% developed HF first, and 21% were diagnosed with both on the same day. A new diagnosis of HF was associated with incident AF at a rate of 5.4% per year, whereas a new diagnosis of AF was associated with incident HF at a rate of 3.3% per year.[11] In a more contemporary analysis of the FHS, AF and HF subtypes were specifically evaluated.[12] This study demonstrated that patients with HFpEF were more likely to have prevalent AF preceding their HF diagnosis than patients with HFrEF, and patients with a new diagnosis of AF were more likely to develop incident HFpEF than incident HFrEF. Furthermore, prevalent AF predicted the development of incident HFpEF but not incident HFrEF. These data suggest that AF may have a particularly close role to play in the pathophysiology of HFpEF.

PATHOPHYSIOLOGY OF ATRIAL FIBRILLATION–HEART FAILURE

Fig. 3 shows the inextricable pathophysiological relationship between HF and AF. The development of the 2 conditions is driven by several common risk factors. Once developed, the 2 conditions have the potential to interact with each other in a vicious cycle.

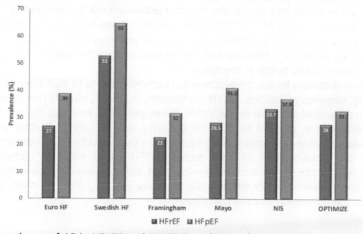

Fig. 2. Prevalence of AF in HFpEF and HFrEF. Prevalence of AF in HFrEF and HFpEF in major HF registries. There is increased prevalence of AF associated with HFpEF in comparison with HFrEF. NIS, National Inpatient Sample; OPTIMIZE, Organized Program to Initiate Life Saving Treatment in Hospitalized Patients with Heart Failure.

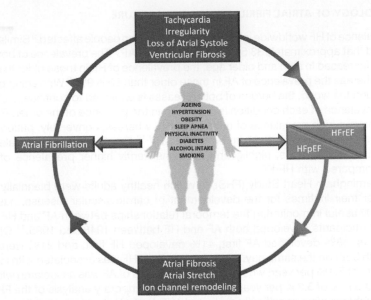

Fig. 3. AF interacts with HFrEF and HFpEF in a vicious cycle. Both AF and HF share common risk factors that lead to their development. AF and HF are then able to induce and perpetuate each other in a vicious cycle.

SHARED RISK FACTORS

Many of the risk factors underlying the development of AF and HF (both HFrEF and HFpEF) are shared (**Fig. 4**). As the general population around the world becomes increasingly older, sedentary, and obese, the prevalence of AF and HF continues to rise. These risk factors cause significant hemodynamic shifts, cardiac inflammation, atrial and ventricular fibrosis, macrovascular and microvascular ischemia, and arterial stiffening, leading to important changes in atrial and ventricular function.

Substantial research has shown the effect of untreated risk factors on the development of atrial disease and AF.[13–16] The importance of these risk factors, and in particular obesity, has been further highlighted by evidence showing that atrial disease can be reversed by aggressive treatment of risk factors through lifestyle modifications as well as by medical and surgical therapies.[17,18]

Similarly, risk factors for the development of both HFrEF and HFpEF also include aging, obesity, sedentary lifestyles, and hypertension. In HFrEF, obesity has been shown to result in a twofold increase in risk of HF development,[19] whereas the overweight/obese phenotype is present in 80% of patients with HFpEF.[20] Further evidence from long-term follow-up registry data has shown that obesity is a comparable risk factor for the development of both incident HFrEF and HFpEF.[10] Interestingly, although obesity increases risk of HF development, substantial evidence exists to suggest that the presence of obesity actually reduces the long-term mortality of these conditions; the so-called "obesity paradox."[21]

HEART FAILURE PROMOTES INCIDENT ATRIAL FIBRILLATION

Both animal and human studies have provided evidence for the mechanistic links between prevalent HF and incident AF. These mechanisms include (1) activation of the

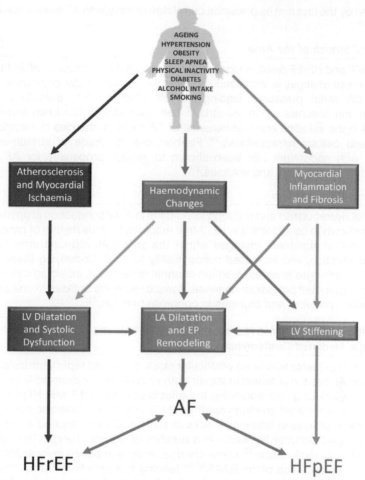

Fig. 4. Similar risk factors underlie the development of AF, HFrEF, and HFpEF. Shared risk factors cause significant alterations in cardiac hemodynamics, myocardial ischemia, and myocardial inflammation. These important changes lead to structural changes of the myocardium that can lead to HFrEF, HFpEF, or AF. AF, atrial fibrillation; EP, electrophysiological; LA, left atrium; LV, left ventricle; HFpEF, heart failure with preserved ejection fraction; HFrEF, heart failure with reduced ejection fraction.

renin-angiotensin-aldosterone system (RAAS), (2) mechanical stretch of the left atrium, and (3) electrophysiological remodeling of the atria.

Neurohormonal Activation and Atrial Fibrosis

The RAAS is a key modulator of the electrophysiological properties of the atria. HF results in activation of the RAAS in response to underperfusion of the kidneys. Activation of RAAS has been shown in animal models to promote fibrosis within the atria, partly mediated by the proinflammatory cytokine transforming growth factor-β.[22] Evidence for this association is strengthened by the fact that interstitial fibrosis appears to be significantly reduced by inhibitors of the RAAS, such as enalapril, candesartan, and spironolactone.[23–25] The pathophysiological importance of this atrial fibrosis is highlighted by the fact that its presence correlates directly with AF recurrence after AF ablation.[26]

Mechanical Stretch of the Atria

Both HFpEF and HFrEF result in significant hemodynamic alterations within the heart. One of the key changes is increased end-systolic left ventricular pressures. This increases left atrial pressures leading to left atrial stretch, activating stretch-dependent ion channels within the atria.[27] Left atrial stretch has been shown to be important in the initiation and maintenance of AF through changes in electrical conduction and cellular refractoriness.[28] Furthermore, blockade of stretch-activated channels with gadolinium has been shown to reduce propensity for AF despite increased atrial pressures and volumes.[29]

Ion Channel Dysregulation

Ion channel dysregulation and resulting alterations in atrial conduction properties have also been shown to be important in HF. Atrial mapping in sinus rhythm of patients with HFrEF identified significant changes within the atria with reduced atrial voltages, slowed conduction, and increased susceptibility to AF.[30] Underlying these electrophysiological changes is widespread ion channel remodeling, including dysregulation of voltage-dependent potassium channels, inward rectifying potassium channels, calcium handling proteins, and changes in connexin function.[31]

ATRIAL FIBRILLATION PROMOTES INCIDENT HEART FAILURE
Tachycardia-Mediated Cardiomyopathy

AF commonly presents with rapid ventricular rates. Sustained rapid ventricular rates in response to AF has the potential to impair both systolic and/or diastolic left ventricular (LV) function, inducing and worsening the effects of both HFrEF and HFpEF.

Tachycardia-mediated cardiomyopathy (TMC) specifically refers to the reversible systolic dysfunction seen following weeks of sustained and untreated elevated heart rates. Prolonged tachycardia results in a number of cellular changes that contribute to this LV systolic dysfunction.[32] These changes include impaired myocardial contractile function, upregulation of the RAAS[33,34] leading to a proinflammatory response,[35] fluid accumulation and dysfunctional hypertrophy of ventricular myocytes,[36] dysregulation of cellular calcium handling,[37] and alterations in the extracellular matrix.[38] In addition, significant hemodynamic changes further contribute to LV dysfunction with tachycardia causing increased LV wall stress, raised LV filling pressures, and increased afterload due to increased systemic vascular resistance.[39–41]

Importantly, these changes appear to be temporary, with restoration of sinus rhythm associated with normalization of hemodynamics and with normalization of LV function occurring within weeks. However, there is evidence to suggest that chronic changes within the ventricular myocardium may persist following TMC; increased collagen deposition, LV stiffness, and impaired diastolic function have been noted in animal studies of TMC,[38,42] whereas long-term follow-up of patients with previous TMC suggests an increased propensity for these patients to develop recurrent HF and even sudden death.[43,44]

Irregular Ventricular Rhythm

There is growing evidence to suggest that irregular R-R intervals in AF also impair LV function irrespective of tachycardia. In patients with persistent AF in whom the heart rate is adequately controlled, regularization of the heart rhythm with either restoration of sinus rhythm or atrioventricular (AV) node ablation and pacing has been shown to improve ejection fraction in selected patients with HFrEF.[45,46] On a cellular level, animal studies have demonstrated that irregular cycle lengths result in abnormal calcium handling and therefore impaired cardiac myocyte function.[47]

Loss of Atrial Systole

In sinus rhythm, coordinated atrial systole contributes to approximately 20% of cardiac output by increasing ventricular filling during ventricular diastole. Loss of atrial systole caused by AF consequently results in impaired systolic function due to reduced stroke volume according to the Frank-Starling mechanism.[48] Furthermore, impaired LV filling during diastole results in diastolic dysfunction, raised left atrial pressures, and resultant symptoms of HFpEF.[49]

Ventricular Fibrosis

Cardiac MRI studies have identified diffuse ventricular fibrosis in patients with AF in the absence of any other cause.[50] This ventricular fibrosis has a dose-dependent relationship with AF; the greater the burden of AF, the greater the degree of fibrosis.[50] Ventricular fibrosis has a detrimental effect on both systolic and diastolic function and therefore has a potential impact in both HFrEF and HFpEF.[51]

PROGNOSTIC IMPLICATIONS OF ATRIAL FIBRILLATION–HEART FAILURE
Mortality

Although individual studies have demonstrated conflicting results regarding the impact of prevalent AF on all-cause mortality in HFrEF, a number of meta-analyses have now been performed confirming an overall increased long-term risk of between 17-40%.[52–54] **Table 1** shows that the pattern is similar with HFpEF, with most, but not all, randomized controlled trials (RCTs) and registries demonstrating a statistically significant increased risk of long-term all-cause mortality. In addition, there are conflicting data regarding whether AF is more dangerous in HFrEF or HFpEF; a meta-analysis pooling comparative risk estimates for all-cause mortality in AF-HFrEF and AF-HFpEF suggested that AF-HFrEF carried greater risk.[55] However, this study was limited by variable definitions of HFpEF with some studies defining patients with ejection fractions of 40% as HFpEF. On the other hand, a number of other studies have suggested that risk of all-cause mortality may rise with increasing ejection fractions in HF.[56,57]

Interestingly, developing incident AF after a diagnosis of either HFrEF or HFpEF appears to confer a much greater risk of long-term all-cause mortality than prevalent AF (AF before HF diagnosis).[54] The reasons for this remain unclear, although several mechanisms have been postulated: (1) new AF is more likely to be poorly rate-controlled than established AF, (2) risks associated with potent antiarrhythmic medications may be highest during the initiation phase, (3) over-anticoagulation or under-anticoagulation is more likely when newly prescribed compared with established regimens, and (4) a sudden change from sinus rhythm to AF is less likely to be hemodynamically tolerated in the failing heart when compared with ongoing long-standing AF.[58]

Stroke

AF is associated with a fivefold increase in risk of cerebral thromboembolism, independent of hypertension and age.[59] Studies from the pre-anticoagulation era show that congestive cardiac failure may elevate this risk of stroke,[60] although other studies demonstrate no significant association.[61,62] These conflicting data likely expose a lack of uniformity in the definition of HF in these studies. Indeed, when HF is defined purely

Table 1
Association of prevalent and incident AF in HFpEF with all-cause mortality

Study	Study Type	Population	Number of HFpEF Participants	Average Follow-up, y	Effect of Prevalent AF on Risk of All-Cause Mortality (Adjusted HR)	Effect of Incident AF on Risk of All-Cause Mortality (Adjusted HR)
TOPCAT 2018[97]	RCT	• At least 1 sign/symptom of HF • LVEF >45% • >50 y • Controlled systolic BP • K <5 • GFR >30	1765	2.9	• 1.34 (1.09–1.65)	• 2.53 (1.80–3.55)
CHARM 2006[56]	RCT	• Symptomatic HF • NYHA II-IV • LVEF >40%	7599	3.1	• 1.37 (1.06–1.79)	• Odds ratio (unadjusted) – 2.57 (1.70–3.90)
I-PRESERVE 2014[98]	RCT	• Symptomatic HF (NYHA II-IV) • LVEF >45% • >1 hospitalization previous 6 mo	4128	4.4	• 1.23 (0.99–1.54)	• Not reported
PRESERVE 2012[99]	RCT	• >1 HF hospitalization OR >3 ambulatory HF visits • LVEF >50%	14,295	1.8	• 1.11 (1.03–1.20)	• 1.62 (1.42–1.84)
Zakeri et al,[100] 2013	Registry	• Olmstead County HF surveillance study cohort • LVEF >50%	939	4.3	• 1.27 (1.06–1.51)	• 2.22 (1.73–2.84)
Sartipy et al,[68] 2017	Registry	• Swedish HF • Registry • Clinician-judged HF • EF >50%	9595	2.2	• 1.11 (1.02–1.21)	• Not reported
Zafrir et al,[69] 2018	Registry	• HF Long-Term Registry of the ESC • LVEF >50%	3879	1	• 1.20 (0.95–1.50)	• Not reported

| Santhanakrishnan et al,[12] 2016 | Registry | • Framingham Heart Study participants 1980–2012 • LVEF >45% | 309 | 3.6 (+/−3.4) | • 1.33 (0.97–1.83) • 1.58 (1.08–2.3) |
| Rusinaru et al,[101] 2008 | Registry | • HF admissions in Somme region • LVEF >50% | 368 | 5 | • 1.19 (0.89–1.6) • Not reported |

Large RCTs and HF registries providing risk estimates for all-cause mortality in patients with AF and HFpEF. Most studies suggest that prevalent AF increases risk of all-cause mortality in HFpEF but risk is significantly higher in incident AF than prevalent AF.

Abbreviations: AF, atrial fibrillation; BP, blood pressure; EF, ejection fraction; ESC, European Society of Cardiology; GFR, glomerular filtration rate; HF, heart failure; HFpEF, heart failure with preserved ejection fraction; HR, hazard ratio; LVEF, left ventricular ejection fraction; NYHA, New York Heart Association; RCT, randomized controlled trial.

as a moderate-to-severe reduction in LVEF, the risk of stroke is more than doubled (2.5x higher).[63] On the other hand, when the HF definition includes clinician-judged symptoms or previously documented history, the association with stroke often disappears.[64]

Data on the risk of stroke in AF-HFpEF from the pre-anticoagulation era are limited. However, recent studies have attempted to define the risk in patients with AF-HFpEF, albeit in largely anticoagulated populations. The CODE-AF registry of 10,697 Korean patients with AF showed that patients with AF-HFpEF were at significantly increased risk of stroke compared with patients with AF in the absence of HF.[65] On the other hand, the similarly sized US-based ORBIT-AF registry identified that there was no independent increased stroke risk in patients with HFpEF, albeit in a cohort with lower overall stroke rates.[66] Other studies have identified that there is no significant difference in risk of stroke between AF-HFrEF and AF-HFpEF.[55,67,68]

Overall, the data therefore suggest that the presence of HFrEF may increase the risk of stroke in patients with AF, depending on the definition of HFrEF used. Data in HFpEF are limited and more studies are required to further define this risk.

ATRIAL FIBRILLATION AND HEART FAILURE WITH MIDRANGE EJECTION FRACTION

In 2016, the European Society of Cardiology introduced the concept of HF with midrange ejection fraction (HFmrEF). These are patients with symptoms and signs of HF, ejection fraction between 40% and 49%, and elevated natriuretic peptides with evidence of structural heart disease or diastolic dysfunction. This additional classification of HF was an acknowledgment that a gray zone existed between HFrEF and HFpEF. Interestingly, studies have since shown that this group of patients demonstrate characteristics and prognoses that are intermediate between HFrEF and HFpEF. Indeed, the prevalence of AF in HFmrEF, and the risk of all-cause mortality of AF-HFmrEF, appears to lie somewhere between the prevalence and mortality in HFrEF and HFpEF.[68,69]

MANAGEMENT OF ATRIAL FIBRILLATION–HEART FAILURE

Optimal management of AF-HF mirrors the management of AF alone with 4 key principles; anticoagulation, rhythm control, rate control, and risk factor management (RFM). However, HFrEF and HFpEF differ entirely in pathophysiology and responses to treatment and must, therefore, be considered as separate entities when considering management. Although the evidence supporting various management options is significantly more advanced in AF-HFrEF, the evidence-base for AF-HFpEF continues to grow.

MANAGEMENT OF ATRIAL FIBRILLATION–HEART FAILURE WITH REDUCED EJECTION FRACTION
Anticoagulation

Anticoagulation has been extensively shown to effectively reduce the risk of stroke in patients with AF by up to 68%.[61] Current clinical guidelines propose anticoagulation according to the presence of risk factors. The CHADS2Vasc risk score is in widespread use to assist in anticoagulation decision-making.[70] Congestive cardiac failure, defined loosely as "signs/symptoms of HF or objective evidence of reduced LVEF," forms part of this risk stratification tool. Given that anticoagulation is generally recommended for patients with a CHADS2Vasc score of 1 or more, any patient with a diagnosis of AF-HFrEF would, by definition, warrant anticoagulation according to clinical guidelines. Adequately anticoagulated patients with AF-HFrEF have reduced incidence of ischemic stroke compared with non-anticoagulated patients with AF-

HFrEF.[64] In addition, anticoagulated patients with AF-HFrEF have equivalent adjusted stroke risks to adequately anticoagulated patients with AF-only, with no significant difference in bleeding.[64,71–74] Therefore, although strong evidence for an increased adjusted stroke risk with AF-HFrEF compared with AF-only may be lacking, anticoagulation of these cohorts reduces overall stroke incidence and does not appear to cause significant harm.

In terms of choice of anticoagulant to use in patients with AF-HFrEF, substudies of the major direct oral anticoagulant (DOAC) RCTs have shown that each DOAC (Apixaban, Dabigatran, Rivaroxaban, and Edoxaban) is at least as safe as warfarin in this population, with some showing superiority in terms of reduced risk of stroke[71,72] and major bleeding.[71,72,74]

Pharmacological Rhythm Versus Rate Control

Although anticoagulation in AF-HFrEF is universally expected in the absence of contraindications, the choice between rate control or rhythm control remains guided by patient symptoms and physician preferences. The reason for this is the absence of clear data supporting one strategy above the other. The AF-CHF trial randomized patients with AF and either symptomatic HF (New York Heart Association class II-IV) with LVEF less than 35% or asymptomatic HF with recent decompensation or LVEF less than 25% to a strategy of rate control or rhythm control.[75] Rhythm control strategies included electrical cardioversion and/or pharmacologic rhythm control (mainly involving amiodarone) whereas rate control involved beta-blockers and/or digoxin and/or device implantation with AV node ablation. The study showed that there was no benefit of rhythm control over rate control in terms of the risk of cardiovascular mortality, all-cause mortality, stroke, and worsening HF after 3 years of follow-up.

A cautious approach should be taken in interpreting this study, however. First, 21% of the patients starting in the rhythm control group crossed-over to the rate control group because of a failure to maintain sinus rhythm. Second, 82% of the patients in the rhythm control group were treated with amiodarone compared with just 7% in the rate control group. Amiodarone has been shown in observational studies to increase risk of all-cause mortality and noncardiac mortality and may have neutralized any potential benefits associated with rhythm control.[76,77] Therefore, although the AF-CHF trial showed that pharmacologic rhythm control was not superior to rate control strategies in the AF-HFrEF population, these findings should not be generalized to include nonpharmacological methods for rhythm control, such as catheter ablation.

Catheter Ablation

Two of the main advantages of catheter ablation over pharmacologic rhythm control for treatment of AF are the lower long-term AF recurrence rates and the reduced need for toxic antiarrhythmic drugs such as amiodarone. Catheter ablation is now established as first-line therapy for patients with symptomatic AF in the absence of structural heart disease, and in recent years there has been growing interest in its potential utility for patients with AF-HFrEF. A number of RCTs have been published investigating the effect of catheter ablation on patients with AF-HFrEF (**Table 2**). In general, these studies provide consistent evidence that catheter ablation is more effective than medical rate control in improving LVEF, quality of life, and exercise tolerance. Whether this translates to long-term prognostic benefits remains unclear, with previous evidence suggesting that long-term maintenance of sinus rhythm is poor after catheter ablation for AF-HFrEF. However, the CASTLE-AF trial did show cardiovascular mortality benefits of ablation at 36 months.[78] On the other hand, these trials also suggest that patients with HFrEF are at higher risk of peri-procedural complications

Table 2
Major RCTs investigating outcomes of catheter ablation in patients with HFrEF

Study, Year	Population	Intervention	Comparator	Follow-up, mo	Outcomes
Khan et al,[82] 2008	• Symptomatic AF • NYHA II–III • EF <40% • OMT	PVI (n = 41)	AV node ablation and BiV pacing (n = 40)	6	With PVI: • Improved MLHF score • Longer 6MWT • Improved EF
MacDonald et al,[102] 2011	• Persistent AF • NYHA II–IV • EF <35% • OMT	RFA PVI ± Linear ± CFAEs (n = 22)	Medical rate control (n = 19)	9.7 (RFA group), 6.9 (control group)	With RFA • Radionuclide EF improved • CMR EF not improved • MLHF and 6MWT not improved
Jones et al,[103] 2013	• Persistent AF • NYHA II–IV • EF <35% • OMT	RFA PVI ± Linear ± CFAEs (n = 26)	Medical rate control (n = 26)	12	With RFA • Improved peak oxygen consumption • Improved MLHF • Nonsignificant trend to improved LVEF • Nonsignificant trend to improved 6MWT
Hunter et al,[104] 2014	• Persistent AF • NYHA II–IV • EF <50% • Adequate ventricular rate control	RFA PVI ± CFAEs ± Linear (n = 26)	Medical rate control (n = 24)	6	With RFA • Improved LVEF • Improved peak oxygen consumption • Improved MLHF
Di Biase et al,[105] 2016	• Persistent AF • Dual chamber ICD/CRT-D • NYHA II–IV • EF <40% • OMT	RFA PVI +/PW + CS ± SVC ± CFAE (n = 102)	Amiodarone (n = 101)	24	With RFA • Improved freedom from AF • Reduced unplanned hospitalization • Lower all-cause mortality • Improved LVEF • Improved MLHF • Improved 6MWT

Prabhu et al,[46] 2017	• Persistent AF • NYHA II-IV • EF <45% (on CMR) • Absence of CAD • Absence of any other cause of HF	RFA PVI +/PW (n = 33)	Ongoing medical rate control (n = 33)	6	With RFA • Improved LVEF • Improved NYHA class
Marrouche et al,[78] 2018	• Paroxysmal or persistent AF • NYHA II-IV • LVEF <35% • ICD or CRT-D	RFA PVI ± additional at operator discretion	Medical therapy (rate or rhythm control)	37.8	With RFA • Reduced composite all-cause mortality and HF hospitalization • Reduced all-cause mortality • Reduced cardiovascular mortality • Reduced HF hospitalization • Improved LVEF

Abbreviations: 6MWT, 6-min walk test; AF, atrial fibrillation; AV, atrioventricular; BiV, biventricular; CAD, coronary artery disease; CFAE, complex fractionated atrial electrograms; CMR, cardiac MRI; CRT-D, cardiac resynchronization therapy and defibrillator; CS, coronary sinus; EF, ejection fraction; HF, heart failure; ICD, implantable cardiac defibrillator; MLHFQ, Minnesota Living with Heart Failure Questionnaire; NYHA, New York Heart Association; OMT, optimal medical treatment; PVI, pulmonary vein isolation; PW, posterior wall; RCT, randomized controlled trial; RFA, radiofrequency ablation; SVC, superior vena cava.

compared with non-HFrEF patients, perhaps highlighting the increased fragility of this population. Further evidence is required to assess the balance between efficacy and safety of catheter ablation in this population.

A major difficulty in the design and interpretation of these trials involving AF-HFrEF is the heterogeneity in underlying HF etiology. Many of these studies recruited a mix of ischemic and nonischemic patients with HF, and interpreted the results to reflect HF as an entirety. However, there is evidence to suggest that efficacy rates of catheter ablation may diverge according to etiology. The CAMERA-MRI RCT recruited patients with nonischemic cardiomyopathy only and used cardiac MRI to establish the presence of ventricular fibrosis before intervention (catheter ablation or continued medical rate control).[46] Absence of ventricular fibrosis implicated arrhythmia-induced cardiomyopathy as the underlying etiology. The results showed that an absence of ventricular fibrosis predicted greater improvements in LVEF in the catheter ablation arm and ventricular fibrosis volume inversely correlated with absolute improvement in LVEF. This study therefore emphasizes the need for further stratification of the HFrEF population, both in the design of future trials as well as considering management for individual patients

Rate Control

The AF-CHF trial showed that, for patients with AF-HFrEF, controlling heart rate to less than 80 beats per minute at rest or less than 110 beats per minute during exertion was equal to restoration of sinus rhythm in terms of long-term mortality.[75] On the other hand, the RACE II trial showed that there was no significant mortality or morbidity benefit associated with a strict rate control strategy (resting heart rate [HR] <80 beats per minute) compared with a lenient strategy (resting HR <110 beats per minute).[79] Rate control is therefore an appropriate strategy for patients with AF-HFrEF but target HR remains unclear.

Strategies for rate control in the HFrEF population include medications such as beta-blockers and digoxin or pacemaker implantation and AV node ablation. The Swedish HF Registry provides evidence for the efficacy of beta-blockers in this population with the associated reduction in HR linked to a significant reduction in mortality.[80] Digoxin, on the other hand, has not been shown to be efficacious in the AF-HFrEF population but is often used empirically on the basis that it has proven benefit in patients with HFrEF and sinus rhythm.[81]

AV node ablation is established as an option for rate control in AF-HFrEF, albeit an inferior option to AF ablation as seen in the PABA-CHF trial.[82] In general, it is a strategy that is used as a last resort when attempts at rhythm control and medical rate control have failed. This is because it necessitates prior implantation of a pacemaker, on which the patient will be dependent. In patients with HFrEF and heart block, the BLOCK-HF study showed that biventricular pacing was superior to right ventricular pacing, regardless of baseline QRS duration.[83] A number of observational studies have shown the significant mortality and symptomatic benefits of AV node ablation and biventricular pacemaker implantation compared with medical rate control, and this has been confirmed in meta-analyses.[83,84] However, HF etiology remains an important factor with evidence to suggest that patients with ischemic cardiomyopathy may respond less well compared with those with nonischemic cardiomyopathy.[85]

Risk Factor Management

RFM is an essential component of the management of AF. Numerous studies provide evidence that aggressive monitoring and treatment of the risk factors described previously improve sinus rhythm maintenance, AF-related symptoms, and quality of life.[14–16,18,86,87] Particular benefits have been seen with simple lifestyle modifications resulting in significant weight loss. However, data in the AF-HFrEF population are lacking. Cardiac rehabilitation has proven beneficial in the overall HF population, in terms of reducing hospitalizations and improving quality of life, albeit in the absence of proven benefit on mortality.[88] However, significant barriers to lifestyle modifications in the HFrEF cohort exist, with patients more likely to be elderly and frail and resistant to change because of psychosocial and behavioral issues.[88] Furthermore, there is evidence to suggest that being overweight or obese may confer a survival benefit to patients with HFrEF compared with normal-weight patients with HFrEF.[21] Further studies are required to investigate the association between aggressive RFM and outcomes in the AF-HFrEF population.

MANAGEMENT OF ATRIAL FIBRILLATION–HEART FAILURE WITH PRESERVED EJECTION FRACTION
Anticoagulation

Patients with AF-HFpEF generally have higher CHADS2Vasc scores because they are more likely to be women, elderly, and have associated comorbidities such as hypertension and diabetes.[89] Therefore, regardless of the diagnosis of AF-HFpEF, these patients often warrant anticoagulation. Despite this, the AF-HFpEF cohort has been found to be under-anticoagulated compared with patients with HFrEF, with the difference most pronounced in those with CHADS2Vasc scores of 1 or 2.[89] This perhaps reflects the difficulty in diagnosis of HFpEF and the lack of clarity on its contribution to the CHADS2Vasc scoring system. As with AF-HFrEF, the major DOAC trials showed that anticoagulated patients with AF-HFpEF had adjusted stroke rates similar to patients with AF-only without a significantly increased risk of bleeding.[71]

Rate Versus Rhythm Control

Unlike AF-HFrEF, there are no RCTs available to compare the efficacy of rhythm control versus rate control in the AF-HFpEF population. Clinical guidelines do not specifically propose one strategy over the other. A recently published retrospective analysis of the Get With the Guidelines HF Registry suggested that rhythm control may confer a modest mortality benefit in comparison with rate control.[90] However, this study was significantly limited by a weak definition of HFpEF using EF alone, weak definition of rate control based purely on documented use of beta-blockers or calcium-channel blockers, and an inability to monitor the success or failure of each strategy with follow-up electrocardiogram or Holter.

Catheter Ablation

Currently, only observational studies investigating the efficacy of catheter ablation in AF-HFpEF have been published.[91–96] Most of these studies defined HFpEF simply as HF symptoms and signs in the absence of depressed LV function, thereby likely including a substantial proportion of patients without true HFpEF. Overall, these studies have shown that long-term freedom from AF after catheter ablation is lower in patients with AF-HFpEF compared with patients with AF-only, and is similar to rates in AF-HFrEF populations.[91,92,95,96] One study specified echocardiographic evidence of LV diastolic failure as an inclusion criterion for the HFpEF group, and this showed that freedom from AF rates were intermediate between the AF-only group and the AF-HFrEF group.[92] A further single-arm observational study demonstrated that diastolic function may improve following catheter ablation in HFpEF; however, at this stage there is insufficient evidence to support catheter ablation for AF-HFpEF. Well-designed RCTs with clearly defined patients with HFpEF are required to further understand the importance of catheter ablation treatment in this population.

SUMMARY

AF and HF have similar risk factors, frequently coexist, and potentiate each other in a vicious cycle. AF appears to play a particularly important role in the pathophysiology of HFpEF. Evidence suggests that the presence of AF in both HFrEF and HFpEF increases the risk of all-cause mortality as well as stroke in these conditions, and is particularly problematic when AF is incident. Growing evidence suggests that catheter ablation may be an effective strategy in controlling symptoms and improving quality of life in patients with AF-HFrEF, although further evidence to help stratify the patients most likely to respond is needed. Evidence for mortality benefits remains tenuous at this stage. Strong data guiding management of AF-HFpEF are also lacking largely due to its challenging diagnosis. Therefore, although the dangers of these coexistent conditions are clear, improving outcomes associated with them requires further careful investigation.

CLINICS CARE POINTS

- Patients with HF are 10 times more likely to develop AF than those without HF.
- HF patients who develop AF have 17-40% increased risk of all-cause mortality compared to those without AF.
- Catheter ablation for AF-HFrEF improves symptoms and quality of life and may have mortality benefits.
- Optimal management to improve long-term prognosis in patients with AF-HFpEF has yet to be established.

FINANCIAL DISCLOSURES

Dr. J. Ariyaratnam is supported by the Australian Government Research Training Program Scholarship from the University of Adelaide. Dr D. Lau is supported by the Robert J. Craig Lectureship from the University of Adelaide. Dr P. Sanders is supported by a Practitioner Fellowships from the National Health and Medical Research Council of Australia and by the National Heart Foundation of Australia. Dr Kalman is supported by a Practitioner Fellowship from the National Health and Medical Research Council of Australia.

CONFLICT OF INTEREST DISCLOSURES

Dr P. Sanders reports having served on the advisory board of Medtronic, Abbott Medical, Boston Scientific, CathRx, and PaceMate. Dr P. Sanders reports that the University of Adelaide has received on his behalf lecture and/or consulting fees from Medtronic, Abbott Medical, and Boston Scientific. Dr P. Sanders reports that the University of Adelaide has received on his behalf research funding from Medtronic, Abbott Medical, Boston Scientific, and MicroPort.

REFERENCES

1. Chugh SS, Havmoeller R, Narayanan K, et al. Worldwide epidemiology of atrial fibrillation: a global burden of disease 2010 study. Circulation 2014;129(8): 837–47.
2. Savarese G, Lund LH. Global public health burden of heart failure. Card Fail Rev 2017;3(1):7–11.

3. Bursi F, Weston SA, Redfield MM, et al. Systolic and diastolic heart failure in the community. JAMA 2006;296(18):2209–16.

4. Pieske B, Tschöpe C, de Boer RA, et al. How to diagnose heart failure with preserved ejection fraction: the HFA-PEFF diagnostic algorithm: a consensus recommendation from the Heart Failure Association (HFA) of the European Society of Cardiology (ESC). Eur J Heart Fail 2020;22(3):391–412.

5. Lam CS, Rienstra M, Tay WT, et al. Atrial fibrillation in heart failure with preserved ejection fraction: association with exercise capacity, left ventricular filling pressures, natriuretic peptides, and left atrial volume. JACC Heart Fail 2017; 5(2):92–8.

6. Ponikowski P, Anker SD, AlHabib KF, et al. Heart failure: preventing disease and death worldwide. ESC Heart Fail 2014;1(1):4–25.

7. Redfield MM, Jacobsen SJ, Burnett JC Jr, et al. Burden of systolic and diastolic ventricular dysfunction in the community: appreciating the scope of the heart failure epidemic. JAMA 2003;289(2):194–202.

8. Go AS, Hylek EM, Phillips KA, et al. Prevalence of diagnosed atrial fibrillation in adults: national implications for rhythm management and stroke prevention: the AnTicoagulation and Risk Factors in Atrial Fibrillation (ATRIA) Study. JAMA 2001;285(18):2370–5.

9. Ling LH, Kistler PM, Kalman JM, et al. Comorbidity of atrial fibrillation and heart failure. Nat Rev Cardiol 2016;13(3):131–47.

10. Brouwers FP, de Boer RA, van der Harst P, et al. Incidence and epidemiology of new onset heart failure with preserved vs. reduced ejection fraction in a community-based cohort: 11-year follow-up of PREVEND. Eur Heart J 2013; 34(19):1424–31.

11. Wang TJ, Larson MG, Levy D, et al. Temporal relations of atrial fibrillation and congestive heart failure and their joint influence on mortality: the Framingham Heart Study. Circulation 2003;107(23):2920–5.

12. Santhanakrishnan R, Wang N, Larson MG, et al. Atrial fibrillation begets heart failure and vice versa: temporal associations and differences in preserved versus reduced ejection fraction. Circulation 2016;133(5):484–92.

13. Abed HS, Wittert GA, Leong DP, et al. Effect of weight reduction and cardiometabolic risk factor management on symptom burden and severity in patients with atrial fibrillation: a randomized clinical trial. JAMA 2013;310(19):2050–60.

14. Pathak RK, Elliott A, Middeldorp ME, et al. Impact of CARDIOrespiratory FITness on arrhythmia recurrence in obese individuals with atrial fibrillation: the CARDIO-FIT Study. J Am Coll Cardiol 2015;66(9):985–96.

15. Pathak RK, Middeldorp ME, Lau DH, et al. Aggressive risk factor reduction study for atrial fibrillation and implications for the outcome of ablation: the ARREST-AF cohort study. J Am Coll Cardiol 2014;64(21):2222–31.

16. Pathak RK, Middeldorp ME, Meredith M, et al. Long-term effect of goal-directed weight management in an atrial fibrillation cohort: a long-term follow-up study (LEGACY). J Am Coll Cardiol 2015;65(20):2159–69.

17. Donnellan E, Wazni OM, Elshazly M, et al. Impact of bariatric surgery on atrial fibrillation type. Circ Arrhythm Electrophysiol 2020;13(2):e007626.

18. Middeldorp ME, Pathak RK, Meredith M, et al. PREVEntion and regReSsive Effect of weight-loss and risk factor modification on Atrial Fibrillation: the REVERSE-AF study. Europace 2018;20(12):1929–35.

19. Kenchaiah S, Evans JC, Levy D, et al. Obesity and the risk of heart failure. N Engl J Med 2002;347(5):305–13.

20. Haass M, Kitzman DW, Anand IS, et al. Body mass index and adverse cardio-vascular outcomes in heart failure patients with preserved ejection fraction: results from the Irbesartan in Heart Failure with Preserved Ejection Fraction (I-PRESERVE) trial. Circ Heart Fail 2011;4(3):324–31.

21. Oreopoulos A, Padwal R, Kalantar-Zadeh K, et al. Body mass index and mortality in heart failure: a meta-analysis. Am Heart J 2008;156(1):13–22.

22. Li D, Shinagawa K, Pang L, et al. Effects of angiotensin-converting enzyme inhibition on the development of the atrial fibrillation substrate in dogs with ventricular tachypacing-induced congestive heart failure. Circulation 2001;104(21): 2608–14.

23. Kumagai K, Nakashima H, Urata H, et al. Effects of angiotensin II type 1 receptor antagonist on electrical and structural remodeling in atrial fibrillation. J Am Coll Cardiol 2003;41(12):2197–204.

24. Milliez P, Deangelis N, Rucker-Martin C, et al. Spironolactone reduces fibrosis of dilated atria during heart failure in rats with myocardial infarction. Eur Heart J 2005;26(20):2193–9.

25. Sakabe M, Fujiki A, Nishida K, et al. Enalapril prevents perpetuation of atrial fibrillation by suppressing atrial fibrosis and over-expression of connexin43 in a canine model of atrial pacing-induced left ventricular dysfunction. J Cardiovasc Pharmacol 2004;43(6):851–9.

26. Marrouche NF, Wilber D, Hindricks G, et al. Association of atrial tissue fibrosis identified by delayed enhancement MRI and atrial fibrillation catheter ablation: the DECAAF study. JAMA 2014;311(5):498–506.

27. Sachs F. Stretch-activated ion channels: what are they? Physiology (Bethesda) 2010;25(1):50–6.

28. Solti F, Vecsey T, Kekesi V, et al. The effect of atrial dilatation on the genesis of atrial arrhythmias. Cardiovasc Res 1989;23(10):882–6.

29. Bode F, Katchman A, Woosley RL, et al. Gadolinium decreases stretch-induced vulnerability to atrial fibrillation. Circulation 2000;101(18):2200–5.

30. Sanders P, Morton JB, Davidson NC, et al. Electrical remodeling of the atria in congestive heart failure: electrophysiological and electroanatomic mapping in humans. Circulation 2003;108(12):1461–8.

31. Nattel S, Maguy A, Le Bouter S, et al. Arrhythmogenic ion-channel remodeling in the heart: heart failure, myocardial infarction, and atrial fibrillation. Physiol Rev 2007;87(2):425–56.

32. Gopinathannair R, Etheridge SP, Marchlinski FE, et al. Arrhythmia-induced cardiomyopathies: mechanisms, recognition, and management. J Am Coll Cardiol 2015;66(15):1714–28.

33. Spinale FG, de Gasparo M, Whitebread S, et al. Modulation of the renin-angiotensin pathway through enzyme inhibition and specific receptor blockade in pacing-induced heart failure: I. Effects on left ventricular performance and neurohormonal systems. Circulation 1997;96(7):2385–96.

34. Travill CM, Williams TD, Pate P, et al. Haemodynamic and neurohumoral response in heart failure produced by rapid ventricular pacing. Cardiovasc Res 1992;26(8):783–90.

35. Bradham WS, Bozkurt B, Gunasinghe H, et al. Tumor necrosis factor-alpha and myocardial remodeling in progression of heart failure: a current perspective. Cardiovasc Res 2002;53(4):822–30.

36. Spinale FG, Holzgrefe HH, Mukherjee R, et al. Angiotensin-converting enzyme inhibition and the progression of congestive cardiomyopathy. Effects on left ventricular and myocyte structure and function. Circulation 1995;92(3):562–78.

37. Cory CR, McCutcheon LJ, O'Grady M, et al. Compensatory downregulation of myocardial Ca channel in SR from dogs with heart failure. Am J Physiol 1993; 264(3 Pt 2):H926–37.

38. Spinale FG, Tomita M, Zellner JL, et al. Collagen remodeling and changes in LV function during development and recovery from supraventricular tachycardia. Am J Physiol 1991;261(2 Pt 2):H308–18.

39. O'Brien PJ, Ianuzzo CD, Moe GW, et al. Rapid ventricular pacing of dogs to heart failure: biochemical and physiological studies. Can J Physiol Pharmacol 1990;68(1):34–9.

40. Ohno M, Cheng CP, Little WC. Mechanism of altered patterns of left ventricular filling during the development of congestive heart failure. Circulation 1994;89(5): 2241–50.

41. Seymour AA, Burkett DE, Asaad MM, et al. Hemodynamic, renal, and hormonal effects of rapid ventricular pacing in conscious dogs. Lab Anim Sci 1994;44(5): 443–52.

42. Spinale FG, Zellner JL, Johnson WS, et al. Cellular and extracellular remodeling with the development and recovery from tachycardia-induced cardiomyopathy: changes in fibrillar collagen, myocyte adhesion capacity and proteoglycans. J Mol Cell Cardiol 1996;28(8):1591–608.

43. Nerheim P, Birger-Botkin S, Piracha L, et al. Heart failure and sudden death in patients with tachycardia-induced cardiomyopathy and recurrent tachycardia. Circulation 2004;110(3):247–52.

44. Watanabe H, Okamura K, Chinushi M, et al. Clinical characteristics, treatment, and outcome of tachycardia induced cardiomyopathy. Int Heart J 2008;49(1): 39–47.

45. Natale A, Zimerman L, Tomassoni G, et al. Impact on ventricular function and quality of life of transcatheter ablation of the atrioventricular junction in chronic atrial fibrillation with a normal ventricular response. Am J Cardiol 1996;78(12): 1431–3.

46. Prabhu S, Taylor AJ, Costello BT, et al. Catheter ablation versus medical rate control in atrial fibrillation and systolic dysfunction: the CAMERA-MRI study. J Am Coll Cardiol 2017;70(16):1949–61.

47. Ling LH, Khammy O, Byrne M, et al. Irregular rhythm adversely influences calcium handling in ventricular myocardium: implications for the interaction between heart failure and atrial fibrillation. Circ Heart Fail 2012;5(6):786–93.

48. Mitchell JH, Gupta DN, Payne RM. Influence of atrial systole on effective ventricular stroke volume. Circ Res 1965;17:11–8.

49. White CW, Kerber RE, Weiss HR, et al. The effects of atrial fibrillation on atrial pressure-volume and flow relationships. Circ Res 1982;51(2):205–15.

50. Ling LH, Kistler PM, Ellims AH, et al. Diffuse ventricular fibrosis in atrial fibrillation: noninvasive evaluation and relationships with aging and systolic dysfunction. J Am Coll Cardiol 2012;60(23):2402–8.

51. Liu T, Song D, Dong J, et al. Current understanding of the pathophysiology of myocardial fibrosis and its quantitative assessment in heart failure. Front Physiol 2017;8:238.

52. Cheng M, Lu X, Huang J, et al. The prognostic significance of atrial fibrillation in heart failure with a preserved and reduced left ventricular function: insights from a meta-analysis. Eur J Heart Fail 2014;16(12):1317–22.

53. Mamas MA, Caldwell JC, Chacko S, et al. A meta-analysis of the prognostic significance of atrial fibrillation in chronic heart failure. Eur J Heart Fail 2009;11(7): 676–83.

54. Odutayo A, Wong CX, Williams R, et al. Prognostic importance of atrial fibrillation timing and pattern in adults with congestive heart failure: a systematic review and meta-analysis. J Card Fail 2017;23(1):56–62.

55. Kotecha D, Chudasama R, Lane DA, et al. Atrial fibrillation and heart failure due to reduced versus preserved ejection fraction: a systematic review and meta-analysis of death and adverse outcomes. Int J Cardiol 2016;203:660–6.

56. Olsson LG, Swedberg K, Ducharme A, et al. Atrial fibrillation and risk of clinical events in chronic heart failure with and without left ventricular systolic dysfunction: results from the Candesartan in Heart failure-Assessment of Reduction in Mortality and morbidity (CHARM) program. J Am Coll Cardiol 2006;47(10): 1997–2004.

57. Pai RG, Varadarajan P. Prognostic significance of atrial fibrillation is a function of left ventricular ejection fraction. Clin Cardiol 2007;30(7):349–54.

58. Anter E, Jessup M, Callans DJ. Atrial fibrillation and heart failure: treatment considerations for a dual epidemic. Circulation 2009;110(18):2516–25.

59. Wolf PA, Dawber TR, Thomas HE Jr, et al. Epidemiologic assessment of chronic atrial fibrillation and risk of stroke: the Framingham study. Neurology 1978; 28(10):973–7.

60. Benjamin EJ, Levy D, Vaziri SM, et al. Independent risk factors for atrial fibrillation in a population-based cohort. The Framingham Heart Study. JAMA 1994; 271(11):840–4.

61. Risk factors for stroke and efficacy of antithrombotic therapy in atrial fibrillation. Analysis of pooled data from five randomized controlled trials. Arch Intern Med 1994;154(13):1449–57.

62. Hart RG, Pearce LA, McBride R, et al. Factors associated with ischemic stroke during aspirin therapy in atrial fibrillation: analysis of 2012 participants in the SPAF I-III clinical trials. The Stroke Prevention in Atrial Fibrillation (SPAF) Investigators. Stroke 1999;30(6):1223–9.

63. Echocardiographic predictors of stroke in patients with atrial fibrillation: a prospective study of 1066 patients from 3 clinical trials. Arch Intern Med 1998; 158(12):1316–20.

64. Friberg L, Lund LH. Heart failure: a weak link in CHA2 DS2 -VASc. ESC Heart Fail 2018;5(3):231–9.

65. Chung S, Kim TH, Uhm JS, et al. Stroke and systemic embolism and other adverse outcomes of heart failure with preserved and reduced ejection fraction in patients with atrial fibrillation (from the COmparison study of Drugs for symptom control and complication prEvention of Atrial Fibrillation [CODE-AF]). Am J Cardiol 2020;125(1):68–75.

66. Cherian TS, Shrader P, Fonarow GC, et al. Effect of atrial fibrillation on mortality, stroke risk, and quality-of-life scores in patients with heart failure (from the outcomes registry for better informed treatment of atrial fibrillation [ORBIT-AF]). Am J Cardiol 2017;119(11):1763–9.

67. Sobue Y, Watanabe E, Lip GYH, et al. Thromboembolisms in atrial fibrillation and heart failure patients with a preserved ejection fraction (HFpEF) compared to those with a reduced ejection fraction (HFrEF). Heart Vessels 2018;33(4): 403–12.

68. Sartipy U, Dahlstrom U, Fu M, et al. Atrial fibrillation in heart failure with preserved, mid-range, and reduced ejection fraction. JACC Heart Fail 2017;5(8): 565–74.

69. Zafrir B, Lund LH, Laroche C, et al. Prognostic implications of atrial fibrillation in heart failure with reduced, mid-range, and preserved ejection fraction: a report

from 14 964 patients in the European Society of Cardiology Heart Failure Long-Term Registry. Eur Heart J 2018;39(48):4277–84.

70. Lip GY, Nieuwlaat R, Pisters R, et al. Refining clinical risk stratification for predicting stroke and thromboembolism in atrial fibrillation using a novel risk factor-based approach: the euro heart survey on atrial fibrillation. Chest 2010; 137(2):263–72.

71. McMurray JJ, Ezekowitz JA, Lewis BS, et al. Left ventricular systolic dysfunction, heart failure, and the risk of stroke and systemic embolism in patients with atrial fibrillation: insights from the ARISTOTLE trial. Circ Heart Fail 2013;6(3):451–60.

72. Ferreira J, Ezekowitz MD, Connolly SJ, et al. Dabigatran compared with warfarin in patients with atrial fibrillation and symptomatic heart failure: a subgroup analysis of the RE-LY trial. Eur J Heart Fail 2013;15(9):1053–61.

73. van Diepen S, Hellkamp AS, Patel MR, et al. Efficacy and safety of rivaroxaban in patients with heart failure and nonvalvular atrial fibrillation: insights from ROCKET AF. Circ Heart Fail 2013;6(4):740–7.

74. Magnani G, Giugliano RP, Ruff CT, et al. Efficacy and safety of edoxaban compared with warfarin in patients with atrial fibrillation and heart failure: insights from ENGAGE AF-TIMI 48. Eur J Heart Fail 2016;18(9):1153–61.

75. Roy D, Talajic M, Nattel S, et al. Rhythm control versus rate control for atrial fibrillation and heart failure. N Engl J Med 2008;358(25):2667–77.

76. Qin D, Leef G, Alam MB, et al. Mortality risk of long-term amiodarone therapy for atrial fibrillation patients without structural heart disease. Cardiol J 2015;22(6): 622–9.

77. Steinberg JS, Sadaniantz A, Kron J, et al. Analysis of cause-specific mortality in the atrial fibrillation follow-up investigation of rhythm management (AFFIRM) study. Circulation 2004;109(16):1973–80.

78. Marrouche NF, Brachmann J, Andresen D, et al. Catheter ablation for atrial fibrillation with heart failure. N Engl J Med 2018;378(5):417–27.

79. Van Gelder IC, Groenveld HF, Crijns HJ, et al. Lenient versus strict rate control in patients with atrial fibrillation. N Engl J Med 2010;362(15):1363–73.

80. Li SJ, Sartipy U, Lund LH, et al. Prognostic significance of resting heart rate and use of β-blockers in atrial fibrillation and sinus rhythm in patients with heart failure and reduced ejection fraction: findings from the Swedish heart failure registry. Circ Heart Fail 2015;8(5):871–9.

81. The effect of digoxin on mortality and morbidity in patients with heart failure. N Engl J Med 1997;336(8):525–33.

82. Khan MN, Jaïs P, Cummings J, et al. Pulmonary-vein isolation for atrial fibrillation in patients with heart failure. N Engl J Med 2008;359(17):1778–85.

83. Mustafa U, Atkins J, Mina G, et al. Outcomes of cardiac resynchronisation therapy in patients with heart failure with atrial fibrillation: a systematic review and meta-analysis of observational studies. Open Heart 2019;6(1):e000937.

84. Ganesan AN, Brooks AG, Roberts-Thomson KC, et al. Role of AV nodal ablation in cardiac resynchronization in patients with coexistent atrial fibrillation and heart failure a systematic review. J Am Coll Cardiol 2012;59(8):719–26.

85. Sohinki D, Ho J, Srinivasan N, et al. Outcomes after atrioventricular node ablation and biventricular pacing in patients with refractory atrial fibrillation and heart failure: a comparison between non-ischaemic and ischaemic cardiomyopathy. Europace 2014;16(6):880–6.

86. Pathak RK, Evans M, Middeldorp ME, et al. Cost-effectiveness and clinical effectiveness of the risk factor management clinic in atrial fibrillation: the CENT study. JACC Clin Electrophysiol 2017;3(5):436–47.

87. Middeldorp ME, Ariyaratnam J, Lau D, et al. Lifestyle modifications for treatment of atrial fibrillation. Heart 2020;106(5):325–32.

88. Long L, Mordi IR, Bridges C, et al. Exercise-based cardiac rehabilitation for adults with heart failure. Cochrane Database Syst Rev 2019;1(1):Cd003331.

89. Contreras JP, Hong KN, Castillo J, et al. Anticoagulation in patients with atrial fibrillation and heart failure: insights from the NCDR PINNACLE-AF registry. Clin Cardiol 2019;42(3):339–45.

90. Kelly JP, DeVore AD, Wu J, et al. Rhythm control versus rate control in patients with atrial fibrillation and heart failure with preserved ejection fraction: insights from Get with the guidelines-heart failure. J Am Heart Assoc 2019;8(24): e011560.

91. Black-Maier E, Ren X, Steinberg BA, et al. Catheter ablation of atrial fibrillation in patients with heart failure and preserved ejection fraction. Heart Rhythm 2018; 15(5):651–7.

92. Cha YM, Wokhlu A, Asirvatham SJ, et al. Success of ablation for atrial fibrillation in isolated left ventricular diastolic dysfunction: a comparison to systolic dysfunction and normal ventricular function. Circ Arrhythm Electrophysiol 2011;4(5):724–32.

93. Elkaryoni A, Al Badarin F, Spertus JA, et al. Comparison of the effect of catheter ablation for atrial fibrillation on all-cause hospitalization in patients with versus without heart failure (from the nationwide readmission database). Am J Cardiol 2020;125(3):392–8.

94. Ichijo S, Miyazaki S, Kusa S, et al. Impact of catheter ablation of atrial fibrillation on long-term clinical outcomes in patients with heart failure. J Cardiol 2018; 72(3):240–6.

95. Jayanna MB, Mohsen A, Inampudi C, et al. Procedural outcomes of patients with heart failure undergoing catheter ablation of atrial fibrillation. Am J Ther 2019; 26(3):e333–8.

96. Vecchio N, Ripa L, Orosco A, et al. Atrial fibrillation in heart failure patients with preserved or reduced ejection fraction. prognostic significance of rhythm control strategy with catheter ablation. J Atr Fibrillation 2019;11(5):2128.

97. Cikes M, Claggett B, Shah AM, et al. Atrial fibrillation in heart failure with preserved ejection fraction: the TOPCAT trial. JACC Heart Fail 2018;6(8):689–97.

98. Oluleye OW, Rector TS, Win S, et al. History of atrial fibrillation as a risk factor in patients with heart failure and preserved ejection fraction. Circ Heart Fail 2014; 7(6):960–6.

99. McManus DD, Hsu G, Sung SH, et al. Atrial fibrillation and outcomes in heart failure with preserved versus reduced left ventricular ejection fraction. J Am Heart Assoc 2013;2(1):e005694.

100. Zakeri R, Chamberlain AM, Roger VL, et al. Temporal relationship and prognostic significance of atrial fibrillation in heart failure patients with preserved ejection fraction: a community-based study. Circulation 2013;128(10):1085–93.

101. Rusinaru D, Leborgne L, Peltier M, et al. Effect of atrial fibrillation on long-term survival in patients hospitalised for heart failure with preserved ejection fraction. Eur J Heart Fail 2008;10(6):566–72.

102. MacDonald MR, Connelly DT, Hawkins NM, et al. Radiofrequency ablation for persistent atrial fibrillation in patients with advanced heart failure and severe left ventricular systolic dysfunction: a randomised controlled trial. Heart 2011; 97(9):740–7.

103. Jones DG, Haldar SK, Hussain W, et al. A randomized trial to assess catheter ablation versus rate control in the management of persistent atrial fibrillation in heart failure. J Am Coll Cardiol 2013;61(18):1894–903.
104. Hunter RJ, Berriman TJ, Diab I, et al. A randomized controlled trial of catheter ablation versus medical treatment of atrial fibrillation in heart failure (the CAM-TAF trial). Circ Arrhythm Electrophysiol 2014;7(1):31–8.
105. Di Biase L, Mohanty P, Mohanty S, et al. Ablation versus amiodarone for treatment of persistent atrial fibrillation in patients with congestive heart failure and an implanted device: results from the AATAC Multicenter randomized trial. Circulation 2016;133(17):1637–44.

Atrial Fibrillation in Valvular Heart Disease

Bobby John, MBBS, MD, DM, PhD, FHRS[a,b,c,]*, Chu-Pak Lau, MD[d]

KEYWORDS

- Atrial fibrillation • Rheumatic heart disease • Remodeling • Embolism

KEY POINTS

- Atrial fibrillation in rheumatic heart disease increases the embolic risk several folds compared with the nonvalvular group.
- Prompt identification of atrial fibrillation and institution of oral anticoagulation is imperative to reduce morbidity and mortality.
- Identification of a high-risk subset that is prone to develop atrial fibrillation may prevent its devastating complications.
- Substrate maintaining atrial fibrillation may be reversible in the early stages.

PREVALENCE OF RHEUMATIC HEART DISEASE

The prevalence of rheumatic heart disease (RHD) declined in the developed world after the industrial revolution.[1,2] However, it continues to be a major health problem in the developing world. Even in developed countries, pockets of indigenous population may remain affected, as for example, in the aboriginal population of Australia and the New Zealand Maori.[3] It is estimated that 15.6 million suffer from RHD and 3%.0 to 7.5% of all strokes in developing countries are directly related to RHD.[4–6]

The 3 main factors that have been reported to determine the prevalence of RHD in a community are (1) the environmental factors; (2) virulence of the organism, that is, Group A *Streptococcus*; and (3) the host. Lower socioeconomic status and overcrowding are associated with higher prevalence of RHD, especially in children living in households of more than 8. The virulence of the organism contributed to the resurgence of rheumatic fever in the United States.[7,8] Racial difference in prevalence of

This article originally appeared in *Cardiac Electrophysiology Clinics*, Volume 13, Issue 1, March 2021.

[a] James Cook University, Townsville, Australia; [b] Cardiology Unit, Townsville University Hospital, 100 Angus Smith Drive, Douglas, Queensland 4814, Australia; [c] Christian Medical College, Vellore, India; [d] Department of Medicine, Queen Mary Hospital, The University of Hong Kong, Suite 1301-3, Central Building, 1 Pedder Street, Central, Hong Kong
* Corresponding author. Cardiology Unit, Townsville University Hospital, 100 Angus Smith Drive, Douglas, QLD 4814, Australia.
E-mail address: bobby.john@health.qld.gov.au

Clinics Collections 13 (2023) 375–388
https://doi.org/10.1016/j.ccol.2023.02.013

RHD within the same geographic location has been observed, but has been attributed to the difference in exposure and treatment rather than genetic susceptibility.[9] In a recent survey, the prevalence of RHD in the aboriginal population was 11.8 per 1000 and 6.5 per 1000 in the Maori population of New Zealand.[3,10] Comparable findings were noted in the Indian population, where the prevalence was 6 per 1000.[11]

The estimated prevalence of RHD in a community depends on the size of the population that has been studied, in addition to the definition, method used to confirm the diagnosis, and the period in which it was undertaken. This was evident in a study conducted by Jose and Gomathi[12] that included 229,829 school-going children. Of the 374 children who were diagnosed by auscultation to have heart disease, only 41.8% (157) were diagnosed to have RHD on color Doppler study, emphasizing that both the population studied and diagnostic tool used would change the prevalence.[12]

An extensive study that uses echocardiogram as the diagnostic tool would involve tremendous financial resource and skilled personal, thus limiting the number of subjects who could be screened. A systematic review by Noubiap and colleagues[13] found that when the auscultatory method was used to screen the population and further confirmation was carried out using echocardiogram, the cumulative prevalence per 1000 was 6.3 (95% confidence interval [CI] 4.02–9.21) in a total population of 774,073, as opposed to 21.23 per 1000 (95% CI 15.26–28.94) using echocardiogram but with screening of a far smaller population of 296,909. This suggests the limitations of auscultation as a tool and also at the same time, the sensitivity of echocardiogram to diagnose borderline cases that may not necessarily progress to chronic RHD with the attendant structural changes. The review highlighted that only 11.3% (95% CI 6.9–16.5) progressed to definite RHD.[13]

PREVALENCE OF ATRIAL FIBRILLATION IN RHEUMATIC HEART DISEASE

Prevalence of the arrhythmia in the rheumatic population is widely variable. This is primarily because of differing periods of study, diagnostic methods used, and the country in which it was reviewed.

Diker and colleagues[14] in 1995, in a retrospective study using echocardiographic criteria, evaluated 1100 patients in Turkey and reported it in 29% of patients with pure mitral stenosis and in 58% of those with mitral stenosis in conjunction with other valvular disease. The prevalence among those with pure aortic valve disease was rare; none seen in those with aortic regurgitation and 5% in those with aortic stenosis.[14] Okello and colleagues,[15] in a cross-sectional study of 309 patients with newly diagnosed RHD attending a tertiary hospital in Africa, found the overall prevalence of atrial fibrillation (AF) was 13.9%. Among these, AF was most prevalent in those with mitral regurgitation (81.4%) and mitral stenosis (58.1%), whereas it was not common in aortic regurgitation (32.6%) and none found in patients with aortic stenosis.[15] Negi and colleagues,[16] while studying 1918 consecutive patients attending a tertiary hospital in India, found that those with tricuspid regurgitation had the highest prevalence of AF (34.9%) as compared with mitral stenosis (31.7%) and mitral regurgitation (25.3%). There was no association of AF with aortic valve disease in this study.

INCIDENCE OF ATRIAL FIBRILLATION IN RHEUMATIC HEART DISEASE

Longitudinal studies of patients with mitral stenosis determining the incidence of AF are very few and far between. One of the earliest studies was done in a Swedish cohort by Olesen.[17] He followed a cohort of patients with isolated mitral stenosis with a mean age of 41.5 (range 14–73) years from 1932 to 1951 and found a prevalence of 57%.[17] In this study, the diagnosis of mitral stenosis was based solely on clinical examination and later confirmed at autopsy in some. The largest series was published by Paul Wood[18] in 1954 involving 300 patients. He reported an incidence of 40%, of which 5% were paroxysmal episodes. It is likely that the incidence of paroxysmal AF was underestimated in this study for lack of very close follow-up.

SEQUEL OF ATRIAL FIBRILLATION

AF in the rheumatic population heralds in greater morbidity and mortality as compared with the nonrheumatic population. It is not uncommon for patients to become symptomatic for the first time with the onset of AF; acute pulmonary edema, as a result of fast ventricular rate and abbreviated diastolic filling time, being one such example.[19] It precipitates cardiac failure and increases mortality.[20,21] The most devastating complication is systemic embolization with 18.0% ± 6.8% of patients having left atrial thrombus.[22] Coulshed and colleagues,[23] in an extensive study involving 737 patients with predominant mitral stenosis, found that 32% of patients with AF developed systemic embolism in contrast to 8% in the sinus rhythm group. The most common site of embolization was the cerebral circulation, being found in 60% to 75%.[18,24] Unlike the nonrheumatic population, AF conferred 17.5-fold increased risk for stroke as opposed to the fivefold risk in the former.[25] Notably, stroke occurs in a much younger population with consequent loss of man power and resultant burden on the economy. In addition, AF is associated with poorer outcome after surgical valvular intervention.

ASYMPTOMATIC ATRIAL FIBRILLATION IN RHEUMATIC HEART DISEASE

Silent AF poses a great risk for thromboembolic events as revealed in a study by Coulshed and colleagues.[23] More than 20% of patients with RHD presenting with ischemic stroke for the first time, were in sinus rhythm.[23] Therefore, it has become apparent that they were not truly in sinus rhythm but would have periods of AF that predisposed them to embolic events. In a cohort of 179 patients who were in sinus rhythm at presentation, 27% had AF lasting 30 seconds recorded on 24-hour ambulatory electrocardiogram monitor.[26] When a broader class of supraventricular arrhythmias were included, such as paroxysmal atrial tachycardia, multifocal atrial tachycardia, and flutter in addition to AF, the number who suffered from the rhythm disturbance was higher; approaching more than 50%.[27] It was even more remarkable to note that 95% of these patients were asymptomatic.[27] These patients, although asymptomatic, remained at risk for embolic complications.

PREDICTORS FOR ATRIAL FIBRILLATION IN RHEUMATIC HEART DISEASE

Publications related to predictors for AF in native rheumatic valvular disease are scant (Table 1). Age at presentation has been an important determinant for prevalence of AF. In a number of studies, it has been consistently found that patients older than 50 years have a high prevalence, between 33% and 57%.[16,28–34]

It would be intuitive to consider functional symptom class to correlate with AF, as it would reflect deleterious hemodynamic effects of the arrhythmia and also duration of the disease in the subject. However, there have been differing observations. Almost one-third of patients who have New York Heart Association (NYHA) class II or more symptoms have been found to have AF in a registry of almost 2000 patients.[16] Kabukcu and colleagues[35] made similar observations in 92 patients. Those with AF were most often in NYHA Class III (74% vs 22%) compared with subjects who maintained sinus rhythm.[35] However, a study of 650 patients undergoing mitral valve intervention in France did not find functional class as a significant predictor for AF.[36]

Table 1
Published predictors of atrial fibrillation occurrence in rheumatic mitral stenosis

Risk Factors	Remarks	
Age, y[16,28-34]	<40	21%
	40–54	59%
	55–69	73%
	≥70	85%[34]
NYHA Class[16,35]	≥NYHA Class II increase risk	
Left atrium diameter[14,37,38]	>4 cm	54%[37]
Valve calcification[36,39]		
Valve area[38,40]	<1 cm^2[38,40]	
Mitral valve gradient[14]	>10 mm Hg	
Pulmonary artery hypertension[38]		

Abbreviation: NYHA, New York Heart Association.

Left atrial diameter on echocardiogram has shown to be an important parameter to predict AF. Henry and colleagues[37] reported a prevalence of 54% when the left atrial diameter was greater than 4.0 cm. This was further corroborated by Diker and colleagues,[14] in which mean left atrial dimension of 5.7 ± 1.2 cm (P<.0001) was found in those with AF. Recent studies, from India have reported left atrial dimension greater than 22 mm/m^2 and presence of spontaneous echo contrast as significant risk factors for AF and consequently ischemic stroke.[38]

Valve calcification is found in 35% of patients with mitral valve disease and its prevalence increases with age.[39] It is an important marker for embolic events and may well be a manifestation of the length of time the disease process has been established.[23,36] A multivariate analysis including 650 patients found mitral valve calcification as a significant predictor for AF.[36]

There are conflicting reports on the presence of pulmonary hypertension and mitral valve gradient as predictors for AF. Diker and colleagues[14] found that mean mitral valve gradient of 9.5 ± 6.1 mm Hg was strongly associated with AF (P<.05). Gupta and colleagues,[38] in a case-control design, noted that presence of pulmonary hypertension (75% vs 42.5%, P = .003) conferred higher risk for ischemic stroke. However, Kabukcu and colleagues[35] did not find a correlation with hemodynamic derangements and AF. Similarly, Negi and colleagues[16] in a multivariate analysis did not observe pulmonary hypertension to be a contributor for AF, but tricuspid regurgitation was an important determinant.

The severity of mitral valve stenosis has correlated with AF. Mitral valve area less than 1.0 cm^2 has been found in most patients with AF in a cross-sectional study done in India.[38,40]

STRUCTURALLY REMODELING IN MITRAL STENOSIS

Interstitial fibrosis, degenerative remodeling, and inflammation are hallmarks of pathologic changes in the rheumatic atria.[41-46] The differences in pathology relate to the age of the patient, the site of sampling, and the severity of mitral stenosis. The upstream changes related to elevated atrial pressure in mitral stenosis are not uniform. It affects each of the atria differently and some parts more than others. Shenthar and colleagues[41] studied patients with isolated mitral stenosis undergoing open heart surgery. Intraoperative biopsies of 5 different sites from both atria were sampled. Although interstitial fibrosis was found in all sites, endocardial inflammation was most common in the left atrial appendage. Advanced matrix and subendocardial remodeling was found more extensively in the left atrium than the right atrium by Park and colleagues.[46] On electron microscopy, cells affected by AF revealed widespread loss of contractile elements with marked areas of sarcoplasmic vacuolation.[45] Myocytolysis was seen as opposed to myocyte hypertrophy and glycogen deposition in sinus rhythm.[41]

Fibrogenesis is a complex process. It occurs consequent to deposition of extracellular matrix and activity of connective tissue growth factor. Studies have confirmed that transforming growth factor-β1 (TGF-β1) plays a pivotal role in differentiation of cardiac myofibroblast. TGF-β1 results in phosphorylation of focal adhesion molecule (FAK) and its downstream effects are mediated by AKT/S6K signaling pathway. This was evidenced by suppression of α-smooth muscle actin expression in TGF-β1–induced fibroblasts with FAK and AKT inhibitors in an animal model.[44] In addition, calreticulin and integrin-alpha5 expression has been found to correlate with AF among patients with RHD.[47]

Remodeling of connexins have been explored as another mechanism of AF in patients with RHD. Samples of right atrial appendage were examined. The collagen volume fraction of type 1 (CVF-1) was significantly increased whereas the volume fraction of connexin-43 was reduced in AF, suggesting its role in arrhythmogenesis.[42]

Immunohistochemistry, quantitative real-time polymerase chain reaction, and Western blotting have been used to evaluate the signaling pathway in fibrosis related to RHD.[43] Alpha-actin-2 was upregulated via the TGF-β1/Smad pathway in patients with AF secondary to RHD compared with those in sinus rhythm with congenital heart disease. Angiotensin II/Rac1/STAT3 signaling is the other putative pathway to induce atrial fibrosis in this subset of patients.[48]

ELECTROANATOMICAL REMODELING OF THE ATRIA IN RHEUMATIC MITRAL STENOSIS

Chronic mitral stenosis results in left atrial "stretch" due to elevated pressure. Although left atrial enlargement due to stretch per se may be sufficient to explain the increase in AF in this population, rheumatic process affecting the atrium also results in significant electrical remodeling, thereby creating the substrate for atrial arrhythmias. Dilatation and pressure on the PVs and elsewhere may also increase their firing and serve as triggers. This electrical remodeling has been validated in patients who were undergoing percutaneous mitral commissurotomy (PTMC). The control population consisted of patients who underwent transseptal puncture for ablation of left side accessory pathways.[49]

Patients with mitral stenosis demonstrated the following abnormalities compared with controls (**Fig. 1**):

i. Marked conduction abnormalities within the atria characterized by regions of double potentials, fractionated electrograms, prolonged conduction times, and P-wave duration, and site-specific conduction delay.
ii. No change or an increase in effective refractory period (ERP) with no change in heterogeneity of ERP and preservation of rate adaptation of ERP. This finding is consistent with prior studies evaluating clinical substrates for AF but in contrast to the remodeling attributed to AF itself.
iii. Sinus node remodeling characterized by prolongation of the corrected sinus node recovery times.

Potentially as a consequence of these abnormalities, patients with mitral stenosis developed AF more frequently.

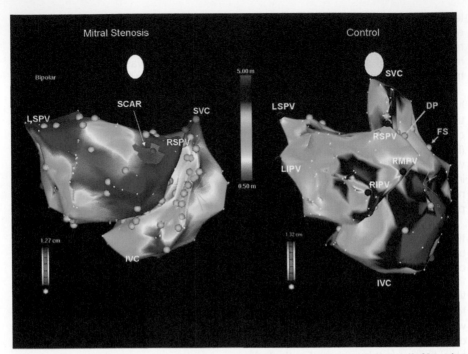

Fig. 1. Electroanatomic bipolar voltage map of a patient with mitral stenosis (*left*) and a representative age-matched control (*right*). Both atria are oriented in the posterior-anterior projection and are of similar scale. The color scale is identical in both images with red representing low voltage areas (≤0.5 mV) and purple being voltages ≥5 mV. The patient with MS (*left image*; left atrium 120 mL, right atrium 58 mL) has a much larger atria than the control patient (left atrium 80 mL, right atrium 100 mL). In addition to having greater regions of low voltage (*red*), the patient with mitral stenosis has regions of spontaneous scar (*gray*), and evidence of conduction abnormalities in the form of fractionated signals (FS; *pink tags*) and double potentials (DS; *blue tags*).

Importantly, although these abnormalities were observed within both atria, their extent was greater in the left atrium than the right atrium. Thus, the electrical substrate for AF in patients with MS is related to the structural abnormalities and the associated widespread and site-specific conduction abnormalities rather than the changes observed in atrial refractoriness.

ACUTE EFFECTS REVERSAL OF CHRONIC ATRIAL STRETCH REVERSAL ON LEFT AND RIGHT ATRIAL ELECTRICAL REMODELING

As demonstrated, severe mitral stenosis results in significant electrical and electroanatomic remodeling of the atria. PTMC has been established to reverse the hemodynamic effects of the stenosed valve with marked reduction in left atrium size and pressure. The effect of acute pressure reduction following PTMC is associated with the following electrophysiological changes (**Fig. 2**):

i. An almost instantaneous reduction in P-wave duration (PWD) suggesting a global improvement in atrial conduction.

ii. Although there was no change in conduction time as evaluated along linearly placed catheters, there was improvement observed in site-specific conduction

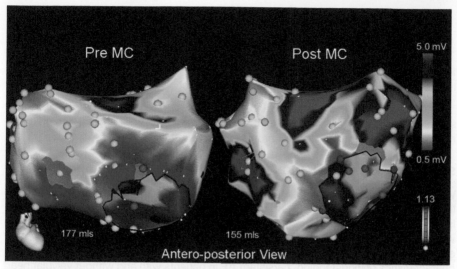

Fig. 2. Electroanatomic voltage map of the left atrium before and immediately after MC. Left is before and the right is after MC. Note the increase in voltage at all sites in left atrium with decrease in volume.

along the crista terminalis. In particular, there was significant improvement in conduction across this structure while pacing from the left atrium.
iii. There was no significant change in atrial refractoriness.
iv. Improvement in bipolar voltage in both the left atrium and right atrium with no regional specificity.
v. Increased conduction velocity in both the left atrium and right atrium with no regional specificity.

In another study involving 12 patients with mitral stenosis in sinus rhythm following PTMC, there was reduction of conduction delay (CD) and the index of heterogeneity (CoV) of ERP with homogeneous increase in regional ERPs.[50] On the other hand, in those patients with more severe mitral stenosis and AF cardioverted at the time of PTMC, both ERP and CD were unaffected after acute left atrium pressure reduction, suggesting chronic changes had already been established. However, both the vulnerability for AF induction and CoV of CD were reduced, suggesting stretch played an important role in AF induction. It is likely that rheumatic process or AF itself has made the atrial substrate more valuable in addition to pressure effect.

These findings suggest that the electroanatomic substrate predisposing to atrial arrhythmias due to chronic atrial stretch may be at least partially reversible with treatments directed at the stretch stimulus before it is established. Importantly, it demonstrates marked improvement in the structural and conduction abnormalities that are considered important elements of the AF substrate. Despite these limited changes, there was a trend for reduced vulnerability for AF.

LONG-TERM EFFECTS OF CHRONIC ATRIAL STRETCH REVERSAL

The long-term effects of chronic stretch reversal were characterized by performing high-density electrophysiological and electroanatomic mapping of the atria 6 months after MC. It revealed the following:

i. Progressive structural changes, which were characterized by a reduction in atrial size and an improvement in the bipolar voltage.
ii. There was widespread and site-specific improvement in conduction velocity associated with a significant reduction in the PWD.
iii. Reduction in atrial refractoriness.
iv. As a result of these changes, there was a reduction in the vulnerability for AF.

These findings stress the importance of treatment directed at reversal of stretch stimulus with progressive reversal of the abnormal electrophysiological and electroanatomic changes consequent to chronic stretch.[51]

SPATIOTEMPORAL ORGANIZATION AND ELECTROGRAM FRACTIONATION

With the increasing recognition that the sources maintaining persistent AF may not be limited to the posterior left atrium, this study sought to determine the bi-atrial characteristics of longstanding, persistent AF in valvular heart disease, a common substrate in which the mechanisms of AF remain incompletely characterized.[52] Using high-density endocardial mapping, the spatiotemporal organization and electrogram fractionation characteristics of longstanding, persistent AF in patients with and without valvular heart disease were compared. Twenty patients with (n = 10) and without (n = 10) valvular heart disease due to mitral stenosis underwent bi-atrial, high-density contact-mapping during AF. Complex fractionated atrial electrograms were quantified using previously validated software, and activation frequencies and electrical organization characterized by spectral analysis. Slower activation frequencies ($P = .01$) and less fractionation ($P<.001$) was present in valvular AF (**Fig. 3**). Areas of greatest frequency and fractionation were located in the right atrium of valvular AF ($P = .005$ both), whereas these were in the left atrium in nonvalvular AF ($P<.01$ both). Similarly, most high-frequency "clusters" were in the right atrium in valvular AF (82%) as opposed to the left in nonvalvular AF (76%). A right-to-left gradient in organization index was additionally present in valvular AF ($P = .001$). The study suggests that a distinct substrate underlying longstanding, persistent AF is seen in patients with valvular heart disease. In a unique subgroup of patients, dominant right atrial sources were maintaining AF. These observations propose a potential role for ablation within the right atrium beyond current individual, but as yet suboptimally identified, patients who require ablation beyond the left atrium.[52]

REMODELING OF PULMONARY VEINS DUE TO CHRONIC STRETCH

The pulmonary vein has been established as a common source of trigger for AF.[53,54] It possesses distinct properties that promote arrhythmogenesis.[55,56] Pacemakerlike potential and spontaneous after depolarizations have been observed within the pulmonary vein, suggesting focal activity may play an important role in the arrhythmogenesis[57,58]; however, the anatomic structure of the pulmonary vein has been shown to promote heterogeneous conduction implicating reentry, as an alternative mechanism.[56,59] This is further supported by the finding that the pulmonary veins in patients with AF have been noted to possess distinctive electrophysiological properties characterized chiefly by abbreviation of ERP and delay in conduction.[60]

Elimination or isolation of pulmonary vein triggers are the main targets of catheter AF ablation; however, there are very few publications of the PV in AF. Although atrial stretch can lead to atrial electrophysiology change and PV firing, much less is known for RHD.[61,62] The electrophysiological properties of the pulmonary veins in RHD with mitral stenosis (n = 12; 29 ± 7 years) was compared with control group formed by those undergoing left-sided accessory pathway ablation (n = 12; 31 ± 7 years) using

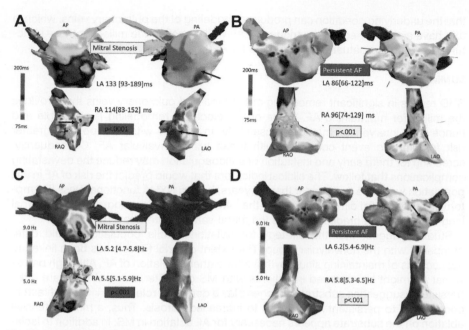

Fig. 3. (*A, B*) Bi-atrial complex fractionated electrograms during AF in valvular and nonvalvular heart disease. High-density color maps demonstrating complex fractionated electrogram during longstanding, persistent AF in a patient with valvular heart disease as compared with the nonvalvular heart disease. Note that areas of fractionation (*red color*) are clustered more often in the right atrium compared with the left atrium in mitral stenosis. (*C, D*) Bi-atrial activation frequencies during AF in valvular and nonvalvular heart disease. High-density color maps demonstrating activation frequencies during longstanding, persistent AF in a patient with valvular heart disease as compared with the nonvalvular heart disease. Note that areas of high frequency (*blue/purple color*) are clustered more often in the right atrium compared with the left atrium in mitral stenosis.

multi-electrode basket to perform high-density mapping using the NavX system.[63] The ERP proximal/distal; conduction time (CT); intrapulmonary vein conduction block (CB; $\geq$30 ms between adjacent poles) resulting in circuitous conduction during the drive (S_1) and preexcited stimulus (S_2); and intrapulmonary vein voltage were determined. Acute stretch was induced in the control group by simultaneous right ventricle and pulmonary vein pacing. This resulted in ERP shortening (240 $\pm$ 33–225 $\pm$ 39 ms; P = .03), prolonged CT with S_2, which increased further with stretch (77 $\pm$ 30–88 $\pm$ 37 ms; P = .02). Intrapulmonary vein CB became prominent with S_2 and accentuated with stretch (40 $\pm$ 23–59 $\pm$ 32 ms; P<.0001). The changes were not site specific. On the other hand, chronic pressure-overload stretch, as seen in mitral stenosis, resulted in following:

i. Marked structural remodeling characterized by a greater region demonstrating low voltage.

ii. Prolongation of the pulmonary vein refractory period.

iii. Conduction slowing and block that was evident in some cases even during sinus rhythm.

These findings implicate stretch as cause for heterogeneous conduction abnormalities within the pulmonary vein that support reentry. Importantly, it provides evidence that the underlying condition can produce remodeling of the pulmonary veins, which in turn have a direct effect on the triggers of AF while creating the milieu for these structures to act as perpetuators or substrate for AF.

SUMMARY

RHD results in significant remodeling of the atria and pulmonary veins that provides the milieu for maintaining AF. Some of the electrical remodeling is reversible and hence early intervention may prove useful. AF in patients with RHD poses a greater risk for embolic event compared with those with nonvalvular AF. Consequently, screening for them early and institution of anticoagulation may reduce the devastating complications that follow. The clinical indicators that would predict the risk of AF in this population would be those older than 50 years, having NYHA functional class II symptoms, with left atrial dimension greater than 4.0 cm on echocardiogram in parasternal long-axis view and gradients across the mitral valve greater than 10 mm Hg.

Studies suggest that the strategy for ablation in this population would differ compared with the nonvalvular group. The extent of atrial fibrosis has been linked to the success of maintaining sinus rhythm after catheter ablation of AF. Although paroxysmal AF might be recorded in patients with MS on Holter, most of them are often persistent, suggesting substrate changes play a dominant role.[26] It is likely that factors contributing to persistent AF will lead to increased fibrosis. Thus, a more extensive ablation on the substrate appears necessary for AF ablation in MS. In addition to isolation of pulmonary veins, targeting complex fractionated electrograms in the right atrium may prove to be efficacious in maintaining sinus rhythm in this population. The 2017 American Heart Association/American College of Cardiology guidelines suggest a full bi-atrial maze procedure at the time of valvular surgery, compared with a lesser ablation procedure, in patients with chronic permanent AF. In addition, molecules that inhibit downstream signaling pathways for fibrogenesis may retard the development of substrate that promotes AF in this vulnerable group.

DISCLOSURE

This study was supported in part by Grant-in-Aid (G.08A.3646) from National Heart foundation of Australia and Indo-Australian strategic research grant (DBT/Indo-Aus/03/16/08); Ministry of Science and Technology, India.

REFERENCES

1. Gordis L. The virtual disappearance of rheumatic fever in the United States: lessons in the rise and fall of disease. T. Duckett Jones memorial lecture. Circulation 1985;72(6):1155–62.
2. WHO programme for the prevention of rheumatic fever/rheumatic heart disease in 16 developing countries: report from Phase I (1986-90). WHO Cardiovascular Diseases Unit and principal investigators. Bull World Health Organ 1992;70(2):213–8.
3. Carapetis JR, Wolff DR, Currie BJ. Acute rheumatic fever and rheumatic heart disease in the top end of Australia's Northern Territory. Med J Aust 1996; 164(3):146–9.
4. Awada A. Stroke in Saudi Arabian young adults: a study of 120 cases. Acta Neurol Scand 1994;89(5):323–8.
5. Banerjee AK, Varma M, Vasista RK, et al. Cerebrovascular disease in north-west India: a study of necropsy material. J Neurol Neurosurg Psychiatry 1989;52(4): 512–5.

6. Luijckx GJ, Ukachoke C, Limapichat K, et al. Brain infarct causes under the age of fifty: a comparison between an east-Asian (Thai) and a western (Dutch) hospital series. Clin Neurol Neurosurg 1993;95(3):199–203.
7. Veasy LG, Wiedmeier SE, Orsmond GS, et al. Resurgence of acute rheumatic fever in the intermountain area of the United States. N Engl J Med 1987;316(8):421–7.
8. Veasy LG, Tani LY, Daly JA, et al. Temporal association of the appearance of mucoid strains of *Streptococcus pyogenes* with a continuing high incidence of rheumatic fever in Utah. Pediatrics 2004;113(3 Pt 1):e168–72.
9. Carapetis JR, Currie BJ, Mathews JD. Cumulative incidence of rheumatic fever in an endemic region: a guide to the susceptibility of the population? Epidemiol Infect 2000;124(2):239–44.
10. Talbot RG. Rheumatic fever and rheumatic heart disease in the Hamilton health district: I. An epidemiological survey. N Z Med J 1984;97(764):630–4.
11. Padmavati S. Rheumatic heart disease: prevalence and preventive measures in the Indian subcontinent. Heart 2001;86(2):127.
12. Jose VJ, Gomathi M. Declining prevalence of rheumatic heart disease in rural schoolchildren in India: 2001-2002. Indian Heart J 2003;55(2):158–60.
13. Noubiap JJ, Agbor VN, Bigna JJ, et al. Prevalence and progression of rheumatic heart disease: a global systematic review and meta-analysis of population-based echocardiographic studies. Sci Rep 2019;9(1):17022.
14. Diker E, Aydogdu S, Ozdemir M, et al. Prevalence and predictors of atrial fibrillation in rheumatic valvular heart disease. Am J Cardiol 1996;77(1):96–8.
15. Okello E, Wanzhu Z, Musoke C, et al. Cardiovascular complications in newly diagnosed rheumatic heart disease patients at Mulago Hospital, Uganda. Cardiovasc J Afr 2013;24(3):80–5.
16. Negi PC, Sondhi S, Rana V, et al. Prevalence, risk determinants and consequences of atrial fibrillation in rheumatic heart disease: 6 years hospital based- Himachal Pradesh- Rheumatic Fever/Rheumatic Heart Disease (HP-RF/RHD) Registry. Indian Heart J 2018;70(Suppl 3):S68–73.
17. Olesen KH. The natural history of 271 patients with mitral stenosis under medical treatment. Br Heart J 1962;24:349–57.
18. Wood P. An appreciation of mitral stenosis. Part I. Clinical features. Br Med J 1954;1(4870):1051–63, contd.
19. Selzer A, Cohn KE. Natural history of mitral stenosis: a review. Circulation 1972;45(4):878–90.
20. Selzer A. Effects of atrial fibrillation upon the circulation in patients with mitral stenosis. Am Heart J 1960;59:518–26.
21. Gajewski J, Singer RB. Mortality in an insured population with atrial fibrillation. JAMA 1981;245(15):1540–4.
22. Davison G, Greenland P. Predictors of left atrial thrombus in mitral valve disease. J Gen Intern Med 1991;6(2):108–12.
23. Coulshed N, Epstein EJ, McKendrick CS, et al. Systemic embolism in mitral valve disease. Br Heart J 1970;32(1):26–34.
24. Casella L, Abelmann WH, Ellis LB. Patients with mitral stenosis and systemic emboli; hemodynamic and clinical observations. Arch Intern Med 1964;114:773–81.
25. Wolf PA, Dawber TR, Thomas HE Jr, et al. Epidemiologic assessment of chronic atrial fibrillation and risk of stroke: the Framingham study. Neurology 1978;28(10):973–7.

26. Karthikeyan G, Ananthakrishnan R, Devasenapathy N, et al. Transient, subclinical atrial fibrillation and risk of systemic embolism in patients with rheumatic mitral stenosis in sinus rhythm. Am J Cardiol 2014;114(6):869–74.

27. Ramsdale DR, Arumugam N, Singh SS, et al. Holter monitoring in patients with mitral stenosis and sinus rhythm. Eur Heart J 1987;8(2):164–70.

28. Hernandez R, Banuelos C, Alfonso F, et al. Long-term clinical and echocardiographic follow-up after percutaneous mitral valvuloplasty with the Inoue balloon. Circulation 1999;99(12):1580–6.

29. Wang A, Krasuski RA, Warner JJ, et al. Serial echocardiographic evaluation of restenosis after successful percutaneous mitral commissurotomy. J Am Coll Cardiol 2002;39(2):328–34.

30. Multicenter experience with balloon mitral commissurotomy. NHLBI balloon valvuloplasty registry report on immediate and 30-day follow-up results. The National Heart, Lung, and Blood Institute Balloon Valvuloplasty Registry Participants. Circulation 1992;85(2):448–61.

31. Palacios IF, Sanchez PL, Harrell LC, et al. Which patients benefit from percutaneous mitral balloon valvuloplasty? Prevalvuloplasty and postvalvuloplasty variables that predict long-term outcome. Circulation 2002;105(12):1465–71.

32. Tomai F, Gaspardone A, Versaci F, et al. Twenty year follow-up after successful percutaneous balloon mitral valvuloplasty in a large contemporary series of patients with mitral stenosis. Int J Cardiol 2014;177(3):881–5.

33. Neumayer U, Schmidt HK, Fassbender D, et al. Early (three-month) results of percutaneous mitral valvotomy with the Inoue balloon in 1,123 consecutive patients comparing various age groups. Am J Cardiol 2002;90(2):190–3.

34. Nunes MC, Nascimento BR, Lodi-Junqueira L, et al. Update on percutaneous mitral commissurotomy. Heart 2016;102(7):500–7.

35. Kabukcu M, Arslantas E, Ates I, et al. Clinical, echocardiographic, and hemodynamic characteristics of rheumatic mitral valve stenosis and atrial fibrillation. Angiology 2005;56(2):159–63.

36. Acar J, Michel PL, Cormier B, et al. Features of patients with severe mitral stenosis with respect to atrial rhythm. Atrial fibrillation in predominant and tight mitral stenosis. Acta Cardiol 1992;47(2):115–24.

37. Henry WL, Morganroth J, Pearlman AS, et al. Relation between echocardiographically determined left atrial size and atrial fibrillation. Circulation 1976;53(2):273–9.

38. Gupta A, Bhatia R, Sharma G, et al. Predictors of ischemic stroke in rheumatic heart disease. J Stroke Cerebrovasc Dis 2015;24(12):2810–5.

39. Kitchin A, Turner R. Calcification of the mitral valve. Results of valvotomy in 100 cases. Br Heart J 1967;29(2):137–61.

40. Sharma SK, Verma SH. A clinical evaluation of atrial fibrillation in rheumatic heart disease. J Assoc Physicians India 2015;63(6):22–5.

41. Shenthar J, Kalpana SR, Prabhu MA, et al. Histopathological study of left and right atria in isolated rheumatic mitral stenosis with and without atrial fibrillation. J Cardiovasc Electrophysiol 2016;27(9):1047–54.

42. Luo MH, Li YS, Yang KP. Fibrosis of collagen I and remodeling of connexin 43 in atrial myocardium of patients with atrial fibrillation. Cardiology 2007;107(4):248–53.

43. Zhang L, Zhang N, Tang X, et al. Increased alpha-actinin-2 expression in the atrial myocardium of patients with atrial fibrillation related to rheumatic heart disease. Cardiology 2016;135(3):151–9.

44. Zhang P, Wang W, Wang X, et al. Focal adhesion kinase mediates atrial fibrosis via the AKT/S6K signaling pathway in chronic atrial fibrillation patients with rheumatic mitral valve disease. Int J Cardiol 2013;168(4):3200–7.

45. Sharma S, Sharma G, Hote M, et al. Light and electron microscopic features of surgically excised left atrial appendage in rheumatic heart disease patients with atrial fibrillation and sinus rhythm. Cardiovasc Pathol 2014;23(6):319–26.

46. Park JH, Lee JS, Ko YG, et al. Histological and biochemical comparisons between right atrium and left atrium in patients with mitral valvular atrial fibrillation. Korean Circ J 2014;44(4):233–42.

47. Zhao F, Zhang S, Shao Y, et al. Calreticulin overexpression correlates with integrin-alpha5 and transforming growth factor-beta1 expression in the atria of patients with rheumatic valvular disease and atrial fibrillation. Int J Cardiol 2013;168(3):2177–85.

48. Xue XD, Huang JH, Wang HS. Angiotensin II activates signal transducers and activators of transcription 3 via Rac1 in the atrial tissue in permanent atrial fibrillation patients with rheumatic heart disease. Cell Biochem Biophys 2015;71(1):205–13.

49. John B, Stiles MK, Kuklik P, et al. Electrical remodeling of the left and right atria due to rheumatic mitral stenosis. Eur Heart J 2008;29(18):2234–43.

50. Fan K, Lee KL, Chow WH, et al. Internal cardioversion of chronic atrial fibrillation during percutaneous mitral commissurotomy: insight into reversal of chronic stretch-induced atrial remodeling. Circulation 2002;105(23):2746–52.

51. John B, Stiles MK, Kuklik P, et al. Reverse remodeling of the atria after treatment of chronic stretch in humans: implications for the atrial fibrillation substrate. J Am Coll Cardiol 2010;55(12):1217–26.

52. John B, Wong CX, Stiles MK, et al. Differences in left to right atrial gradient of spatiotemporal organization and fractionation in patients with valvular and non valvular atrial fibrillation. Heart Rhythm 2009;6(5):S9.

53. Haissaguerre M, Jais P, Shah DC, et al. Spontaneous initiation of atrial fibrillation by ectopic beats originating in the pulmonary veins. N Engl J Med 1998;339(10):659–66.

54. Chen SA, Hsieh MH, Tai CT, et al. Initiation of atrial fibrillation by ectopic beats originating from the pulmonary veins: electrophysiological characteristics, pharmacological responses, and effects of radiofrequency ablation. Circulation 1999;100(18):1879–86.

55. Verheule S, Wilson EE, Arora R, et al. Tissue structure and connexin expression of canine pulmonary veins. Cardiovasc Res 2002;55(4):727–38.

56. Hocini M, Ho SY, Kawara T, et al. Electrical conduction in canine pulmonary veins: electrophysiological and anatomic correlation. Circulation 2002;105(20):2442–8.

57. Cheung DW. Pulmonary vein as an ectopic focus in digitalis-induced arrhythmia. Nature 1981;294(5841):582–4.

58. Chen YJ, Chen SA, Chen YC, et al. Electrophysiology of single cardiomyocytes isolated from rabbit pulmonary veins: implication in initiation of focal atrial fibrillation. Basic Res Cardiol 2002;97(1):26–34.

59. Ho SY. Pulmonary vein ablation in atrial fibrillation: does anatomy matter? J Cardiovasc Electrophysiol 2003;14(2):156–7.

60. Jais P, Hocini M, Macle L, et al. Distinctive electrophysiological properties of pulmonary veins in patients with atrial fibrillation. Circulation 2002;106(19):2479–85.

61. Tse HF, Pelosi F, Oral H, et al. Effects of simultaneous atrioventricular pacing on atrial refractoriness and atrial fibrillation inducibility: role of atrial mechanoelectrical feedback. J Cardiovasc Electrophysiol 2001;12(1):43–50.

62. Walters TE, Lee G, Spence S, et al. Acute atrial stretch results in conduction slow-ing and complex signals at the pulmonary vein to left atrial junction: insights into the mechanism of pulmonary vein arrhythmogenesis. Circ Arrhythm Electrophy-siol 2014;7(6):1189–97.
63. John B, Brooks AG, Kuklik P, et al. Effect of acute and chronic stretch on the pul-monary veins in humans: implications for arrhythmogenic triggers. Circulation 2008;118(8):S591.

The Cardiorenal Syndrome in Heart Failure

Maria Rosa Costanzo, MD, FESC

KEYWORDS

- Cardiorenal syndrome • Heart failure • Diuretics • Ultrafiltration • Acute kidney injury
- Worsening renal function • Creatinine • Fluid overload

KEY POINTS

- The heart and the kidney are highly interdependent in health and disease.
- In acute heart failure, transient elevations of serum creatinine represent a physiologic response to fluid removal and should not trigger discontinuation of symptom-improving and/or life-saving decongestive therapies.
- Accurate quantitative measurement of fluid volume is vital to individualizing therapy for patients with congestive heart failure.
- The inherent diuretic unresponsiveness of patients with fluid-overloaded heart failure should stimulate investigation of alternative decongestive therapies.
- Investigation of new fluid-management technologies should focus on safety, ease of use, candidates' selection, and cost.

INTRODUCTION

This discussion is focused on the interactions during acute and chronic heart failure (HF) between heart and kidney, which are highly interdependent in health and disease. In normal individuals the kidney depends on the blood flow and perfusion pressure provided by the heart, whose performance is contingent on the kidney's regulation of the body's content of salt and water.[1] In HF, fluid overload produces mutually harmful and self-perpetuating interactions between the heart and the kidney, which lead to deterioration of both organs and increased morbidity and mortality. The term "cardiorenal syndrome" has evolved to encompass all maladaptive relationships between

This article previously appeared in *Cardiology Clinics*, Volume 40, Issue 2, May 2022.
This article originally appeared in *Heart Failure Clinics*, Volume 16, Issue 1, January 2020.
Disclosures: Dr M.R. Costanzo receives consulting honoraria from CHF-Solutions, Fresenius, Abbott, Medtronic, Boston Scientific, and Axon Technologies. Dr M.R. Costanzo's Institution, the Advocate Heart Institute, receives research grant funding from Abbott, Boehringer Ingelheim, V-Wave Medical, and Merck.
Heart Failure Research, Advocate Heart Institute, Edward Hospital Center for Advanced Heart Failure, 801 South Washington Street, Naperville, IL, USA
E-mail address: mariarosa.costanzo@advocatehealth.com

Clinics Collections 13 (2023) 389–413
https://doi.org/10.1016/j.ccol.2023.02.003

heart and kidney occurring with diverse and sometimes overlapping diseases.[1] Although countless articles have attempted to capture the diagnosis, pathophysiology, prognosis, and treatment of the cardiorenal syndrome, knowledge gaps persist in all these areas.

EPIDEMIOLOGIC AND PROGNOSTIC CONSIDERATIONS

Approximately 50% of patients with chronic HF with both reduced and preserved left ventricular ejection fraction (LVEF) have an estimated glomerular filtration rate (eGFR) of less than 60 L/min/1.73 m^2, consistent with underlying chronic kidney disease.[2] Multivariate analyses from the SOLVD (Study of Left Ventricular Dysfunction) trials first demonstrated that moderate renal insufficiency (defined as eGFR <60 mL/min/1.73 m^2 by the Cockroft-Gault equation) was associated with increased risk for all-cause mortality, pump-failure death, and the combined end point of death or hospitalization for HF.[3] Among 372 patients enrolled in the Second Prospective Randomized Study of Ibopamine on Mortality and Efficacy, eGFR, and not LVEF, had the greatest prognostic value: subjects in the lowest eGFR quartile (<44 mL/min) had almost 3-times the mortality risk (relative risk, 2.85; P<.001) of those in the highest quartile (>76 mL/min).[4] These findings have been repeatedly confirmed.[2]

Unlike chronic HF, the significance of renal function changes in acute HF remain controversial because of the assumption that "increased serum creatinine (sCr)/cystatin C," "worsening renal function" (WRF), and "acute kidney injury" (AKI) are different names of the same pathologic entity.[5] In fact, transient sCr increases may represent a benign, and potentially reversible hemodynamically driven reduction in GFR, reflective of effective decongestion, which portends improved outcomes.[6] In aggressively diuresed patients, increases in either sCr or markers of tubular damage were poorly correlated with each other and with diuretic effect, and may have worsened patients' outcomes by triggering premature discontinuation of decongestive therapies.[7] Assessment of renal status by sCr is not straightforward, because defective excretion of sCr can result from extrarenal hypovolemia, impaired blood perfusion, intrinsic kidney etiology, or postrenal disease.[8] It is implausible, therefore, that creatinine, an end product of muscle catabolism freely filtered by the glomerulus and secreted by the tubule, can discriminate between causes of renal dysfunction. Although measurement of sCr is cheap, widely available, and standardized, its disadvantages include the many inducers of elevated sCr, and the numerous conditions affecting its non-GFR determinants (renal reserve, muscle metabolism, protein intake, volume of distribution, medications, and extrarenal degradation).[8] Equations estimating GFR using sCr have variable bias across populations and are imprecise despite standardization of sCr assays and inclusion of age, sex, race, and body size as surrogates for creatinine generation.[8] These equations assume that sCr is a steady-state marker of creatinine production and disposal, conditions that do not apply to AKI or HF. An alternative to creatinine, cystatin C, is a protein produced in all nucleated cells and distributed in extracellular fluid. It is freely filtered and mostly reabsorbed and catabolized by the proximal tubule. Although not affected by modifiers of sCr, smoking, inflammation, adiposity, thyroid diseases, malignancy, and glucocorticoids influence cystatin C levels, diminishing their value as a measure of renal excretory performance.[8] Estimation of GFR using creatinine, cystatin C, or both have not been validated in acutely ill patients.[9] It is disappointing, therefore, that the severity of AKI is classified by changes in sCr or cystatin C.[8,10] A patient may have tubular damage without significant changes in sCr because of renal reserve. Conversely, the correlation of an increase in sCr levels with better outcomes during HF treatment suggests that elevation of this analyte identifies physiologic, volume-sensitive responses to diuretics, rather than AKI.[6]

Advances in kidney transcriptomics and urinary proteomics suggest that kidney genes and their encoded proteins can be specific for certain stimuli and cellular targets. Serum creatinine is not in this category because it can be similarly elevated in different experimental and clinical situations. Different genetic signatures are activated by renal ischemia versus volume depletion in both animal models and patients with a broad range of illnesses.[11,12] The intrinsic characteristics of sCr (delayed, insensitive, not specific to tubular damage) contrast with the genetic responses of the kidney (rapid, sensitive, cell- and stimulus-specific).[11,13,14] Therefore, an obvious question is why biomarkers of tubular injury are not widely used in patients with decompensated HF to distinguish true AKI from changes in renal clearance resulting from diuresis-driven hemoconcentration. In predictive modeling, the performance of AKI biomarkers is undermined by both use of sCr as the "gold standard" comparator and disregard for disease prevalence in the target population.[14] Assuming that, at a certain cutoff value, sCr is 90% sensitive and 90% specific and disease prevalence is 20%, a new biomarker with 100% sensitivity and 100% specificity may seem to have only 69% sensitivity and 97% specificity compared with the "imperfect gold standard."[14] Therefore, changes in acute HF therapy based only on sCr increases may trigger adjustment or discontinuation of symptom-improving and/or life-saving antineurohormonal drugs and prevent effective decongestion.[5,15] Mounting evidence shows that unresolved congestion trumps renal function as a predictor of poor HF outcomes.[5–7,15]

MECHANISMS OF FLUID ACCUMULATION IN HEART FAILURE AND THE CARDIORENAL SYNDROME

In chronic HF, renal retention of sodium and water causes intravascular and interstitial fluid-volume expansion and redistribution. Renal sodium excretion decreases early in response to an absolute or relative decrease in cardiac output (CO), which reduces arterial filling and, consequently, effective circulating blood volume (BV).[16,17] The resulting alteration of baroreceptor activity produces neurohormonal activation, which enhances renal sodium and water reabsorption. Although sympathetic-driven vasoconstriction initially maintains organ perfusion, concomitant gradual fluid accumulation in the interstitium produces a compensatory and sustained expansion of plasma volume (PV). Because with lower CO less than 30% to 40% of total BV resides in the arterial circulation, volume must expand to preserve tissue perfusion.[16] When this compensatory mechanism becomes maladaptive, volume overload and organ congestion ensue (Fig. 1). Hypervolemia leads to increased cardiac filling pressures and later to clinical congestion, which often becomes apparent after retention of several liters of fluid. Because diuretics incompletely eliminate fluid excess, a vicious circle occurs whereby a partial response to treatment triggers gradual reaccumulation and redistribution of fluid, leading to recurrent HF decompensation.[5,15,18–21] In untreated patients with symptomatic systolic dysfunction, indicator dilution techniques showed that interstitial and intravascular volumes expand proportionately (33%–35% above normal).[16] Normally, fluid retention expands PV because of low interstitial compliance. When this increases in HF, the interstitium can accommodate a greater amount of fluid volume, which persists after clinical congestion appears resolved.[20,22,23] Reduced effective circulating BV and systemic blood pressure lower capillary hydrostatic pressure, facilitating fluid shifts from the interstitial to the intravascular compartment. Conversely, abnormal capillary endothelial permeability, coupled

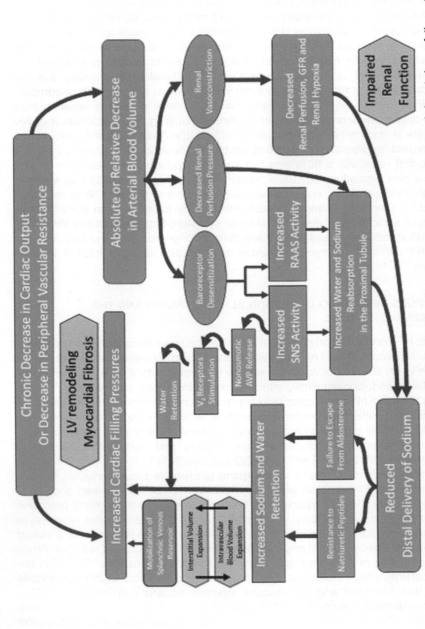

Fig. 1. Interactions between the heart and the kidney leading to volume expansion and congestion in acute and chronic heart failure. AVP, arginine vasopressin; GFR, glomerular filtration rate; LV, left ventricle; RAAS, renin-angiotensin-aldosterone system; SNS, sympathetic nervous system; V₂ Receptors, vasopressin receptors type 2.

with reduced plasma oncotic pressure from albumin loss, promotes fluid shifts from the intravascular to the interstitial compartment.[19,20] Diuretic response becomes inadequate when the ratio of interstitial volume to PV exceeds by severalfold the normal 3:1 to 4:1 ratio (**Fig. 2**). Persistent hypervolemia can progress to acute HF decompensation when sympathetic-mediated vasoconstriction causes transfer of up to 1 L of fluid from the splanchnic venous reservoir into the central circulation.[18,23–27] Importantly, red blood cell volume can also contribute to volume overload. In HF, polycythemia is often masked by a low hemoglobin or hematocrit level owing to dilution in an expanded PV. In chronic HF, polycythemia is a physiologic response to low CO, tissue hypoxia, impaired oxygen exchange, and acidosis. With polycythemia, diuretics may enhance thrombotic risk and myocardial work because of increased blood viscosity.[28–30] These facts underscore that accurate quantitative measurement of both red blood cell volume and PV are vital to the individualization of therapy for patients with congestive HF.

Methods for assessing fluid volume are described later in this article.

PATHOPHYSIOLOGIC EVENTS IN THE KIDNEY IN THE SETTING OF HEART FAILURE

The kidney filtration function is the sum of single nephrons' GFR. This depends on the area and permeability characteristics of the glomerular membrane and Starling forces in the glomerular capillary, and Bowman's space favoring and opposing filtration. Normal single-nephron GFR and filtration fraction (FF) are 40 to 70 mL/min and 20% to 25%, respectively. When renal blood flow (RBF) is high, the glomerular capillary colloid osmotic pressure (πGC) increases slowly from the proximal to the distal end of the glomerular capillary and a filtration pressure gradient persists over the length of the capillaries. When RBF decreases, the PV exposed to the filtration pressure gradient per area unit of the capillary wall is smaller. The faster increase of πGC along the glomerular capillary results in an increased πGC at the level of the efferent arteriole and, hence, an increase in FF. This will attenuate the absolute drop in a single nephron's GFR, independent of changes in glomerular capillary hydrostatic pressure. However, when the maximum FF of ~60% is achieved, a further decrease in RBF causes single-nephron GFR to drop linearly so that the filtration pressure gradient cannot be maintained over the length of the glomerular capillary (wasted capillary). These mechanisms are amplified by the neurohormonal activation occurring in HF.[31]

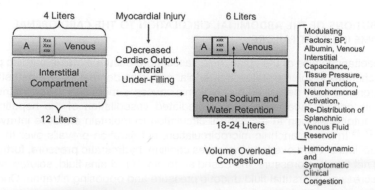

Fig. 2. Mechanisms of interstitial and intravascular volume expansion in chronic heart failure. BP, blood pressure; CO, cardiac output. (*From* Miller WL. Fluid volume overload and congestion in heart failure. time to reconsider pathophysiology and how volume is assessed. Circ Heart Fail. 2016;9:e002922; with permission.)

In the proximal tubules, different transporters mediate active movement of sodium across their luminal side. However, because the proximal tubular epithelium is leaky, back flux occurs and net sodium reabsorption depends on passive Starling forces between peritubular capillaries and interstitium. These processes can occur independent of, but are exaggerated by, neurohumoral activity. In HF, because of increased FF, peritubular capillary colloid osmotic pressure is higher, which stimulates sodium and water reabsorption. Moreover, owing to fluid overload and encapsulation of the kidney, interstitial fluid hydrostatic pressure and peritubular capillary hydrostatic pressure both increase, whereas interstitial fluid colloid osmotic pressure decreases because of removal of interstitial proteins by increased lymph flow (Q_L). This further facilitates net sodium and water reabsorption.[31]

Normally, the macula densa senses increased chloride delivery because active chloride transport triggers metabolism of adenosine triphosphate (ATP) to adenosine, which has a paracrine vasoconstrictive effect on the afferent arteriole. This tubule-glomerular feedback protects the nephron from hyperfiltration. In HF, diminished chloride delivery to the macula densa caused by increased proximal reabsorption stimulates nitric oxide synthetase I and cyclo-oxygenase-2, and release of nitric oxide and prostaglandin E_2. The latter 2 act on the granulosa cells of the afferent arteriole, causing renin release and vasodilation resulting from relaxation of smooth muscle cells. Renin activates angiotensin II, which initiates a vicious cycle of neurohumoral activation and further sodium and water retention. Notably, loop diuretics inhibit the $Na^+/K^+/2Cl^-$ cotransporter, further reducing intracellular chloride levels in the macula densa and thus escalating renin secretion.[31]

The distal convoluted tubules and collecting ducts reabsorb only $\leq 10\%$ of the total amount of sodium filtered by the glomerulus. Distal fractional sodium reabsorption rates vary according to tubular flow rate, and aldosterone and arginine vasopressin levels.[32–34] In normal subjects, high doses of aldosterone initially increase renal sodium retention so that the volume of extracellular fluid is increased by 1.5 to 2 L. However, renal sodium retention then ceases, sodium balance is re-established, and no edema occurs. This escape from mineralocorticoid-mediated sodium retention depends, at least in part, on an increase in delivery of sodium to aldosterone's site of action in the collecting ducts. Owing to increased proximal sodium reabsorption, such escape fails to occur in HF patients, who continue to retain sodium in response to aldosterone. Hence, substantial natriuresis can be expected in HF with mineralocorticoid antagonists.[35]

CONTRIBUTIONS OF THE ABDOMINAL CIRCULATION TO THE CARDIORENAL SYNDROME IN HEART FAILURE

The capacitance veins of the splanchnic vasculature ensure a stable cardiac preload despite changes in volume status. If arteriolar perfusion decreases, sympathetic stimulation from centrally perceived hypovolemia causes α-mediated vasoconstriction of splanchnic capacitance veins and β_2-mediated vasodilation of the hepatic veins, causing autotransfusion to the central circulation to maintain effective intravascular volume.[27,36] In the splanchnic microcirculation, net filtration prevails over the length of the capillaries. Fluid overload increases capillary hydrostatic pressure, further augmenting net filtration pressure. Increased abdominal Q_L drains fluid, solutes, and proteins, decreasing interstitial fluid oncotic pressure and opposing filtration. Once Q_L is maximal and interstitial compliance increases, protein-rich edema compresses lymphatics, further impairing Q_L and promoting fluid accumulation.[36–38]

In the liver, adenosine, continuously produced from ATP by hepatocytes, accumulates in the perisinusoidal space and is drained by lymphatics. When portal blood flow is reduced by α-receptor–mediated vasoconstriction, Q_L decreases and intrahepatic adenosine concentrations increases. The resulting stimulation of hepatic afferent nerves, which are synapsed with renal efferent nerves, promotes further sodium retention.[36]

The spleen also contributes to the regulation of intravascular volume. Because splenic sinusoids are permeable to plasma proteins, their colloid osmotic pressure is the same as that of the lymphatic matrix, so that fluid transport between the 2 spaces is determined by differences in hydrostatic pressure. Transient splanchnic venous system congestion results in increased hydrostatic pressure in the splenic sinusoids. Therefore, more fluid is drained to the lymphatic matrix and buffered in the splenic lymphatic reservoirs. However, with increased cardiac filling pressures and atrial natriuretic peptide production, splenic arterial vasodilation and venous vasoconstriction facilitate fluid shifts into the perivascular splenic third space. This leads to perceived central hypovolemia and further neurohumoral activation.[36] Moreover, overload of the lymphatic system results in interstitial edema.

The countercurrent system of the intestinal microcirculation allows extensive exchange between arterioles and venules. Therefore, oxygen short-circuits from arterioles to venules, creating a gradient with the lowest oxygen partial pressure at the villus tip. In HF, the low-flow state in the splanchnic microcirculation caused by hypoperfusion, increased venous stasis, and sympathetically mediated arteriolar vasoconstriction increases oxygen exchange between arterioles and venules, augmenting the gradient between the villus base and tip. The resulting ischemia causes loss of the intestinal barrier function of the epithelial cells, which permits lipopolysaccharide and endotoxin, produced by gram-negative bacteria in the gut lumen, to enter the systemic circulation and further increase generalized inflammation and hemodynamic abnormalities.[39]

METHODS FOR THE ASSESSMENT OF FLUID VOLUME IN THE CARDIORENAL SYNDROME OCCURRING IN HEART FAILURE
Blood Volume Measurement and the Indicator Dilution Principle

Indicator dilution techniques measure an unknown volume when a known volume of a known concentration of a tracer is added to an unknown volume of fluid.[40] After complete mixing, the concentration of the tracer is measured in a sample taken from the unknown volume. The size of the unknown volume is inversely proportional to the concentration of the tracer in the sample because the latter becomes progressively more diluted as the size of the unknown volume increases. This can be calculated as $C_1V_1 = C_2V_2$, where C_1 is the concentration of tracer injected, V_1 is the volume of tracer injected, C_2 is the concentration of the tracer in a sample from the unknown volume, and V_2 is the unknown volume. Nuclear medicine techniques can accurately measure a radioisotope tracer concentration in fluid samples using the indicator dilution technique, which allows assessment of PV with [131]iodine-tagged human serum albumin. A propensity-score control matching analysis by demographics, comorbidity, and time of treatment was performed in 245 consecutive HF admissions undergoing BV analysis and controls derived from the Center for Medicare and Medicaid data and matched 10:1 for demographics, comorbidity, and year of treatment. Decongestion strategy targeted total BV to 6%–8% above patient-specific norm.[41] Compared with controls, subjects receiving BV analysis-guided therapy experienced lower 30-day readmissions (12.2% vs 27.7%, $P<.001$), 30-day mortality (2.0% vs 11.1%, $P<.001$), and 1-year mortality (4.9% vs 35.5%, $P<.001$) rates.[41] Independent validation that increased adoption of BV analysis provides incremental benefit with a favorable cost-benefit profile is required.

Bioelectrical Impedance Analysis Methods

The human body is akin to a conducting cylinder.[42] Both intracellular fluid and extracellular fluid are ionic solutions and are therefore good electricity conductors (low impedance to passage of an alternating current). The protein-lipid-protein layers of cell membranes function as capacitors. Bone and adipose tissue act as resistors (high impedance to the passage of an alternating current). Therefore, living soft tissues form a complex network of resistive and capacitive conductors arranged in parallel and in series. When an alternating current is applied to them, bioelectrical impedance depends on tissue composition and the current's frequency. Driving electrodes deliver the alternating current while sensing electrodes measure the voltage according to Ohm's law:

$$V = (R + X_c)I$$

where V is the voltage, I is the current, and $R + X_c$ is the complex impedance consisting of resistance (R) and reactance (X_c), which accounts for the movement of electrons determined by the characteristics of the tissue where they reside.[42] In humans, driving and sensing electrodes can be placed sufficiently far apart to measure whole-body impedance, or closer to each other to measure impedance of a body segments. Alternating current can be applied at single (50 kHz), dual (50 and 200 kHz), or multiple frequencies (5–1000 kHz).

A device manufactured by RSMM (Tel Aviv, Israel) that measures net lung impedance was used in a single-blind 2-center trial (NCT01315223) wherein 256 HF patients with LVEF ≤35%, New York Heart Association (NYHA) class II to IV, and a recent HF hospitalization were randomized to controls (clinical assessment alone) or to a lung impedance-guided therapy group.[43] Net lung impedance typically decreased 3 weeks before hospitalization. Over 48 months, compared with controls, the monitored group had fewer hospitalizations (rate per patient-year follow-up: 1.03 vs 1.68, hazard ratio [HR] 0.66, 95% confidence interval [CI] 0.59–0.74, P<.001) and deaths (HR 0.52, 95% confidence interval 0.35–0.78, P = .002).[43] The study's limitations include possible influence of treatment assignment on hospitalization, no independent adjudication of events, and a high event rate (0.94/patient-year) in a population with 50% of subjects being NYHA class II.[44]

Bioreactance

Bioreactance measures phase shifts of the electrical currents traversing the thorax and may provide a more accurate estimation of hemodynamics thanks to its higher signal-to-noise ratio. Preliminary investigations suggest that bioreactance methods can discriminate between cardiac and noncardiac dyspnea, assess the efficacy of ultrafiltration (UF) during hemodialysis, and predict fluid responsiveness in spontaneously breathing patients.[42]

Pulmonary Artery Pressure Sensors

Elevated cardiac filling pressures increase the risk for hospitalizations and mortality.[45,46] Regardless of LVEF, filling pressures gradually increase more than 2 weeks before HF-related hospitalizations.[47,48] In the CHAMPION trial (CardioMEMS Heart Sensor Allows Monitoring of Pressure to Improve Outcomes in Class III Heart Failure), HF treatment guided by pulmonary artery (PA) pressures measured by the CardioMEMS sensor was associated with a reduction in HF hospitalization rates of 28% and 37% at 6 and 15 months, respectively, compared with clinical management.[49,50] The CHAMPION-HF trial algorithm recommended use of sequential doses of diuretics and vasodilators to lower and maintain the PA diastolic pressure below 20 mm Hg and provided guidance for de-escalation of diuretics if the filling pressures were low, to prevent hypovolemia and renal dysfunction.[51] More than twice as many medication changes (both increases and decreases) occurred in the active monitoring group compared with the blind therapy group. Although the average diuretic doses from baseline to 6 months were higher in the active monitoring group, the eGFR was similar in the 2 arms, indicating that the decrease in HF hospitalizations because of PA pressure–guided therapy did not occur at the expense of WRF.[50,51] A recent CHAMPION-HF analysis showed that hemodynamically guided HF management also reduces mortality in patients with reduced LVEF receiving guideline-directed medical therapy, highlighting the important synergy of hemodynamic and neurohormonal targets of HF therapy.[52] The PA pressure–guided therapy had similar benefits in subjects with preserved and reduced LVEF.[53] The favorable outcomes of CHAMPION-HF have been replicated in clinical practice.[54,55] The Hemodynamic-GUIDEd Management of Heart Failure (GUIDE-HF) trial (NCT03387813) is testing the effects of PA pressure–guided therapy in broader HF populations.

Data from Cardiac Implanted Electronic Devices

Approximately 40% of HF patients with reduced LVEF receive a cardiac implantable electronic device (CIED). Some CIEDs can estimate thoracic fluid content when a small alternating current passes between the case and the lead. The greater is the amount of fluid in the path of the electrical impulse, the lower the measured impedance.[56] Studies using this feature have yielded conflicting results.[57] More recent analyses have assessed whether combinations of CIEDs data are superior to measurement of a single variable in risk-stratifying HF patients. To develop the Heart-Logic alert algorithm, available in the COGNIS (Boston Scientific, St Paul, MN) CIED, data from multiple device sensors were used in combination with clinical baseline and HF events data. Initial analyses identified heart sounds (S1 and S3), thoracic impedance, respiration, heart rate, and activity as predictive of an HF event.[58] Changes in these features from each patient's baseline were aggregated and weighted based on an individual's daily risk for worsening HF. The HeartLogic index is updated daily, and an alert is issued when the nominal threshold of 16 is crossed.[58] In the Multisensor Chronic Evaluation in Ambulatory Heart Failure Patients (MultiSENSE) study, this alert index forecasted HF events with a 70% sensitivity and a median of 34-day warning.[58] The ongoing Multiple Cardiac Sensors for the Management of Heart Failure (MANAGE-HF) study compares remote monitoring with versus without HeartLogic alerts to drive HF care (NCT03237858). However, the data obtainable from CIEDs have limitations: (1) estimation only of fluid in the thorax; (2) imprecise quantitation of excess volume and its changes with fluid removal; (3) applicability only to patients with CIED indications, which excludes patients preserved LVEF, constituting greater than 50% of the HF population.[59]

Ultrasound Methods

Lung ultrasonography

Lung ultrasonography (LUS) can assess extravascular lung water (ELW), determined by lung permeability and cardiac filling pressures, with the analysis of B-line artifacts.[60] These are discrete vertical hyperechoic reverberation artifacts that arise from the pleural line, extend to the bottom of the ultrasound screen, and move with lung sliding.[60] Comparison with data from computed tomography and invasive hemodynamics confirms a direct relationship between B lines and ELW. LUS can be performed with any type of echography device at any transducer frequency, is reproducible, and is easy to learn.[60] In one meta-analysis, 3 or more B lines in 2 or more bilateral lung zones were diagnostic for pulmonary edema (sensitivity, 94%; specificity, 92%).[60] A B-line score cutoff of ≥15 is significantly correlated with clinical congestion scores, E/E' ratio, natriuretic peptide levels, increased LV filling pressure, larger LV volumes, LV mass index, left atrial volume index, tricuspid regurgitation velocity, and estimated systolic PA pressure.[60] In 6 studies including 438 acutely decompensated HF patients, B lines decreased as early as 3 hours after therapy initiation and were cleared within 4 days.[61] A decrease of 2.7 B lines occurs with every 500 mL of fluid removed by UF.[62] In HF patients, the number of B lines is correlated with natriuretic peptide levels.[63,64] However, because B lines lack specificity, because those caused by edema versus interstitial fibrosis are similar, they must be considered in the context of clinical, hemodynamic, and echocardiographic assessments.

Inferior vena cava ultrasonography

The diameter of the inferior vena cava (IVC) changes with respiration, reflecting the elasticity of this capacitance vessel. In spontaneously breathing subjects, intrathoracic pressure decreases during inspiration, thereby increasing venous return and causing collapse of the IVC. During expiration, venous return decreases, leading to increased IVC diameter.[65] In acutely decompensated HF, when volume overload dilates the IVC to the limits of its elasticity, respirations produce only minimal changes in IVC diameter.[65] A respiratory variation of IVC diameter of ≤15% was highly sensitive and specific for the diagnosis of acutely decompensated HF.[66] Ultrasonography of the IVC is a rapid, simple, and noninvasive method for bedside monitoring of intravascular volume during UF and adjustment of fluid-removal rate. Accuracy of IVC measurements is influenced by the patient's position and ability to follow instructions as well as intraobserver and interobserver variability.

Biomarkers

The use of natriuretic peptides to assess and guide the treatment of fluid overload is not recommended, given the multiple causes of increased levels of these biomarkers.[67,68] Removal of fluid to achieve prespecified natriuretic peptide levels is untested in acute HF. The limitations of sCr as a biomarker of AKI during fluid removal have been previously discussed.

The staggering number of HF rehospitalizations underscores the inability to accurately estimate fluid excess and determine when euvolemia has been achieved. The most accurate method to measure extracellular fluid is BV analysis. Unfortunately, this approach is not widely used because of the perceived complexity and lack of studies correlating BV analysis with other measures of fluid-volume assessment (hematocrit, biomarkers, hemodynamics, and bioelectrical impedance). All bioelectrical impedance or bioreactance methods lack rigorous comparison with invasive hemodynamics; therefore, their accuracy in quantifying fluid excess and changes with treatment remains unknown. Therapy guided by implanted PA pressure sensors is associated with reductions in rehospitalizations regardless of LVEF, with a pointer toward decreased mortality in NYHA class III HF patients. Although risk scores from CIED data may forecast HF events with enough warning to avert hospitalizations, they cannot provide quantitation of fluid volume and be used in patients without CIED indications. Ultrasound methods have not been meaningfully compared with other methods of fluid-volume determination. Owing to the multitude of factors contributing to their elevation, biomarkers such as natriuretic peptides cannot precisely quantitate fluid excess or guide HF therapy. The use of elevation in sCr, WRF, and AKI as interchangeable terms causes premature discontinuation of decongestive therapies and the resulting poorer outcomes in hospitalized HF patients.

The initial step is to confirm the ability of BV analysis to quantitate fluid excess and diagnose the achievement of euvolemia after treatment; BV analysis should then be compared with methods that can performed easily, serially, and inexpensively: hemodynamically guided therapy can be used for early detection of fluid overload and prevention of HF hospitalizations; CIED data may forecast the risk of HF events early enough to trigger interventions to prevent HF decompensation; and noninvasive wearable devices detecting variables similar to those obtainable from CIEDs may soon become available for all HF patients, regardless of LVEF. As for CIED-derived risk indices, those from wearable devices must provide targets sufficiently specific to trigger appropriate therapies.

REFRACTORINESS TO DIURETICS IN HEART FAILURE

Still the cornerstone of decongestive therapy, diuretics' effectiveness decreases with progression of HF.[69,70] Impaired absorption, decreased RBF, azotemia, and proteinuria result in reduced diuretic concentrations in the tubular lumen[70] (**Fig. 3**). Definitions of diuretic resistance include: persistent congestion despite escalating diuretic doses equivalent to ≥80 mg/d furosemide; amount of sodium excretion as a percentage of filtered load less than 0.2%; and failure to excrete ≥90 mmol of sodium within 72 h of a 160-mg twice-daily furosemide dose. Metrics of diuretic response include: weight loss per 40 mg of furosemide or equivalent; net fluid loss per milligram of loop diuretic; and urinary sodium-to-urinary furosemide ratio.[70] Hallmarks of diuretic resistance are insufficient symptom relief, higher risk of in-hospital HF worsening, increased mortality after discharge, and a 3-fold increase in rehospitalization rates.[70,71] Among more than 50,000 patients enrolled in the ADHERE (Acute Decompensated Heart Failure National

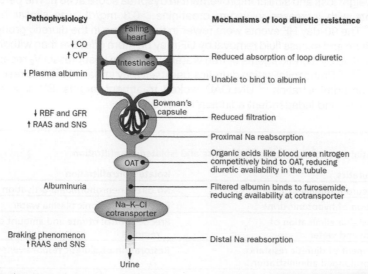

Fig. 3. Mechanisms of diuretic unresponsiveness in patients with heart failure. CO, cardiac output; CVP, central venous pressure; GFR, glomerular filtration rate; OAT, organic anion transporter; RAAS, renin-angiotensin-aldosterone system; RBF, renal blood flow; SNS, sympathetic nervous system. (*From* ter Maaten JM, Valente MA, Damman K, et al. Diuretic response in acute heart failure—pathophysiology, evaluation, and therapy. Nat Rev Cardiol 2015;12:184–92; with permission.)

Registry) study, only 33% lost ≤2.27 kg (5 lb), and 16% gained weight during hospitalization.[72] With conventional diuretic therapies, nearly 50% of hospitalized HF patients are discharged with residual fluid excess.[72] Regardless of diuretic strategy, 42% of acutely decompensated HF subjects in the DOSE (Diuretic Optimization Strategies Evaluation) trial reached the composite end point of death, rehospitalization, or emergency department visit at 60 days.[73] Vasopressin and adenosine-A1 receptor antagonists, exogenous natriuretic peptides, and low-dose dopamine, studied as complement or replacement for diuretics, decrease short-term fluid overload but fail to improve long-term outcomes.[74–76] Therefore, there is an unmet clinical need for more effective fluid-removal methods for HF patients (**Table 1**).

EXTRACORPOREAL ULTRAFILTRATION

Ultrafiltration consists of the production of plasma water from whole blood across a semipermeable membrane (hemofilter) in response to a transmembrane pressure gradient. Newer, simplified UF devices afford the advantages of small size, portability, low blood-flow rates, extracorporeal BV less than 50 mL, and a wide range of UF rates (0–500 mL/h) without requiring cannulation of a central vein and stay in intensive care units.[5]

As ultrafiltrate is isotonic to plasma, approximately 134 to 138 mmol of sodium is removed with each liter of ultrafiltrate.[77] Knowledge that refill of the intravascular space from the interstitium decreases as fluid is removed led to the hypothesis that UF initiation before reduction of capillary refill by previously administered diuretics might decongest HF patients more effectively than intravenous loop diuretics. Hence, in the UNLOAD (Ultrafiltration vs Intravenous Diuretics Decompensated Heart Failure) trial, randomization occurred within 24 h of hospitalization, and after a maximum of 2 intravenous doses of loop diuretic.[78] Compared with standard care, the UF group had greater weight loss and similar improvement in dyspnea score at 48 h. The percentage of patients with increases in serum creatinine ≥0.3 mg/dL was similar between groups.[78] The 90-day HF events were fewer in the UF than in the diuretic group. Total body sodium and excess fluid removal by UF may be more effective than withdrawal of hypotonic fluid by diuretic agents or free water by arginine vasopressin V_2 receptor antagonists.[73–76] Prehospitalization diuretics use itself may impair natriuretic response to intravenous administration.[70] UNLOAD lacked treatment targets, BV assessments, cost analysis, and independent adjudication of events.

Table 1
Differential characteristics of loop diuretics and isolated ultrafiltration

Loop Diuretics	Isolated Ultrafiltration
Direct neurohormonal activation	No direct neurohormonal activation
Elimination of hypotonic urine	Removal of isotonic plasma water
Unpredictable elimination of sodium and water	Precise control of rate and amount of fluid removal
Development of diuretic resistance with prolonged administration	Restoration of diuretic responsiveness
Risk of hypokalemia and hypomagnesemia	No effect on plasma concentration of potassium and magnesium
Peripheral venous access	Peripheral or central venous catheter
No need for anticoagulation	Need for anticoagulation
No extracorporeal circuit	Need for extracorporeal circuit

The CARRESS-HF (Cardiorenal Rescue Study in Acute Decompensated Heart Failure) trial compared a fixed UF rate of 200 mL/h with stepped pharmacologic therapy (adjustable doses of intravenous loop diuretics, thiazide diuretics, vasodilators, and inotropes) in acutely decompensated HF patients with prerandomization increase in sCr.[79] CARRESS-HF's primary end point was the bivariate change in serum creatinine and body weight from baseline to 96 h.[79] According to CARRESS-HF's design, this assumes that weight loss is a measurement of effective fluid removal and that an increase in sCr represents AKI. In CARRESS-HF, both groups lost an equivalent amount of weight, but greater increases in sCr occurred with UF.[79] Although more patients in the UF group experienced serious adverse events, the high crossover rate in CARRESS-HF intention-to-treat analysis impairs their adjudication to one or the other therapy.[79] A per-protocol analysis including only patients who had ultrafiltrate collected if randomized to UF, or no ultrafiltrate collected if randomized to the pharmacologic arm, revealed that UF was associated with higher net fluid loss ($P = .001$) and weight reduction ($P = .02$).[80,81]

In the CUORE (Continuous Ultrafiltration for Congestive Heart Failure) trial, UF-treated patients had a lower incidence of HF rehospitalizations through 1 year than those receiving standard care, despite similar weight loss at discharge. In CUORE, diuretics were continued during UF in the belief that this approach enhances natriuresis.[82] In previous studies, diuretics were stopped during UF to give patients a "diuretic holiday," during which loop diuretic–induced neurohormonal activation is absent.[78,83,84]

The hypothesis of the AVOID-HF (Aquapheresis vs Intravenous Diuretics and Hospitalization for Heart Failure) trial was that patients hospitalized for HF and treated with adjustable UF would have a longer time to first HF event within 90 days than those receiving adjustable intravenous loop diuretics.[85] The trial was terminated unilaterally by the sponsor (Baxter Healthcare, Deerfield, IL) after enrollment of 224 patients (27.5% of the planned sample). Detailed algorithms guided investigators on how to adjust both therapies according to patients' vital signs, renal function, and urine output.[85] The adjustable UF group had a trend to longer time to first HF event than patients in the diuretics group (62 vs 34 days; $P = .106$). At 30 days UF patients had significantly fewer independently adjudicated HF and cardiovascular events.[86] Adjustments of UF rates to individual patients' hemodynamics and renal function may explain the lack of differences in sCr between groups, despite greater net fluid loss with UF.[86] Restoration of diuretic responsiveness may be a key mechanism by which UF delays the recurrence of HF events.[86] Serious therapy-related adverse events occurred at higher rates in the UF group than in the diuretics group (14.6% vs 5.4%; $P = .026$).[86] Although in AVOID-HF, UF-related adverse events were fewer than in CARRESS-HF, the excess of UF-related complications is a serious concern.[79,86] More studies are needed to identify strategies that minimize access-related and other potentially preventable complications.[78,86]

The key features of the trials discussed here are summarized in **Table 2**.

The conflicting results from UF studies suggest that patient selection and fluid-removal targets are incompletely understood.[79,86] Practice guidelines recommend that inadequate response to an initial dose of intravenous loop diuretic be treated with an increased dose.[87,88] If this is ineffective, invasive hemodynamic assessment is suggested. Persistent fluid excess can then be treated with the addition of thiazide diuretics, aldosterone antagonists, or continuous intravenous infusion of a loop diuretic. Only if all these measures fail can UF be considered.[87,88] A similar degree of diuretic resistance characterized CARRESS-HF's subjects, whose poor outcomes may be partially related to the lack of therapy adjustment according to individual

Table 2
Overview of selected ultrafiltration clinical trials

Study Name, Publication Year	Patient Population	UF Arm	Comparison Arm	Primary Efficacy End Point	Primary End Point Result	Reported Clinical Outcomes	Mortality	Adverse Events
UNLOAD, 2007[78]	N = 200 Hospitalized with HF, ≥2 signs of fluid overload	Aquadex System 100[a] Mean fluid-removal rate 241 mL/h for 12.3 ± 12 h	Standard care: intravenous diuretics. For each 24-h period at least twice the prehospitalization daily oral dose	Weight loss and dyspnea assessment at 48 h after randomization	Weight loss: 5.0 ± 3.1 (UF) vs 3.1 ± 3.5 kg (standard care), P = .001 Dyspnea score: 5.4 ± 1.1 (UF) vs 5.2 ± 1.2 (standard care), P = .588	90 d: HF rehospitalization: 18% (UF) vs 32% (standard care), P = .022; HR 0.56, 95% CI 0.28–0.51, P = .04 Unscheduled clinic/emergency visits: 21% (UF) vs 44% (standard care), P = .009	90 d: 9(9.6%) UF vs 11 (11.6) standard care	No significant between group differences, except bleeding (1 UF vs 7 standard care, P = .032). UF group: 1 catheter infection, 5 filter clotting events, 1 patient transitioned to hemodialysis due to insufficient response to UF

CARRESS-HF, 2012[29]	N = 188	Hospitalized with HF, ≥2 signs of congestion, and recent ≥0.3 mg/dL sCr increase	Aquadex System 100[a] at a fixed rate of 200 mL/h Median duration 40 h	SPT with intravenous diuretics dosed to maintain urine output 3–5 L/d	Bivariate response of change in sCr and change in weight 96 h after randomization	Mean sCr change: +0.23 ± 0.70 mg/dL (UF) vs −0.04 ± 0.53 mg/dL (SPT) Mean weight loss: 5.7 ± 3.9 (UF) vs 5.5 ± 5.1 kg (SPT), $P = .58$	Crossover: STP: 6 patients (6%) also received UF (2 before 96 h) UF: 8 patients (9%) received diuretics instead of UF; 28 patients (30%) also received diuretics before 96 h 7 d: No difference in death, worsening or persistent HF, hemodialysis, SAE, or crossover (23% UF vs 18% SPT, $P = .45$) 60 d HF hospitalization 26% (UF) vs 26% (SPT) $P = .97$	60 d: 17% UF vs 13% SPT, $P = .47$	60-d SAE: 72% UF vs 57% SPT, $P = .03$, attributed to renal failure, bleeding, or catheter complications

(continued on next page)

Table 2
(continued)

Study Name, Publication Year	Patient Population	UF Arm	Comparison Arm	Primary Efficacy End Point	Primary End Point Result	Reported Clinical Outcomes	Mortality	Adverse Events
CUORE, 2014[82]	N = 56 NYHA III or IV, LVEF ≤40%, ≥4 kg weight gain from peripheral fluid overload, over 2 mo	Dedyca device[b] Mean treatment duration 19 ± 90 h, volume removed 4254 ± 4842 mL	Intravenous diuretics according to guideline recommendations (standard care)	HF rehospitalization at 1 y	3 (11%) UF vs 14 (48%) standard care; HR 0.14, 95% CI 0.04–0.48, P = .002	Length of index hospitalization: 7.4 ± 4.6 (UF) vs 9.1 ± 1.9 d (standard care), P = .23 Combined death or HF rehospitalization HR for UF vs standard care 0.35, 95% CI 0.15–0.69, P = .0035	1-y: 7 (26%) UF vs 11 (38%) standard care, P = .33	Premature clotting of filter in 6 patients
AVOID-HF, 2016[86]	N = 224 Hospitalized with HF; ≥2 criteria for fluid overload; receiving daily oral loop diuretics	AUF with Aquadex FlexFlow System[c]; adjustment per protocol guidelines based on vital signs and renal function	ALD with adjustment per protocol guidelines based on vital signs and renal function Mean furosemide-equivalent dose 271.26 ±	Time to first HF event (HF rehospitalization or unscheduled outpatient or emergency treatment with intravenous loop diuretics or UF) within	25% AUF vs 35% ALD (P = .11); HR 0.66%, 95% CI 0.4–1.1	Length of index hospitalization: median 6 (AUF) vs 5 (ALD) days, P = .106 30-d HF rehospitalizations/d at risk: 11/2876 (AUF) vs 24/2882 (ALD), P = .06 30-d CV rehospitalizations/	90 d 15% AUF vs 13% ALD, P = .83	At least 1 SAE: 66% (AUF) vs 60% (ALD), P = .4 SAEs of special interest: 23% (AUF) vs 14% (ALD), P = .122 Related SAEs: 14.6% (UF) vs 5.4% (ALD), P = .026

| Mean fluid-removal rate 138 ± 47 mL/h for 80 ± 53 h | 263.06 mg for 100 ± 78 h | 90 d of hospital discharge | d at risk: 17/2882 (AUF) vs 33/2891 (ALD), P = .037 For both HF and CV events: fewer patients re-hospitalized; fewer number of days re-hospitalized/d at risk |

Abbreviations: ALD, adjustable loop diuretic agent; AUF, adjustable ultrafiltration; CI, confidence interval; HF, heart failure; HR, hazard ratio; LVEF, left ventricular ejection fraction; NYHA, New York Heart Association; SAE, serious adverse event; sCr, serum creatinine; SPT, stepped pharmacologic therapy; UF, ultrafiltration.
a CHF solutions, Minneapolis, MN, USA.
b Dellco, Mirandola, Italy.
c Baxter International, Deerfield, IL, USA.

patients' characteristics.[79] In AVOID-HF, fine-tuning of UF rates in response to vital signs, renal function, or urine output resulted in greater net fluid loss and was associated with fewer 30-day HF events without a greater increase in sCr levels compared with the diuretics group.[86] Additional investigation of UF as both first-line and rescue therapy is needed, provided that UF rates are individualized.[78,86] Use of UF is not recommended in de novo HF patients who are likely to respond to intravenous diuretics. The lingering question concerns which patients who develop HF decompensation despite daily oral diuretics should be considered for UF instead of intravenous diuretic agents. One important general recommendation is that the chosen initial UF rate should be either maintained or reduced because capillary refill decreases with fluid removal.[5] In general, UF rates of greater than 250 mL/h are not recommended.[85,86] Patients with predominantly right-sided HF or HF with preserved LVEF are exquisitely susceptible to intravascular volume depletion and may only tolerate low UF rates (50–100 mL/h).[89] Clinical experience teaches us that extracorporeal fluid removal is better tolerated when conducted with low UF rates over prolonged periods of time.[5]

A frequently used approach is to compare patients' current weight with that preceding signs and symptoms of congestion and to use this "dry weight" as the fluid removal. No consensus exists on whether removal of only 60% to 80% of excess fluid by UF and continuation of loop diuretics during therapy results in less hemodynamic instability and greater urinary sodium excretion.[82,86]

NOVEL STRATEGIES TO OVERCOME DIURETIC RESISTANCE

Novel methods to decongest diuretic-resistant HF patients with fluid overload and the cardiorenal syndrome are outlined in **Fig. 4**.

Controlled Diuresis

The Reprieve Cardiovascular (Reprieve Cardiovascular, Milford, MA) therapy is designed to maintain venous return in a controlled manner to prevent intravascular hypovolemia and consequent neurohormonal activation. The device replaces a physician-set portion of urine volume generated by the patient in response to diuretics. The partial, controlled replacement of volume may allow intravascular volume to be maintained at an optimal level. Pilot studies with this technology are ongoing in Poland.[90]

Peritoneal Ultrafiltration Methods

Direct peritoneal sodium removal

Traditional peritoneal dialysis solutions have sodium concentrations nearly isotonic to plasma, so that sodium removal is almost entirely driven by solute drag with UF rather than diffusion down a concentration gradient. A novel approach consists in the use of a salt-free peritoneal solution and the eventual combination with a fully implanted, automatic, programmable pump that can be charged transcutaneously, adjusted wirelessly, and equipped with a catheter that can deliver the salt-rich fluid generated by the concentration gradient directly to the bladder. Preclinical studies show that direct peritoneal sodium removal can withdraw large amounts of fluid and sodium with relatively small intraperitoneal volumes.[91]

Hydrostatic pressure gradient ultrafiltration device

This novel approach consists of the implantation of a permeable absorption chamber in the peritoneum. A pump induces a negative hydrostatic pressure in the absorption chamber, triggering UF of fluid through the peritoneal membranes into the chamber. A microcatheter draining fluid from the absorption chamber is routed to a percutaneous

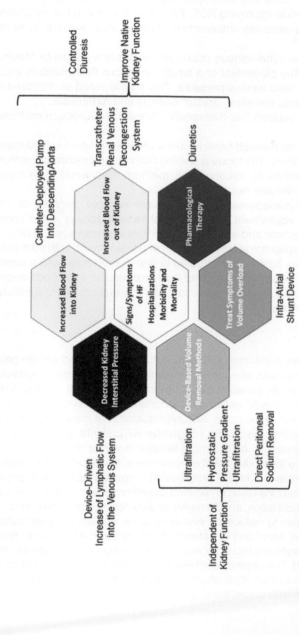

Fig. 4. Novel strategies to overcome diuretic resistance. HF, heart failure.

port. Ongoing work will enable drainage of the accumulated extracellular fluid into the urinary system.[92]

"Decongestive Pumps"

The Aortix device (Procyrion, Houston, TX) is a catheter-deployed pump that is placed in the descending aorta and decouples the heart and the kidneys, with the aim of resting the heart while improving RBF. First-in-man use in patients undergoing high-risk percutaneous coronary intervention showed improvement in hemodynamics and urine output.[93]

The transcatheter renal venous decongestion system (Magenta Medical, Kadima, Israel) consists in the placement of a small continuous flow pump in each renal vein to directly reduce renal venous pressure. This should result in improved responsiveness to diuretics and, therefore, greater diuresis and natriuresis.

Preclinical data support this therapeutic concept. A European multicenter clinical trial is ongoing.[94]

The novel methods outlined herein underscore the evolution in fluid management of congestive HF patients. The focus is shifting from the unpredictable removal of hypotonic fluid by diuretics to decongestive methods that avoid intravascular volume depletion and consequent renal hypoperfusion.

The novel fluid-management methods have variable degrees of invasiveness, ranging from the requirement of a peripheral venous access and a urinary catheter to that for intravascular and intraperitoneal implant procedures. Overall novel fluid-management therapies are at an early stage of development, with some still in preclinical trials and others having been studied in first-in-man trials with a small number of subjects. Further investigation of novel fluid-management methods should focus on assessment of safety, ease of use, candidate selection, reproducibility of effects across HF populations, and costs.

SUMMARY

In HF, fluid overload is the main culprit of mutually harmful and self-perpetuating interactions between the heart and the kidney, which cause disease progression and poor outcomes. In acute HF, transient elevations of sCr represent a physiologic response to fluid removal and should not trigger discontinuation of symptom-improving and/or life-saving decongestive therapies. Accurate quantitative measurement of fluid volume is vital to individualizing therapy for congestive HF patients. BV analysis and PA pressure monitoring appear to be the most reliable methods to assess fluid volume and guide decongestive therapies. Still the cornerstone of decongestive therapy, diuretics' effectiveness decreases with HF progression. Impaired absorption, decreased RBF, azotemia, and proteinuria result in reduced diuretic concentrations in the tubular lumen. Extracorporeal ultrafiltration, an alternative to diuretics, removes fluid isotonic to plasma and has been shown to reduce HF events in some studies. Fluid-removal rates by UF should be adjusted according to patients' hemodynamic and renal profiles. Research on new fluid-management technologies should focus on safety, ease of use, candidate selection, and cost. The urgency of these investigations is underscored by the alarming prognostic and economic implications of recurrent HF hospitalizations, which remain unacceptably high with conventional pharmacologic therapies.

REFERENCES

1. Ronco C, Haapio M, House AA, et al. Cardiorenal syndrome. J Am Coll Cardiol 2008;52:1527–39.

2. Damman K, Valente MA, Voors AA, et al. Renal impairment, worsening renal function, and outcome in patients with heart failure: an updated meta-analysis. Eur Heart J 2014;35:455–69.

3. Dries DL, Exner DV, Domanski MJ, et al. The prognostic implications of renal insufficiency in asymptomatic and symptomatic patients with left ventricular systolic dysfunction. J Am Coll Cardiol 2000;35:681–9.

4. Hillege HL, Girbes AR, de Kam PJ, et al. Renal function, neurohormonal activation, and survival in patients with chronic heart failure. Circulation 2000;102: 203–10.

5. Costanzo MR, Ronco C, Abraham WT, et al. Extracorporeal ultrafiltration for fluid overload in heart failure: current status and prospects for further research. J Am Coll Cardiol 2017;69:2428–45.

6. Brisco MA, Zile MR, Hanberg JS, et al. Relevance of changes in serum creatinine during a heart failure trial of decongestive strategies: insights from the DOSE trial. J Card Fail 2016;22:753–60.

7. Ahmad T, Jackson K, Rao VS, et al. Worsening renal function in acute heart failure patients undergoing aggressive diuresis is not associated with tubular injury. Circulation 2018;137:2016–28.

8. Levey AS, Inker LA. Assessment of glomerular filtration rate in health and disease: a state of the art review. Clin Pharmacol Ther 2017;102:405–19.

9. Bragadottir G, Redfors B, Ricksten SE. Assessing glomerular filtration rate (GFR) in critically ill patients with acute kidney injury–true GFR versus urinary creatinine clearance and estimating equations. Crit Care 2013;17:R108.

10. Kidney Disease: Improving Global Outcomes (KDIGO) Acute Kidney Injury Work Group. KDIGO clinical practice guideline for acute kidney injury. Kidney Int Suppl 2012;2:1–138.

11. Xu K, Rosenstiel P, Paragas N, et al. Unique transcriptional programs identify subtypes of AKI. J Am Soc Nephrol 2017;28:1729–40.

12. Nickolas TL, Schmidt-Ott KM, Canetta P, et al. Diagnostic and prognostic stratification in the emergency department using urinary bio markers of nephron damage: a multicenter prospective cohort study. J Am Coll Cardiol 2012;59:246–55.

13. Barasch J, Zager R, Bonventre JV. Acute kidney injury: a problem of definition. Lancet 2017;389:779–81.

14. Waikar SS, Betensky RA, Emerson SC, et al. Imperfect gold standards for kidney injury biomarker evaluation. J Am Soc Nephrol 2012;23:13–21.

15. Costanzo MR. Verdict in: congestion guilty! JACC Heart Fail 2015;3:762–4.

16. Miller WL. Fluid volume overload and congestion in heart failure. time to reconsider pathophysiology and how volume is assessed. Circ Heart Fail 2016;9: e002922.

17. Schrier RW. Body fluid volume regulation in health and disease: a unifying hypothesis. Ann Intern Med 1990;113:155–9.

18. Rothe CF. Reflex control of veins and vascular capacitance. Physiol Rev 1983;63: 1281–342.

19. Miller WL, Mullan BP. Understanding the heterogeneity in volume overload and fluid distribution in decompensated heart failure is key to optimal volume management: role for blood volume quantitation. JACC Heart Fail 2014;2:298–305.

20. Seymour WB, Pritchard WH, Longley LP, et al. Cardiac output, blood and interstitial fluid volumes, total circulating serum protein, and kidney function during cardiac failure and after improvement. J Clin Invest 1942;21:229–40.

21. Setoguchi S, Stevenson LW, Schneeweiss S. Repeated hospitalizations predict mortality in the community population with heart failure. Am Heart J 2007;154: 260–6.
22. Androne SA, Hryniewicz K, Hudaihed A, et al. Relation of unrecognized hypervolemia in chronic heart failure to clinical status, hemodynamics, and patient outcomes. Am J Cardiol 2004;93:1254–9.
23. Cotter G, Metra M, Milo-Cotter O, et al. Fluid overload in acute heart failure—redistribution and other mechanisms beyond fluid accumulation. Eur J Heart Fail 2008;10:165–9.
24. Metra M, Dei Cas L, Bristow MR. The pathophysiology of acute heart failure—it is a lot about fluid accumulation. Am Heart J 2008;155:1–5.
25. Gheorghiade M, Filippatos G, De Luca L, et al. Congestion in acute heart failure syndromes: an essential target of evaluation and treatment. Am J Med 2006; 119(12 suppl 1).S3 10.
26. Tyberg JV. How changes in venous capacitance modulate cardiac output. Pflugers Arch 2002;445:10–7.
27. Fallick C, Sobotka PA, Dunlap ME. Sympathetically mediated changes in capacitance: redistribution of the venous reservoir as a cause of decompensation. Circ Heart Fail 2011;4:669–75.
28. Sharma R, Francis DP, Pitt B, et al. Haemoglobin predicts survival in patients with chronic heart failure: a substudy of the ELITE II trial. Eur Heart J 2004;25:1021–8.
29. Gagnon DR, Zhang TJ, Brand FN, et al. Hematocrit and the risk of cardiovascular disease—the Framingham study: a 34-year follow-up. Am Heart J 1994;127: 674–82.
30. Androne AS, Katz SD, Lund L, et al. Hemodilution is common in patients with advanced heart failure. Circulation 2003;107:226–9.
31. Verbrugge FH, Dupont M, Steels P, et al. The kidney in congestive heart failure: "are natriuresis, sodium, and diuretics really the good, the bad and the ugly?". Eur J Heart Fail 2014;16:133–42.
32. Lote CJ, Snape BM. Collecting duct flow rate as a determinant of equilibration between urine and renal papilla in the rat in the presence of a maximal antidiuretic hormone concentration. J Physiol 1977;270:533–44.
33. Allen GG, Barratt LJ. Effect of aldosterone on the transepithelial potential difference of the rat distal tubule. Kidney Int 1981;19:678–86.
34. Woodhall PB, Tisher CC. Response of the distal tubule and cortical collecting duct to vasopressin in the rat. J Clin Invest 1973;52:3095–108.
35. Schreier RW, Abraham WT. Hormones and hemodynamics in heart failure. N Engl J Med 1999;341:577–85.
36. Verbrugge FH, Dupont M, Steels P, et al. Abdominal contributions to cardiorenal dysfunction in congestive heart failure. J Am Coll Cardiol 2013;62:485–95.
37. Aukland K, Reed RK. Interstitial-lymphatic mechanisms in the control of extracellular fluid volume. Physiol Rev 1993;73:1–78.
38. Guyton AC. Interstitial fluid pressure. II. Pressure-volume curves of interstitial space. Circ Res 1965;16:452–60.
39. Sandek A, Rauchhaus M, Anker SD, et al. The emerging role of the gut in chronic heart failure. Curr Opin Clin Nutr Metab Care 2008;11:632–9.
40. Manzone TA, Dam HQ, Soltis D, et al. Blood volume analysis: a new technique and new clinical interest reinvigorate a classic study. J Nucl Med Technol 2007; 35:55–63.
41. Strobeck JE, Feldshuh J, Miller WL. Heart failure outcomes with volume-guided management. JACC Heart Fail 2018;6:940–8.

42. Bera TK. Bioelectrical impedance methods for noninvasive health monitoring: a review. J Med Eng 2014. https://doi.org/10.1155/2014/381251.
43. Shotan A, Blondheim DS, Kazatsker M, et al. Non-invasive lung IMPEDANCE-guided preemptive treatment in chronic heart failure patients: a randomized controlled trial (IMPEDANCE-HF trial). J Card Fail 2016;22:713–22.
44. Burkhoff D. Bioimpedance: has its time finally come. J Card Fail 2016;22:723–4.
45. Drazner MH, Rame JE, Stevenson LW, et al. Prognostic importance of elevated jugular venous pressure and a third heart sound in patients with heart failure. N Engl J Med 2001;345:574–81.
46. Zile MR, Bennett TD, St. John Sutton M, et al. Transition from chronic compensated to acute decompensated heart failure: pathophysiological insights obtained from continuous monitoring of intracardiac pressures. Circulation 2008;118:1433–41.
47. Abraham WT, Stough WG, Piña IL, et al. Trials of implantable monitoring devices in heart failure: which design is optimal? Nat Rev Cardiol 2014;11:576–85.
48. Stevenson LW, Zile M, Bennett TD, et al. Chronic ambulatory intracardiac pressures and future heart failure events. Circ Heart Fail 2010;3:580–7.
49. Adamson PB, Abraham WT, Aaron M, et al. CHAMPION trial rationale and design: the longterm safety and clinical efficacy of a wireless pulmonary artery pressure monitoring system. J Card Fail 2011;17:3–10.
50. Abraham WT, Adamson PB, Bourge RC, et al. Wireless pulmonary artery haemodynamic monitoring in chronic heart failure: a randomized controlled trial. Lancet 2011;377:658–66.
51. Costanzo MR, Stevenson LW, Adamson PB, et al. Interventions linked to decreased heart failure hospitalizations during ambulatory pulmonary artery pressure monitoring. JACC Heart Fail 2016;4:333–44.
52. Givertz MM, Stevenson LW, Costanzo MR, et al, on behalf of the CHAMPION Trial Investigators. Pulmonary artery pressure-guided management of patients with heart failure and reduced ejection fraction. J Am Coll Cardiol 2017;70:1875–86.
53. Adamson PB, Abraham WT, Bourge RC, et al. Wireless pulmonary artery pressure monitoring guides management to reduce decompensation in heart failure with preserved ejection fraction. Circ Heart Fail 2014;7:935–44.
54. Heywood JT, Jermyn R, Shavelle D, et al. Impact of practice-based management of pulmonary artery pressures in 2000 patients implanted with the CardioMEMS sensor. Circulation 2017;135:1509–17.
55. Desai AS, Bhimaraj A, Bharmi R, et al. Ambulatory hemodynamic monitoring reduces heart failure hospitalizations in "real-world" clinical practice. J Am Coll Cardiol 2017;69:2357–65.
56. Yu CM, Wang L, Chau E, et al. Intrathoracic impedance monitoring in patients with heart failure: correlation with fluid status and feasibility of early warning preceding hospitalization. Circulation 2005;112:841–8.
57. van Veldhuisen DJ, Braunschweig F, Conraads V, et al, for the DOT-HF Investigators. Intrathoracic impedance monitoring, audible patient alerts, and outcome in patients with heart failure. Circulation 2011;124:1719–26.
58. Boehmer JP, Hariharan R, Devecchi FG, et al. A multisensor algorithm predicts heart failure events in patients with implanted devices: results from the Multi-SENSE Study. JACC Heart Fail 2017;5:216–25.
59. Costanzo MR. The luck of having a cardiac implantable electronic device. Circ Heart Fail 2018. https://doi.org/10.1161/CIRCHEARTFAILURE.118.004894.
60. Price S, Platz E, Cullen L, et al. for the Acute Heart Failure Study Group of the European Society of Cardiology Acute Cardiovascular Care Association

Echocardiography and lung ultrasonography for the assessment and management of acute heart failure. Nat Rev Cardiol 2017;14:422–40.

61. Platz E, Hempel D, Pivetta E, et al. Echocardiographic and lung ultrasound characteristics in ambulatory patients with dyspnea or prior heart failure. Echocardiography 2014;31:133–9.

62. Trezzi M, Torzillo D, Ceriani E, et al. Lung ultrasonography for the assessment of rapid extravascular water variation: evidence from hemodialysis patients. Intern Emerg Med 2013;8:409–15.

63. Volpicelli G, Caramello V, Cardinale L, et al. Bedside ultrasound of the lung for the monitoring of acute decompensated heart failure. Am J Emerg Med 2008;26: 585–91.

64. Gargani L, Frassi F, Soldati G, et al. Ultrasound lung comets for the differential diagnosis of acute cardiogenic dyspnoea: a comparison with natriuretic peptides. Eur J Heart Fail 2008;10:70–7.

65. Guiotto G, Masarone M, Paladino F, et al. Inferior vena cava collapsibility to guide fluid removal in slow continuous ultrafiltration: a pilot study. Intensive Care Med 2010;36:692–6.

66. Blehar DJ, Dickman E, Gaspari R. Identification of congestive heart failure via respiratory variation of inferior vena cava diameter. Am J Emerg Med 2009;27:71–5.

67. Bayes-Genis A, Lupón J, Jaffe AS. Can natriuretic peptides be used to guide therapy? EJIFCC 2016;27:208–16.

68. Felker GM, Ahmad T, Anstronm KJ, et al. Rationale and design of the GUIDE-IT study; guiding evidence based therapy using biomarker intensified treatment in heart failure. JACC Heart Fail 2014;2:457–65.

69. Singh D, Shrestha K, Testani JM, et al. Insufficient natriuretic response to continuous intravenous furosemide is associated with poor long-term outcomes in acute decompensated heart failure. J Card Fail 2014;20:392–9.

70. ter Maaten JM, Valente MA, Damman K, et al. Diuretic response in acute heart failure—pathophysiology, evaluation, and therapy. Nat Rev Cardiol 2015;12: 184–92.

71. Voors AA, Davison BA, Teerlink JR, et al, for the RELAX-AHF investigators. Diuretic response in patients with acute decompensated heart failure: characteristics and clinical outcome—an analysis from RELAX-AHF. Eur J Heart Fail 2014; 16:1230–40.

72. Gheorghiade M, Filippatos G. Reassessing treatment of acute heart failure syndromes: the ADHERE registry. Eur Heart J Suppl 2005;7:B13–9.

73. Felker GM, Lee KL, Bull DA, et al, for the NHLBI Heart Failure Clinical Research Network. Diuretic strategies in patients with acute decompensated heart failure. N Engl J Med 2011;364:797–805.

74. Konstam MA, Gheorghiade M, Burnett JC Jr, et al, for the Efficacy of Vasopressin Antagonism in Heart Failure Outcome Study With Tolvaptan (EVEREST) investigators. Effects of oral tolvaptan in patients hospitalized for worsening heart failure: the EVEREST outcome trial. JAMA 2007;297:1319–31.

75. Massie BM, O'Connor CM, Metra M, et al, for the PROTECT investigators and committees. Rolofylline, an adenosine A1-receptor antagonist, in acute heart failure. N Engl J Med 2010;363:1419–28.

76. O'Connor CM, Starling RC, Hernandez AF, et al. Effect of nesiritide in patients with acute decompensated heart failure. N Engl J Med 2011;365(365):32–43.

77. Ronco C, Ricci Z, Bellomo R, et al. Extracorporeal ultrafiltration for the treatment of overhydration and congestive heart failure. Cardiology 2001;96:155–68.

78. Costanzo MR, Guglin ME, Saltzberg MT, et al, for the UNLOAD trial investigators. Ultrafiltration versus intravenous diuretics for patients hospitalized for acute decompensated heart failure. J Am Coll Cardiol 2007;49:675–83.
79. Grodin JL, Carter S, Bart BA, et al. Direct comparison of ultrafiltration to pharmacological decongestion in heart failure: a per-protocol analysis of CARRESS-HF. Eur J Heart Fail 2018;20:1148–56.
80. Bart BA, Goldsmith SR, Lee KL, et al, for the Heart Failure Clinical Research Network. Ultrafiltration in decompensated heart failure with cardiorenal syndrome. N Engl J Med 2012;367:2296–304.
81. Costanzo MR, Kazory A. Better late than never: the true results of CARRESS-HF. Eur J Heart Fail 2018;20:1157–9.
82. Marenzi G, Muratori M, Cosentino ER, et al. Continuous ultrafiltration for congestive heart failure: the CUORE trial. J Card Fail 2014;20:9–17.
83. Lorenz JN, Weihprecht H, Schnermann J, et al. Renin release from isolated juxtaglomerular apparatus depends on macula densa chloride transport. Am J Physiol 1991;260:F486–93.
84. Schlatter E, Salomonsson M, Persson AE, et al. Macula densa cells sense luminal NaCl concentration via furosemide sensitive $Na^+2Cl^-K^+$ cotransport. Pflugers Arch 1989;414:286–90.
85. Costanzo MR, Negoianu D, Fonarow GC, et al. Rationale and design of the Aquapheresis Versus Intravenous Diuretics and Hospitalization for Heart Failure (AVOID-HF) trial. Am Heart J 2015;170I:471–82.
86. Costanzo MR, Negoianu D, Jaski BE, et al. Aquapheresis versus intravenous diuretics and hospitalizations for heart failure. JACC Heart Fail 2016;4:95–105.
87. Ponikowski P, Voors AA, Anker SD, et al. 2016 ESC guidelines for the diagnosis and treatment of acute and chronic heart failure: the task force for the diagnosis and treatment of acute and chronic heart failure of the European Society of Cardiology (ESC). Developed with the special contribution of the Heart Failure Association (HFA) of the ESC. Eur Heart J 2016;37:2129–200.
88. Yancy CW, Jessup M, Bozkurt B, et al. 2013 ACCF/AHA guideline for the management of heart failure: a report of the American College of Cardiology Foundation/American Heart Association task force on practice guidelines. J Am Coll Cardiol 2013;62:e147–239.
89. Schrier RW, Bansal S. Pulmonary hypertension, right ventricular failure, and kidney: different from left ventricular failure? Clin J Am Soc Nephrol 2008;3:1232–7.
90. Available at: https://reprievecardio.com/. Accessed February 28, 2019.
91. Mahoney D, Rao V, Asher J, et al. Development of a direct peritoneal sodium removal technique with salt-free solution. J Card Fail 2018;24:S34.
92. Feld Y, Hanani H, Costanzo MR. Hydrostatic pressure gradient ultrafiltration device: a novel approach for extracellular fluid removal. J Heart Lung Transplant 2018;37:794–6.
93. Vora AN, Schuyler Jones W, DeVore AD, et al. First-in-human experience with Aortix intraaortic pump. Catheter Cardiovasc Interv 2019;93:428–33.
94. Available at: http://www.magentamed.com/. Accessed February 28, 2019.

Printed and bound by CPI Group (UK) Ltd, Croydon, CR0 4YY

03/10/2024

01040847-0008